Nutrition in Promoting the Public's Health: Strategies, Principles, and Practices

Mildred Kaufman, MS
Professor Emeritus
School of Public Health
University of North Carolina at Chapel Hill
Chapel Hill, NC

JONES AND BARTLETT PUBLISHERS
Sudbury, Massachusetts
BOSTON   TORONTO   LONDON   SINGAPORE

World Headquarters

Jones and Bartlett Publishers	Jones and Bartlett Publishers	Jones and Bartlett Publishers
40 Tall Pine Drive	Canada	International
Sudbury, MA 01776	6339 Ormindale Way	Barb House, Barb Mews
978-443-5000	Mississauga, Ontario L5V	London W6 7PA
info@jbpub.com	1J2	UK
www.jbpub.com	CANADA	

Jones and Bartlett's books and products are available through most bookstores and online book-sellers. To contact Jones and Bartlett Publishers directly, call 800-832-0034, fax 978-443-8000, or visit our website www.jbpub.com.

Substantial discounts on bulk quantities of Jones and Bartlett's publications are available to corporations, professional associations, and other qualified organizations. For details and specific discount information, contact the special sales department at Jones and Bartlett via the above contact information or send an email to specialsales@jbpub.com.

Library of Congress Cataloging-in-Publication Data
Kaufman, Mildred.
Nutrition in promoting the public's health : strategies, principles, and practice / Mildred Kaufman.
    p. ; cm.
Includes bibliographical references.
ISBN-13: 978-0-7637-2840-3
ISBN-10: 0-7637-2840-3
1. Nutrition—United States. 2. Public health—United States.
[DNLM: 1. Nutrition—United States. 2. Public Health—United States. 3. Health Promotion—United States. QU 145 K215n 2006] I. Title.
RA784.K328 2006
362.1—dc22

2006005283

6048

Production Credits
Publisher: Michael Brown
Production Director: Amy Rose
Associate Production Editor: Dan Stone
Associate Editor: Kylah Goodfellow McNeill
Marketing Manager: Emily Ekle
Associate Marketing Manager: Wendy Thayer
Manufacturing and Inventory Coordinator: Amy Bacus
Composition: Auburn Associates, Inc.
Cover Design: Kristin Ohlin
Printing and Binding: Malloy, Inc.
Cover Printing: Malloy, Inc.

Printed in the United States of America
10 09 08 07 06   10 9 8 7 6 5 4 3 2 1

Dedication

This book is dedicated to the memory of Geraldine M. Piper, my role model, mentor, and friend who shared her experiences as a public health nutrition leader, as well as teacher, at the University of Tennessee. It is also dedicated to Dr. Wilson T. Sowder, the Florida State Health Officer who gave support to developing the state's public health nutrition program based on assessed community needs. Lastly, to Dr. Emily Gates who spoke of the children of Florida as "my children."

Table of Contents

Contributors

Charles N. Abernethy, BSEE, PhD, CHFP
Behavioral Implications Management Consultant
University of Phoenix, Westborough, MA

Elaine C. Barnes, MBA, RD
Assistant Health Director, retired
Buncombe County Health Center, Asheville, NC

Cynthia B. Bartosek, MPH, RD, LD
Nutrition Program Director
Palm Beach County Health Department, Riviera Beach, FL

Katherine A. Cairns, MPH, MBA, RD
President/CEO
Summit Health Group, St. Paul, MN

Nancy Chapman, MPH, RD
President
N. Chapman Associates, Inc., Washington, DC

Harriet H. Cloud, MS, RD
Former Director
Nutrition Division Sparks Center for Development and Learning Disorders
Tuscaloosa, AL

Mildred M. Cody, PhD, MS, RD, LD
Associate Professor, Dept. of Nutrition/Dietetics
Georgia State University, Atlanta, GA

Robert Earl, MPH, RD, LD
Senior Director of Nutrition Policy
National Food Processors Association, Falls Church, VA

Maya T. Edmonds, MPH, RD
Burtonsville, MD

Carole B. Garner, MPH, RD, LD
Assistant Professor, College of Public Health
University of Arkansas for Medical Sciences, Little Rock, AR

Betsy Haughton, EdD, RD
Professor, Director of Public Health Nutrition
University of Tennessee, Knoxville, TN

Barbara Frieberg Kamp, MS, RD
Project Coordinator, Nat'l Policy & Resource Center on Nutrition, Physical Activity and Aging
Florida International University, Miami, FL

Mildred Kaufman, MS
Professor Emeritus, Department of Nutrition, School of Public Health
University of North Carolina, Chapel Hill, NC

Alice J. Lenihan, MPH, RD, LDN
Head, Nutrition Svcs. Branch, Women & Children's Health Section
Division of Public Health, Raleigh, NC

Meg Malloy, DrPH, MPH, RD, LDN
Executive Director
NC Prevention Partners, Carrboro, NC

Mary C. Maloney, MPH, RD, LD
Health Services & Facilities Consultant
Florida Agency for Health Care Administration, St. Petersburg, FL

Toni Martin, MPH, RD, LDN
Senior Public Health Nutrition Supervisor
Duval County Health Department,
 Jacksonville, FL

Nicole Olmstead, MPH
Arthritis Program Manager, Office of
 Chronic Disease Prevention and
 Nutrition Services
Arizona Department of Health, Phoenix,
 AZ

Lynn Parker, MS
Director of Child Nutrition Programs and
 Nutrition Policy
Food Research and Action Center
 (FRAC), Washington, DC

**Judith C. Rodriguez, PhD, RD, LD,
 CHE, FADA**
Professor, Chairperson, Department of
 Public Health
Director, BSH Nutrition Program
University of North Florida, Jacksonville,
 FL

Marjorie Scharf, MPH, RD
Public Health Nutrition Consultant
Private Practice
Merion, PA

Sandra B. Sherman, EdD, EdM, MS
Director of Nutrition Education
The Food Trust, Philadelphia, PA

Margaret Tate, MS, RD
Chief, Office of Chronic Disease
 Prevention and Nutrition Services
Arizona Department of Health, Phoenix,
 AZ

Marie Tymrak, MPH, RD
Public Health Nutritionist, Office of
 Chronic Disease Prevention and
 Nutrition Services
Arizona Department of Health, Phoenix,
 AZ

Nancy Wellman, PhD, RD, FADA
Professor of Dietetics and Nutrition
 Director, Nat'l Policy and Resource
 Center on Nutrition, Physical Activity,
 and Aging
Florida International University, Miami,
 FL

Kathie Westpheling, MPH, RD
Executive Director, Association of
 Clinicians for the Underserved (ACU)
Tyson's Corner, VA

Diane R. Wilson, MPH, RD
Co-owner and Vice President, Gulf View
 Consulting, Inc.
Ft. Myers Beach, FL

Foreword

Modern history and the history of contemporary public health is the history of public health nutrition. The description of the "occupational" hazards of sailors related to scurvy in the 1500s and 1600s, and the identification of its "cure" in the 1700s, allowed the great explorations (and sadly war and conquests) of the New World to unfold. Similarly, the recognition of the increasing incidence and causes of rickets in Europe in the early 1600s facilitated the urbanization of the Old World, a prerequisite for the launch of the industrial revolution.

Despite these early empirical findings, it is humbling to note that it wasn't until centuries later, and less than 100 years ago, that luminaries in the science of nutrition postulated and demonstrated the existence of "accessory nutritional elements" (C. A. Pekelharing), "minimal qualitative factors" (Frederick Hopkins), and finally a class of chemical amines vital to the antineuritic affect of specific foods on beriberi—to become known as "vitamines" (Casimir Funk). With these and a host of other findings, the science of nutrition joined that of infectious diseases to establish the framework of modern public health. For nearly a century, these two fields have been inextricably linked to the response to the "Classical Morbidities" and epidemiology of illness and disease that affected humanity.

Having succeeded in understanding and responding to the basic relationship between diet and health, and buoyed by continuing advances in the science of nutrition and infectious diseases over the past 50 years, the success of public health has resulted in a shift in the epidemiology of morbidity and mortality in the developed world. This transition to a "New Morbidity" (Robert Haggerty), characterized primarily by behaviorally determined preventable chronic diseases, is once again demanding a response by public health nutrition. This response will demand a new approach to public health nutrition framed by the core and essential functions of public health and a retooled public health workforce. More so than in the past, where dramatic gains in health could be attained simply through exogenous nutritional supplementation, the epidemiological transition to the New Morbidities will require population-based and clinical approaches to behavior to affect the evolving issues of obesity and nutrition-related chronic diseases.

As such, the importance of this new book on public health nutrition. The success of public health's response to the New Morbidities will depend on an expanded and retooled public health nutritionist workforce. Grounded in the science of nutrition, nutritionists, whether working in clinical or public health venues, will need to be skilled in the behavioral sciences and social marketing to affect the preventable etiologies of obesity and chronic diseases. They will similarly need to be knowledgeable about the genetics of chronic diseases and strategies to mitigate the effect of environment on the expression of the genetic basis of disease.

But, lest the field become the least bit complacent, there is yet another epidemiological transition evolving that will place further demands on public health nutrition, expand the required expertise of nutritionists, and increase the importance of the profession and its relevance to the public's health. Our rapidly expanding understanding of the social and environmental determinism of health is defining the "Millennial Morbidities." While the "Classical Morbidities" related to nutritional deficiencies, the "New Morbidities" relate to the behavior of individuals and populations, the "Millennial Morbidities" relate to the social and environmental determinants of health and illness. The response to the "Millennial Morbidities" will require public health nutritionists to expand their expertise in the social sciences, integrate these sciences into the field of nutrition, and assume new roles in the generation of public policy affecting all areas of society. If we are to succeed in this response, public health nutrition and the public health nutritionists will need to assume new roles and functions in public health and in our communities.

As a final and sobering note to this Foreword, it would be inappropriate not to mention the relevance of this book to the billions of people who live in the developing world. The global relevance of public health nutrition to the "Classical," "New," and "Millennial" morbidities in the developing world cannot be overstated. The opportunity for public health nutritionists to influence the growing health disparities between the Northern and the Southern hemispheres establishes an ethical responsibility for the field to respond. This book will be an important contribution to the future of public health and the relevance of public health nutritionists to global health.

Jacksonville, FL 2006

Jeff Goldhagen, MD, MPH
Medical Director
Duval County Health Department

Acknowledgements

Many thanks to the contributing chapter authors who made this book possible and whose names are listed elsewhere, and especially to Diane R. Wilson, who was always able to give extra assistance, when needed. Diane K. Faulkner is greatly appreciated for her editorial knowledge and skills to quickly prepare the manuscript into its final form to submit for publication. And many thanks to Edwinna Green for her word processing.

CHAPTER 1

Practice as a Public Health Professional

Mildred Kaufman

Reader Objectives

- Define public health and its three levels of prevention.
- Discuss the three core governmental public health functions and the ten essential public health services.
- Compare and contrast the public health approach to the medical care model.
- List the health, technological, societal, and economic trends that affect the public's health.
- Discuss the contributions of nutrition and dietary behavior changes to reversing the major public health problems.
- Assess competencies as a public health nutritionist, and write a personal career development plan.

DEFINE PUBLIC HEALTH

"Obesity kills more Americans than cigarettes!" proclaims a billboard along a busy city street. "Overcoming Obesity in America" heralds the cover of a special issue of a popular news magazine.[1] "Fighting Flab in Arkansas: Fried Chicken Becomes the Devil's Food" heads an article in another news magazine that continues to relate how the state's governor had a health scare that motivated him to lose 100 pounds in a year through diet and exercise. And now he is on a campaign to have his state's people emulate him, anticipating that slimming them down will result in significant savings in Medicaid costs.[2] A Centers for Disease Control and Prevention (CDC) press release dated January 24, 2004, proclaims "Obesity Costs States Billions in Medical Expenses." This figure is based on a study by researchers at RTI International and the CDC that estimates

U.S. medical expenditures attributable to obesity reached $75 billion in 2003 and that taxpayers financed about half of these costs through Medicare and Medicaid.[3]

Consequently, public health and public health nutrition issues are hitting the headlines and present public health nutritionists with new challenges and opportunities for leadership.

In 1920, C.E.A. Winslow defined public health as "the science and art of preventing disease, prolonging life and efficiency through organized community effort, so organizing these benefits as to enable every citizen to realize his birthright of health and longevity."[4] In 1978 the World Health Organization (WHO) revised its 1946 definition of health as "not merely the absence of disease but a state of complete physical, mental, and social well-being" to "a level of health that permits people to lead socially and economically productive lives."[5] In 1988, the Institute of Medicine of the National Research Council defined the mission of public health as "fulfilling society's interest in assuring conditions in which people can be healthy."[6]

Community health is profoundly affected by the collective beliefs, attitudes, and behaviors of everyone who lives in the community.[7] The health of individuals living in every community in every state and territory determines the health status of the nation. Environmental factors and individual behaviors are responsible for an estimated 70% of all premature deaths in the United States. Developing and implementing policies and preventive interventions that effectively address these determinants of health can reduce the burden of illness, enhance the quality of life, and increase longevity.[8]

Assuring the health of the public means reaching the whole population with prevention strategies. It differs from the medical care model of one-to-one diagnosis and treatment of sick individuals who present with observable symptoms. Examples of time-tested public health strategies that reach everybody in the community include providing a safe water and food supply; fortification of table salt with iodine to prevent goiter; bread and cereal enrichment with thiamin, riboflavin, niacin, iron, and folic acid to prevent pellagra, beriberi, iron deficiency anemia, and neural tube defects; fortification of milk with vitamins A and D, originally to prevent rickets and now to prevent osteoporosis; and adding fluorides to community drinking water to reduce dental caries. Each of these strategies was a response to commonly observed nutrition-related health problems in the population.

In 1994, the U.S. Department of Health and Human Services convened a public health functions steering committee with representatives from the major public health constituencies. This committee expanded on the three core governmental public health functions of *assessment, policy development* and *assurance* and organized them into 10 essential public health services:

"*Assessment*
 1. Monitor health status to identify community health problems.
 2. Diagnose and investigate health problems and health hazards in the community.

Policy development
3. Inform, educate, and empower people about health issues.
4. Mobilize community partnerships to identify and solve health problems.
5. Develop policies and plans that support individual and community health efforts.

Assurance
6. Enforce laws and regulations that protect health and ensure safety.
7. Link people to needed personal health services, and assure the provision of health care when otherwise unavailable.
8. Assure a competent public health and personal health care workforce.
9. Evaluate effectiveness, accessibility, and quality of personal and population-based health services.

Serving all functions
10. Research for new insights and innovative solutions to health problems."[9]

These 10 essential public health services are proposed as responsibilities of the public health infrastructure. This infrastructure includes the tax-supported state and local public health departments in partnership with nongovernment agencies and organizations that provide any of these services. *Healthy People 2010* envisions environmental health, occupational health and safety, mental health, and substance abuse as integral parts of public health. Service providers, such as managed care organizations, hospitals, nonprofit corporations, schools, faith organizations, and businesses, can support the public health infrastructure as partners.[10]

VIEW THE COMMUNITY AS THE "PATIENT"

The official (tax-supported) public health department views its whole community, whether it is a district, city, county, tribe, state, or nation, as its "patient" using epidemiological data. Public health departments strive to promote health and prevent communicable and chronic diseases by doing the following:

- Directing programs and funds to the priority health problems and high-risk populations identified through a community needs assessment
- Reaching out with services based on research evidence to target those people who are particularly vulnerable to disease because of inadequate income, education, ethnicity, heredity, age, lifestyle, or food insecurity
- Marketing a healthy lifestyle as a shared value for all of the people who live in their community
- Collaborating with other health and human service professionals, educators, policy makers, legislators, community leaders, business executives, interested public citizens, and consumers to make wise use of available resources
- Monitoring statistical data, program evaluations, and consumer satisfaction surveys to be certain that the public health system is responding to current and anticipated needs

SPECTRUM OF PREVENTION

Traditionally, public health workers have classified disease prevention into three levels from wellness to final disease. This concept can be viewed as a seamless spectrum.

Primary prevention or *health promotion* eliminates or reduces potential risk factors among the whole population. Primary prevention efforts work to change the environment in ways that will enhance and maintain wellness and improve the quality of life and productivity of the people, thus reducing their needs for costly medical care. Health promotion should be part of national, state, and local health agendas. Health promotion or primary prevention efforts are enhanced through partnerships between the public health agency and cooperative extension offices, the food distribution system, mass media, schools, houses of worship, work sites, gyms, recreation centers, clubs, and social groups. Although important at any age of life, health promotion directed to children, youth, and families has the greatest potential for "adding life to years" as well as "years to life." To promote wellness, nutritionists educate and persuade the public to use the current *Dietary Guidelines for Americans 2005* to select their daily meals and snacks. Nutritionists consult with food processors, food marketers, and restauranteurs to modify their formulas, recipes, and menus and to control portion sizes using dietary guidelines to offer the population more tasty health-promoting foods (Chapter 18).

Secondary prevention, also known as *clinical preventive services* or *primary medical care,* appraises and reduces health risks by screening and early treatment before observable signs and symptoms of disease appear. The goal is to reduce risk among those people who may be susceptible to a health problem because of family history (genetics), lifestyle, environment, or age. Secondary prevention services include screening, detection, early diagnosis, treatment, and follow-up. These services are offered by the tax-supported public health agencies as well as by primary health care centers, primary care practitioners, or managed care organizations. For secondary prevention, nutritionists continue to urge members of the public to follow the *Dietary Guidelines for Americans 2005* as they choose foods from the supermarket, fast-food takeout, or their favorite restaurant. Nutritionists also counsel individual clients who require medical nutrition therapy prescribed by a health care provider as part of medical treatment.

Tertiary prevention or *tertiary medical care* is treatment and rehabilitation for persons who have a diagnosed health condition that requires medical treatment and follow-up. Its goal is to prevent or delay disability, pain, suffering, and premature death. Tertiary care is usually provided by community health care centers, managed health care organizations, university medical centers, hospital outpatient and inpatient facilities, home health agencies, rehabilitation facilities, extended care facilities, private physicians in specialty practices, or hospices. These resources are disproportionately used by older persons.[11] As in secondary prevention, nutritionists and dietitians counsel patients to follow the *Dietary*

Guidelines for Americans 2005 and any medical nutrition therapy prescribed by their health care provider.

A strong federal, state, and local public health infrastructure responds to acute and chronic threats to community health. The infrastructure is the foundation for planning, delivering, and evaluating public health services. It requires a well-organized structure; a knowledgeable and highly skilled interdisciplinary work force, and reliable and accessible data and information systems to document public health services. Applied research as an integral part of the public health infrastructure identifies opportunities to improve community health, to strengthen information systems and organizations, to monitor the quality and impact of services, and to make more cost-effective and efficient use of resources.[12]

TRENDS THAT IMPACT THE PUBLIC'S HEALTH

Public health workers monitor health and disease trends by collecting, analyzing, and interpreting the data for their communities to be sure that programs and services reflect local needs. Some discouraging trends include the following:

- Over half of the adults in the United States are estimated to be overweight or obese. Being overweight or obese vies with tobacco use as the leading health indicator in *Healthy People 2010.*[13]
- By 2025, almost 20% of the U.S. population is expected to be older than age 65, the age group in which about two thirds of chronic disabling conditions occur.[14]
- The proportion of the population who are Hispanic, African-American, Asian-American, or Native American is expected to grow from 28% in 2000 to 32% by 2010. Pervasive inequities and institutional racism identified in the health care system often result in unequal and unacceptable treatment to patients who belong to racial and ethnic minorities.[15]
- When population data are analyzed by gender, race and ethnicity, income and education, and sexual orientation, disparities in health are noted. Deficits in health literacy contribute to complications of chronic diseases among people unable to read instructions and understand their prescribed treatment. Further disparities are found for younger people who are disabled and for populations in rural areas.[16]
- An estimated 44 million persons under age 65 years are not covered by health insurance, including 11 million uninsured children.[17]

Work of public health professionals is enhanced by applying evidence-based public health practice, which means more rigorous scientific scrutiny for efficacy and effectiveness of community-based interventions as modeled on the work of the U.S. Preventive Services Task Force. This task force is reviewing the most frequently used clinical preventive services to differentiate what works from what does not. Adopting the recommended guidelines can raise the standards of practice for clinical preventive services to selected age groups.

Increased access and use of personal computers and the Internet by professionals and the public offers ever-expanding access to unlimited health information. The Internet offers opportunities to network with others with similar health concerns and to mobilize concerned professionals and consumers to influence health policy and legislation. Health and nutrition information currently at the fingertips of Internet users is empowering. However, some information may be misleading, erroneous, and even dangerous if users are not given adequate guidance to discriminate between fact and fiction.[18]

With advances in genomics, some diseases may be detected at the gene level permitting preventive treatment long before disease actually presents symptoms. However, genetic research raises many scientific and ethical questions.[19]

HISTORY OF OFFICIAL PUBLIC HEALTH AND PUBLIC HEALTH NUTRITION

State, city, and county governments became actively involved in public health during the late 1800s when it became necessary to organize community efforts against epidemics of communicable diseases, to assure safe water and food supplies, and to establish proper sewage disposal. In the late 1800s and early 1900s, application of the emerging sciences of bacteriology and epidemiology brought the devastating epidemics of fatal contagious diseases under control through vaccines developed for their prevention and in later years with antibiotics developed for their treatment. Some epidemics of seemingly communicable diseases such as pellagra, rickets, and scurvy were found by epidemiologists to be due to nutrient deficiencies readily treated first by improved diets and then by specific vitamins identified in the early 1900s. The ultimate public health response was specific food enrichment or fortification legislation.

As successes were achieved with many of the communicable and nutrient deficiency diseases, federal, state, and local public health agencies moved forward to reduce maternal and infant mortality and morbidity. In the 1930s through Title V of the Social Security Act, federal funds became available to state health departments to employ nutritionists as consultants to public health physicians and nurses and as educators to mothers and families.

Maternal and child health continues as a public health priority, Now primary prevention focuses on family planning, preconceptional care, reproductive health, and early prenatal care. Health needs of women with high-risk pregnancies (particularly teenagers), low birth weight infants, and children with developmental disabilities demand secondary preventive strategies. Nutritionists have been increasingly employed to develop nutrition services in maternal and child health (see Chapter 8). Since 1974, by far the largest numbers of public health and community nutrition personnel have been employed through funds available from the U.S. Department of Agriculture to state, local, and tribal health agencies for the popular Supplemental Nutrition Program for Women, Infants, and Children (WIC) (see Chapter 8).

In the 1950s, official public health agencies began to observe the growing health and economic burden on society of an aging population, and the needs to prevent, control, and delay chronic diseases (e.g., heart disease, stroke, cancer, diabetes, kidney disease, osteoporosis, and arthritis) became a priority. Many state and local health departments have employed nutritionists to develop primary prevention strategies and provide or arrange for physician-prescribed medical nutrition therapy (see Chapters 9, 10, and 11). Successive surgeon general's reports in the 1970s and 1980s, followed by *Healthy People 1990, Healthy People 2000,* and *Healthy People 2010,* reported health status data and published measurable objectives. These objectives have been used to set the agendas for national, state, and local public health initiatives. Since the 1980s *Dietary Goals* and the successive revisions of the *Dietary Guidelines* have focused attention on the chronic disease risks of the pervasive popular American diet, which is high in calories, sodium, saturated fat, and alcohol while it is low and often even lacking in nutrient-dense, lower-calorie foods such as reduced-fat dairy products, fruits and vegetables, dried beans, nuts, and whole grains. These excesses and deficiencies have been linked to obesity, hypertension, heart disease, stroke, diabetes, and some types of cancers. The federal government has supported state and local health departments by providing grants-in-aid; setting standards and guidelines; offering technical assistance, consultation, and training; developing and distributing educational materials for professional and public education; developing and managing data systems; and supporting basic and applied research.

NUTRITION IN PUBLIC HEALTH

Early nutrition efforts in public health focused on control of single nutrient deficiency diseases such as scurvy, beriberi, pellagra, and rickets. This was followed by the contributions of nutrition to the health of pregnant women, their growing infants, and children. Now there is compelling scientific evidence that documents the relationships of multiple, often interacting dietary components to the prevention and dietary management of some of today's most serious, costly, disabling, and killing conditions. Conditions cited in *Healthy People 2010* were most clearly associated with dietary factors. Obesity and being overweight are now compellingly associated with many of the leading diseases causing death in the United States. Poor diet and lack of sufficient physical activity have even placed with tobacco use among the actual causes of death in the United States in 2000. Those causes of death specifically tied to obesity and being overweight in *Healthy People 2010* are:

- Hypertension
- Coronary heart disease
- Type 2 diabetes
- Cancer, particularly breast and colorectal cancers
- Stroke
- Osteoarthritis

Dietary Goals and *Dietary Guidelines for Americans* have been published, revised, and widely distributed by the United States Departments of Agriculture and Health and Human Services for over 25 years. Yet, the popular American diet is still excessively high in calories and saturated fats, trans fats, refined sugar, and sodium contributing to the current epidemic of obesity and overweight Americans and the resulting diseases and disabilities previously listed. The proportion of meals and snacks eaten or prepared away from home increased by more than two thirds from 1977 to 1995: from 16% of all meals in 1977 to 27% of all meals con- sumed in 1995.[20] Most foods prepared away from home contain excessive amounts of fat, particularly saturated fats and trans fats, plus refined sugar and salt. Most people consume more calories when they eat away from home. Meals and snacks that children purchase in school also are high in saturated fats and sugar.[21] Although research is identifying the role of antioxidants and other nutri- ents in fruits, vegetables, dried beans, and whole grains, these are the very foods most frequently found to be lacking in meals most commonly eaten by both adults and children.

Never before has there been greater challenge and opportunity for public health nutritionists to demonstrate their knowledge and skills by taking the lead in addressing life-threatening public health problems. Collaborating with their public health colleagues, nutritionists must vigorously and visibly promote the healthy eating and physical activity essential to primary prevention efforts directed to the population as a whole.

Public health nutritionists keep pace with the emerging nutrition research and incorporate what is applicable as the evidence base for public health promotion programs (Chapter 2). They assess food and nutrition needs and problems among the population of their communities (Chapters 3 and 4). Bringing these issues to the attention of their administrators, community leaders, consumers, policy mak- ers, and legislators, nutritionists participate in establishing policy and proposing needed legislation (Chapters 5, 6, and 7). Nutritionists incorporate cost-effective and consumer-friendly nutrition interventions to promote and protect the public's health throughout the lifespan (Chapters 8, 9, and 10); vulnerable populations receiving primary care (Chapter 11); and children and older adults who live in group care facilities (Chapter 12). Public health nutritionists collaborate with environmentalists and the food industry to assure that everyone has access to safe, nutritious affordable food. (Chapter 13). Nutritionists mobilize support as they design, implement, and evaluate programs and services in their jurisdiction to address the priority health needs related to food, nutrition, and diet (Chapter 14). Nutritionists sharpen their skills to market nutrition services to the public (Chapter 15), manage data (Chapter 16), and manage money (Chapter 17). Nutritionists motivate and educate school children and adults of all ages through innovative programs in schools, libraries, gyms, houses of worship, food markets, restaurants, civic and social clubs, mass media, and all other channels that they can use to establish contact with large numbers of people (Chapter 18).

To achieve the most with a productive, creative workforce, it is necessary to employ qualified staff and effectively supervise public health nutrition personnel (Chapters 19 and 20), partner with colleagues within the agency and the community (Chapters 21), and network face to face and on the Internet (Chapter 22). To survive in a competitive world requires administrative support (Chapter 23), always pursuing excellence (Chapter 24), and anticipating the future (Chapter 25).

ESSENTIAL KNOWLEDGE AND SKILLS FOR PUBLIC HEALTH NUTRITION PRACTICE

As the community's and agency's nutrition experts, practitioners in public health nutrition must understand, interpret, and apply current research from nutrition science and medical nutrition therapy to people of all educational levels. Nutritionists' audiences include those with limited health literacy and those who speak and read different languages. Nutritionists must be equally knowledgeable in the theory and practice of changing eating behavior and know how to reach and motivate hard-to-reach populations. To address the needs of all of the people in the community, the public health nutritionist must additionally possess the knowledge and skills used by their public health colleagues including:

- Biostatistics—Collecting, compiling, analyzing, and interpreting demographic (population characteristics), health, nutrition assessment, and food consumption data
- Epidemiology and nutritional epidemiology—Applying health, nutritional status, and disease distribution patterns in the population and studying trends over time
- Health behavior—Understanding personal, interpersonal, and community influences on individual and population behavior and applying tested models to design successful interventions to guide individuals and communities to make positive changes in eating and exercise
- Policy, planning, and administration—Collaborating with colleagues, administrators, and policy makers to plan, organize, manage, market, and

evaluate nutrition services and programs as a component of the health improvement plan for the community
- Environmental science—Identifying the biological and chemical factors that affect the quality and safety of the air, water, and food supply

Self-assessment provides the baseline for each nutritionist to periodically review and update a professional career development plan. Keeping pace with advances in nutrition science research and public health practice requires a life-long plan for learning through continuing education (on-the-job and academic course work), use of consultants, technical assistance, and research to function as a respected leader and resource on the interdisciplinary public health team and in the community. The Commission on Dietetic Registration (CDR) *Professional Development Portfolio Guide* provides examples of self-assessment for the public health nutritionist on its Web site www.cdrnet.org. The examples assess individual competencies in the five areas essential to excel in the practice of public health nutrition:

1. Nutrition science and dietetic practice
2. Communication
3. Public health science and practice
4. Management
5. Policy, legislation, and advocacy

Public health/community nutritionists further earn the respect and admiration of their public health colleagues, the media, and the people in their community when they "practice what they preach." This includes role modeling desirable body weight achieved by following *Dietary Guidelines for Americans* and pursuing a regular exercise routine. The chapters in this handbook challenge each nutritionist employed in public and community health to be among those taking the lead to promote the public's health in this new century.

POINTS TO PONDER

- How should tax dollars be allocated between population-based health promotion programs (including nutrition interventions) and medical care to high-risk populations lacking health insurance?
- How should the public health nutritionist prioritize time and effort between work in the community and in the health agency primary care clinics?
- What competencies are most important for the nutritionist working in public health?
- What gaps in educational backgrounds can be filled by on-the-job continuing education and which educational deficits require supervised clinical and public health experience and/or advanced academic course work?

HELPFUL WEB SITES

Commission on Dietetic Registration: www.cdrnet.org

NOTES

1. Overcoming obesity in America [Cover]. *Time.* June 7, 2004.
2. Fighting flab in Arkansas. *The Economist.* June 12, 2004;29.
3. Winslow CEA. The untilled field of public health. *Modern Medicine.* March 1920; 2:183.
4. Whaley RF, Haskin TJ. *A Textbook of World Health.* New York, NY: Parthenon; 1995.
5. Institute of Medicine. *The Future of Public Health.* Washington, DC: National Academy Press; 1988:7.
6. US Department of Health and Human Services. *Healthy People 2010,* 2nd ed. McLean, Va: International Medical Publishing; 2002:3.
7. US Department of Health and Human Services. *Healthy People 2010: Understanding and Improving Health.* Washington, DC: US Department of Health and Human Services; 2000:3,18.
8. Institute of Medicine. *The Future of the Public's Health in the 21st Century.* Washington, DC: National Academy Press; 2001:99.
9. US Department of Health and Human Services. *Healthy People 2010.* 2nd ed. McLean, Va: International Medical Publishing; 2002:23–3.
10. Turnock B. *Public Health: What It Is and How It Works.* 2nd ed. Sudbury, Mass: Jones and Bartlett Publishers; 2001:89–90.
11. US Department of Health and Human Services. *Healthy People 2010.* 2nd ed. McLean, Va: International Medical Publishing; 2002:23–3,23–4.
12. US Department of Health and Human Services. *Healthy People 2010.* 2nd ed. McLean, Va: International Medical Publishing; 2002:29.
13. Institute of Medicine. *The Future of the Public's Health in the 21st Century.* Washington, DC: National Academies Press; 2001:232.
14. Institute of Medicine. *The Future of the Public's Health in the 21st Century.* Washington, DC: National Academies Press; 2001:36.
15. US Department of Health and Human Services. *Healthy People 2010.* 2nd ed. McLean, Va: International Medical Publishing; 2002:11–16.
16. US Department of Health and Human Services. *Healthy People 2010.* 2nd ed. McLean, Va: International Medical Publishing; 2002:45.
17. Turnock B. *Public Health: What It Is and How It Works.* 2nd ed. Sudbury, Mass: Jones and Bartlett Publishers; 2001:266–269.
18. Institute of Medicine. *The Future of the Public's Health in the 21st Century.* Washington, DC: National Academies Press; 2001:17,38.

19. Institute of Medicine. *The Future of the Public's Health in the 21st Century.* Washington, DC: National Academies Press; 2001:37.

20. US Department of Health and Human Services. *Healthy People 2010.* 2nd ed. McLean, Va: International Medical Publishing; 2002:19–30.

BIBLIOGRAPHY

Commission on Dietetic Registration. Professional development portfolio guide, public health nutritionist. Available at: http://www.cdrnet.org.

Institute of Medicine. *The Future of the Public's Health in the 21st Century.* Washington, DC: National Academies Press; 2003.

Kaufman M, ed. *Nutrition in Public Health: A Handbook for Developing Programs and Services.* Rockville, Md: Aspen Publishers; 1990.

Scuthchfield FD, Keck CW, eds. *Principles of Public Health Practice.* 2nd ed. Clifton Park, NY: Thomson Delmar Learning; 2003.

Turnock BJ. *Public Health, What It Is and How It Works.* 2nd ed. Sudbury, Mass: Jones and Bartlett Publishers; 2004.

US Department of Health and Human Services. *Healthy People 2010.* 2nd ed. McLean, Va: International Medical Publishing Inc: 2002.

US Department of Health and Human Services. *Healthy People 2010: Understanding and Improving Health.* Washington, DC: US Department of Health and Human Services; 2000.

US Preventive Services Task Force. *Guide to Clinical Preventive Services.* 2nd ed. McLean, Va: International Medical Publishing Inc; 1996.

CHAPTER 2

Establish the Evidence Base for Nutrition Practice

Judith C. Rodriguez

Reader Objectives

- Identify the methods, applications, and issues related to nutrition research.
- Describe the basis, uses, and limitations of the dietary recommendations and guidelines to apply in public health nutrition practice.
- Discuss the impact of nutrition trends (e.g., weight loss diets) and research issues (e.g., nutrigenomics) on public health nutrition practice.
- Develop benefit–risk and evidence-based approaches to select public health nutrition interventions and disseminate information to diverse populations.
- List and access some of the resources public health nutritionists can use to keep up with current research.

NUTRITION EXPERTISE IN PUBLIC HEALTH

"Should I stop eating carbohydrates in order to lose weight?" "If both of my parents are fat, is there any use for me to try to lose weight?" These are among the common questions addressed to public health nutritionists every day. The public relies heavily on the ability of nutrition professionals to translate current scientific information into accurate, relevant, and consumer-friendly messages.[1]

Public health nutritionists contribute to their health agency's mission, policies, and programs when they provide technical assistance and expertise in accessing, evaluating, and applying science-based information from a wide range of reliable sources. They train other public health personnel and plan, design, implement,

13

and evaluate programs[2] to promote health and contribute to primary, secondary, and tertiary disease prevention at each stage of the life span.[3,4]

Public health nutritionists are the authoritative resource professionals on food, nutrition, and diet to promote the health of the people in their communities. They advocate on behalf of consumers and agencies for local, state, and national nutrition policies (see Chapters 5, 6, and 7).[5] Nutritionists collaborate with print and broadcast media reporters to assure that the nutrition, diet, and health information they disseminate to the public is based on sound, current research evidence. Nutritionists are challenged with growing opportunities to advise food processors, food marketers, and food service directors to offer the people they serve food choices to promote more healthy diets. Nutritionists collaborate and educate administrators, colleagues, staff, and consumer groups on the contributions of healthy food in maintaining a desirable weight, promoting health, and preventing many chronic diseases.

A nutritionist's credibility in these roles is established by demonstrating the ability to interpret up-to-date scientific data, adjusting the message as the public becomes more science literate and as more nutrient labeling and claims appear on food packaging and in advertisements for food products. Public health nutritionists are called upon to provide guidelines to evaluate available information, a particularly important task at a time of ever-changing information. The public is increasingly bombarded with conflicting, often misleading and biased, nutrition information from a variety of sources. Every nutritionist must possess the self-confidence to take an informed stand on controversial issues and use a common-sense approach to translate nutrition science findings into useful consumer education.

Nutrition research has made great strides ranging from the first identification of the essential vitamins and trace minerals to the current use of social marketing to promote healthy foods and to inform the public of the role of diet in promoting health and preventing obesity and related chronic diseases. Nutrition science continues to evolve with many unanswered questions and continuing controversies. The researchers' view of the "half-empty cup" of knowledge inspires continuing scientific pursuits. Nutrition practitioners are the optimists who interpret the "half-full cup" of research information to benefit the health and quality of life of the people in their communities.[6]

Research as the Base for Practice

To respond effectively to questions from professional colleagues, consumers, the public, and clients, nutrition professionals must integrate the current research findings in food science, nutrition, dietetics, human physiology, chemistry, biochemistry, medicine, education, marketing, economics, and personal and group behavior. They interpret findings from a rich history and from the continuing evolution of scientific research.

After identifying and describing the major nutrients, scientists quantified basic human requirements for each of these nutrients. Balance studies determined protein and mineral needs. Vitamin requirements were estimated using growth studies and tissue saturation tests. The research included food analysis and studies of human digestion, absorption, and metabolism, as well as specific nutrient needs and studies of nutrient deficiency diseases and their prevention and cure.

Nutrition science is grounded in research methods that identify nutrients, human nutrient needs, and nutrient composition of foods, as well as disease prevention and treatment through medical nutrition therapy. Nutrition research studies range from evaluating programs that promote healthy eating behaviors to identifying and integrating the impact of technological changes. Today some studies test the application of behavioral models to promote healthy food choices and try to analyze an array of increasingly complex issues.

Nutrition science integrates research findings from the natural, behavioral, health, and related sciences. A number of investigative designs can be used in research related to nutrition, diet, and health. Practitioners must understand the different research designs and their constraints. To critically evaluate research findings and determine their potential applications, practitioners need to know that research is synonymous with the scientific method and is founded on the requirement of replication. Well-designed research starts with a clearly articulated hypothesis, question, or problem that is then subdivided into smaller and more manageable units.[7] Well-designed research follows systematic procedures to collect and analyze the data. Basic research is usually conducted in a laboratory and seeks new knowledge. Applied research is usually conducted in field settings and tests interventions, programs, or initiatives.

Epidemiological research includes nutritional epidemiology. Epidemiologists observe and document naturally occurring patterns in the frequency, distribution, and determinants of health and disease in populations. In correlational and ex post facto (causal-comparative) designs, data are analyzed to observe whether differences in one variable are related to differences in other variables.[8] This enables researchers to compare a population's diet, related characteristics, and health and disease patterns. Several classic nutrition studies and subsequent scientific developments resulted from epidemiological studies. For example, a study done in the southeastern United States attributed pellagra to the lack of niacin and tryptophan in the region's then commonly consumed corn-based diet. Observations of lower heart disease rates among Eskimos compared to other ethnic groups led to subsequent findings of the beneficial effects of a diet rich in omega-3 fatty acids.[9] Ecological research collects statistical data and analyzes it for associations between disease, exposure parameters, and disease rates of groups or populations in different countries or geographic regions or within a specified time period.[10] Areas of concern in epidemiological research are:

- Were the appropriate questions asked?
- Were the correct population groups selected?

- Were the factors under study the correct ones to be studying?
- Are the dietary factors under study actually the attributable causes?
- Have any unidentified but important associations been omitted or missed?[11]

Survey research describes and measures selected characteristics to provide a statistical profile of a defined population.[12] The United States National Nutrition Monitoring System (see Chapter 16) includes a number of surveys that provide baseline and comparative data collected using representative probability or purposive samples. *Monitoring* involves intermittent data collection. *Surveillance* is continuous data collection. These systems track the health status of the community to facilitate a prompt response. The National Nutrition Monitoring and Related Research Program (NNMRRP) periodically collects, analyzes, and reports five major types of data:

- Food supply determinations, such as the *US Food and Nutrition Supply Series*
- Food and nutrition consumption data, such as *5-A-Day for Better Health*, the *Nationwide Food Consumption Survey*, and the *Continuing Survey of Food Intake by Individuals*
- Nutrition statistics and related health measures, such as the Pediatric Nutrition Surveillance System and *National Health and Nutrition Examination Survey (NHANES)*
- Food composition and nutrient databases, such as the *National Nutrient Data Bank*[13]
- Knowledge, attitude, and behavior data, such as the *Diet and Health Knowledge Survey* and the *Behavioral Risk Factor Surveillance System.*[14,15]

The Behavioral Risk Factor Surveillance System collects data from all 50 states, as well as Puerto Rico, Guam, and the District of Columbia. It includes a fixed core of questions and two other rotating cores of questions. For example, Rotating Core 2 includes questions on fruits and vegetable consumption, physical activity, and weight control.[16] These data are also used to periodically set and measure progress toward achieving health goals and objectives as in *Healthy People 2000* and *Healthy People 2010.*

Areas of concern in survey research are the sample, validity, and reliability of the survey instrument and survey process; the response rate; and potential biases. For example, does the probability sample used for *National Health and Nutrition Examination Survey* characterize the overall United States population, and is it adjusted for age, gender, ethnic, and economic distribution of a particular area?[17] If a survey is based on a convenience sample, the data only describes the specific population surveyed and may have limited application to the population as a whole.

A form of applied research commonly used by public health professionals is program evaluation. Public health programs usually focus on the assessed health problems and needs of the population who live or work within a geographically defined area. Health promotion and disease prevention initiatives targeted to people in their natural environment provide an ideal setting to evaluate large-scale food and nutrition interventions and to measure achievement of national, state, and local health goals and objectives. Public health nutritionists should participate in demonstration or pilot projects that are part of policy initiatives. This permits programs that are both specific for and sensitive to local communities, and simultaneously allows for evaluation of models and concepts that may have broad-based application.[18] This may include a community intervention trial or study that determines the effectiveness of a program.[19]

Formative evaluation collects and analyzes data to provide continuing feedback while a program is in progress. This permits midcourse improvements while the program and activities are in progress. Summative evaluation is retrospective, usually collecting data at the beginning and end of the program, and compares information about the performance up to the time when the evaluation is completed. Program evaluation may focus on outcome or utilization. It may include evaluation standards of utility, feasibility, propriety, and accuracy.[20]

An experiment is a precise investigation to test a hypothesis. The investigation involves two or more variables. The independent variable is tested through one or a series of controlled settings using nonrandomized or randomized sampling methods. The dependent variable is influenced by the independent variable. Nonrandomized experimental designs include the observational cohort study in which the population of interest is selected and followed over a specified period of time to record subsequent occurrences of disease. In the retrospective case control study, a group of people in whom the disease is already present is matched to a comparable control group for such characteristics as age, gender, race, and ethnicity.

The gold standard of cause–effect research is the true experimental study. This includes animal and metabolic studies and clinical trials. Animal studies are commonly used in experimental nutrition research because the genetic backgrounds of the laboratory animals are known or easy to determine. Under laboratory conditions, the food and nutrient intakes of the animals can be controlled or manipulated to study the variables of interest. All aspects of the animals' growth, development, health, and reproductive outcomes can be observed. Small animals can be observed over several generations and their tissues examined after their death in a shorter time period than is possible in human research.

In metabolic studies and in clinical trials that use human subjects, blinding is a desirable element of experimental research. In a blind study, the subjects do not know whether they are in the experimental or control (placebo) group. In a double-blind study, neither the subjects nor the investigators who collect the data know which subjects are in the experimental or control group.

Balance studies, which may involve small animals or humans, are primarily used in nutrition research to determine the levels of nutrient intake needed to achieve equilibrium between intake and output. The results from studies using laboratory animals are interpreted carefully and can be used as a basis to pursue further research. Findings may not be easily generalized from nonhumans to humans or when the experimental group does not represent the total population in terms of age, ethnicity, or socioeconomic status.[21]

A common experimental nutrition research method, the randomized clinical trial, uses small numbers of human subjects and runs for a short period. Randomized clinical trials are used to test dietary interventions to control kinds and amounts of foods, formula diets, or formulated food products. If the experimental group is fed a formulated diet and compared to a control group, it is called a metabolic study. In animal studies rats, mice, rabbits, guinea pigs, dogs, sheep, and monkeys are selected for characteristics known to be most similar to humans in terms of digestion, absorption, and metabolism.[22]

Meta-analysis compares the results of various studies. This type of analysis can only be done when data from many investigations are available. This research involves complex statistical analysis of results from a combination of experimental and ex post facto studies to determine if they provide predictable results. The current emphasis is to use statistical methods to estimate heterogeneity among studies.[23]

Nutrition science is grounded in research methods to identify nutrients, nutrient needs, composition of foods, and their contributions to human health, growth, and development throughout the life span. This includes evaluating the effectiveness of medical nutrition therapy to treat major chronic diseases. Today nutrition science is broader based than it was in its founding years, and the expectations and standards for the conduct of research are more rigorous.[24,25,26]

Issues and Problems Related to Nutrition Research Methods

Three common factors limit human nutrition research studies:

1. Cost
2. Obtaining diverse human subjects that meet the inclusion criteria such as finding comparable control and experimental groups
3. Including minority or underrepresented populations.[27]

Large population samples or studies involving many geographical areas are costly. Small experiments may need expensive equipment or supplies. It may be difficult to get participants to adhere to the diet or there may be large subject dropout rates.[28] If the separation between the control and experimental groups is not maintained there can be some group crossover or contamination effects. If there is selection or researcher bias or faulty randomization or design the results can be incorrect and misinterpreted.[29,30] A qualitative study is flexible, open ended, and evolving but challenging to design. Data may possibly be misinterpreted, and it may be easy to lose focus. Well-designed research plans attempt to identify potential problems and incorporate processes to minimize anticipated problems.

Although randomized controlled trials are considered the ideal for clinical research, these trials may not be appropriate for public health investigations. Evaluation of large-scale public health programs that involve multiple and complex variables are challenging and require a variety and combination of investigative methods.[31]

Research Evidence for Dietary Recommendations

How does a public health nutritionist decide how to respond to questions? A primary function of official public health agencies is to protect the health of its citizens. This protection includes formulating health and nutrition policies, initiatives, and practices based on sound science. Initially public health protections focused on sanitation and treatment of nutrient deficiency diseases.[32] This function has evolved into the current interests in the contributions of diet and nutrition to promote the quality of life and prevent chronic diseases. A timely example is to fortify foods with folic acid to prevent the birth of infants with neural tube defects.[33] Another use of this systematic and analytical review of the evolving scientific literature is to develop recommended nutrient intake standards and national dietary guidelines.[34]

Research and Nutrient Density

The concept of nutrient density is an example of how basic research including investigations of food composition and human nutrient needs is used in public health practice. Nutrient density is the ratio of the amount of one or various nutrients to the total calories provided by the food. It is usually expressed as the amount of the nutrient per 1000 kcal of energy. This index of nutritional quality (INQ) is widely used in public health nutrition education.[35] Nutrient density facilitated the shift from recommending foods to overcome dietary deficiencies to suggesting foods to promote health and avoid over consumption of energy.[36]

DIETARY RECOMMENDATIONS

The United States Department of Agriculture (USDA) first published dietary recommendations in 1917 and has done so periodically since that time. The Food and Nutrition Board (FNB), a unit of the Institute of Medicine (IOM) of the National Academy of Sciences (NAS), was established in the 1940s to study and to provide judgment on nutrition issues related to the health of the public. The first recommended nutrient levels, the Recommended Dietary Allowances (RDAs), published by the National Research Council of the National Academy of Science (1943) were quantifications based on epidemiological, clinical, and laboratory research about human nutrient needs. The Basic 7 Food Groups plan, classified foods by their nutrient composition and recommended daily minimum numbers of servings for each of the food groups.[37] Since the 1940s the Food and Nutrition Board meets intermittently to review the emerging scientific data and to update the daily nutrient intake recommendations. These values are used to set nutrient standards and facilitate dietary planning, including development of those used in public health nutrition programs and policies.[38]

History of the DRIs

Historically, the RDAs, developed specifically for United States population groups, were nutrient reference values to use to provide the base for dietary guidelines. The early emphasis was to prevent nutrient deficiency diseases and recommend adequate consumption of specific essential nutrients. A "margin of safety" was added for all nutrients except calories. As scientific data on the minimum, optimal, and excessive intake levels of some nutrients became available, it was periodically necessary to update the recommendations. These reviews and changes have not always been easily achieved through broad consensus. For example, the publication of the 10th edition of the RDAs was delayed due to several policy and science issues.[39,40]

Continuing advances in nutrition research have now led to a complex set of nutrient recommendations that specify three different quantities of calories and essential nutrients needed by healthy American males and females at different ages, growth rates, and activity levels. Using current scientific evidence, the Dietary Reference Intakes (DRIs) were eventually developed and published, and the RDAs became a category within the DRIs.[41,42] DRIs are reference values used for populations of both the United States and Canada.

The DRIs include the following:

- Estimated Average Requirements (EAR)
- Estimated Energy Requirements (EER)
- Recommended Dietary Allowances (RDA)
- Adequate Intakes (AI)
- Acceptable Macronutrient Distribution Range (AMDR)
- Tolerable Upper Intake Level (UL)

Figure 2–1 graphically compares the risks of inadequate or the risks of excess intakes for the EAR, RDA, and UL.

Daily Reference Values (DRVs) were developed to use for nutrient labeling and are based on an established 2000 or 2500 calories in a daily diet.[43] Current dietary reference intakes also include data from research reports for bioactive compounds, such as phytoestrogens, other phytochemicals, and carnitine. The role of alcohol in health and disease is also discussed. To update information go to http://www.nal.usda.gov.

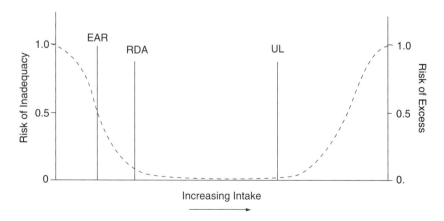

Figure 2–1 Graphic Illustration of the Relationship Between the Estimated Average Requirement (EAR), Recommended Dietary Allowance (RDA), and Tolerable Upper Intake Level (UL). *Source:* Institute of Medicine. *Dietary Reference Intakes Applications in Dietary Assessment.* Washington, DC: National Academies Press; 2000.

Applications of the DRIs

As knowledge about specific nutrient requirements grows, so do the opportunities to apply these findings to populations served by public health programs. The DRIs are quantitative recommendations of nutrient needs and recommended intakes that represent scientific consensus. These recommendation are used as the foundation of federal nutrition policies and the vehicle for the federal agencies to speak with one voice on nutrition and health.[44] Applications and uses fall into two general categories: diet assessment and diet planning.

Diet assessment applications are used to determine the possible adequacy or inadequacy of dietary intakes of populations of public health concern. Diet assessment applications are also used to measure progress of public health interventions to change consumer food choices. Although this conceptual framework appears simple, it is complex, and public health nutritionists should recognize that the applications differ according to whether they are used for an individual or for population groups.

For individuals, uses of DRIs include the following:

- EARs and RDAs to determine diet adequacy and appropriateness to life stage and gender
- AI to plan intake at or above the adequate level
- UL to determine if an individual is at potential risk of adverse effect[45]

For groups, use of DRIs include the following:

- EARs to determine the prevalence or percentage of the population subgroups at risk for inadequate intake. The references provide baseline data to determine risk of inadequate intake; to compare nutrient intakes by mean, median, and distributions for population subgroups; to identify changes in food consumption patterns that might reduce or increase the risk of inadequate intake; and to monitor changes over time.
- Determination of mean AI at one point in time and for comparison purposes
- ULs to determine potential risk of adverse effects or percentage of the population subgroups at risk for excessive intake at one point or over time
- Estimating or monitoring the potential of the food supply to meet the nutritional needs of the population[46]

Diet planning applications are used to plan nutrient intakes for individuals or groups. The nutritionist follows a systematic or schematic decision-making plan. Dietary references are used to develop the USDA food plans. The Thrifty Food Plan is used as the basis for the Food Stamp Program. The moderate and liberal food plans are used as the basis for military food allowances, which must be adjusted for different field conditions or during peacetime, overseas, or war. Figure 2–2 presents schematic decision tree for dietary planning of nutrient intake for an individual as a group.

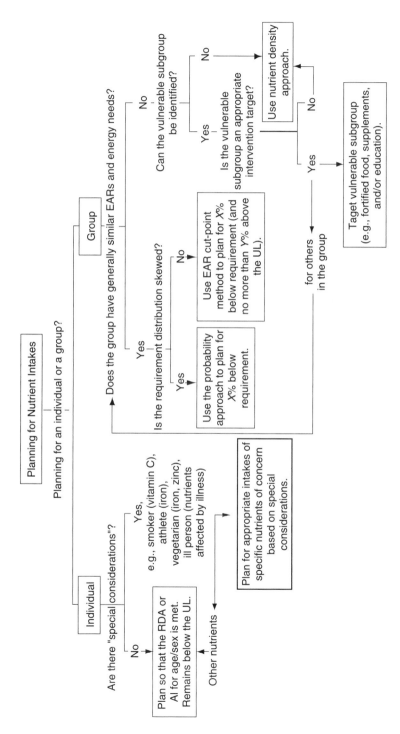

Figure 2–2 Schematic Decision Tree for Dietary Planning. *Source:* National Academy of Sciences. http://books.nap.edu/catalog/10609.html.

Box 2–2   Uses of DRIs for Planning Intakes of Apparently Healthy Individuals and Groups

For an Individual

EAR[a]: Should not be used as an intake goal for the individual

RDA: Plan for its intake; usual intake at or above this level has a low probability of inadequacy.

AI: Plan for this intake; usual intake at or above this level has a low probability of inadequacy.

UL: Plan for usual intake below this level to avoid potential risk of adverse effects from excessive nutrient intake.

For a Group

EAR[a]: Use to plan for an acceptably low prevalence of inadequate intakes within a group.

RDA: Should not be used to plan intakes of groups

AI[b]: Plan for mean intake at this level; mean usual intake at or above this level implies a low prevalence of inadequate intakes.

UL: Use in planning to minimize the proportion of the population at potential risk of excessive nutrient intake.

[a]In the case of energy, an EER is provided. The EER is the dietary energy intake that is predicted (with variance) to maintain energy balance in a healthy adult of a defined age, gender, weight, height, and level of physical activity. In children and pregnant and lactating women, the EER includes the needs associated with deposition of tissues or secretion of milk at rates consistent with good health. For individuals, the EER represents the mid-point of a range within which an individual's energy requirements are likely to vary. As such, it is below the needs of half the individuals with the specified characteristics and exceeds the needs of the other half. Body weight should be monitored and energy intake adjusted accordingly.

[b]The AI should be used with less confidence if it has not been established as a mean intake of a healthy group.

Another application is to establish nutrient standards to design meal patterns that provide a specified percentage of the dietary reference standards for federal food programs such as the National School Lunch Program, the Child and Adult Care Feeding Program, the Summer Food Service Program, and Older Americans Act Congregate and Home Delivered Meal Program. The nutrient standards are also used to evaluate and modify nutrient content of prescribed food packages for the Special Supplemental Nutrition Program for Women, Infants, and Children (WIC), the Commodity Supplemental Food Program, and the Food Distribution Program on Indian Reservations. The USDA's low-cost food plan is used for financial planning in bankruptcy cases. Federal, state, and local government agencies can use the reference standards to design, operate, and evaluate their food and nutrition assistance programs. Scientific and regulatory agencies can use these references to formulate standards and regulations to ensure that foods are safe and appropriately marketed and advertised.

The food industry uses the standards as a guide to develop, modify, produce, enrich, and/or fortify their products. The reference intakes are used to monitor trends, evaluate changes, identify the contribution of nutrients by specific foods or food groups, and determine the potential of the food supply to meet the nutritional needs of the population.

Reference standards can be used to assist individuals or groups to select healthy foods as they plan their meals. These standards are used to educate individuals and groups about the most nutrient-dense foods and health-promoting food consumption patterns. When using the dietary references to plan diets for groups, the dietary goals must be identified or selected, the target usual nutrient intake distribution must be estimated, menus must be planned to achieve that target, and the results of the plan must be assessed. If the plan is for a nonhomogeneous group, special needs must be considered.[47]

Individuals can use the standards to decide what kinds and amounts of foods to eat each day. The goal for individual diet planning is to use the references to achieve a low probability of nutrient inadequacy. The AI is used when there is not sufficient evidence to establish an EAR or RDA. The AI is the target used to minimize the risk of inadequacy. However, when planning intake based on the energy need of individuals the goal is to determine the level that minimizes the risks of inadequacy or excess. In this way, individual total energy expenditure (TEE) and energy needs related to gender, age, height, and weight, and activity level constitute the needed estimated energy requirement (EER).[48]

Table 2–1 displays the Dietary Reference Intake for 14 specified nutrients for specified age groups from infancy (0–6 months) to older adults (over 70 years).

Daily Nutrient Values on Food Labels

Federal law now requires that specified nutrients be listed on the food label in terms of the percentage of the daily value provided by a standard serving of the food. This nutrient information enables consumers to make informed food choices to select their total daily diet. These daily values for nutrients are based on two sets of reference values, the Daily Reference Values (DRVs) and the Reference Daily Intake (RDIs). RDI values are the same as the US RDA's 1968 highest recommended levels found in the US Recommended Daily Allowances (US RDA).[49]

The DRVs have an important regulatory role as the basis for calculating the percentage of the daily values used on the nutrition facts section of food labels (Figure 2–3).

In the 10th edition published in 1998 DRVs were established for fat, carbohydrates, cholesterol, and fiber, nutrients for which there were no previous stan-

Table 2-1 Dietary Reference Intakes (RDIs)

Life-Stage Group	Recommended levels for individual intake (a)													
	Calcium (mg/d)	Phosphorus (mg/d)	Magnesium (mg/d)	Vitamin D^bc (μg/d)	Fluoride (mg/d)	Thiamin (mg/d)	Riboflavin (mg/d)	Niacin^d (mg/d)	Vitamin B_6 (mg/d)	Folate^e (μg/d)	Vitamin B_{12} (μg/d)	Pantothenic acid (mg/d)	Biotin (μg/d)	Choline^f (mg/d)
Infants														
0–6 mo.	210*	100*	30*	5*	0.01*	0.2*	0.3*	2*	0.1*	65*	0.4*	1.7*	5*	125*
7–12 mo.	270*	275*	75*	5*	0.5*	0.3*	0.4*	4*	0.3*	80*	0.5*	1.8*	6*	150*
Children														
1–3 y	500*	460	80	5*	0.7*	0.5	0.5	6	0.5	150	0.9	2*	8*	200*
4–8 y	800*	500	130	5*	1*	0.6	0.6	8	0.6	200	1.2	3*	12*	250*
Males														
9–13 y	1300*	1250	240	5*	2*	0.9	0.9	12	1.0	300	1.8	4*	20*	375*
14–18 y	1300*	1250	410	5*	3*	1.2	1.3	16	1.3	400	2.4	5*	25*	550*
19–30 y	1000*	700	400	5*	4*	1.2	1.3	16	1.3	400	2.4	5*	30*	550*
31–50 y	1000*	700	420	5*	4*	1.2	1.3	16	1.3	400	2.4	5*	30*	550*
51–70 y	1200*	700	420	10*	4*	1.2	1.3	16	1.7	400	2.4 (g)	5*	30*	550*
> 70 y	1200*	700	420	15*	4*	1.2	1.3	16	1.7	400	2.4 (g)	5*	30*	550*
Females														
9–13 y	1300*	1250	240	5*	2*	0.9	0.9	12	1.0	300	1.8	4*	20*	375*
14–18 y	1300*	1250	360	5*	3*	1.0	1.0	14	1.2	400 (h)	2.4	5*	25*	400*
19–30 y	1000*	700	310	5*	3*	1.1	1.1	14	1.3	400 (h)	2.4	5*	30*	425*
31–50 y	1000*	700	320	5*	3*	1.1	1.1	14	1.3	400 (h)	2.4	5*	30*	425*
51–70 y	1200*	700	320	10*	3*	1.1	1.1	14	1.5	400	2.4 (g)	5*	30*	425*
> 70 y	1200*	700	320	15*	3*	1.1	1.1	14	1.5	400	2.4 (g)	5*	30*	425*

26

Pregnancy														
< 18 y	1300*	1250	400	5*	3*	1.4	1.4	18	1.9	600 (i)	2.6	6*	30*	450*
19–30 y	1000*	700	350	5*	3*	1.4	1.4	18	1.9	600 (i)	2.6	6*	30*	450*
31–50 y	1000*	700	360	5*	3*	1.4	1.4	18	1.9	600 (i)	2.6	6*	30*	450*
Lactation														
< 18 y	1300*	1250	360	5*	3*	1.5	1.6	17	2.0	500	2.8	7*	35*	550*
19–30 y	1000*	700	310	5*	3*	1.5	1.6	17	2.0	500	2.8	7*	35*	550*
31–50 y	1000*	700	320	5*	3*	1.5	1.6	17	2.0	500	2.8	7*	35*	550*

Footnotes

(a) Recommended Dietary Allowances (RDAs) are presented in bold type and Adequate Intakes (AIs) in ordinary type followed by an asterisk (*). RDAs and AIs may both be used as goals for individual intake. RDAs are set to meet the needs of almost all (97% to 98%) individuals in a group. For healthy breast-fed infants, the AI is the mean intake. The AI for other life-stage and gender groups is believed to cover needs of all individuals in the group, but lack of data or uncertainty in the data prevent being able to specify with confidence the percentage of persons covered by this intake.

(b) As cholecalciferol. I μg cholecalciferol = 40 IU vitamin D.

(c) In the absence of adequate esposure to sunlight.

(d) As niacin equivalents (NE). 1 mg niacin = 60 mg tryptothan; 0 to 6 mo = preformed niacin (not NE).

(e) As dietary folate equivalent (DFE). I DFE = 1 μg food folate = 0.6 μg folic acid (from fortified food or supplement) consumed with food = 0.5 μg synthetic (supplemental) folic acid taken on an empty stomach.

(f) Although AIs have been set for choline, there are few data to assess whether a dietary supply of choline is needed at all stages of the life cycle, and it may be that the choline requirement can be met by endogenous synthesis at some of these stages.

(g) Because 10% to 30% of older people may malabsorb food-bound vitamin B_{12}, it is advisable for those older than 50 years to meet their RDA mainly by consuming foods fortified with vitamin B_{12} or a supplement containing vitamin B_{12}.

(h) In view of evidence linking folate intake with neural tube defects in the fetus, it is recommended that all women capable of becoming pregnant consume 400 μg synthetic folic acid from fortified foods and/or supplements in addition to intake of food folate from a varied diet.

It is assumed that women will continue consuming 400 μg folic acid until their pregnancy is confirmed and they enter prenatal care, which ordinarily occurs after the end of the periconceptional period—the critical time for formation of the neural tube.

Source: Food and Nutrition Board—National Academy of Sciences, 1998.

Nutrition Facts
Serving Size 1/2 cup (114 g)
Servings Per Container 4

Amount Per Serving	
Calories 90	Calories from Fat 30
	% Daily Value*
Total Fat 3 g	5%
Saturated Fat 0g	0%
Cholesterol 0mg	0%
Sodium 300 mg	13%
Total Carbohydrate 13 g	4%
Dietary Fiber 3g	12%
Sugars 3g	
Protein 3g	
Vitamin A 80% •	Vitamin C 60%
Calcium 4% •	Iron 4%

* Percent Daily Values are based on a 2,000 calorie diet. Your daily values may be higher or lower depending on your calorie needs.

		Calories 2,000	2,500
Total Fat	Less than	55g	80g
Sat Fat	Less than	20 g	25g
Cholesterol	Less than	300mg	300mg
Sodium	Less than	2,400mg	2,400mg
Total Carbohydrate		300g	375g
Dietary Fiber		25g	30g

Calories per gram:
Fat 9 • Carbohydrate 4 • Protein 4

Figure 2–3 Nutrition Facts Panel. *Source:* Food and Drug Administration.

dards. For labeling purposes, 2000 calories has been established as the reference, partly because it is a round number to make it easy for consumers to calculate individual nutrient needs. DRVs for cholesterol, sodium, and potassium are the same for all calorie levels. DRVs for some nutrients represent the upper limit considered desirable because of the links between these specific nutrients and certain chronic diseases, such as the association of excess saturated and trans fat to increased risk of heart disease or excess sodium linked to a heightened risk for high blood pressure. The DRVs suggest a desirable goal, such as for fiber or protein, or a healthy maximum as, for total fat.

Since 1996 the Food and Drug Administration (FDA) has set standards for the claims about nutritional values that can be made on restaurant menus. If claims such as *low fat* or *heart healthy* are made on a restaurant menu, the restaurateur must be able to demonstrate reasonable evidence of the basis for the claim.

DIETARY GUIDELINES FOR THE PUBLIC

The Department of Health and Human Services (DHHS) and the Department of Agriculture (USDA) jointly publish and periodically update the *Dietary Guidelines for Americans.* These *Dietary Guidelines* are designed to help consumers make healthy food choices, control weight, promote health, and reduce the risk and incidence of some chronic diseases. Designed for the general population, the

Dietary Guidelines are useful for individual as well as institutional meal planning and as a guide for the food industry. The guidelines are periodically revised and updated. The following summarize the nine major messages in the *Dietary Guidelines for Americans* 2005:[50]

- Consume a variety of foods within and among the basic food groups while staying within energy needs.
- Control calorie intake to manage body weight.
- Be physically active every day.
- Increase daily intake of fruits and vegetables, whole grains, and nonfat or low-fat milk and milk products.
- Choose fats wisely for good health.
- Choose carbohydrates wisely for good health.
- Choose and prepare foods with little salt.
- If you drink alcoholic beverages, do so in moderation.
- Keep food safe to eat.[50]

See Appendix A for the DHHS/USDA *Dietary Guidelines for Americans 2005*. For more information see *Dietary Guidelines* in the Helpful Web Sites section at the end of this chapter.

The *Dietary Guidelines for Americans 2005* are the basis of the U.S. Food Guide Pyramid. The food guide pyramid uses narrative with pictorial food illustrations to help consumers choose healthy foods and support nutrient recommendations. USDA food guides began with the early food guides (1894–1940), the World War I canning and gardening posters (1917–1918), and Early World War II Guides (1941–1942). A post-WWII food guide was the Basic 7 Food Guide (1943–1955). In 1957, the US Department of Agriculture Four Food Groups used the then current RDAs to propose four rather than seven foods groupings. The Basic Four Food Guide and Hassle-Free Food Guide proposed that foods that primarily contributed kilocalories and insignificant amounts of any of the micronutrients did not fit into the four categories. The Pattern for Daily Food Choices (1984) included the US Food Guide Pyramid.[51,52] Food guides have limitations. These guides continue to be revised and updated as educational tools for healthy populations. Table 2–2 compares and contrasts the emphasis of dietary guidelines from 1980 through 2000.

Dietary guidelines for the public attempt to translate current nutrition science into practical food consumption guidelines. These recommendations are revised and reissued about every five years to provide a quicker response to public health goals and to better educate people to choose nutrient-dense foods. Extensive research as well as social, political, and economic implications and national health goals are used to develop guidelines. The early guidelines did not emphasize the maintenance of ideal body weight or consumption of a variety of foods. Over the years, the emphasis of the guidelines has shifted from eat more to eat less.[53,54,55,56] Recent guidelines emphasize physical fitness as well as choosing nutrient dense foods.

Table 2-2 Dietary Guidelines for Americans, 1980 to 2000

1980	1985	1990	1995	2000	
7 guidelines	7 guidelines	7 guidelines	7 guidelines	10 guidelines, clustered into 3 groups	
Eat a variety of foods	Eat a variety of foods	Eat a variety of foods	Eat a variety of foods		
Maintain ideal weight	Maintain desirable weight	Maintain healthy weight	Balance the food you eat with physical activity—maintain or improve your weight	Aim for a healthy weight	*Aim for Fitness*
				Be physically active each day	
				Let the Pyramid guide your food choices	*Build a Healthy Base*
Avoid too much fat, saturated fat, and cholesterol	Avoid too much fat, saturated fat, and cholesterol	Choose a diet low in fat, saturated fat, and cholesterol			
Eat foods with adequate starch and fiber	Eat foods with adequate starch and fiber	Choose a diet with plenty of vegetables, fruits and grain projects	Choose a diet with plenty of grain products, vegetables, and fruits	Choose a variety of grains daily, especially whole grains	
				Choose a variety of fruits and vegtables daily	
				Keep food safe to eat	
			Choose a diet low in fat saturated fat, and cholesterol	Choose a diet that is low in saturated fat and cholesterol and moderate in total fat	*Choose Sensibly*
Avoid too much sugar	Avoid too much sugar	Use sugars only in moderation	Choose a diet moderate in sugars	Choose beverages and foods to moderate your intake of sugars	
Avoid too much sodium	Avoid too much sodium	Use salt and sodium only in moderation	Choose a diet moderate in salt and sodium	Choose and prepare foods with less salt	
If you drink alcohol, do so in moderation	If you drink alcoholic beverages, do so in moderation	If you drink alcoholic beverages, do so in moderation	If you drink alcoholic beverages, do so in moderation	If you drink alcoholic beverages, do so in moderation	

Source: Center for Nutrition Policy and Promotion, USDA, May 30, 2000.

Applications of Dietary Guidelines

Dietary guidelines and food guides translate nutrient recommendations into popular advice about foods to meet the needs of most healthy individuals in the target population. Nutrition professionals use the guidelines to help consumers identify specific behaviors, help set local policies, design educational materials, and develop educational campaigns that include messages, recipes, or menus.[57] The guidelines translate nutrition-related health goals into servings of nutrient-dense foods that fit into local and cultural food preferences. The recommendations provide the food industry with a framework for production and marketing initiatives. The guidelines also can provide a database to study trends and changes in food consumption.

Limitations of Dietary Recommendations, Guidelines, and Guides

Public health nutritionists and other nutrition educators must understand that there are limitations to the use of dietary references, guidelines, and food guides. Dietary references are estimates based on the professional judgment of the scientists appointed to the review committees as they evaluate and interpret the existing research evidence. Each committee weighs similar as well as different factors to estimate adequacy. This may include the amount needed to prevent disease, the levels needed for tissue saturation, and possible toxicity. Their usual process is to establish the criterion of adequacy and then set the recommended intake at $+2$ standard deviations (SD) from the mean so that only a few individuals are expected to have a higher requirement.[58] The RDAs were not intended to be used as standards to assess the adequacy of any one individual's nutrient intake or risk of malnutrition. However, nutrition practitioners frequently have used the RDAs for that purpose. Anthropometric measurements and clinical and biochemical determinations should be used in conjunction with a nutrient analysis of food intake to assess an individual's nutritional status. It may be difficult to develop food guides that meet the RDAs and AIs for all nutrients and also consider the Tolerable Upper Intake Level (UL). Despite controversy over various political and food industry influences on the development of food guides, research indicates that the pictorial representation of the US Food Guide Pyramid does convey proportionality and moderation.[59]

NUTRITION SCIENCE VS NUTRITION POLICY

The ultimate purpose of science is to apply information gained to better the quality of human life. Nutrition is the basic and applied science of food and diet-related behaviors. Nutrition science continues to evolve, but despite the advances in evidence-based research, problems of over- and underconsumption, access, availability, and numerous related issues continue. In the United States, while hunger and undernutrition persist in some populations, overweight and obesity are now the urgent public health problems that connect individuals and their communities through a complex web of political, economic, ethnic, and sociodemographic factors.

Nutrition science research should provide the evidence to create and implement policy. Nutrition policy (see Chapters 5 and 6) uses these scientific findings to establish goals, objectives, and related interventions to promote the health and nutritional status of the population. Public health nutritionists improve the health of the public when they develop, implement, and evaluate nutrition policies and programs.[60] To establish effective and predictable outcomes, policies must be based on sound science. This includes the scientific evidence that relates nutrients to human needs, to health promotion and disease progression, to individual and group behaviors, to economic and consumption patterns, and to communication and marketing. Nutrition policies in the United States stand on four elements:

- Food assistance, which began with distribution of agricultural food surpluses to needy low-income individuals and families
- Education, as exemplified by the succeeding updated editions of the *Dietary Guidelines* and the related graphic such as the U.S. Food Guide Pyramid
- Nutrient labeling of packaged food products
- Nutrition research[61]

The four important steps necessary to improve nutrition policies in the United States are improved nutrition education; maternal, infant and child nutrition; research; and providing the resources needed to carry out comprehensive health policy initiatives.[62] Developing goals and policies requires evidence-based risk–benefit analysis and informed and unbiased professional judgments.

Risk–Benefit Analysis and Professional Judgment

Despite many commonalities, there is a range of individual variability that influences nutrient needs. Nutritionists and dietitians would prefer absolute proof of beneficial outcomes as their evidence to make dietary recommendations. In the real world, before they take action they must analyze existing information and apply their professional judgment to weigh the potential risks and benefits indicated by the available evidence—all the while demanding continued research.[63]

Professional judgment combined with evaluation of the current scientific evidence is used to establish nutrient guidelines to plan programs for the public, to consult with food processors, and to counsel clients requiring medical nutrition therapy. For example, vitamin A has a range of intakes that confer optimal function. An intake below this range for vitamin A imposes risk for various deficiency-related diseases. Exceeding the optimal physiological range can impose risk, thus suggesting a cautious approach to excessive intake.[64] It is often difficult for researchers to distinguish between normal nutrition requirements to promote health and maximum function and the requirement to prevent specified chronic diseases. There is also some controversy concerning the potential harm and benefits of large doses of some nutrients, and whether the physiological effect of these doses should be considered pharmacological rather than normal nutrition. Nutrition professionals must consider the potential benefits of large doses of some nutrients, such as vitamin C, in which the interaction between ascorbic acid and nitrates and/or nitrites prevents formation of carcinogenic nitrosamines.[65] Current research findings suggests a more liberal approach with water-soluble vitamin C than with fat-soluble vitamin A.[66] Nutritionists must know the guidelines and understand the rationales that support their recommendations.

A purist's nutrition perspective is that policies and programs should be based solely on the most current nutrition research findings. Food and nutrition policies have a cultural context and result from multiple social, economic, and political influences. Policy makers are also influenced by many more powerful factions that promote their special interests. This has been an historical fact, but growing public awareness of this issue increasingly creates controversy related to dietary recommendations guidelines and policies. Books and articles published since the year 2000 document the impact of special interest groups on formulation of national health and nutrition policies. These publications have become popular reading not only among nutrition professionals, but also among the concerned public. Public health nutritionists must respond to nutrition-related questions providing the consensus of scientific evidence for their responses.

DIETARY RECOMMENDATIONS FOR THE PUBLIC

In the mid 1900s, epidemiological evidence correlated obesity and overweight with dietary factors that contributed to the increasing prevalence of many chronic diseases recognized as major public health problems. Scientific developments in the 1900s shifted the focus of national health goals, from prevention of nutrient deficiency and infectious diseases to primary prevention—especially the promotion of optimal health and the prevention of chronic diseases. Nutritionists now urge Americans to change their eating habits. The current messages to the public are: avoid overweight and obesity; reduce intakes of total, trans, and saturated fats; reduce intakes of cholesterol, sugar, and salt/sodium; and increase consumption of fruits, vegetables, whole grains, and complex carbohydrates.

In the 1950s the Framingham Heart Study became a seminal source of empirical evidence supporting the role of lifestyle, including diet, in cardiovascular health.[67] The Bureau of Nutrition in the New York City Department of Health tested the fat- and cholesterol-controlled *Prudent Diet*.[68] The American Heart Association, using data based on epidemiological, clinical, and animal studies, published eight dietary guidelines to reduce intake of foods containing animal fats[69] (see Chapter 9).

In 1977 the Senate Select Committee on Nutrition and Human Needs published their staff report, *Dietary Goals for the United States*, which focused on the prevention of chronic degenerative diseases. In 1989, the National Research Council published *Diet and Health: Implications for Reducing Chronic Disease Risk*, which thoroughly reviewed the research literature then available and provided an analysis of the dietary risk factors contributing to specific chronic diseases. The report emphasized the currently prevalent chronic diseases—heart disease, certain forms of cancer, diabetes, and obesity. The report proposed the need to use a health promotion and primary disease prevention approach.[70]

Dietary guidelines are published not only by government agencies, but also by several of the disease-specific voluntary health agencies. These disease-specific guidelines create more public awareness of the role of diet in the prevention and medical nutrition therapy of the disease of their concern. Public health nutritionists must be familiar with all of these guidelines and their rationales. The American Cancer Society's goal is to decrease cancer risk through a variety of preventive behaviors, including diet. Their guidelines are based on current research related to cancer prevention and health promotion (see Chapter 9).

Eat a variety of healthful foods with an emphasis on plant sources: five or more servings of a variety of vegetables and fruits, and choose whole grains in preference to processed grains and sugars. Limit consumption of red meats, especially when it is processed or high in fat. Choose foods that maintain a healthful weight. Maintain a healthful weight throughout life with emphasis on caloric balance and weight loss if currently overweight or obese. Adopt a physically active lifestyle with emphasis on engaging in at least moderate activity for 30 minutes or more on five or more days of the week to reduce the risk of breast and colon cancer. If you drink alcoholic beverages, limit consumption.

Variations from the federal government guidelines is logical as the goals of the American Cancer Society highlight the scientific findings that support the role of phytochemicals in cancer prevention and role of dietary fats as risk factors in various types of cancers.[71]

The American Heart Association's Dietary Guidelines for Healthy Adults are designed to minimize the risk of cardiovascular disease by helping to reduce three of the major risk factors for heart attack or the risk of stroke (high blood cholesterol, high blood pressure, and excess body weight). These guidelines include: a healthy eating pattern selecting foods from all major food groups, maintaining a healthy body weight and a desirable blood cholesterol and lipoprotein profile, and desirable blood pressure.[72] An important guideline of the American Heart Association has been to maintain a total fat intake of less than 30% of total daily calories, with saturated fats comprising less than one third of that total fat. These guidelines are based on scientific data concerning diet and risk, and promote such protective factors as soluble fibers, omega-3 fatty acids, folate, vitamin B_6, and vitamin B_{12}, vitamin E, soy protein, isoflavones, and the use of alcohol in moderation.

The National Heart, Lung, and Blood Institute's Adult Treatment Panel III (ATPIII) includes detailed dietary and treatment guidelines. This third report by the Expert Panel on Detection, Evaluation, and Treatment of High Blood Cholesterol in Adults is the National Cholesterol Education Program's (NCEP's) updated, evidence-based clinical guidelines for cholesterol testing and management. In the report, recommendations, or "Therapeutic Lifestyle Changes (TLC)," are directed to high-risk and moderately at-risk individuals.[73]

Nutrition and Diet Objectives in *Healthy People 2000* and *Healthy People 2010*

Late in the 1900s the National Institutes of Health sponsored several conferences focused on the chronic diseases observed to have the greatest impact on the public's health. The conferees studied the research evidence ranging from relationships of nutritional status and specific dietary factors to the health status and chronic disease occurrence in the US population. The first published nutrition-related objectives were based on the recommendations summarized in the *Surgeon General's Report on Nutrition and Health* and the Institute of Medicine's National Academy of Sciences' report, *Diet and Health*. These recommendations were then stated as measurable objectives to be achieved through population-based public health programs. Healthy People 2000 included 17 nutrition objectives. *Promoting Health/Preventing Disease: Year 2000 Objectives for the Nation* listed 24 objectives to challenge nutritionists charged with promoting the public's health.[74]

Healthy People 2010, launched in January 2000 by the Department of Health and Human Services, organizes 467 objectives into 28 focus areas. Where baseline data and credible sources are available, the objectives are stated in measurable terms. Of the 28 focus areas, the following 13 include objectives to be directly or indirectly achieved by interventions that require changes in dietary behavior:

- Arthritis, osteoporosis, and chronic back conditions
- Cancer
- Chronic kidney disease
- Diabetes
- Food safety
- Health communication
- Heart disease and stroke

- HIV/AIDS
- Maternal, infant, and child health
- Nutrition and overweight
- Oral health
- Physical activity and fitness
- Substance abuse

These 28 focus areas are linked to the nation's 10 leading health indicators.[75]

Leading health indicators listed in *Healthy People 2010* were determined from surveillance and monitoring data. These indicators are based on their relevance, ability to motivate action, and the availability of data to monitor progress. The Leading Health Indicators include the following:

1. Physical activity
2. Overweight and obesity
3. Tobacco use
4. Substance abuse
5. Responsible sexual behavior
6. Mental health
7. Injury and violence
8. Environmental quality
9. Immunization
10. Access to health care[76]

These Leading Health Indicators are the major public health challenges of the new century—obesity, heart disease, stroke, diabetes, cancer, osteoporosis, low birth weight, birth defects, and HIV/AIDS. All are directly or indirectly related to, or impacted by, nutrition and food choices (see Chapter 1).

To measure and achieve the nation's nutrition objectives requires funding strong basic and applied nutrition research programs, a national nutrition monitoring system, nutrition information and education programs for the public, and intensive efforts to implement and monitor achievements.[77]

Priority Issues That Require Further Research

The American Dietetic Association (ADA) states, "Research is the foundation of the profession and provides the basis for practice, education, and policy." These are the nine priority research areas they recommend:

- Prevention and treatment of obesity and associated chronic diseases
- Effective nutrition and lifestyle change interventions
- Translation of research into nutrition interventions and programs
- Effective nutrition indicators and outcome measures
- Dietetics education and retention

- Delivery and payment for dietetic services
- Access to safe and secure food supply
- Customer satisfaction
- Nutrients and gene expression[78]

Emerging trend data list a wide range of promising issues for which additional research evidence is still required:

Antioxidants The well-known nutrients that have demonstrated evidence of antioxidant functions include vitamin C, vitamin E, vitamin B_6, beta-carotene and other carotenoids, iron, zinc, and selenium. An increasing number of phytochemicals may also play some role in antioxidant function.

Fats Increasing research must distinguish between beneficial and harmful types of fats. Future research to differentiate benefits of polyunsaturated (omega-6 and omega-3) and monounsaturated fats continue to be a major research area, as do the harmful effects of trans and saturated fats. Other research areas include: relationship of, and levels of, saturated fat that contribute to heart disease risk; the impact of replacing saturated fats with monounsaturated fats on low-density lipoprotein (LDL) and triglyceride levels; and the role of trans fats in increasing LDL and increasing HDL (high-density lipoprotein) levels.

Fiber The relationship of low dietary fiber intake and increased risk for heart disease as well as suggesting that more dietary fiber may help promote weight control and prevent colon cancer are hopeful. The Institute of Medicine report *Dietary Reference Intakes for Energy, Carbohydrate, Fiber, Fat, Fatty Acids, Cholesterol, Protein, and Amino Acids* defines total fiber as the combination of dietary and functional fiber. There needs to be more work for systematic adoption of these definitions. Nutritionists must help consumers to identify ways to increase their fiber intake and interpret information concerning fiber content on food labels.[79]

Genetically Modified Foods This is among the most controversial issues public health nutritionists encounter. There are strong pro and con opinions concerning the safety of genetically modified foods in the food supply. Biotechnology is a complex issue with a potentially significant impact on consumers, food producers, and processors. Biotechnology has demonstrated potential to increase efficiency of food production and to enhance the quality, nutritional value, and variety of foods. However, public fears persist about its potential risks. On a philosophical and personal level, some consider genetically modifying agricultural products to be "tampering with nature." Nutritionists must carefully evaluate pro and con data concerning genetic modification and integrate research evidence that considers the empirical information, as well as respecting the values of their clients.[80]

Glycemic Index   This ranks individual foods based on their potential to raise blood glucose levels in the body. To date, this ranking is based on preliminary data on individual foods. Most foods are eaten accompanied by or in combination with other foods. There is insufficient research to systematically apply the concept of glycemic index to dietary management. Although some nutritionists use this preliminary data as a basis to recommend increased use of complex and less processed carbohydrates, more research is needed to empirically and systematically apply the use of the glycemic index. Public health nutritionists must track developments as well as popular trends and fads concerning the use of this concept to work effectively with the public.[81]

Medical Nutrition Therapy   The American Dietetic Association takes the position that medical nutrition therapy (MNT) and lifestyle counseling are essential parts of the care process prescribed to manage and treat specific diseases, including obesity, diabetes mellitus, hypertension, hyperlipidemias, osteoporosis, cardiovascular disease, and cerebrovascular disease. MNT is also important in treatment of other chronic conditions, including inflammatory bowel syndrome and other conditions that affect the gastrointestinal tract, Parkinson's disease, seizure disorders that respond to a ketogenic diet, chronic obstructive pulmonary disease, congestive heart failure, renal and liver disease, cancer, and immune system diseases. There should be a team approach to the care of patients who receive both MNT and pharmacotherapy. Empirical data documents that MNT improves health outcomes and speeds recovery, with fewer complications. Patients with heart disease and diabetes who regularly receive medical nutrition therapy require fewer high-cost hospital stays, surgeries, and medications. More health insurance plans including Medicare now pay for medical nutrition therapy prescribed for obesity, diabetes, and renal disease. Registered dietitians must continue to use research evidence to demonstrate the cost-effectiveness of medical nutrition therapy.[82]

Minerals   There is growing interest in the contributions of calcium to bone health as well as its potential role in previously unknown functions, such as in fat lipolysis. Publications reporting new research findings must be monitored continuously by nutritionists considering potential application to critical public health issues, including weight management. Selenium continues to be investigated for its antioxidant properties, protective potential, and possible impact on chronic diseases.[83]

Nutraceuticals   The lack of a universally accepted definition for nutraceuticals, also referred to as *functional foods*, confuses many consumers. These substances or parts of foods considered to provide health or medical benefits blur the line between the use of foods for normal nutrition or for pharmacological treatment. More research must identify the physiologically active components, health benefits, and risks of individual functional foods so that these foods are more clearly defined. The Food and Drug Administration (FDA) has expanded its role in regulating functional foods over the past years. However, this term remains confusing and continues to be a challenge to nutritionists.[84,85]

Phytochemicals   Numerous types of phytochemicals in foods may have health benefits. Anthocyanins and coumarins may have anticancer and cardioprotective properties. Capsaicin may be an antioxidant. Various citrus flavonoids may protect against harmful free radicals. Catechins, ellagic acid, lignans, limonene, phytosterols, quercetin, some sulfur compounds, and glucosinolates may have anticancer properties. Isoflavonoids may have anticancer functions, decrease menopausal symptoms, and promote bone health. Reservatrol and saponins may protect against harmful blood cholesterol levels. Much of this research is preliminary. Future research should provide more definitive data.

Phytoestrogens   These are naturally occurring phenolic plant compounds present in beans, cabbage, soybeans, and grains. They are structurally similar to estrogen and estradiol. Classes of phytoestrogens are lignans and isoflavones. Isoflavones include genistein and daidzein. Research has largely focused on isoflavones, which may help suppress or inhibit normal estrogen thus reducing menopausal symptoms, risk of breast cancer, and osteoporosis.

Phytosterols   Plant sterols and plant stanols, collectively known as phytosterols, have chemical structures similar to that of cholesterol. But phytosterols block dietary cholesterol from absorption into the bloodstream. Both the phytosterols and dietary cholesterol are excreted in waste matter. Plant sterols and stanols are being incorporated into functional foods such as vegetable oils. The extent of their benefits, which may include prevention of heart disease and management of blood glucose, needs further research.

Vitamins   Based on research findings, at any point in time different vitamins capture researchers' interest. Folic acid is among the vitamins currently receiving their interest, particularly its relationship to bioavailability, its synthetic form and its implications for food fortification, and its relationship to chronic conditions, not just the prevention of neural tube defects.[86]

Water   The Dietary Reference Intakes for electrolytes and water, published early in 2004, changed the long-standing guideline of six to eight glasses of water each day. New guidelines state that the vast majority of healthy people adequately meet their hydration needs by letting thirst be their guide. They now recommend about 2.7 liters of total water from all beverages and foods for women and about 3.7 liters of total water for men.[87] This challenges public health nutritionists, who must satisfactorily respond to questions and comments about this new information from clients and the public and explain the scientific basis for these changes.

IMPACT OF NUTRIGENOMICS ON PUBLIC HEALTH NUTRITION PRACTICE

Genomics is the use of genetic information for a variety of purposes that range from improving the quantity and quality of food production to the prevention of disease.[88] *Nutrigenomics* is the term used for the science of nutrition and genetics. Functional genomics links a function to a gene or a dysfunction to a disease[89] This emerging science investigates how genetics and nutrition affect health, either by changing the genetic structure or through gene expression. This data presents previously unavailable research with applications to nutrition practice. Nutrigenomics will provide information on how genetic variation influences health through diet–gene interactions. It will enable nutritionists to use results of diagnostic tests to individually customize medical nutrition therapy. An anticipated contribution of nutrigenomics is to use genetic information to develop food and dietary guidelines as shown in Figure 2–4.

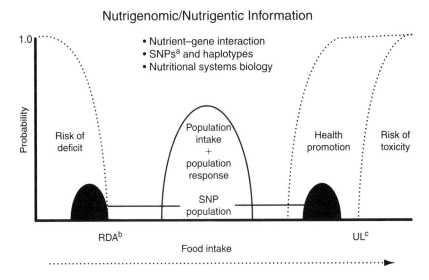

Figure 2–4 Integration of new genetic information into the development of food-based dietary guidelines. [a]SNP = single nucleotide polymorphism, [b]RDA = Recommended Dietary Allowance, [c]UL = Upper limits.
Source: Gillies PJ. Nutrigenomics: the Rubicon of molecular nutrition. *J Am Diet Assoc.* 2003;103:S50–S55.

Genomics raises many ethical, legal, and social issues.[90] These include privacy and fair use of information; ensuring informed consent for genetic testing and research; consumer consent and access to registries, archived data, and specimens; questions about the best way to integrate related techniques into the clinical setting; educating the public about the purposes, benefits, and risks of genetic testing; population access to testing opportunities; potential stigmatization as a consequence of test results; and access to appropriate services based on test findings.[91] The expected growth of nutrigenomics companies, especially those accessed through the Internet, will increase the need for public health nutritionists to educate and counsel the public. This is especially important when results of a genetics test has implications for nutrition-related disease risk requiring medical nutrition therapy.[92]

Despite the increasing body of knowledge, many unanswered questions and continually emerging controversies persist. Other issues that concern the public and need further investigation are: the impact of changes in the health care system; the increasing cost of health care; the increasing diversity of the population; the increasing variety of foodstuffs, increasing knowledge, interest, and expectations by the public; and changing meal and snack patterns and lifestyle behaviors.

Evaluate Research as the Evidence Base for Practice

Public health practitioners must have a research agenda to build an evidence base to guide policy.[93] To meet the challenges, goals, and quality improvement expectations of public health programs and services, there are increasing expectations for evidence-based strategies[94] that have evolved from clinical practice. Evidence-based medicine is a flow process that evaluates clinical knowledge, patient preferences, and best research evidence to make clinical decisions. The key difference between a clinical and public health evidence-based process are the type and volume of data and settings.[95]

Evidence-based practice helps the public health professional decide how to decide.[96] This approach maximizes the potential for success when applying or implementing public health nutrition initiatives. An evidence-based approach requires the practitioner to do the following:

1. Identify and quantify the problem or issues.
2. Formulate each issue as a question.
3. Search and find the research evidence and options.
4. Analyze, evaluate, and interpret the research findings.
5. Determine the impact of the data application.
6. Make decisions and recommendations.
7. Specify and prioritize the strength of the evidence.

8. Develop and evaluate interventions.
9. Disseminate findings.[97,98]

This approach ensures that current, credible, and consistent research evidence is evaluated for applications in public health programs and services. This systematic problem-solving approach must be used to critically address problems and provide the evidence base for nutrition education to the public and for cost-effective medical nutrition therapy when prescribed for patients in their treatment plan.

APPLY EVIDENCE-BASED PRACTICE TO THE OBESITY CRISIS

The obesity pandemic is an epidemic in the United States.[99,100] Using body mass index (BMI) standards, data for 2004 indicate that only 42% of American adults are at their healthy weight. The obesity rate is even higher in several population subgroups, such as African-Americans, Hispanics, and some Native Americans. The overall rate of obesity in the population continues to increase.

Obesity and overweight are now recognized as major public health problems. This demands aggressive public health action related to prevention, intervention, and research.[101,102] This requires federal, state, and local public health agencies to broaden their mission from traditional indigent health care services to health promotion and the primary prevention of obesity-related chronic diseases by directing prevention messages to all population segments—affluent and indigent, males and females, young and old.[103]

Given the current obesity epidemic, the most common questions posed to public health nutritionists relate to weight loss or management. The large number of popular diets generally can be grouped into a few specific categories or descriptors. Popular plans have one or more of the following characteristics:

- Nutrient restricted or nutrient focused (e.g., low-carbohydrate diet, very low-calorie diet, low-fat diet, high-protein diet)
- Food limited or food focused (e.g., grapefruit diet, wine lover's diet, lollipop diet, rice diet)
- Food-nutrient groupings (e.g., exchange lists)
- Celebrity or lifestyle focused (e.g., the famous model's diet)
- Behavior focused (e.g., behavior modification, cognitive restructuring)
- Physical activity

Evaluate the Research Evidence to Support Popular Weight Loss Diets

Over time, popular fad weight-loss diets come and go. Public health nutritionists must provide weight management advice that is nutritionally sound and evidence based.[104,105] The challenge to nutritionists is that the research evidence may conflict with what appeals to the public. Public health nutritionists must take the existing research data and repackage and promote it to appeal to the public's continuing search for a "quick fix."[106,107,108,109]

The Role of Public Health Professionals in Promoting Safe Weight Management and Loss

Primary, secondary, and tertiary prevention and treatment of obesity and overweight is a national public health priority. Public health nutritionists must take leadership to advocate for economic and workplace incentives. They must garner support to fund community-based nutrition and physical fitness programs and encourage other health professionals to take active leadership to prevent and treat obesity as a major risk to the public's health.[110]

MONITOR NUTRITION RESEARCH FOR PUBLIC HEALTH APPLICATIONS

The American public spends over $30 billion annually on medical and nutritional health fraud and quackery. The sale of unproven weight loss programs and products and sports drinks have soared. How does a public health nutritionist respond to a client who asks about the latest weight loss fad, popular diet, or media report about scientific findings? How does the public health nutritionist use the information explosion, sort it, evaluate it, and resynthesize it into manageable messages that the public will understand and use?

State and local public health agency offices should maintain a variety of authoritative, peer-reviewed resources, including current editions of nutrition science textbooks; current editions of national reports, such as health goals and monitoring and surveillance reports; the current dietary guidelines of the US government, major health organizations, and voluntary health agencies; position statements of professional organizations; and key nutrition, public health, and medical journals. The Internet enables public health nutritionists to access a wide variety of journals, reports, and databases. A basic skill for the practitioner is to navigate the World Wide Web for reliable resources and to distinguish between peer-reviewed (refereed) and biased sources of information.[111]

Authoritative Sources of Nutrition Research Information

Many of the US national nutrition monitoring system databases and related reports are readily available through the official government Web sites. The Centers for Disease Control & Prevention (CDC), in cooperation with state and local health departments, maintains many reliable information-gathering systems.[112] This includes mortality and morbidity data and information concerning participation in a variety of health and nutrition programs. The CDC's National Center for Health Statistics (CDC/NCHS) publishes an annual report *Health, United States*. The US Census Bureau gathers demographic data useful for community needs assessments (see Chapter 3). *FedStats*, an Internet-based official statistical information site of the federal government, provides information or links to a variety of data sources from more than 100 federal agencies.[113] Many food- and nutrition-related sources can be accessed through the US Agricultural Research Service. Health information can be obtained through the federal Human Resources and Services Administration (HRSA) of the Department of Health and Human Services.

Because nutrition is a multidimensional discipline, public health nutritionists must be resourceful in gathering scientific information and not limit their searches to food and nutrition sites. Some publications that are sources of research-based information include:

- Medical nutrition therapy and clinical interventions: *Circulation, Diabetes Care, Journal of the American Dietetic Association, Journal of the American Medical Association, American Journal of Clinical Nutrition, Preventive Medicine, Lancet, New England Journal of Medicine, Topics in Clinical Nutrition*
- Population-based studies: *American Journal of Public Health, Journal of Clinical Epidemiology, Journal of Epidemiology and Community Health, Preventive Medicine*
- Nutrition and natural sciences: *Human Biology, Microbiology, Genetics*
- Food composition, food safety, and food science and technology: *Food Safety, Food Technology, Food Science*
- Food production, access, and policy: *Agriculture Outlook, National Food Review*
- Food economics and consumer behavior: *Family Economics and Nutrition Review, Journal of Family and Consumer Science*
- Counseling, pedagogy, and andragogy: *Health Education Research, Health Education and Behavior, Journal of Nutrition Education and Behavior, Journal of Counseling and Development*
- Belief, behaviors, psychology, and sociology: *American Journal of Health Behavior, Developmental Psychology, Health Psychology, Journal of Health and Social Behavior, Journal of Religion and Health, Journal of Social Issues, Journal of Social Psychology, Medical Anthropology Quarterly, Social Science and Medicine*
- Gender- and age-related literature: *American Journal of Dis Child, Journal of Pediatrics, Age and Aging, Aging, Journal of American Geriatrics Society, Journal of Gerontology*

- Multiculturalism and ethnicity: *Amerasia Journal, Ethnicity and Disease, Ethnicity and Health, Hispanic Journal of Behavioral Science, Journal of Afro-American Issues, Journal of Ethnic and Migration Studies, Journal of the Black Nurses Association, Journal of Multicultural Counseling and Development*
- Complementary health: *Journal of Alternative Complementary Medicine, National Center for Complementary and Alternative Medicine* (http://nccam.nih.gov)

Results of studies published in these and other peer-reviewed professional journals are readily accessible through online databases. Another source of information are research reports produced by trade associations, research companies, and industry such as the Food Marketing Institute. The information must be carefully evaluated. These data may include surveys concerning dietary habits, purchasing patterns, or values and food-related attitudes of diverse or select market segments.

The large number of sources and quality of information[114] increase the possibility that some research findings may be misinterpreted, misapplied, or incorrect. Nontraditional data sources require careful scrutiny. Public health nutritionists must be on the front lines in evaluating the source of research funding and possible conflicts of interests. Other ethical issues include the exclusion of some high-risk population groups in studies as well as protection of confidentiality in Web-based surveys and the maintenance of objective research records.

Evidence-based practice requires the nutrition professional to continuously monitor developments in nutrition and related sciences. Information about the latest findings can be obtained by reading current professional journals, attending professional conferences or seminars, and consulting other professionals. Public health nutritionists should review and periodically update their professional development plans to sharpen their critical thinking skills, to carefully review research methodologies as well as to acquire, evaluate, and resynthesize new scientific information and emerging issues. The ability to weigh the evidence and build self-confidence in professional judgment can be developed with a well-designed and implemented professional development plan. The public health nutritionist is a communicator of research to the public.[115] To communicate evidence-based information, the nutritionist must keep these questions in mind:

- Have the research methods and conclusions been peer reviewed?
- Are important facts and key information about the study disclosed?
- Will the communication enhance public understanding of the relationship of nutrition and diet to health?
- How can the scientific findings be translated into a manageable, appropriate, applicable, and positive context useful to the target population?

POINTS TO PONDER

- What scientific evidence justifies the inclusion of nutrition in the planning and implementing of community chronic disease risk-reduction programs?
- How can professional judgment and scientific data be used to determine whether or not to promote the consumption of phytochemicals or use of low-carbohydrate diets?
- Why should public health nutritionists question whether scientific findings under debate have any special interest funding or commercial biases that might account for the divergent opinions?
- How can the public be educated about the science-based versus popular diet trends and popular theories concerning weight control?
- How can public health nutritionists compare, contrast, evaluate, and reconcile dietary guidelines being promoted by different official and voluntary health agencies?

HELPFUL WEB SITES

American Cancer Society: www.cancer.org
American Heart Association: www.americanheart.org
American Public Health Association food and nutrition section:
   www.aphafoodandnutrition.org
American Public Health Association policy statements:
   www.apha.org/legislative/policy/policies.htm
Centers for Disease Control and Prevention, Division of Nutrition and
   Physical Activity: Programs and Campaigns:
   www.cdc.gov/nccdphp/dnpa/ npa-proj.htm
Centers for Disease Control National Center for Health Statistics:
   www.cdc.gov.nchs
Dietary Guidelines for Americans 2005:
   www.health.gov/dietaryguidelines/dga2005/report/HTML/A_Exec
   Summary.htm
Food and Drug Administration: Food labeling and restaurant Menu
   Regulations: www:fda.gov
Healthy People: www.healthypeople.gov
Health-related quality of life data: www.cdc.gov/hrqol
Institute of Medicine Dietary Reference Intakes for vitamin C, vitamin
   E, selenium, and carotenoids for 8/3/2000:
   www.iom.edu/report.asp?id= 511
National Agricultural Library: www.nal.usda.gov
National Center for Complementary and Alternative Medicine:
   www.nccam.nih.gov

National Heart, Lung, and Blood Institute: www.nhlbi.nih.gov
National Library of Medicine: www.nlm.nih.gov
Official federal government statistics: www.fedstats.gov/aboutfedstats.html
USDA Agricultural Statistical Services: www.usda.gov.nass
U.S. Census Bureau: www.census.gov

NOTES

1. American Dietetic Association. Position of the American Dietetic Association: the role of dietetics professionals in health promotion and disease prevention. *J Am Diet Assoc.* 2002;102:1680.

2. Lin BH, Smallwood D, Hamilton W, Rossi PH. Research designs for assessing the USDA's food assistance and nutrition programs outcomes, part 2: impact evaluation of demonstrations. *Nutr Today.* 2004;39:40–45.

3. Endres JB. *Community Nutrition.* Upper Saddle River, NJ: Merrill Publishing; 1999.

4. Kaufman M. *Nutrition in Public Health.* Rockville, Md: Aspen Publishers; 1990.

5. Kaufman M. *Nutrition in Public Health.* Rockville, Md: Aspen Publishers; 1990:15.

6. Kaufman M. *Nutrition in Public Health.* Rockville, Md: Aspen Publishers; 1990:15.

7. Heaney RP, Dougherty CJ. *Research for Health Professionals Design, Analysis, and Ethics.* Ames, Ia: Iowa State University Press; 1988.

8. Leedy PD, Ormrod JE. *Practical Research Planning and Design.* New York, NY: Macmillan Publishing Co; 2005.

9. Kaufman M. *Nutrition in Public Health.* Rockville, Md: Aspen Publishers; 1990.

10. Kaufman M. *Nutrition in Public Health.* Rockville, Md: Aspen Publishers; 1990: 16,17.

11. Kaufman M. *Nutrition in Public Health.* Rockville, Md: Aspen Publishers; 1990:16.

12. Leedy PD, Ormrod J.E. *Practical Research Planning and Design.* New York, NY: Macmillan Publishing Co; 2005.

13. Stumbo P, Chenard CA, Hemingway DL. Plowing through the data: harvesting knowledge from food composition tables. *The Digest.* 2004;39:1–3.

14. Boyle MA. *Community Nutrition in Action.* Belmont, Calif: Thomson Wadsworth; 2003.

15. *3 Report on Nutrition Monitoring in the United States.* Vol 1. Washington, DC: US Government Printing Office; 1995.

16. *3 Report on Nutrition Monitoring in the United States.* Vol 1. Washington, DC: US Government Printing Office; 1995:10.

17. Kaufman, M. *Nutrition in Public Health.* Rockville, Md: Aspen Publishing; 1990.

18. Issel ML. *Health Program Planning and Evaluation.* Sudbury, Mass: Jones and Bartlett Publishers; 2004.

19. Blumenthal DJ, DiClemente RJ, eds. *Community-Based Health Research.* New York, NY: Springer Publishing Co; 2004.

20. Issel ML. *Health Program Planning and Evaluation.* Sudbury, Mass: Jones and Bartlett Publishers; 2004.

21. Kaufman M. *Nutrition in Public Health.* Rockville, Md: Aspen Publishers; 1990.

22. Kaufman M. *Nutrition in Public Health.* Rockville, Md: Aspen Publishers; 1990:18.

23. Stangl DK, Berry DA, eds. *Meta-Analysis in Medicine and Health Policy.* New York, NY: Marcel Dekker Inc; 2000.

24. American Dietetic Association. Position of the American Dietetic Association: the role of dietetics professionals in health promotion and disease prevention. *J Am Diet Assoc.* 2002;102:1680.

25. Holland WW, Detels R, Knox G, Breeze E, eds. *Oxford Textbook of Public Health, Volume 1 History, Determinants, Scope and Strategies.* New York, NY: Oxford University Press; 1984.

26. American Dietetics Association. Position of the American Dietetic Association: food and water safety. *J Am Diet Assoc.* 2004;103:1203.

27. Scott BS. Project Impact. Increasing minority participation and awareness of clinical trials. *Closing the Gap.* August 2003;8.

28. Heaney RP, Dougherty CJ. *Research for Health Professionals Design, Analysis, and Ethics.* Ames, Ia: Iowa State University Press; 1988.

29. Heaney RP, Dougherty CJ. *Research for Health Professionals Design, Analysis, and Ethics.* Ames, Ia: Iowa State University Press; 1988.

30. Neutens JJ, Rubinson L. *Research Techniques for the Health Sciences.* San Francisco, Calif: Pearson Education Inc; 2002.

31. Victora CG, Habicht J-P, Bryce J. Evidence-based public health: moving beyond randomized trials. *Am J Public Health.* 2004;94:400–405.

32. Laidlaw SH. Supplements: folic acid and female health. *Nutr Complementary Care.* 2004;6:72.

33. Smith Edge, M. Promoting healthful diets from a public perspective. *J Am Diet Assoc.* 2004;104:827–831.

34. Cooper MJ, Zlotkin SH. An evidence-based approach to the development of national dietary guidelines. *J Am Diet Assoc.* 2004;103(Suppl 2):S28.

35. Kaufman M. *Nutrition in Public Health.* Rockville, Md: Aspen Publishing; 1990.

36. Kaufman M. *Nutrition in Public Health.* Rockville, Md: Aspen Publishing; 1990:26.

37. Kaufman M. *Nutrition in Public Health.* Rockville, Md: Aspen Publishing; 1990:27.

38. Kaufman M. *Nutrition in Public Health.* Rockville, Md: Aspen Publishing; 1990:19, 20.

39. Kaufman M. *Nutrition in Public Health.* Rockville, Md: Aspen Publishing; 1990:20.

40. Nestle M. *Food Politics.* Berkeley, Calif: University of California Press; 2002.

41. Eldridge AL. Comparison of 1989 RDAs and DRIs for water-soluble vitamins. *Nutr Today.* 2004;39:88–93.

42. Nestle M. *Food Politics*. Berkeley, Calif: University of California Press; 2002.

43. Center for Nutrition Policy and Promotion [CNPP]. *Using Food Labels to Follow the Dietary Guidelines for Americans. A Reference*. Alexandria, Va: CNPP; 1994. USDA/CNPP Agricultural Information Bulletin 704.

44. McMurry KY. Setting dietary guidelines: the U.S. process. *J Am Diet Assoc.* 2003;103(Suppl 2):S10–S17.

45. Institute of Medicine. *Dietary Reference Intakes: Applications in Dietary Assessment.* Washington, DC: National Academies Press; 2003.

46. Institute of Medicine. *Dietary Reference Intakes: Applications in Dietary Assessment.* Washington, DC: National Academies Press; 2003.

47. Institute of Medicine. *Dietary Reference Intakes: Applications in Dietary Planning.* Washington, DC: National Academies Press; 2003.

48. Institute of Medicine. *Dietary Reference Intakes: Applications in Dietary Planning.* Washington, DC: National Academies Press; 2003.

49. http://www.cfsan.fda.gov/~dms/fdnewlab.html. Accessed November 10, 2004.

50. http://www.health.gov/dietaryguidelines/dga2005/report/HTML/A_ExecSummary. htm. Accessed Nov. 10, 2004.

51. Food and Nutrition Information Center. Historical food guides background and development. Available at: http://www.nal.usda.gov/fnic/history/index.html. Accessed May 29, 2004.

52. Hogbin M, Lyon J, Davis C. Comparison of dietary recommendations using the dietary guidelines for Americans as a framework. *Nutr Today.* 2003;38:203–217.

53. Nestle M. *Food Politics*. Berkeley, Calif: University of California Press; 2002.

54. Schneeman B. Evolution of the dietary guidelines. *J Am Diet Assoc.* 2003;103(Suppl 2):S5–S9.

55. Tillotson JE. Pandemic obesity: what is the solution? *Nutr Today.* 2004;39:6–9.

56. Arias DC. Politics outweighing science in policy decisions, report says. *The Nation's Health.* April 2004:1.

57. Hogbin M, Lyon J, Davis C. Comparison of dietary recommendations using the dietary guidelines for Americans as a framework. *Nutr Today.* 2003;38:203–217.

58. Kaufman M. *Nutrition in Public Health*. Rockville, Md: Aspen Publishers; 1990.

59. Nestle M. *Food Politics*. Berkeley, Calif: University of California Press; 2002.

60. Bronner F, ed. *Nutrition Policy in Public Health*. New York, NY: Springer Publishing Co; 1997.

61. Smith Edge, M. Promoting healthful diets from a public perspective. *J Am Diet Assoc.* 2004;104:827–831.

62. Smith Edge, M. Promoting healthful diets from a public perspective. *J Am Diet Assoc.* 2004;104:827–831.

63. U.S. Department of Health and Human Services. *Healthy People 2010,* 2nd ed, McLean, VA. International Medicine Publishing; 2002.

64. U.S. Department of Health and Human Services. *Healthy People 2010,* 2nd ed, McLean, VA. RG-1 and RG-2, International Publishing; 2002.

65. Kaufman M. *Nutrition in Public Health.* Rockville, Md: Aspen Publishers; 1990:24,26.

66. http://www.nhlbi.nih.gov/about/framingham/timeline.htm

67. Kaufman M. *Nutrition in Public Health.* Rockville, Md: Aspen Publishers; 1990:31.

68. Kaufman M. *Nutrition in Public Health.* Rockville, Md: Aspen Publishers; 1990:31.

69. Kaufman M. *Nutrition in Public Health.* Rockville, Md: Aspen Publishers; 1990:36.

70. Kaufman M. *Nutrition in Public Health.* Rockville, Md: Aspen Publishers; 1990:36.

71. http://www.cancer.org/docroot/MED/content/MED_2_1X_American_Cancer_Society_guidelines_on_diet _and_cancer_prevention.asp

72. http://www.americanheart.org/presenter.jhtml?identifier=1330

73. Grundy SM. et al. Executive Summary of the Third Report of the National Cholesterol Education Program (NCEP) Expert Panel on Detection, Evaluation, and Treatment of High Blood Cholesterol in Adults (Adult Treatment Panel III). *JAMA.* 2001;285:2486–2497.

74. Kaufman M. *Nutrition in Public Health.* Rockville, Md: Aspen Publishers; 1990.

75. http://www.healthypeople.gov

76. http://www.healthypeople.gov

77. Kaufman M. *Nutrition in Public Health.* Rockville, Md: Aspen Publishers; 1990.

78. http://www.eatright.org/Member/Files/ResearchBrief.pdf

79. http://www.iom.edu/report.asp?id=4340,9/5/2002

80. American Dietetic Association. Position paper of the American Dietetic Association: biotechnology and the future of food. *J Am Diet Assoc.* 1995;95:1429–1432.

81. American Dietetic Association. The Glycemic Index, What is it? Available at: http://www.eatright.org/Public/NutritionInformation/index_19161.cfm. Accessed August 5, 2005.

82. American Dietetic Association. Position paper of the American Dietetic Association: integration of medical nutrition therapy and pharmacotherapy. *J Am Diet Assoc.* 2003;103:1363–1370.

83. Institute of Medicine. IOM dietary reference intakes for vitamin c, vitamin e, selenium, and carotenoids. Available at: http://www.iom.edu/report.asp?id=8511. Accessed August 3, 2000.

84. American Dietetic Association. ADA functional foods position statement. Available at: http://www.eatright.org/Public/Other/index_adap1099.cfm. Accessed August 5, 2004.

85. Hasler CM. Functional foods: benefits, concerns, and challenges – a position paper from the American Council on Science and Health. *J Nutr.* 2002;132:3772–3781.

86. Institute of Medicine. IOM dietary reference intakes for folate and other b vitamins. Available at: http://www.iom.edu/project.asp?id=4015. Accessed April 1998.

87. http://www.iom.edu/report.asp?id=184952/11/04

88. Gillies PJ. Nutrigenomics: the Rubicon of molecular nutrition. *J Am Diet Assoc.* 2003;103:S50–S55.

89. De Busk R. *Genetics: The Nutrition Connection.* Chicago, Ill: American Dietetic Association; 2003.

90. Khoury MJ, Burke W, Thomson, EJ, eds. *Genetics and Public Health in the 21st Century.* New York, NY: Oxford University Press; 2000.

91. Jackson K. Nutrigenomics: it's in the genes. *Today's Dietitian.* 2003;5:27–29.

92. Jackson K. Nutrigenomics: it's in the genes. *Today's Dietitian.* 2003;5:27–29.

93. Institute of Medicine. *The Future of the Public's Health in the 21st Century.* Washington, DC: National Academies Press; 2003.

94. Brownson RC, Baker EA, Leet TL, Gillespie KN. *Evidence-Based Public Health.* New York, NY: Oxford Press; 2003.

95. Brownson RC, Baker EA, Leet TL, Gillespie KN. *Evidence-Based Public Health.* New York, NY: Oxford Press; 2003.

96. Shanklin C. Evidence-based practice: practice based on evidence. Right? *ADA Times.* January 12, 2003:1,3.

97. Shanklin C. Evidence-based practice: practice based on evidence. Right? *ADA Times.* January 12, 2003:1,3.

98. Brownson RC. Baker EA, Leet TL, Gillespie KN. *Evidence-Based Public Health.* New York, NY: Oxford Press; 2003.

99. Tillotson JE. Pandemic obesity: what is the solution? *Nutr Today.* 2004;39:6–9.

100. Flegal KM, Carroll MD, Ogden CL, Johnson CL. Prevalence and trends in obesity among U.S. adults, 1999–2000. *JAMA.* 2002;288:1723–1727.

101. Meerschaert CM. The obesity solution. *Today's Dietitian.* 2004;6:30–33.

102. Tillotson JE. Pandemic obesity: what is the solution? *Nutr Today.* 2004;39:6–9.

103. HHS tackles obesity. *FDA Consumer.* 2004;38:14–16.

104. Bravata DM, Sanders L, Huang J, Krumholz HM, Olkin H, Gardner CD. Efficacy and safety of low-carbohydrate diets: a systematic review. *JAMA.* 2003;289:1837.

105. Yancy WS Jr, Olsen MK, Guyton JR, Bakst RP, Westman EC. A low-carbohydrate, ketogenic diet versus a low-fat diet to treat obesity and hyperlipidemia: a randomized, controlled trial. *Ann Intern Med.* 2004;140:769.

106. Zeph B. Effects of an Atkins type diet on weight loss in the obese. *Am Fam Phys.* 2004;69:176.

107. Bronner F, ed. *Nutrition Policy in Public Health.* New York, NY: Springer Publishing Co; 1997.

108. Bravata DM, Sanders L, Huang J, Krumholz HM, Olkin H, Gardner CD. Efficacy and safety of low-carbohydrate diets: a systematic review. *JAMA.* 2003;289:1837.

109. Improving public understanding. Guidelines for communicating emerging science on nutrition, food safety, and health. *J Natl Cancer Inst.* 1998;90:194–199.

110. Coile RD. *Futurescan 2003. A Forecast of Health Care Trends 2003–2007.* Chicago, Ill: Health Adm. Press; 2003.

111. Bouchoux A, ed. Highway to health: cruising for accurate information on the Web. *Food Insight.* September/October 2003:1–4.

112. Holland WW, Detels R, Knox G, Breeze E, eds. *Oxford Textbook of Public Health, Volume 3 Investigative Methods in Public Health.* New York, NY: Oxford University Press; 1985.

113. Federal statistics Web site. Available at: http://www.fedstats.gov/aboutfedstats.html. Accessed May 21, 2004.

114. Improving public understanding. Guidelines for communicating emerging science on nutrition, food safety, and health. *J Natl Cancer Inst.* 1998;90:194–199.

115. Myers E. Systems for evaluating nutrition research for nutrition care guidelines: Do they apply to population dietary guidelines? *J Am Diet Assoc.* 2003;103(Suppl 2):S34–S41.

BIBLIOGRAPHY

American Dietetic Association. Position paper of the American Dietetic Association: biotechnology and the future of food. *J Am Diet Assoc.* 1995;95:1429–1432.

American Dietetic Association. Position paper of the American Dietetic Association: food and water safety. *J Am Diet Assoc.* 2004;103:1203.

American Dietetic Association. Position paper of the American Dietetic Association: integration of medical nutrition therapy and pharmacotherapy. *J Am Diet Assoc.* 2003; 103:1363–1370.

American Dietetic Association. Position paper of the American Dietetic Association: the role of dietetics professionals in health promotion and disease prevention. *J Am Diet Assoc.* 2002;102:1680.

American Dietetic Association Standards of Professional Practice. Available at: http://www.eatright.org/Public/GovernmentAffairs/98_9468.cfm. Accessed June 6, 2004.

Arias DC. Politics outweighing science in policy decisions, report says. *The Nation's Health.* April 2004:1.

Blumenthal DJ, DiClemente RJ, eds. *Community-Based Health Research.* New York, NY: Springer Publishing Co; 2004.

Bouchoux A, ed. Highway to health: Cruising for accurate information on the Web. *Food Insight.* September/October 2003:1–4.

Boyle MA. *Community Nutrition in Action.* Belmont, Calif: Thomson Wadsworth; 2003.

Bravata DM, Sanders L, Huang J, Krumholz HM, Olkin H, Gardner CD. Efficacy and safety of low-carbohydrate diets: a systematic review. *JAMA.* 2003;289:1837.

Bronner F, ed. *Nutrition Policy in Public Health.* New York, NY: Springer Publishing Co; 1997.

Brownson RC, Baker EA, Leet TL, Gillespie KN. *Evidence-Based Public Health.* New York, NY: Oxford Press; 2003.

Center for Nutritional Policy and Promotion [CNPP]. Table of dietary guidelines for Americans, 1980–2000. Available at: http://www.usda.gov/cnpp/Pubs/DG2000/Dgover.PDF. Accessed May 29, 2004.

Center for Nutrition Policy and Promotion [CNPP]. *Using Food Labels to Follow the Dietary Guidelines for Americans. A Reference.* Alexandria, Va: CNPP; 1994. USDA/CNPP Agricultural Information Bulletin 704.

Coile RD. *Futurescan 2003. A Forecast of Health Care Trends 2003–2007.* Chicago, Ill: Health Adm. Press; 2003.

Cooper MJ, Zlotkin SH. An evidence-based approach to the development of national dietary guidelines. *J Am Diet Assoc.* 2004;103:S28.

De Busk R. *Genetics: The Nutrition Connection.* Chicago, Ill: American Dietetic Association; 2003.

Eldridge AL. Comparison of 1989 RDAs and DRIs for water-soluble vitamins. *Nutr Today.* 2004;39:88–93.

Endres JB. *Community Nutrition.* Upper Saddle River, NJ: Merrill Publishing; 1999.

Fairchild AL, Bayer R. Ethics and the conduct of public health surveillance. *Science.* 2004;303:631.

Federal statistics Web site. Available at: http://www.fedstats.gov/aboutfedstats.html. Accessed May 21, 2004.

Flegal KM, Carroll MD, Ogden CL, Johnson CL. Prevalence and trends in obesity among U.S. adults, 1999–2000. *JAMA.* 2002;288:1723–1727.

Food and Nutrition Board - National Academy of Sciences. Dietary Reference Intakes (RDIs). 1998. Available at: http://www.utexas.edu/courses/ntr311/nutinfo/RDIchart.html. Accessed May 31, 2004.

Food and Nutrition Information Center. Historical food guides background and development. Available at: http://www.nal.usda.gov/fnic/history/index.html. Accessed May 29, 2004.

Gillies PJ. Nutrigenomics: the Rubicon of molecular nutrition. *J Am Diet Assoc.* 2003; 103:S50–S55.

Grundy SM, et al. Executive Summary of the Third Report of the National Cholesterol Education Program (NCEP) Expert Panel on Detection, Evaluation, and Treatment of High Blood Cholesterol in Adults (Adult Treatment Panel III) *JAMA.* 2001;285: 2486–2497.

Hasler CM. Functional foods: benefits, concerns, and challenges – a position paper from the American Council on Science and Health. *J Nutr.* 2002;132:3772–3781.

Heaney RP, Dougherty CJ. *Research for Health Professionals Design, Analysis, and Ethics.* Ames, Ia: Iowa State University Press; 1988.

HHS Tackles Obesity. *FDA Consumer.* 2004;38:14–16.

Hogbin M, Lyon J, Davis C. Comparison of dietary recommendations using the dietary guidelines for Americans as a framework. *Nutr Today.* 2003;38:203–217.

Holland WW, Detels R, Knox G, Breeze E, eds. *Oxford Textbook of Public Health, Volume 1 History, Determinants, Scope and Strategies.* New York, NY: Oxford University Press; 1984.

Holland WW, Detels R, Knox G, Breeze E, eds. *Oxford Textbook of Public Health, Volume 3 Investigative Methods in Public Health.* New York, NY: Oxford University Press; 1985.

Improving public understanding. Guidelines for communicating emerging science on nutrition, food safety, and health. *J Natl Cancer Inst.* 1998;90:194–199.

Institute of Medicine. *Dietary Reference Intakes Applications in Dietary Assessment.* Washington, DC: National Academies Press; 2000.

Institute of Medicine. *The Future of the Public's Health in the 21st Century.* Washington, DC: National Academies Press; 2003.

Issel ML. *Health Program Planning and Evaluation.* Sudbury, Mass: Jones and Bartlett Publishers; 2004.

Jackson K. Nutrigenomics: it's in the genes. *Today's Dietitian.* 2003;5:27–29.

Khoury MJ, Burke W, Thomson EJ, eds. *Genetics and Public Health in the 21st Century.* New York, NY: Oxford University Press; 2000.

Laidlaw SH. Supplements: folic acid and female health. *Nutr Complementary Care.* 2004;6:72.

Leedy PD, Ormrod JE. *Practical Research Planning and Design.* New York, NY: Macmillan Publishing Co; 2005.

Lin BH, Smallwood D, Hamilton W, Rossi PH. Research designs for assessing the USDA's food assistance and nutrition programs outcomes, part 2: impact evaluation of demonstrations. *Nutr Today.* 2004;39:40–45.

McMurry KY. Setting dietary guidelines: the U.S. process. *J Am Diet Assoc.* 2003;103 (Suppl 2):S10–S17.

Meerschaert CM. The obesity solution. *Today's Dietitian.* 2004;6:30–33.

Myers E. Systems for evaluating nutrition research for nutrition care guidelines: Do they apply to population dietary guidelines? *J Am Diet Assoc.* 2003;103(Suppl 2):S34–S41.

National Center for Complementary and Alternative Medicine Web site. Available at: http://nccam.nih.gov. Accessed November 10, 2004.

National Heart, Lung, and Blood Institute. Framingham Heart Study timeline. Available at: http://www.nhlbi.nih.gov/about/framingham/timeline.htm. Accessed December 5, 2005.

Nestle M. *Food Politics.* Berkeley, Calif: University of California Press; 2002.

Neutens JJ, Rubinson L. *Research Techniques for the Health Sciences.* San Francisco, Calif: Pearson Education Inc; 2002.

Schneeman B. Evolution of the dietary guidelines. *J Am Diet Assoc.* 2003;103(Suppl 2):S5–S9.

Scott BS. Project Impact. Increasing minority participation and awareness of clinical trials. *Closing the Gap.* August 2003:8.

Shanklin C. Evidence-based practice: practice based on evidence. Right? *ADA Times.* January 12, 2003:1,3.

Smith Edge M. Promoting healthful diets from a public perspective. *J Am Diet Assoc.* 2004;104:827–831.

Stangl DK, Berry DA, eds. *Meta-Analysis in Medicine and Health Policy.* New York, NY: Marcel Dekker Inc; 2000.

Stumbo P, Chenard CA, Hemingway DL. Plowing through the data: harvesting knowledge from food composition tables. *The Digest.* 2004;39:1–3.

3 Report on Nutrition Monitoring in the United States. Vol 1. Washington, DC: U.S. Government Printing Office; 1995.

Tillotson JE. Pandemic obesity: What is the solution? *Nutr Today.* 2004;39:6–9.

Tulchinsky TH, Varavikova EA. *The New Public Health.* New York, NY: Academic Press; 2000.

US Department of Health and Human Services. Executive summary of dietary guidelines. Available at: http://www.health.gov/dietaryguidelines/dga2005/report/HTML/A_Exec Summary.htm. Accessed Nov. 10, 2004.

Victora CG, Habicht J-P, Bryce J. Evidence-based public health: moving beyond randomized trials. *Am J Public Health.* 2004;94:400–405.

Yancy WS Jr, Olsen MK, Guyton JR, Bakst RP, Westman EC. A low-carbohydrate, ketogenic diet versus a low-fat diet to treat obesity and hyperlipidemia: a randomized, controlled trial. *Ann Intern Med.* 2004;140:769.

Zeph B. Effects of an Atkins type diet on weight loss in the obese. *Am Fam Phys.* 2004;69:176.

CHAPTER 3

Assess the Community's Needs for Nutrition Services

Toni Martin

Reader Objectives

- Understand the purpose and use of the community assessment.
- Understand the several health-planning models available and their community assessment approaches.
- Recognize that the obesity epidemic needs to drive the community assessment process.
- Understand and know how to obtain qualitative (subjective) and quantitative (objective) data.
- Know how and when to mobilize various stakeholders in the community assessment.

COMMUNITY NEEDS ASSESSMENT

Community needs assessment is used to identify and prioritize health needs and health problems in the community. A variety of tools or instruments may be used. Essential elements are community engagement and collaborative participation. Community assessment is one of the three core governmental public health functions. The two essential assessment services are considered to be:

1. Monitor health status to identify community health problems.
2. Diagnose and investigate health problems and health hazards in the community.[1]

Communities are defined as groups of people who share common characteristics. The community of interest used in planning public health programs usually has geographic boundaries. It is frequently a designated jurisdiction such as a zip code, neighborhood, census track, village, town, city, state, tribe, or nation. Within these boundaries, the official or tax-supported health agency has mandated responsibilities to assure services to protect and promote the health of the people who live, work, or visit within it.

A community may also be defined as a group of people who share common needs or interests. The principles of community assessment also may be applied to a clinic, catchment area, parish, school district, or to a target population that share similar problems such as the same disease or disability. The process of assembling and analyzing both subjective observations and objective statistics to profile community needs and concerns may be called:

- Community assessment
- Needs assessment
- Community profile
- Market research[2]

COMMUNITY HEALTH PLANNING MODELS

During the last two decades there has been increasing leadership from federal agencies and national public health organizations to encourage each state and local public health agency to write its own unique health improvement plan. *Healthy People 2010* sets the objective "to increase the proportion of Tribes, States and the District of Columbia that have a *Health Improvement Plan* linked with their State's plan and increase the proportion of local jurisdictions that each have their own *Health Improvement Plan*.[3] To guide development of these plans, federal agencies have collaborated with national public health organizations to prepare several community health planning models. Each model highlights the assessment of the community needs as they identify their populations' significant health risks and set priorities.

Step-by-step guidance published for local and state public health agencies leads them through their community assessment and to use data to develop their health improvement plan. Public health nutritionists must understand and use these various models, especially the one selected for use by their agency administrators, planners, and community leaders.

Currently, the most widely used models are PATCH (Planned Approach to Community Health); *Healthy Communities 2000: Model Standards*; APEXPH (Assessment Protocol for Excellence in Public Health); MAPP (Mobilizing for Action through Planning and Partnership); and the *Healthy People 2010 Toolkit*. Each of these models emphasizes collaboration, community involvement in the assessment, and policy development assurances.

PATCH (Planned Approach to Community Health)

PATCH was developed in 1983 by the Centers for Disease Control and Prevention (CDC) in partnership with state and local health departments and concerned community planning groups. It was created for use by various partners at the local level. Collaborations included the federal, state, and local governmental public health infrastructure joining with voluntary organizations, academia, and others. It is widely recognized as an effective model to plan, conduct, and evaluate community health promotion and disease prevention programs. PATCH is a practical, community process based on the latest health education, health promotion, and community development knowledge and theories. Many communities use PATCH to prioritize their competing public health concerns, including obesity, cardiovascular disease, HIV, injuries, teenage pregnancy, and access to health care. PATCH lists a sequence of five phases to complete the process, as shown in Figure 3–1. The five phases are repeated with each new public health problem as it emerges, as new target groups are selected, or as new interventions are developed. Although PATCH can be applied to various health problems or communities, the five phases remain the same.

- Phase I: Mobilize the Community—This phase starts as a community organizes to move through the process. The community of interest is defined, participants from the community are recruited, partnerships are formed, and a demographic profile of the community is completed. The demographic profile ensures that the PATCH community-planning group represents the many different socioeconomic and ethnic populations living and working in the community. The community-planning group and steering committee are organized, and working groups are appointed. In this first phase, the media publicizes the PATCH process to help win support, particularly from community leaders.
- Phase II: Collect and Organize Data—This phase begins as the working groups research and analyze data on mortality, morbidity, prevailing opinions of the citizens, and their health behaviors. Qualitative (subjective) data

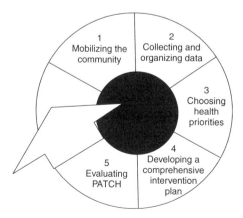

Figure 3–1 The PATCH (Planned Approach to Community Health) model. *Source:* CDC; 1997.

describes or explains health attitudes and practices and can be categorized or ranked but not quantified. Subjective data is obtained by interviewing people who know the community, its history, and past efforts to address health concerns. Quantitative or objective data consists of collecting statistics that can be measured. Examples of quantitative data are vital statistics and results of population health surveys. Community members may identify other sources of local data that should be collected. The community-planning group analyzes the data to list the leading health problems in the community. During this phase, PATCH users also recommend ways to publicize results of this data analysis to the people in their community.

- Phase III: Choose Health Priorities—In this phase behavioral and any additional data collected are presented to the community-planning group. They analyze the social, economic, political, and environmental factors that contribute to behaviors that put their population at risk for disease, injury, disability, and death. Issues are listed in priority order.
- Phase IV: Developing a Comprehensive Intervention Plan—Using information generated in Phases II and III, in Phase IV the planning group chooses, designs, and recommends interventions. They set measurable objectives as they develop the health improvement plan for their community.
- Phase V: Evaluation—Phase V is ongoing in PATCH: It monitors and assesses progress during the five phases to evaluate the effectiveness of the selected interventions. The community-planning group sets criteria to measure achievements and identifies data to be collected. Continuing feedback is publicized to the community to encourage their continuing participation as well as for planners to use to improve program interventions.

PATCH is widely used in states and communities throughout the United States. The time required from assessment to implementation of specific interventions in a PATCH program is usually from 8 to 12 months. PATCH is one of the first community health planning tools to be used as a process for community organization and community needs assessment that emphasizes citizen mobilization and constituency building. PATCH focuses on orienting and training community leaders, public health professionals, and other community members in all aspects of the community needs assessment process. It includes useful documentation and resource materials.[4]

For more information, visit www.cdc.gov/nccdphp/patch/index.html or www.apha.org/ppp/science/guide2.htm.

Healthy Communities 2000: Model Standards

Healthy Communities 2000: Model Standards is a set of health status and process objectives that local public health leaders can adapt to the unique needs of their own community. As a collaborative effort, the American Public Health Association, the Association of State and Territorial Health Officials, the National Association of County Health Officials, the United States Conference of Local Health Officers, the Association of Schools of Public Health, and the Centers for Disease Control and Prevention published *Healthy Communities 2000* in 1991. There are 11 steps to *Healthy Communities 2000: Model Standards*.

Steps of Healthy Communities 2000: Model Standards

1. Assess and determine the role of the health agency. Each community is organized and structured differently, and the specific roles of local public health organizations vary from community to community.
2. Assess the lead health agency's organizational capacity to carry out its role in the community.
3. Develop an agency plan to build organizational capacity by studying the organization's strengths and weaknesses. This step includes developing specific objectives to address the weaknesses identified and to assign responsibilities with a process to track progress over time.
4. Assess the community's organizational and power structures, a long-term and continuous process in which the relationships of all important community stakeholders and partners (e.g., official and voluntary health agencies, providers of health and related services, community organizations, community leaders, interest groups, the media, and the general public) are assessed. This step determines how and under whose sponsorship health planning will take place within the community.
5. Organize the community to build a stronger constituency for public health and establish partnerships with other health agencies. Specific strategies and activities can vary from community to community but generally include hearings, dialogues, discussion forums, meetings, and collaborative planning sessions.
6. Assess community health needs to identify the community's most urgent health problems. This assessment utilizes and combines quantitative information derived from available data sets with qualitative information derived from the community's citizen's perceptions of their problems. Community readiness to work on problems, as their people perceive them, greatly increases the potential for success and support in the community.
7. Determine local priorities and community health resources. After priority health problems are identified, decisions must be made to rank those most important for community action. This requires community participation so that priorities will be owned by the people in the community rather than imposed by the agency. Debate and negotiation are essential.
8. Select outcome objectives. After priorities are selected, a target level must be established to be achieved for each problem. Targets must be achievable

with available resources. Selected community objectives should be linked to national health objectives.

9. Develop intervention strategies. This step specifies strategies and methods to achieve the measurable outcome objectives established for each priority health problem. After consensus is reached on strategies and methods, responsibilities for implementing and evaluating the selected interventions will be assigned.

10. Develop and implement a plan of action. Once interventions are selected, responsibilities are assigned to distribute and coordinate activities among agencies and organizations.

11. Continuous monitoring and evaluation tracks performance related to process and outcome objectives and activity measures over time.[5]

Healthy Communities 2000 provides practical tools to apply the national health objectives to local needs and priorities. It encourages consensus of community leaders who develop local goals, outcome and process objectives, and implementation plans to achieve the objectives.

APEXPH (Assessment Protocol for Excellence in Public Health)

APEXPH (Assessment Protocol for Excellence in Public Health) was developed by the National Association of County and City Health Officials (NACCHO) in 1991 in collaboration with several of the national public health organizations. APEXPH is a tool for organizational self-assessment and improvement for local public health departments. It is a simple tool for community needs assessment. It should focus on community-wide public health practice, including the health department's role in the community and the real and perceived needs of the community leaders and citizens. It guides community planners to assess the population's health needs, set priorities, develop the policies that govern the process, and ensure that identified health needs are addressed. There are three parts to APEXPH:

1. Organizational capacity assessment involves the health department leaders through an internal self-assessment. Together, they study their authority to operate; develop policies; perform community assessment; and manage fiscal, personnel, and other administrative resources. An organizational action plan sets priorities for correcting perceived weaknesses.

2. The community process begins when a community advisory committee is formed to identify priority health problems and set health status goals and objectives. The aim is to mobilize community resources to pursue locally relevant public health objectives that are consistent with the *Healthy People* objectives. The result of this committee's work is a community health

improvement plan based on data and representing the concerns of people of the community.

3. Completing the cycle occurs when the local health department implements the community health improvement plan. The local health official and the agency staff must pull the results of the community health plan together. The product must be studied to make sure their capabilities and resources match the needs identified by community leaders.[6]

APEXPH is a process that local health departments use to assess their capacity to create community partnerships. It studies the health department's administration, organizational structure, and its role in the community. It supports the development of partnerships with collaborating community representatives to identify health problems and develop a priority list. It enables the development of the community plan to improve the ability of the health department to address the community's identified health needs.[7] To learn more, visit www.apha.org/ppp/science/guide2.htm.

MAPP (Mobilizing for Action through Planning and Partnership)

MAPP (Mobilizing for Action through Planning and Partnership) is the newest health planning model and was developed by the National Association of County and City Health Officials (NACCHO) and the CDC in 2000. It provides models to identify and prioritize public health issues, as shown in Figure 3–2. MAPP is a community-wide strategic planning tool to improve community health. It builds on the foundation of the APEXPH to guide local health officials in assessment and planning. The MAPP model involves interconnected and interactive components or steps that need not be conducted in a fixed order. It includes four assessments based on strategic issues usually stated after visioning has taken place and before strategic issues are identified. The four MAPP assessments inform the planning process and the identification of strategic issues. Although the sequencing of the assessments is not relevant to the success of the process, all assessments must be utilized.

- Community themes and strengths assessment identifies issues that interest the people of the community, their perceptions about their quality of life, and the community's assets. It collects input and insights from leaders and constituents throughout the community to understand the issues that the residents feel are most important.
- Local public health system assessment measures the capacity and performance of the local public health system—all organizations and entities that contribute to the public's health. This involves an analysis of mission, vision, and goals with performance measures for the essential public health services. Strengths and areas for improvement are identified.

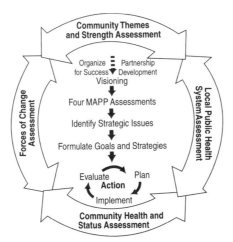

Figure 3–2 The MAPP (Mobilizing for Action through Planning and Partnerships) model. *Source:* NACCHO, CDC; 2000.

- Community health status assessment compiles data about the health status, quality of life, and risk factors in the community. It involves 11 domains: asset mapping, environmental health, socioeconomic, demographic, behavioral risk factors, infectious diseases, sentinel events, social and mental health, maternal and child health, health resource availability, and health status indicators.
- Forces of change assessment identifies elements such as legislation, technology, and other forces that can affect the context in which the community and the public health system operate.

Together these four assessments guide the group to identify strategic issues and to prepare goals, strategies, and information as participants plan for action, implementation, and evaluation. Conducting periodic MAPP assessments can establish a continuing community initiative designed to lead to a healthier community.[8]

For more information, visit: www.naccho.org/documents/MAPP_field_guide2.pdf or www.naccho.org/prod102.cfm.

Healthy People 2010 Toolkit

The *Healthy People 2010 Toolkit* provides guidance for states, territories, and tribes to write their specific *Healthy People 2010* health improvement plans. It consists of seven major action areas derived from the national and state Healthy People 2010 initiatives. With guidance from the Office of Disease Prevention and Health Promotion and the US Department of Health and Human Services (HHS), the Public Health Foundation reviewed year 2000 and year 2010 initiatives and identified seven areas as common elements of most health planning and improvement efforts.

Build the Foundation: Leadership and Structure Effective leaders influence public opinion, mobilize support, engage partners, inspire action, and advocate for the health improvement plan. They also facilitate finding, obtaining, and allocating resources and set policy and assure that objectives are measurable and monitored. An organized and well-defined planning structure positions the planning process for success. Once the state's 2010 goals are envisioned, the authority structure is established. Participants should know their responsibilities in an advisory role and a steering role. Participants should provide informed input on the *Healthy People 2010* planning process, priority areas, target populations, and scope of objectives, marketing, and other aspects of the 2010 community health improvement plan. Members of a steering committee navigate the course of the planning process, establish work groups, determine input processes, and make decisions about the content of the state plan.

Identify and Secure Resources A detailed budget should be developed showing the funding needed to implement the planned activities. There are many options for identifying and securing sufficient resources for planning. One general strategy is to suggest how the goals of the state or local health improvement plan may be aligned with the goals of potential resource funders. This will secure public and private resources. The budget should cover all aspects of the development process, including the resources needed to carry out each of the seven areas outlined in the toolkit.

Identify and Engage Community Partners By establishing effective partnerships with the people and leaders of the community, official public health agencies strengthen their planning process. Community partners can advocate for the goals and objectives of the plan, recruit additional partners, contribute a variety of unique skills and talents, and help monitor progress toward achieving objectives. Community partners consist of representatives of government agencies, businesses, nonprofit organizations, and concerned citizens. *Healthy People 2010* initiatives begin with the commitment to collaborate among a variety of constituencies so that they all can share a claim of ownership of the plan.

Set Health Priorities and Establish Objectives There are many models and resources to help select priorities. To agree on priorities, it is necessary to develop consensus among steering group members on what models to use, and how qualitative data, quantitative data, assets, community opinions, and political agenda will influence setting the priorities.

Obtain Baseline Measures, Set Targets, and Measure Progress Collecting and analyzing quantitative and qualitative data are essential to establish health priorities.

After listing priority health issues and potential indicators, a baseline is set to establish the current situation on each problem or indicator. Targets set the desired amount of change over a specified time interval. Data is collected and analyzed on a schedule to monitor progress toward meeting each objective.

Manage and Sustain the Process   This requires committed leadership and the continuing support of public health administrators and policy makers. Commitment and energy of community partners as they identify needs and set objectives or targets begin the process. Some strategies to sustain the development and implementation process for the health improvement plan include appointing key staff to manage the plan, maintaining open communications between all of the partners, sharing management responsibilities across departments and agencies, and integrating *Healthy People 2010* initiatives into other key health programs and services in the community.

Communicate Health Goals and Objectives   The success of the *Healthy People 2010* process depends on communicating the goals and objectives to the community. This includes identifying the target audiences, constructing clear messages, and effectively communicating these messages to the target audience. Effective communication increases the likelihood of the health improvement plan being accepted and used by the state and community partners.[9]

To learn more, visit www.astho.org or www.naccho.org.

ASSESS THE COMMUNITY NEEDS FOR NUTRITION SERVICES

Conducting an assessment of the community's perceived health and nutrition status and its existing resources is the best and easiest way to start to integrate nutrition services into the state or local health improvement plan. The community assessment process introduces key players and stakeholders in the community to those who have developed or are developing a community health plan. When an agency or organization is revising or updating its health improvement plan, the community assessment is essential to develop effective interventions.[10]

Overweight and obesity are now identified in epidemic numbers both among adults and children and are considered to be major factors contributing to the increased prevalence of costly, killing, and crippling chronic diseases. Thus nutrition and diet are assuming major importance to public health intervention strategies.[11]

For more information, visit: www.cdc.gov/nccdphp/dnpa/obesity/index.htm and www.healthfinder. gov.

The public health nutritionist who participates in the community assessment process focuses on the health issues that relate to nutrition, diet, and food security. Public health nutritionists assume responsibility for collecting, analyzing, and interpreting both the subjective and objective data. Collaboration in data collection and analysis should include partners who share the interests and concerns of the public health nutritionist. These include but are not limited to dietitians in local health care facilities and private practice, food service managers in schools and health care facilities, and cooperative extension agents and their homemaker groups. Other resources include faculty and students in the department of nutrition or dietetics in local universities, community colleges, and dietetic internships programs. Concerned parents, senior citizens, clergy, business leaders, and food banks expand the partnerships interested in health and nutrition as well as food security.[12]

Collecting Nutrition Data

Excessive numbers of obese and overweight men, women, and children are easily observed in their neighborhoods, workplaces, schools, shopping malls, and wherever people of all ages gather. News items highlight the growing market for fashionable plus size clothing for women or that airlines are concerned about rising fuel costs because the numbers of heavier passengers require their planes to utilize more fuel. Thus, subjective observations can be documented with qualitative documentation of obesity and overweight as the major public health and nutrition issue of the new century.

Qualitative or subjective assessment begins with a careful study of the mass media—reading the local newspapers, including those that serve the various neighborhoods or ethnic groups; listening to the area radio stations, including those that target ethnic groups or special interests; and watching local television coverage. Local media usually reflect local values, political views, interests, educational level, and lifestyles including the food choices of their constituents.

By studying media coverage of meetings of local, state, and national governmental bodies, it is possible to determine the emerging issues and to identify the opinion leaders and their opposing views. Public spending priorities show up in coverage of governmental budget hearings. The media presents insights into the local economy and monitors employment and unemployment trends. They report the stresses and tensions among various ethnic, religious, or socioeconomic groups and social issues that arouse human interest. They often report sentinel events, such as stories about families who are hungry or homeless, adults and children with serious illness or disabilities, elderly persons coping with fixed incomes, or the plight of migrant farm workers and the new and changing ethnic groups who have come into the community in recent years. Food and health reports reflect local food tastes, the latest quick fix weight loss diet fads, and the growing public concerns about overweight and obesity, and their interest in fitness, diet, and exercise. Weekly supermarket ads provide information on plentiful foods and their prices. Reports and plans available from community agencies, civic groups, chambers of commerce, or area planning agencies can be obtained to provide additional details on information covered by the media.

To get "in touch" with the community, it is useful to study the map of the jurisdiction with a resident who knows the area. This might be a professional who has had long experience in the agency, a geographer or an anthropologist from a local university, or a well-informed member of the community planning group. This key informant can give history and background information and point out unique characteristics and idiosyncrasies of the geography and the people.

Visits to the various types of food markets and family-type cafeterias or restaurants inform the nutritionist about the prices, quality, and choices of foods available, as well as the preferred regional or ethnic foods. Observing and tasting the menu items featured in restaurants, schools, or group care facilities provides information on popular methods of food preparation, serving sizes, and the use of fats and salt as seasonings. Market or restaurant managers and food service directors can discuss what foods are preferred and any prevailing food beliefs or taboos. Observing the number of overweight and obese children and adults and conversing with many of these people provides insights into their perceptions of health and nutritional status and into their worries and aspirations for themselves and their children. These explorations may provide a sense of the flavor and color of the community life, which is in constant flux. With more people becoming aware of the value of regular exercise, the availability of walking paths, playgrounds, and public and private gyms should be noted.

More structured information gathering might include soliciting community opinions through focus groups, a method used in social marketing.[13]

Perceived problems and needs for public health nutritionists to expand nutrition education and weight management programs and services can be solicited by interviewing professional colleagues in the health agency to ascertain their perspectives on the community.

Health Directors or Administrators, Public Health Physicians, and Health Planners These individuals will express their opinions and priorities regarding the contribution of nutrition services in the health agency's health promotion programs. They can share their knowledge of community health care services and facilities. They know the power structure, elected officials, and leaders. They may provide copies of special studies or surveys of diet-related chronic diseases conducted in the area by federal, state, or local governmental agencies; legislative study groups; contract consultants; or universities. They can provide long- and short-term agency plans, grant proposals, and annual reports with informative statistics and descriptive information.

Health Educators These individuals know community organizations and formal and informal networks. They understand the political system and the power structure. They can identify knowledgeable contacts in state or local government, other health and human service agencies, schools, houses of worship, businesses, and neighborhoods. They may have insight into the concerns about the growing obesity epidemic as well as possible interests in fitness, nutrition, and health of various subpopulations in the area. In their files, they may have useful, up-to-date facts and figures.

Public Health Nurses These individuals know the community through their close contacts with clients, families, schools, industries, clinics, and other health care facilities. Working within agency policies on information privacy and confidentiality, their client and family health records may be reviewed to compile information on the health and nutritional status of the women they serve in the family planning and prenatal clinics; the infants and children receiving well- or ill-child special health care services as WIC participants; the adults seen for chronic disease screening or primary care; the children enrolled in day care or schools; and the chronically ill patients visited for home health services. Client and family records are confidential and must be treated carefully, using only aggregated data and not identifying any individuals.

Environmental Health Specialists and Health Care Facility Inspectors These individuals know the housing conditions in local neighborhoods, including whether kitchens have indoor plumbing, working ranges, and refrigerators. They know the safety of the public and private water supplies. They also can provide information on the safety, sanitation, and quality of the food services in the schools, child day care centers, hospitals, nursing homes, jails and other group care faculties, and in public eating establishments and food markets.

Human Service Agency Directors and Social Workers These individuals know the financial status, food and housing needs, and expenditures of individuals and families. They are aware of the prevalence of personal and family emotional and social stresses, including alcohol and drug abuse; child, spouse, and elder abuse; and special needs of single-parent families. They can describe the ethnic and immigrant status and religious mix and its influences on community relations. They can list and describe the public and private agencies and institutions that provide food and financial assistance, food stamps; emergency food and shelter, and mental health and family counseling to residents, immigrants, and migrants. They know or can advise on how to find out about eligibility and application procedures for the various services and their caseloads.

Hospital Administrators and Their Staff These individuals can provide access to data on hospital discharges and on any existing or anticipated community services. Clinical dietitians can discuss diagnostic categories for patients to whom they provide medical nutrition therapy in the hospital and refer upon discharge to home health agencies.

Health Maintenance Organizations (HMO) Administrators These individuals often have aggregated data on the health status and educational needs of the populations they serve. Dietitians who are employed by HMOs or community health centers may be able to share statistics on age groups and diagnoses of their clients.

School Superintendents and Principals These individuals can approve access to aggregated data from school health records. They can introduce the nutritionist to teachers, school nurses, and school food service directors who observe the health, weight status, and growth of children. They can provide data on participation in school meal programs and on the numbers of free and reduced-priced meals served and nutrition education. Special educators and school counselors and psychologists can describe problems of children who are overweight or obese or who have diabetes, other chronic diseases or developmental disabilities, social and emotional needs, eating disorders, or other nutrition-related health conditions.

Cooperative Extension Specialists These individuals include agronomists who have information on local crops, growing conditions, and family gardens. Cooperative extension home economists know the practices and competencies of area homemakers in meal planning, food purchasing, food preparation, use of food stamps, and other aspects of family life.

Local Television, Radio, or Newspaper Medical or Science Reporters These individuals can share extensive community profiles with useful statistics and human-interest stories.

Local Clergy These individuals may share information on the food security and health status of the people in their congregations. Some of the families in their congregations may use or need to be referred to local soup kitchens, or food pantries.[14]

Table 3–1 is a sample format that can be used to record, organize, and scale the subjective data from various informants.

Collecting, categorizing, and interpreting this data are essential to understand the attitudes, lifestyle, and opinions of the people interviewed. It is used to understand the community and identify any existing barriers. It is important to involve the key stakeholders in the program design, development, implementation, and evaluation to assure the needed commitment of the community from the very beginning of the nutrition needs assessment.[15]

Quantitative or objective assessment collects facts and figures concerning what is known about the community's population in the aggregate compared to what is known about individuals. Readily available demographic statistics may not be specific for nutrition, but can point the nutritionist to populations who may be at risk for nutrition- or diet-related health problems because of age, income,

Table 3–1 Subjective Data Collection Form

Perceived Nutrition Needs in the Community List	Attitude Toward Nutrition Services			Knowledge of Nutrition		
	+	0	–	+	0	–
Clients/Patients						
Public						
Media						
Government officials						
Agency administrators						
Physicians/dentists						
Hospital administrators						
Nurses						
Health educators						
Nutritionists/dietitians						
Agency board members						
Principals/teachers						
Social workers						
Clergy						

Code + = positive, supportive attitude toward nutrition and health services
     0 = neutral or apathetic toward nutrition
     – = negative attitude toward nutrition

Source: Adapted from Kaufman, M. *Nutrition in Public Health: A Handbook for Developing Programs and Services.* Rockville, Md: Aspen Publishers; 1990:52.

education, or diagnosis. Demographic statistics are obtained from publications reporting the national decennial census. As the decade progresses, estimates are projected by the state demographer.

For much of the assessment, the statistic that is the reference point or denominator for comparisons with the other data is the total population or the number of residents who live in the jurisdiction. In areas where the population is seasonally enlarged by an influx of students, summer or winter residents, tourists, or migrant workers who use health and nutrition services, their numbers must be known and factored in. The population figure can be categorized according to the demographic characteristics shown in Table 3–2.

Vital statistics on births and deaths reported to the state health agency are also used in the community assessment. All births and deaths are recorded through a local registrar or clerk, usually in the city or county health department. Because law mandates these registrations, data obtained from birth and death certificates cover virtually the entire population and are a reliable statistical basis for community assessment. Birth certificates record the birth weight of the infant, which can then be used to categorize the infant according to low birth weight (LBW— less than or equal to 2500 grams) or very low birth weight (VLBW—less than or equal to 1500 grams). Birth certificates also classify infants by the gestational age and the age and race of the mother. In many states, the birth attendant's observation of a birth defect is required on the birth certificate. Unfortunately, the attending pediatrician may not always record this or the type of birth defect may not be readily apparent until the infant is older or tested. Death certificates also document neonatal, post neonatal, and infant death rates. Infant birth and death certificates can be linked for such factors as low or very low birth weight, ages of the infants, and ethnicity of the mothers. To compare vital statistics from one geographic area to those of another (i.e., a city or county to the state or nation) or one population to another, various rates are calculated, see Table 3–3.[16]

Table 3–2 Demographic Population Data

Characteristic	Description
Age	Infants, preschool and school age children, adolescents, young, middle-aged and older or elderly adults, the aged, and women of child-bearing years
Gender	Male or female
Ethnicity	White, nonwhite, specifically, African-American, Hispanic, Asian, and American Indian
Education	Number of years of school completed by adults over the age of 18
Income	Numbers or percentages of individuals who live on incomes at various levels above or below the current poverty index
Employment	Number or percentage of the workforce and the unemployed

Source: Adapted from Kaufman M. *Nutrition in Public Health: A Handbook for Developing Programs and Services.* Rockville, Md: Aspen Publishers; 1990:53.

Table 3–3 Calculating Rate to Compare Vital Statistics from One Area or Population to Another

Birth rate =	# of live births _____	× 100
	Population of area	
Fetal mortality rate =	# of fetal deaths _____	× 100
	# of live births + # of fetal deaths in area	
Infant mortality rates =	# of infant deaths _____	× 100
	# of live births in the area	
Death rate	# of deaths _____	× 100
	population of area	

Source: Adapted from Kaufman M. *Nutrition in Public Health: A Handbook for Developing Programs and Services*. Rockville, Md: Aspen Publlishers; 1990:55.

Death certificates provide information on the primary and sometimes secondary cause of death (mortality). Dietary factors are closely associated with 5 of the 10 leading causes of death. These are hypertension, cardiovascular diseases, some forms of cancer, cirrhosis, stroke and, diabetes mellitus. Now that overweight and obesity are considered to be the second of the 10 leading health indicators for *Healthy People 2010*, the rates of these statistics may indicate the extent of this diet-related problem in the local population. The death rates in the community can be then compared with other similar areas—cities, counties, states, and the nation, to observe what trends may be apparent in the population. Trends can also be monitored over time to evaluate the impact of the interventions and education. Assistance in interpreting the data may be obtained from the statisticians and epidemiologists at the local and state health agencies, especially when sorting the data into usable formats. The health statistics used should be from the most recent reported year, but it is important to remember that there can be a two to three year lag time between collecting and reporting of the data. It is important when comparing data with other populations such as local to county, state, or national, the data all needs to be for the same year. It may be necessary to go back several years to make valid comparisons. Most health agencies have collection forms available for use. Tables 3–4, 3–5, and 3–6 are examples of forms that can be used to collect and compare demographic data for a community.

The public health nutritionist may also study specific nutrition and dietary status data available through secondary data sources collected by national and state organizations or by university statisticians experienced in population sampling methodology. The National Health and Nutrition Examination Surveys (NHANES) directed by the National Center for Health Statistics meticulously collects data by administering a battery of nutritional and health status measures to a national probability sample of the population. National survey information may be appropriate to review the nutritional status for large-scale populations. This data needs to be analyzed and interpreted for use in the local area, adjusting the data for age, gender, ethnicity, and income. These statistics make it possible to project the prevalence of obesity and being overweight, impaired growth status, hypertension, high-risk

Table 3–4   Objective Data Collection Form, Example 1

	Leading Causes of Death	Local Rates			State Rates		
		W	NW	Total	W	NW	Total
1.							
2.							
3.							
4.							
5.							
6.							
7.							
8.							
9.							
10.							

Source: Adapted from Kaufman M. *Nutrition in Public Health: A Handbook for Developing Programs and Services.* Rockville, Md: Aspen Publlishers; 1990:57.

serum cholesterol, diabetes, stunted growth, low serum vitamin A and C, and the use of vitamin and mineral supplements.

Disease prevalence (number of people in the population living with communicable or chronic disease) and disease incidence (new cases of disease) are very useful community assessment information for program planning. However, because health care providers are not required to report chronic diseases to the official health agency, the prevalence or incidence data are not easily available. Hospital discharge data can provide useful indicators. Special surveys can be conducted on random

Table 3–5   Objective Data Collection Form, Example 2

Prevalence Rates for Leading Nutrition-Related Health Problems—Synthetic Estimates from NHANES Data	Estimates Rates		
	W	NW	Total
1. Obesity			
2. Cardiovascular disease			
3. Hypertension			
4. Cancer			
5. Stroke			
6. Diabetes			
7. Cirrhosis			
8. Iron deficiency anemia			

Source: Adapted from Kaufman M. *Nutrition in Public Health: A Handbook for Developing Programs and Services.* Rockville, Md: Aspen Publlishers; 1990:57.

Table 3–6 Objective Data Collection Form, Example 3

	Pregnancy Outcome			Perinatal/infant Mortality Rates			
Live births, number	W	NW	Total	Fetal	W	NW	Total
% low birth weight (≤ 2500 gms)				Neonatal			
% mothers ≤ 17 years				Postneonatal			

Source: Adapted from Kaufman M. *Nutrition in Public Health: A Handbook for Developing Programs and Services.* Rockville, Md: Aspen Publlishers; 1990:57.

population samples or samples of convenience. These surveys may not reflect the habits of the population at large, and their development and implementation may be costly. Public health nutritionists may need to conduct surveys of the target population specific to the identified nutritional or health problem that exists in that group.

Public health nutritionists may collect data using the following acceptable parameters:

- Anthropometric or body measurements such as height, weight, body mass index, and head circumference. These measures indicate normal or abnormal growth patterns, under nutrition, overweight, or obesity.
- Biochemical tests most commonly used in public health programs include hemoglobin and/or hematocrit to measure iron nutriture, serum cholesterol, HDL, LDL, and triglycerides to assess cardiovascular disease or blood glucose to screen for diabetes risk and hemoglobin A1C to measure diabetes control.
- Clinical or physical examination for observable signs and symptoms of severe malnutrition as abnormalities of the skin, hair, mouth, eyes, or face.
- Measuring standards for nutrient intake may be completed by the nutrient analysis of dietary intake. This may be obtained by interview, self-administered written questionnaires, a 24-hour or usual day's food intake, or quantified food frequency. These records can be quickly assessed and analyzed by using one of the computerized dietary analysis systems now available. The analysis will provide estimates of usual caloric intake and its distribution, as well as vitamin and mineral intake.
- Individual interviews can determine the economic, social, and environmental factors that influence the client's access to food and resources for food storage and preparation.[17]

For small populations the nutrition information may need to be collected, analyzed, and interpreted by the nutritionist using locally available resources to support the identified needs of the target population. Readily available data are: Nutrition status and nutrition-related health measurements (objective data)

- Overweight and obesity
- Anemia
- Serum cholesterol levels
- Lead screening
- Hypertension

Food and nutrient composition of diets (objective data)

- Intake of total fat, saturated fat, calories, vitamins, and minerals

Knowledge, attitudes, and behavior assessments (subjective data)

- Awareness of the benefits of breast-feeding
- Breast-feeding rates
- Physical activity patterns
- Perceptions of food and nutrition issues

Food composition and nutrition databases (objective data)

- Calorie and nutrient composition for foods, including new and brand-name foods

Food supply determinations (objective data)

- Amount of food available
- Nutrient availability
- Emergency food resources
- Food disappearance data
- Household food expenditures

The total (objective and subjective) data collection, analysis, and interpretation will lead to the needs of the target population; if these needs are perceived, real, or not important; what services are currently available; and the identification of the gaps in services that may or may not be addressing the problems.[18]

A new tool now available to collect a variety of data on populations is the geographic information system (GIS). This system clusters populations based on different demographic data from census records, grocery store purchases, and other resources. The data is processed into color-coded maps to be interpreted. Information about food purchases and products can be programmed to provide information on food behaviors. GIS can provide information on the "healthiness of a neighborhood's food environment." In studies done in the state of Washington, GIS has been used to look at the food environment (what is and is not available), access to food, and relationship with food systems to assist in planning for the improvement in the nutrition status of a population.[19]

To learn about GIS, visit: www.cdc.gov/reproductivehealth/gisatlas/, www.geo data. gov, www.goe-one-stop.gov, or www.tdh.state.tx.us/library/gis.htm.

Another new method used in some areas is the photovoice. People who are the experts on local life use their photographs to raise questions about their communities. Questions such as "Why does this situation exist?" "What can we do about it?" and "How?" are typical. Using their own words and presenting their community's situations to policy makers allows this dialogue to advocate grassroot changes. It contributes to group discussion about community issues and assets. It is designed to reach policy makers and community leaders. Photovoice shows that images carry messages that can influence policy. Citizens can participate in advocating for healthful public policy in the areas where they live.[20]

Inventory Available Resources

Another major component of the community needs assessment is an inventory of existing nutrition and food services by other agencies in the community. This includes the following:

- Medical nutrition therapy (MNT) and basic nutrition education (individual or group) by private practice dietitians or employed by home health agencies or in health care facilities
- Health promotion with weight management, nutrition education, and exercise programs at worksites, senior centers, recreation centers, spas, gyms, outpatient clinics, or rehabilitation sites
- Food stamps, financial aid, emergency food or meals, supplemental foods, food pantries, and food banks that address food insecurity
- Housing and homeless shelters that offer meals and nutrition education
- Nutrition and consumer education and homemaking skills development offered by cooperative extension service
- Mass media nutrition education

An inventory catalogs community agencies to refer clients and respond to the public as needed. All health, human services, education, and voluntary programs that provide food and nutrition services in the community should be listed in this catalog or database. In many communities, this type of health and human services inventory is done by a voluntary agency such as United Way or a city or county government. A telephone number may be available to provide information and referrals to all types of services, agencies, and programs available in the geographical area. The services may range from those that provide basic needs such as emergency food and shelter to referral or information; and advocacy and outreach to specific counseling and treatment. For each service agency, the inventory and database should include the following:

- Name and address of the agency
- Services offered
- Number and types of clients who qualify for the services
- Fee or price of the services, if any
- Number and qualifications of staff employed (professional and paraprofessional)

- Client satisfaction with the services
- Were the program participants included in designing the programs?
- Geographical coverage of the program

The purpose of the inventory is to provide a concise listing of all services available to the varied populations in the community. This inventory also identifies services currently stretched to their capacity and those that may be underutilized. This provides insight into the gaps in availability of needed food assistance and nutrition services. By identifying and listing all food assistance and nutrition service providers in the community needs assessment, nutrition-related health problems and people suffering food insecurity can be detected and publicized. This information can be used to propose solutions to address service gaps.[21]

Establish the Problem List and Set the Priorities

The qualitative data information (perceived or felt need) when merged with the quantitative data (demographics, health statistic, and so on), as shown in Tables 3–3, 3–4, and 3–5, and GIS information—all these taken together display the nutrition problem list for the community. In small areas, the problem list specifying the nutrition and health risks may be community wide. In densely populated urban areas, it may be limited to a census tract, neighborhood, zip code area, ethnic, or age groups where high-risk populations are concentrated. Needs identified should be compared and contrasted with the capacity of existing health and social agencies to determine how the needs might be met or what additional resources may be required.

When several nutrition problems are identified in the assessment process, the question becomes "What health outcome is most important?" Limited resources for any program must be reviewed. The nutritionist should share the findings of the community nutrition needs assessment with other agencies, and the stakeholders in the community. Sharing information and resources can be the first step in building partnerships and coalitions. It can be cost-effective (others having knowledge of funding), prevents duplication of efforts, and promotes cooperation and coordination among agencies and stakeholders.

The community assessment guides and justifies rational choices. It provides the objective and subjective information required to use limited resources to address the most urgent needs of the people who live and work in the community. There is no single ranking method to use to determine which identified nutritional need should be selected over another.[22] The following can provide guidance to rank priorities:

- Community priorities, preferences, and concerns should be given priority.
- Higher priority should be given to common problems than to rare ones.
- Higher priority should be given to serious problems than to less serious ones.
- The health problems of mothers and children that can easily be prevented should have a higher priority than those that are more difficult to prevent.

- Higher priority should be given to the health problems whose frequencies are increasing over time than to those whose frequencies are declining or remaining static.
- There should be research evidence on which to base population prevention interventions.

POINTS TO PONDER

- What criteria should be considered in selecting one of the available health improvement planning models?
- What methods could be used to involve the stakeholders in assessing nutrition, health, and food security issues in their community?
- Consider what strategies the public health nutritionist may need to explore to convince stakeholders in the target population of the implication of the obesity epidemic when they view overweight and obesity as a usual attribute to their population.
- How can public health nutritionists make the most effective use of new tools, such as GIS and photovoice, in their community needs assessment?

HELPFUL WEB SITES

American Public Health Association: www.apha.org
Association of State and Territorial Health Officials: www.astho.org
Census Bureau: www.census.gov
CDC: www.cdc.gov
FedStats: www.fedstats.gov
Geospatial One Stop: www.geodata.gov
Healthfinder: www.healthfinder.gov
National Agricultural Statistics Services: www.usda.gov/nass
National Voice for Local Public Health: www.naccho.org
Texas Department of Health: www.tdh.state.tx.us

NOTES

1. Institute of Medicine. *The Future of the Public Health in the 21st Century.* Washington, DC: National Academies Press; 2003:32.

2. Kaufman M. *Nutrition in Public Health: A Handbook for Developing Programs and Services.* Rockville, Md: Aspen Publishers; 1990:46.

3. US Department of Health and Human Services. *Healthy People 2010,* 2nd ed. McLean, Va: International Medical Publishing Inc; 2002:23–16.

4. http://www.cdc.gov/nccdphp/patch/index.htm. Accessed April 18, 2004.

5. http://www.apha.org/ppp/msmain.htm. Accessed February 25, 2005.

6. http://www.apha.org/ppp/science/theguide.htm, Accessed February 25, 2005.

7. Turnock BJ. *Public Health: What It Is and How It Works.* Gaithersburg, Md: Aspen Publishers; 2001:322.

8. http://www.archiev.naccho.org/documents/MAPP_field_guide2.pdf 2. Accessed February 25, 2005.

9. http://www.healthypeople.gov/state/toolkit/. Accessed February 25, 2005.

10. Kaufman M. *Nutrition in Public Health: A Handbook for Developing Programs and Services.* Rockville, Md: Aspen Publishers; 1990:46.

11. US DHHS. The Surgeon General's call to action to prevent and decrease overweight and obesity. US DHHS, PHS, Office of the Surgeon General, 2001. Available at: http://www.surgeongeneral.govtopics/obesity. Accessed February 25, 2005.

12. Kaufman M. *Nutrition in Public Health: A Handbook for Developing Programs and Services.* Rockville, Md: Aspen Publishers; 1990:47.

13. Kaufman M. *Nutrition in Public Health: A Handbook for Developing Programs and Services.* Rockville, Md: Aspen Publishers; 1990:48–49.

14. Kaufman M. *Nutrition in Public Health: A Handbook for Developing Programs and Services.* Rockville, Md: Aspen Publishers; 1990:50–51.

15. Kaufman M. *Nutrition in Public Health: A Handbook for Developing Programs and Services.* Rockville, Md: Aspen Publishers; 1990:51.

16. Kaufman M. *Nutrition in Public Health: A Handbook for Developing Programs and Services.* Rockville, Md: Aspen Publishers; 1990:55.

17. Kaufman M. *Nutrition in Public Health: A Handbook for Developing Programs and Services.* Rockville, Md: Aspen Publishers; 1990:56–58.

18. Probert K, ed. Moving to the Future: Developing Community-Based Nutrition Services. Washington, DC: Association of State and Territorial Public Health Nutrition Program Directors; 1996:15.

19. Brown D. Mapping the future of dietetics with geographic information systems. *JADA.* 2004;105:727–728.

20. Wang CC, Morrel-Samuels S, Hutchison PM, Bell L, Pestronk M. Flint photovoice: community building among youths, adults and policymakers. *AJPH.* 2004;94: 911–913.

21. Kaufman M. *Nutrition in Public Health: A Handbook for Developing Programs and Services.* Rockville, Md: Aspen Publishers; 1990:58–59.

22. Kaufman M. *Nutrition in Public Health: A Handbook for Developing Programs and Services.* Rockville, Md: Aspen Publishers; 1990:59–61.

BIBLIOGRAPHY

Boyle MA. *Community Nutrition in Action: An Entrepreneurial Approach.* 3rd ed. Belmont, Calif: Thomson-Wadsworth; 2003.

Lee RD, Nieman DC. *Nutritional Assessment*. Madison, Wis: Wm. C. Brown Communications; 1993.

Owen AL, Splett PL, Owen GM. *Nutrition in the Community: The Art and Science of Delivering Services*. 4th ed. Boston, Mass: McGraw-Hill Inc; 1999.

Scutchfield FD, Keck CW. *Principles of Public Health Practice*. Albany, NY: Delmar Publishers; 1997.

CHAPTER 4

Seek the Vulnerable

Lynn Parker

Reader Objectives

- Understand the ways poverty affects an individual's or family's ability to obtain a nutritionally adequate and healthful diet.
- Discuss food insecurity, how it is measured, whom it affects, and its potential consequences.
- Know the basic food and nutrition assistance programs available to vulnerable households, who is eligible, how to apply, and the benefits.
- Understand the role that entitlement status and national nutrition standards play in food assistance programs.
- Suggest ways that public health nutritionists can participate in developing local, state, and national nutrition policies to promote the health and food security of vulnerable individuals and families.

IDENTIFY THE NUTRITIONALLY VULNERABLE

Public health nutritionists are often in the position to seek out and help the most nutritionally vulnerable people in the nation—those with the lowest incomes. Nutritionists frequently encounter individuals or groups of people who must live on very limited amounts of money, incomes so low one might wonder how these households manage to survive in this age when incomes do not keep pace with living costs.

When providing nutrition education and medical nutrition therapy, nutritionists must be sensitive to the extent to which a family's food budget may be limited. Budget, time, and family pressures work against attaining the nutritious foods, healthful diets, and active lives among individuals and families who face special educational, language, and legal barriers. Understanding these paranutritional issues can make public health nutritionists more empathetic, supportive, and effective.

Inability to purchase or obtain enough food can be an invisible problem that makes many families feel ashamed. Many more affluent Americans walk down the street beside a hungry family, stand behind them in a food market checkout line, or sit next to them on a bus and do not know that they are hungry. Low-income neighborhoods often are segregated from more affluent neighborhoods and are less likely to be located in the places where medium or high-income people work and carry on their daily activities. Many people in the United States grow up unaware of the economic deprivation that others in their own city or county suffer.

What Does it Mean to be Low Income?

Low income places individuals and families at risk. It negatively influences their health and places barriers to achieving the optimum quality of life that is possible in the United States. Nutritionists who understand these barriers can be more effective in reaching the vulnerable and helping them to take the fullest advantage of the food assistance and nutrition programs for which most low-income families are eligible.

According to census information, the poverty level in 2003 was $18,810 for a family of four. For current DHHS Poverty Guidelines go to www.aspc.hhs.gov/poverty. The poverty level index, developed in the 1960s, was originally based on the cost of purchasing a very low-cost diet multiplied by three because the cost of food made up one third of household budgets at that time.[1] It has increased since then based on the escalating cost of living. An estimated 12.5% of individuals in the United States live on incomes at or below the poverty level. This translates into 23 million poor adults and 12.9 million poor children—10.7% of the adults in the United States and 17.6% of the children. After steadily decreasing from 1993 to 2000, poverty rates have increased from 9.6% of households in 2000 to 10.8% in 2003.[2] Poverty is especially hard on households headed by single mothers with children (28%), African-American households (24.4%), and Hispanic households (22.5%).[3]

Poverty and food adequacy have a special relationship. Food purchases, although a vital requirement for survival, are unlike other basic need purchases a family makes. Food purchases can be elastic to match the money available to the household. Most families cannot negotiate with landlords on what they pay for rent, with bus drivers on the fare, with gas stations on the price for gas, or with child care providers on the cost of day care. However, the quality and quantity of food in a household can be reduced in order to pay bills that keep a roof over a family's head, ensure transportation to work, and cover the cost of a safe place to leave young children while their parents are at work.

Jobs

The 2004 rate of unemployment was 5.4%,[4] and underemployment affects 10.7% of the workforce.[5] Although there is a reported downward trend in unemployment, many new jobs are entry-level service jobs with low salaries and limited or no benefits such as health insurance, vacation or sick pay, or disability payments. In the United States, 24.2% of low-income households (households with less than $25,000 annual income) do not have health insurance.[6] This strains family budgets in times of medical emergencies and can reduce opportunities for prevention, screening, diagnosis, and early treatment of health problems. Many individuals and families without adequate assistance to pay medical costs must choose between buying prescription medications or sufficient nutritious foods.

The current federal minimum wage of $5.15 per hour translates into $10,300 per year for a full-time worker.[7] This amount of money will not lift a family above the poverty line, making pressures on the food budget even greater. This financial situation often leads low-income wage earners to take on more than one job at a time; this can be physically draining, increase job-related expenses, and limit time to deal with important family issues.

Jobs that pay low wages, besides not providing the usual benefits associated with higher paying jobs, also are not likely to allow employees to take time off for necessary appointments or emergencies. When nutrition program agency hours do not coincide with times individuals are not working, the opportunities to take advantage of program benefits is significantly reduced.

There are added expenses involved with many low-paying jobs. To travel to work, buses are cheaper than cars, but public transportation does not go everywhere and usually takes longer. Public transportation also cannot be relied on for family needs and emergencies during work hours. Cars are expensive to buy, maintain, insure, and fuel. Older cars become less dependable, especially if households must scrimp on maintenance.

When parents are employed, child care is necessary. No-cost child care by family members is not a choice for many because families are often far away from their relatives or other family members are working. Family child care and child care centers offering low-cost or no-cost care are difficult to find. Quality day care that parents can feel good about is still an elusive goal for many, especially for families with low wages.

Housing

Homelessness affects 6.3% of poor people in the United States and represents between 2.3 and 3.5 million adults and children.[8] Without a stable home, it is difficult for homeless families to ensure nutritious foods on a routine basis. Low-income families living in substandard housing may risk food spoilage or loss due to pest infestations and inadequate food preparation and storage facilities. Currently, 14.3 million U.S. households spend more than 50% of their incomes on housing. Three quarters of these families are poor. Another 17.3 million households spend 30% to 50% of their income on housing.[9] Housing costs can account for a large portion of a poor family's budget. High utility costs force many low-income households to choose between spending limited funds on heat or food.

Education

Almost 40% of low-income adults have less than a high school education, compared to 18% of adults with incomes above the poverty line.[10] This may affect their ability to use recipes or read and understand food labels. It reduces their access to educational materials about nutrition, disease prevention, and federal food and nutrition assistance programs. Program application forms may be difficult for them to complete.

Many low-income households have members who understand and speak little to no English. Reaching them may require the help of interpreters or bilingual community health workers. Ensuring that they obtain the food assistance and nutrition program services they need may require some extra effort by nutritionists.

Citizenship Status

Immigrants, legal or undocumented, are reluctant to visit public clinics or government-funded nutrition programs. Many fear that they are ineligible. Others fear that their participation will count against their continued presence in the United States, or that they will be detained by legal authorities regarding citizenship status even if they are legal aliens. Legal aliens are noncitizens with appropriate documents showing their presence in the United States is legal. Some public assistance programs, but not nutrition programs, count as a public charge and work against a person's continued legal presence in the United States. These families may have suffered from severe undernutrition and hunger in their home countries, placing them at greater future risk for health and nutrition problems.

Time

Many families today complain that they do not have enough time to do everything they need and want to do. Low-income parents, especially single parents, often face especially challenging time pressures. When adults work long hours, work more than one job, and face long commutes, time and energy are in short supply. To prepare meals, single mothers must purchase, prepare, serve, and clean up after working long hours. They often must leave their neighborhoods to shop at lower cost, higher-quality supermarkets. This takes a significant amount of time and energy, while tired, hungry young children beg for food and attention. Time for homework and play must be scheduled, plus all the other daily responsibilities to maintain an ordered and positive family life. It is a very challenging life for those seeking to raise happy, healthy children and provide them with nutritious meals and an opportunity for physically active play.

These realities of poverty translate into a difficult environment to achieve sufficient and healthy family meals.

HUNGER IN THE UNITED STATES

In 1967, the Field Foundation funded a group of physicians to travel to the poorest sections of the United States to document the health and living conditions of children from poor families. A personal communication from R. Rosso described to the Food Research and Action Center these physicians report to Congress: "Wherever we went and wherever we looked, whether it was the rural south, Appalachia, or an urban ghetto, we saw children in significant numbers who were hungry and sick, children for whom hunger was a daily fact of life and sickness in many forms, an inevitability. The children we saw were more than just malnourished. They were hungry, weak, apathetic. Their lives are being shortened. They are visibly and predictably losing their health, their energy, their spirits. They are suffering from hunger and disease, and directly or indirectly, they are dying from them—which is exactly what 'starvation' means." These physicians were shocked to find nutritional deficiency diseases among the families they visited that they only would have expected to see in developing nations.

Responding to these reports and many other reports and studies at the time, Congress expanded the Food Stamp Program and the National School Lunch Program to assure that children from low-income families received free or reduced price meals. They legislated new programs: the School Breakfast Program; programs to feed school children during the summer (Summer Food Service Program) and preschool children in child care settings (Child and Adult Care Food Program); and the Special Supplemental Nutrition Program for Women, Infants, and Children (WIC) (see Chapter 8).

Ten years later, in 1977, the Field Foundation sent the medical team to visit the same low-income areas of the country. After these visits, they reported to the Congress: "Our first and overwhelming impression was that there are far fewer grossly malnourished people in this country today than there were 10 years ago. Malnutrition has become a subtler problem. In the Mississippi Delta, in the coal fields of Appalachia and in coastal South Carolina—where visitors 10 years ago could quickly see large numbers of stunted, apathetic children with swollen stomachs and the dull eyes and poorly healing wounds characteristic of malnutrition—such children are not seen in such numbers. Even in areas which did not command national attention 10 years ago, many poor people have food and look better off. This change does not appear to be due to an overall improvement in living standards or to a decrease in joblessness in those areas. In fact, the facts of life for Americans living in poverty remain as dark or darker than they were 10 years ago. But in the area of food, there is a difference. The Food Stamp Program, the nutritional component of Head Start, school lunch and breakfast programs, and to a lesser extent, (i.e., the program did not expand broadly until after 1974 because the funds were impounded until then by the federal government), the Women, Infant, Children (WIC) feeding programs have made the difference."[11]

Since 1977, food and nutrition assistance programs have expanded significantly. After-school snacks and suppers have been added in some communities, as well as emergency food programs that supply commodities to food banks for use by food pantries and soup kitchens. These programs still are not reaching everyone in need, but they have grown over the years and have continued to make a positive difference in the lives of low-income people.

Today, hunger looks different than it did in 1967. Because of food and nutrition assistance programs, physicians and nutritionists rarely see severe nutritional deficiency diseases. However, food insufficiency due to limited income is still present in the United States. It shows itself in lower-quality diets resulting from limited resources for food, households reducing the quantity of food consumed or skipping meals because of lack of money, children not eating enough or adults not eating at all, and people losing weight involuntarily due to lack of food. It translates into concerns that food will run out before resources can be found to purchase more.

The inability to consistently meet basic food needs because of lack of financial or other resources is now known as *food insecurity*. This term refers to the hunger now seen in the United States—chronic, intermittent food insufficiency due to lack of resources. This definition moves away from hunger that is measured clinically with blood values for nutrients and measurements of height and weight. It relies on self-reported feelings, household situations, and coping strategies employed to stave off hunger pangs among both adults and children in the household.

On an annual basis since 1995, the U.S. Bureau of Census and the U.S. Department of Agriculture (USDA) have conducted a nationally representative survey of food insecurity as part of the Census Bureau's Current Population Survey (CPS). The survey results are derived from a core module of questions asking about each household's food security status. According to USDA's most recent report, 11.1% of households in the United States were food insecure at some time in 2002, an increase from 10.7% in 2001.[12] The surveys show the characteristics that place households at greatest risk of food insecurity:

- Incomes below the poverty line
- Households with children, especially those headed by a single woman
- African-American and Hispanic households
- Households in central cities or rural areas, and those living in the South and Southwest.[13]

The developers of the scale used to distinguish food-insecure households from food-secure households, using the module of questions in the CPS, found that food insecurity was a process that was managed by a household: "In this process, households first note serious inadequacy in their food supply, feel anxiety about the sufficiency of their food to meet basic need, and make adjustments to their food budget and food served. As the situation becomes more severe, adults reduce their food intake and experience hunger, but they spare their children this experience. In the third stage, children also suffer reduced food intake and hunger, and adults' reductions in food intake are more dramatic."[14]

Researchers are discovering that food insecurity has negative consequences for individuals. Children from food-insecure households have trouble learning and are more likely to become ill. There appear to be negative mental health consequences for both adults and children who reside in food-insecure households. Food insecurity has been shown to be associated with inadequate dietary intakes of some nutrients.

HUNGER AND OBESITY

Food insecurity also has been shown in national and state survey data and a study in rural New York State to be associated with obesity among low-income women.[15,16,17] Researchers believe this counterintuitive consequence may result from the way low-income women cope with inadequate resources for food in order to ensure that their families do not feel hungry.[18]

Hunger and obesity appear to be paradoxical phenomena that exist in many low-income households. Low-income households face many of the same challenges as more affluent households in the prevention of obesity—the American sedentary lifestyle, the ubiquity of low-cost but high-calorie foods, and the impact of food advertising campaigns. The poor face another layer of unique obesity precursors, including less opportunities for physical activity, the lack of safe places for children to play after school and during the summer months, inaccessibility to high-volume, lower-cost food markets with a good quality and variety of fruits and vegetables, and the inadequacy or lack of affordable preventive health care. These families face the most severe limitations on their food budgets during the last one or two weeks of every month. When resources are limited, families first cut quality and next quantity. Adults take the brunt of the inadequacy until forced by economic circumstances to cut quality and then quantity of foods for children as well.

To address the national obesity problem, policy makers must understand the real-life circumstances of low-income households and the continuing importance of nutrition programs to fill food budget gaps. Nutrition programs can be part of the solution to preventing obesity. Recent research on low-income food insecure girls in elementary school showed they were less likely to be overweight when they participated in the Food Stamp Program, the School Breakfast Program, the School Lunch Program, or any combination of these programs.[19]

FEDERALLY FUNDED FOOD ASSISTANCE AND NUTRITION PROGRAMS

One of the most direct solutions to food insecurity is to ensure that households and individuals take full advantage of the food assistance and nutrition programs for which they are eligible, including the Food Stamp Program, the WIC Program (see Chapter 8), the School Breakfast and Lunch Programs, the Summer Food Service Program, and the Child and Adult Care Food Program.

Public health nutritionists need to understand two vital concepts that underlie the food assistance and nutrition programs: entitlement and nutrition standards. All of these programs operated under the auspices of the U.S. Department of Agriculture are entitlement programs, except WIC. Entitlement means that all schools and eligible sponsors, including all children in their care, can participate in these programs. There are no limits in the number that can participate—all who are eligible and desire to participate can. In the case of the Food Stamp Program, this means that all eligible families can participate in the program if they wish. As the population in need of nutrition programs increases, federal funding for these programs must increase, by law, to meet the need and allow the participation of all those eligible and wishing to participate. During times of economic downturn, this has ensured that there is a national safety net that acts as a food security floor. WIC is a discretionary program and its funding does not automatically grow with need, but rather must go through a special congressional approval process every year.

National nutrition standards are also a key component of all of these programs. These standards ensure that benefits reflect the consensus on good nutrition. The standards protect funding because reductions in funding for these programs would make it difficult to meet the prescribed nutrition guidelines. They also ensure that a child in New England or the Southeast or the West has the same access to the basics of good nutrition.

Because nutrition programs have the potential for improving health and well-being, public health nutritionists who work with vulnerable individuals and families must know these programs and encourage and help all who need these benefits to participate.

Food Stamp Program

The Food Stamp Program provides monthly funding to qualifying low-income households to purchase food. The program has a significant positive effect on overall dietary quality for those who participate. According to a USDA analysis of national food consumption data, for each dollar in food stamps that a household receives, the household's Healthy Eating Index score (an indicator of overall dietary quality) goes up—the higher the level of food stamps, the greater the positive nutritional effect.[20] An analysis of the same national food consumption data showed that participation in the Food Stamp Program has a significant, positive impact on intakes of iron, vitamin A, thiamin, niacin, and zinc among children 1 to 4 years of age.[21]

The Food Stamp Program operates through state and local social service departments and provided funds for food to 24 million people in 2004.[22] According to the most recent analysis available, the program is only reaching a little over half of the people who are eligible, 54% in 2002.[23] Individuals apply as members of a household. They fill out an application, have an interview with a food stamp employee, and provide some documentation of selected information on the application. To be eligible for food stamps, a household must have a gross income below 130% of the poverty level (about $24,000 for a family of four), and a net income after deductions below the poverty line. Also, any property owned cannot be worth more than the food stamp resource limit. If anyone in a household is receiving benefits funded by a state's public assistance program for families and/or SSI, the household is automatically eligible to participate in the Food Stamp Program. Households that receive food stamps have to comply with the Food Stamp Program's work requirements, although there are exemptions in certain circumstances such as a mother caring for a very young child or being pregnant.[24]

The food stamp office must provide food stamp benefits to an eligible household within 30 calendar days from the date of application. However, when an eligible household has very little income, benefits must be received within seven calendar days of the application date. This is called *expedited service*.

When determined eligible, households now receive an electronic card similar to a bank debit card. The card can be used to purchase foods in stores approved to take food stamps. The value of the food stamps a household receives depends largely on the household's income after housing, medical, and child care costs are taken into account. At a maximum, a household with four people receives up to $499 per month. Because benefits go down as income rises, average benefits are about 90 cents per person per meal. Only 24.4% of food stamp households actually receive the full food stamp allotment for their family size.[25]

Because almost all people with low incomes and limited resources are eligible for food stamps, low-income clients should be encouraged to apply for the Food Stamp Program. Reasons that eligible households do not apply often include lack of information or misconceptions about eligibility or how to apply or concerns about how they will be treated at the food stamp office. It is important for potential clients to know that they do not have to be on public assistance to be eligible for food stamps. Many people who have low wages are eligible for food stamps. Some college students and noncitizens can get food stamp benefits. Homeless people are eligible for food stamps as well. Many local organizations offer to screen potential food stamp applicants to give them a sense of whether they are eligible, to make them more comfortable with the process, and to ease the application process by reviewing it and letting them know the types of documentation they require.

Public health nutritionists must know the special rules that cover immigrant families. Although undocumented immigrants cannot receive food stamps for themselves, all citizen children residing with them are eligible. Many legal immigrants are eligible: all refugees and asylees, all legal immigrant adults who have been in the United States for five or more years, and all legal immigrant children ages 18 and under, regardless of date of entry. Language barriers, welfare reform legislation that changed the rules about eligibility and sponsor liability, and fears that food stamp benefits could be counted against families as a public charge have combined to dampen immigrant food stamp participation rates. Fortunately, USDA rules make clear that the Food Stamp Program does not count as a public charge program.

Special Supplemental Nutrition Program for Women, Infants, and Children

Because the Special Supplemental Food Program for Women, Infants, and Children (WIC) has played an enormous role in the public health nutrition system, most public health nutritionists are familiar with the program and encourage pregnant and breast-feeding mothers to apply for themselves and/or their young children. Many women in need or whose children are in need may not think they are eligible and should be encouraged to apply for program benefits.

Family income for WIC eligibility is 185% of the poverty level and significantly higher than that for the Food Stamp Program. There are no limits on assets as there are in the Food Stamp Program. Immigrant status does not affect eligibility. The WIC program does not make an immigrant a public charge. Some immigrant clients are wary of participating in WIC regardless of their legal status. These concerns should not keep families away from a program that has demonstrated such a difference in the health of women, infants, and children. All women, infants, and children who are eligible for the program due to low income and nutritional risk may participate.

Since its inception in 1974, WIC has been the most studied nutrition program. Numerous studies affirm its positive impact on pregnancy outcomes, anemia prevalence, growth of young children, and dietary intake of mothers and children. New research indicates that WIC helps to prevent young children from becoming overweight.[26] The combination of WIC's nutritious supplemental food package, nutrition education provided to mothers (including breast-feeding support), referrals to health care, and its impact on getting pregnant women into early prenatal care add up to a package of services that has been shown to save $1.92 to $4.21 in health care expenses for every WIC dollar spent.[27]

Although administered by the U.S. Department of Agriculture, WIC is operated at the state and local levels through public health agencies. Eligible individuals must be a pregnant or postpartum woman, infant or child under 5 years of age; low-income; and nutritionally at risk and certified by a health professional to have problems such as inadequate weight gain during pregnancy, growth problems in infants and children, or inadequate dietary patterns. In 2004, WIC served 7.85 million women, infants, and children each month.[28]

Eligible individuals receive a WIC food package that consists of a packet of vouchers or an electronic card to use at a store to purchase specific nutrient-dense foods. The contents of the food package are chosen to supplement the diets of women, infants, or young children, providing them with foods rich in the nutrients that they are likely to be lacking. Currently, the food packages have a national average value of $38 per month, which can be an incentive to attract low-income mothers to health clinics for prenatal and well-baby care.[29] (See Chapter 8 for additional information on WIC.)

Child Nutrition Programs

School breakfast and lunch programs, the Summer Food Service Program, and the Child and Adult Care Food Program are administered by the U.S. Department of Agriculture. These programs provide reimbursements to schools and other sponsors to pay for children's meals and snacks and are governed by nutrition standards. Their standards delineate the kinds and quantities of food that must be served to meet children's daily nutrition requirements and to be reimbursable.

These programs have been shown to make a difference in children's dietary patterns, as well as their ability to learn. Children who participate in school lunch and breakfast programs consume more fruits, vegetables, and milk and less sweetened beverages.[30] School breakfast has been shown to improve children's academic achievement.[31] USDA evaluations of the Summer Food Service Program demonstrate that children receive one third or more of their daily nutritional needs from Summer Food Program lunches, and that 95% of summer food programs have activities for children associated with the food program.[32] The Child and Adult Care Food Program improves the nutritional value and healthfulness of meals served to preschoolers and may reduce rates of illness.[33]

Recent innovations should further improve the nutrition benefits provided by these programs. As part of the reauthorization of the child nutrition programs by Congress in 2004, all school districts offering these programs are now required to develop wellness policies. These policies cover the type and level of nutrition education and physical education that must be provided to students. Rules govern the sale and offering of foods in the school during the school day. These policies must be in place by the beginning of school year 2006–2007. The law also requires that district stakeholders be involved in the process of reviewing and developing these policies. Stakeholders include parents, students, and representatives of the school food authority, the school board, school administrators, and the public. Public health nutritionists have the opportunity to shape school nutrition policies and help school officials by offering their nutrition expertise.

Another important child nutrition program development is a USDA-administered voluntary gold and silver certification program. This provides incentives of special certification to schools meeting specific standards that promote a positive nutrition environment for children. The standards include:

- Provision of nutrition education
- Frequent serving of fresh fruits, vegetables, and whole grains
- Opportunities for physical activity
- Nutrition-related limitations on foods sold in competition with the school breakfast and lunch programs

Schools aspiring to this designation must apply to the state education agency and show evidence that they meet the standards. Public health nutritionists can make schools aware of this program and help them to meet the standards.

Small farmers have also become involved in improving the nutritional quality and attractiveness of school meals. Many schools have set up procurement relationships with local farmers to ensure a steady supply of local fresh produce for their nutrition programs. Schools report that students like fresh produce. The use of local products can be used to plan lessons on where food comes from and how it is grown.

A fresh fruit and vegetable pilot program in selected schools in each of eight states and three Indian reservations provides school children with fresh fruits and vegetables every school day. Special emphasis is to serve children in low-income areas. These fruits and vegetables are offered during times of the day when nutrition programs are not available.

Low-income parents who have difficulty purchasing enough nutritious food for their families should be encouraged to take advantage of the child nutrition programs. Assisting them to apply could make the difference between adequate and inadequate diets for these families.

School Lunch

Almost all schools in the United States participate in the federal School Lunch Program, and every child in each of these schools is eligible to participate in the program. Children can receive free meals if their family incomes are below 130% of the poverty level for their family size, or children can receive reduced price meals (only up to $.40 in cost) if family incomes are 185% of the poverty level. Children whose family incomes are higher than 185% are charged more for the lunch, a cost set by the school. The school is reimbursed by the U.S. Department of Agriculture through the state education agency for all meals at varying rates, even those purchased by students not from low-income families. The school also receives a certain amount of commodities for each lunch served.

Students receive an application for free and reduced-price meals at the beginning of the school year. Recent changes in the law allow a family to complete one application with all their children listed, rather than completing multiple applications. The school informs the family about whether their children are eligible for free or reduced-price meals. If families enter a school later in the year or become eligible for free or reduced-price meals later in the year, they can ask the school to provide them with an application. Three percent of applications are verified every year by the school to ensure that families are actually eligible. If a family's application is chosen for verification, they will receive a notice from the school asking for information they need to supply to confirm their child's eligibility for free or reduced-price meals.

Families who participate in the Food Stamp Program or public assistance programs need only write their case number on the school lunch application. Participation in these programs makes children automatically eligible for free school meals. Many schools are working with local food stamp offices on direct certification. Where direct certification is used, households participating in the Food Stamp Program are notified that their children are automatically eligible for free school meals without having to apply for the program.

To ensure that poor children are not singled out or feel stigmatized in the lunchroom, schools are required to implement measures that do not distinguish free or reduced-price meal participants from those who pay the *full* price. Schools use punch cards or PIN numbers rather than exchanging cash on the lunch line.

School Breakfast

The School Breakfast Program is offered in over three fourths of the schools that have a lunch program. When children apply for free and reduced-price meals, they are also applying for the School Breakfast Program. The same rules about not sin-gling out children in the lunch program also apply to the breakfast program. Because breakfast program expansion traditionally has been targeted to low-income neighborhoods, over 80% of children eating a school breakfast receive free and reduced-price meals.[34] This is starting to change, however, as more parents work, and work hours and commutes to work become longer. With increasing awareness of the positive role eating breakfast in the morning has in improving children's ability to learn and do well on tests, many schools are marketing the breakfast program to all families, regardless of income. Some schools are institut-ing *universal* breakfast programs where breakfast is free of charge to all children.

Summer Food Service Program

When school closes for the summer, poor families who depend on school meals during the school year face the prospect of having to stretch their limited food budgets even further for the summer months. America's Second Harvest, a national network of food banks, reports that their members see an increase in fam-ilies with children during the summer months.[35,36,37] They attribute this increase to the lack of availability of school meals. In addition, parents must find affordable, dependable care for their children during the summer so that they will be safe, have fun, and continue to learn and be physically active. The Summer Food Service Program plays an important role in fulfilling that need. This program pro-vides reimbursements for meals and snacks to schools, parks and recreation departments, and nonprofit community-based sponsors (e.g., YMCA's, churches, Boys and Girls Clubs, Kid Cafes) who serve children during the summer. To oper-ate the Summer Food Service Program, schools and sponsors must serve neigh-borhoods that are largely low income. At least 50% percent of the children must be eligible for a combination of both free and reduced-price meals. All children attending the sites, regardless of family income, receive free meals and/or snacks.

State education agencies can provide information about where the summer food sites will be and what summer recreation and education programs they offer. Public health nutritionists can provide a list of sites and should encourage their clients to seek out these programs during the summer months. They can visit some of the sites and may be able to offer future training for sponsors on improving food quality or provide assistance with planning summer curricula and activities.

Child and Adult Care Food Program

More and more families are depending on family child care homes and child care centers to care for and feed their young children while they are at work. A substantial number of the meals and snacks consumed by very young children are provided by child care providers. The Child and Adult Care Food Program (CACFP) reimburses for nutritious meals and snacks offered in a number of different settings: preschool family child care and child care centers, including Head Start; after school programs; homeless, domestic violence, and youth runaway shelters; and day care programs for adults (usually the elderly) who cannot take care of themselves during the day while their families work.

Although administered by the U.S. Department of Agriculture, CACFP is managed by a state's department of education or other state agency. At the local level, the program is operated by child care centers, Head Start programs, and organizations called *sponsors* who work with family child care homes. A family child care home is a child care program that takes place in a provider's home. Sponsors are nonprofit organizations that recruit, train, monitor, and support family child care homes for CACFP. Like the school lunch, breakfast, and summer food programs, eligible homes and centers must be allowed to participate in CACFP, and all children in their care must be served.

Immigrant status does not affect a family's eligibility. Participation in CACFP does not count as a public charge. In CACFP, families do not pay directly for meals, but centers and homes receive higher levels of reimbursement for serving low-income children. CACFP reimbursements and technical assistance can mean the difference between children receiving high-fat foods and carbonated beverages versus meals that include nutritious fruits, vegetables, and milk.

CACFP also pays for after-school snacks in low-income areas where over 50% percent of children are eligible for free and reduced-price meals. After-school suppers are available in low-income neighborhoods in seven states—Delaware, Illinois, Michigan, Missouri, New York, Oregon, and Pennsylvania. All eligible sites and the children they serve may participate in these programs.

CACFP also provides reimbursements for meals and snacks served to low-income children up to 18 years of age living in homeless shelters, domestic violence shelters, and shelters for runaway youth. These reimbursements, and the nutrition standards required by the program, can make a significant difference in the nutritional quality of the meals served and allow shelter funds to be used for other important services. Many shelter providers are unaware of the availability of these benefits, and public health nutritionists can provide information about CACFP to them.

Emergency Food Programs

Many public health nutritionists know about food pantries and soup kitchens in their communities. These programs are operated by private nonprofit groups often associated with faith-based organizations. Emergency food sites offer grocery bags or meals a certain number of times per month for emergency needs and to supplement inadequate food budgets. Sometimes they require some type of identification and proof that the individuals seeking their services meet the agency's eligibility guidelines or have been referred by a social service agency. Public health nutritionists should maintain lists of local pantries and soup kitchens and their guidelines to assist families in emergencies.

A unique emergency food provider of special interest to public health nutritionists is Boston Medical Center's Grow Clinic that serves children suffering from failure to thrive. This clinic has an onsite food pantry to help families with emergency food needs and also assists families to determine their eligibility for federal nutrition programs and how to apply.

ASSIST THE VULNERABLE THROUGH PUBLIC POLICY

Public health nutritionists have the challenging opportunity to help vulnerable clients improve their nutritional status, health, and food security. On an individual basis, they can diagnose food insecurity and assist clients to locate, apply for, and take advantage of the food assistance and nutrition programs available. On a policy level, public health nutritionists can use what they learn from clients and what they know about nutrition programs and food insecurity in their community to work to improve local, state, and national policies that help the nutritionally vulnerable in our nation.

Policy means to look beyond helping to solve the day-to-day, individual food and nutrition problems on a one-on-one basis, or in a group learning setting, and to think about what can be done to solve, or even prevent, nutrition problems on a broader scale, in ways that change the "system" and in ways that can improve the lives of many more people.

Usually policy, in one way or another, involves government at some level, because local, state, and national laws, regulations, policies, and guidelines keep current practices in place and often must be changed in order to institute new and better practices.

This author had a professor who had been a psychologist at a state mental hospital. He worked long and hard there to help and heal each one of his patients. He said that he felt that he was at the end of an assembly line that was delivering injured people to him, and his job was to do the best he could to put them back together. He yearned to get to the front of the assembly line, to stop the emotional injuries from happening in the first place. Getting to the front of the assembly line is "policy." Work in policy requires one to transcend the routine, the personal, and the individual, and take a bird's-eye view, at the world in which one is working. This viewpoint can help public health nutritionists advocate for changes that can improve many people's lives.

Public Health Nutritionists Can Improve the Lives of Low-Income Clients

Make your client's real needs the focus of your efforts. Often, professionals think about, and have to think about, issues from the perspective of how it will affect our agency or how it will affect our own convenience. Try thinking about issues from your low-income clients' perspective. What will make a positive difference for them? What is most important to them? Learn everything you can about the nutrition programs in your community. Visit some of the programs to see how they operate. Introduce yourself to the people who run them and alert them to your desire to refer your clients to them. Participate in community and state meetings about nutrition, hunger, and poverty to learn about the issues in your community, and meet some of the health and nutrition leaders. Your knowledge of these programs will not only help the individuals and families you work with, but they will also give you an understanding of how well the programs operate in your community. Knowing all the players in the nutrition program community in your area will place you in a position to be called on to speak about health and nutrition problems in your community and potential policy solutions. You will also place yourself in a position of potential leadership on important issues. Figure out how to be a policy leader within the constraints of your agency. Watch what others do and how they do it. Share ideas with those of similar mind in your agency. Learn the written and unwritten rules. Think about ways to engage in nutrition policy that involve your agency leadership and bring important resources or desired positive attention to what your agency does.

As an individual, and/or as a member of your professional organizations, learn about and meet your local, state, and national government officials and members of Congress and their staff members. Find out what they think about and what they do on issues related to nutrition programs and poverty. Let them know about the importance of nutrition programs to your clients. Follow legislative and regulatory developments, and learn the most effective times and ways to comment, give your ideas, or send messages of support for legislation. (See Chapters 5, 6, and 7)

POINTS TO PONDER

- What is the role, of the public health nutritionist in dealing with the problem of food insecurity?
- How can a local public health nutritionist become involved in policy issues affecting federal food assistance and nutrition programs for vulnerable people?
- How should a public health nutritionist respond to inquiries about the increasing rate of obesity among low-income women participating in food assistance and nutrition programs and whether or not such programs should change benefits to overweight and obese participants?

- What public policy initiatives or legislation could a public health nutrition-ist recommend to a member of Congress working to improve the health and nutrition of people with low incomes?

NOTES

1. De Navas-Walt C, Proctor BD, Mills RJ. *Current Population Reports, P60-226, Income, Poverty and Health Insurance Coverage in the United States: 2003.* Washington, DC: US Census Bureau; 2004.

2. Koerner BI. How the Feds define poverty: What's food got to do with it? *Slate.* Available at: http://slate.msn.com/id/21081341. Accessed October 13, 2004.

3. De Navas-Walt C, Proctor BD, Mills RJ. *Current Population Reports, P60-226, Income, Poverty and Health Insurance Coverage in the United States: 2003.* Washington, DC: US Census Bureau; 2004.

4. De Navas-Walt C, Proctor BD, Mills RJ. *Current Population Reports, P60-226, Income, Poverty and Health Insurance Coverage in the United States: 2003.* Washington, DC: US Census Bureau; 2004.

5. US Department of Labor. Bureau of Labor Statistics Web page. Available at: http://www.bls.gov. Accessed October 14, 2004.

6. Bernstein J, Michel L. *Labor Market Left Behind: Evidence Shows that Post-Recession Economy Has Not Turned into a Recovery for Workers.* Washington, DC: Economic Policy Institute; 2003.

7. De Navas-Walt C, Proctor BD, Mills RJ. *Current Population Reports, P60-226, Income, Poverty and Health Insurance Coverage in the United States: 2003.* Washington, DC: US Census Bureau; 2004.

8. Food Research and Action Center. *State of the States: 2005, A Profile of Food and Nutrition Programs Across the Nation.* Washington, DC: Food Research and Action Center; 2005.

9. Urban Institute. Millions still face homelessness in a booming economy. [press release]. Washington, DC: February 1, 2000. Available at: http://www.urban.org/urlprint.cfm?ID=6972. Accessed October 8, 2004.

10. Joint Center for Housing Studies of Harvard University. *The State of the Nation's Housing: 2003.* Cambridge, Mass: Graduate School of Design, John F. Kennedy School of Government; 2003.

11. Rosso R. Analysis of March 2004 Current Population Survey data, Food Research and Action Center. Washington, DC: personal communication; October 13, 2004.

12. Kotz N. *Hunger in America: The Federal Response.* New York, NY: The Field Foundation; 1979:8–9.

13. Kotz N. *Hunger in America: The Federal Response.* New York, NY: The Field Foundation; 1979:8–9.

14. Nord M, Andrews M, Carlson S. *Household Food Security in the United States, 2002.* Washington, DC: Economic Research Service/USDA; 2003.

15. Nord M, Andrews M, Carlson S. *Household Food Security in the United States, 2002.* Washington, DC: Economic Research Service/USDA; 2003.

16. Hamilton WL, Cook JT, Thompson WW, et al. *Household Food Security in the United States in 1995: Summary Report of the Food Security Measurement Project.* Alexandria, Va: Food and Consumer Services, USDA; 1997.

17. Townsend MS, Peerson J, Love B, Achterberg C, Murphy SP. Food insecurity is positively related to overweight in women. *J Nutr.* 2001;131:2880–2884.

18. Adams EJ, Grummer-Strawn L, Chavez G. Food insecurity is associated with increased obesity in California women. *J Nutr.* 2003;133:1070–1074.

19. Olson CM. Nutrition and health outcomes associated with food insecurity and hunger. *J Nutr.* 1999;131:521S–524S.

20. Olson C. The relationship between hunger and obesity: what do we know and what are the implications for public policy? [paper]. Washington, DC: Roundtable on Understanding the Paradox of Hunger and Obesity, Food Research and Action Center; November 2004.

21. Jones SJ, Jahns L, Lanaia BA, Haughton B. Lower risk of overweight in school-aged food insecure girls who participate in food assistance. *Arch Pediatr Adolesc Med.* 2003;157:780–784.

22. Basiotis PP, Kramer-LeBlanc CS, Kennedy ET. Maintaining nutrition security and diet quality: The role of the Food Stamp Program and WIC. *Fam Econ Nutr Rev.* 1998;11:4–16.

23. Cook JT, Sherman LP, Brown JL. *Impact of food stamps on the dietary adequacy of poor children.* Medford, Mass: Center on Hunger Poverty and Nutrition Policy, Tufts University, School of Nutrition; 1995.

24. US Department of Agriculture, Food and Nutrition Service. Food Stamp Program annual summary. Available at: http://www.fns.usda.gov/pd/fssummar.htm. Accessed August 12, 2005.

25. Cunnyngham K. *Trends in Food Stamp Program Participation Rates: 1999–2002,* Alexandria, Va: USDA Food and Nutrition Service, Office of Analysis, Nutrition, and Evaluation; 2004.

26. Parker L. A safety net for very young children. *The Nutrition of Very Young Children, Zero to Three.* 2000;21:29–36.

27. Cunnyngham K, Brown B. *Characteristics of Food Stamp Households: Fiscal Year 2003,* Alexandria, Va: USDA Food and Nutrition Service, Office of Analysis, Nutrition, and Evaluation; 2004.

28. Bitler MP, Currie J. *Medicaid at Birth, WIC Take Up, and Children's Outcomes,* Institute for Policy Research; 2004.

29. Mathematica Policy Research Inc. *The Savings in Medicaid Costs for Newborns and Their Mothers from Prenatal Participation in the WIC Program, Vol. 1.* Alexandria, Va: USDA Food and Nutrition Service, Office of Analysis, Nutrition, and Evaluation; 1990.

30. USDA Food and Nutrition Service. *Program and Information Report (Key Data) U.S. Summary, FY 2004-FY2005.* Alexandria, Va: USDA Food and Nutrition Service; 2005.

31. USDA Food and Nutrition Service. *Program and Information Report (Key Data) U.S. Summary, FY 2004-FY2005.* Alexandria, Va: USDA Food and Nutrition Service; 2005.

32. Gleason P, Suitor C. *Children's Diets in the Mid-1990s: Dietary Intake and Its Relationship with School Meal Participation.* Alexandria, Va: USDA Food and Nutrition Service, Office of Analysis, Nutrition, and Evaluation; 2001.

33. Murphy JM, Pagano ME, Nachmani J, Sperling P, Kane S, Kleinman RE. The relationship of school breakfast to psychosocial and academic functioning, *Arch Pediatr Adolesc Med.* 1998;152:899–907.

34. Gordon A, Briefel R, Needels K, et al. *Feeding Low-Income Children When School Is Out – The Summer Food Service Program: Final Report.* Washington, DC: USDA Economic Research Service; 2003.

35. Bruening K, Gilbride JA, Passanante MR, McClowry S. Dietary intake and health outcomes among young children attending 2 urban day-care centers. *J Am Diet Assoc.* 1999;99:1529–1535.

36. Food Research and Action Center. *School Breakfast Scorecard: 2004, Fourteenth Annual Status Report on the School Breakfast Program.* Washington, DC: Food Research and Action Center; 2004.

37. America's Second Harvest. *Hunger in America 2001: America's Second Harvest Third National Hunger Study.* Chicago, Ill: America's Second Harvest; 2001.

CHAPTER 5

Develop Agency, Community, and State Nutrition Policies

Nancy Chapman and Maya T. Edmonds

Reader Objectives

- Define policy, and discuss its importance for public health nutrition.
- Describe the players, process, and intent of policy making at the agency, local, and state levels.
- List the steps to formulate successful policy.
- Identify leadership roles for the public health nutritionist in formulating, implementing, and evaluating policy.
- Give some examples of how nutritionists influence policy.

DEFINE POLICY

A policy is a statement of principle or intent that guides the selection of priorities. Policies set the direction of programs and actions of an individual, organization, or government. Values, convictions, and beliefs form the basis for a policy statement.

Carefully formulated policies assure consistent actions and prevent shortsighted or impulsive decisions. Mission statements, position papers, policy and procedure manuals, protocols, office rules, and written memorandums from administrators or program managers convey policies within an organization. Local ordinances and state and federal laws and regulations articulate formal policies of governments.

A policy is not a plan for action, nor is it an anticipated outcome of an action, although policy statements may include these elements. Without clear, comprehensive policies that are written and communicated to those who are affected by them, actions can be narrow, fragmented, inconsistent, and even contradictory. The absence of a well-articulated guiding statement impairs the assessment of programs or initiatives that are implemented.

The process of establishing policy differs according to the individual or group formulating it, the position of the policy maker in the power structure, and the number of people or the size of the population whose lives or work will be affected. Policies provide the framework to do the following:

- Select priorities from competing options.
- Guide plans for programs, services, products, or campaigns.
- Set standards for measuring the quality of programs, services, or products.
- Specify eligibility criteria and benefit levels for target populations of programs.
- Allocate funds.
- Select and deploy personnel.
- Generate revenue for projects, programs, or organizational work.
- Set directions and priorities for research and development.

IMPORTANCE OF POLICIES

Agency administrators, as well as local, state, and federal governments, generate policies to address specific concerns appropriate to or associated with the agency's mission. Because policies have far-reaching influence, nutritionists must understand policy, how policies have evolved, their current intent, and implications for the future. By working with other interested groups and broadening their networks or coalitions, nutritionists can be effective in promoting and protecting the public's health through public policy.

To initiate or change a policy requires knowing (1) its importance to the policy maker(s), (2) who benefits, and (3) why it was initiated and adopted. A historical review of nutrition services, education, food assistance, food safety, nutrition research, and monitoring offers insights for answering these questions. The evidence base for public health and nutrition practice (see Chapter 2) should provide a foundation for nutrition and health policies. Policy making should balance scientific evidence with the values, priorities, needs, and concerns of stakeholders and constituents. Policy makers are always constrained by budget realities.

AGENCY POLICY

Although authority and funding for many public health nutrition programs originate in Washington, DC, agency administrators and local and state government officials can authorize additional funds and programs to address observed community needs. Many policies originate at the program level as the nutrition staff and agency administrators develop their strategic plans, operational plans, and protocols for delivering services and write grant proposals for innovative new programs.

Public health nutritionists participate in developing agency policy when they do the following:

- Assess their community's food, nutrition, and health needs and present these findings to program directors, agency administrators, and boards.
- Recommend programs using results of assessments.
- Monitor and report their agency's progress in meeting nutritional objectives.
- Establish policies, procedures, and protocols for nutrition services for their agency.
- Adopt national model standards for their nutrition services such as those in *Healthy People 2010*.

To accomplish these tasks requires understanding the formal and informal power structures and policy-making processes in the agency. It is important to know the values and priorities of administrators or officials who make the overall policies of which nutrition policies are a part. Public health nutrition programs and services are often affected by agency, local, state, and federal policies not specific to food or nutrition, such as personnel policies or policies on health professional training, health care financing, or public assistance.

LOCAL POLICY

With the diversity of local political structures in the United States, nutritionists must investigate the workings of their own local governments. Many states have strong county governments with elected boards of commissioners or supervisors who pass ordinances and approve the county budget. Where the county government is responsible for public health services, the county commissioners usually appoint the county manager and the county's board of health.

In large cities, a city council promulgates local ordinances, budgets local revenues, and appoints the city board of health. An elected mayor or appointed city manager administers the daily activities of the city. The county or city board of health appoints the chief health official, who may or may not be a health professional. The agency health official is responsible for local public health policy. In these agencies, the nutritionist should advise the health official and the board of health on nutrition policy. *Moving to the Future: Developing Community-Based Nutrition Services* provides a framework of reference for organizing and implementing community-based nutrition services.

In states where there are no official local public health agencies, the state health agency may provide services through district or regional offices. Another model is for the state health agency to contract with local hospitals, health centers, or other institutions to provide health and nutrition services. When a locality lacks a public health official or when the local health agency does not employ a nutritionist, nutritionists employed by the state health agency or other community agencies must build coalitions to advance nutrition policies.

STATE POLICY

State government policy-making structures and processes closely parallel those of the federal government. State government officials are usually accessible and usually look to the state health agency's public health nutrition staff as their experts on the nutritional status of the people in their communities.

State Legislature

Every state, except Nebraska which has a unicameral legislature, has two houses of elected legislators. State senates and houses of representatives or general assemblies function through a committee and subcommittee system, much like the US Congress. To influence nutrition policy it is essential to understand the state legislative process and to know the key committees and the legislators on those committees who are responsible for health, nutrition, food, professional licensure, budget, personnel, education, and consumer affairs. The nutritionist should consult the legislative liaison on the state health agency staff for guidance on how to participate in the process within agency policy. The legislative liaisons for the state public health or state dietetic associations are other useful resource persons.

State Executive Branch

The governor is the state's chief executive officer who directs the state agencies responsible for administering programs and allocating resources. These include both state revenues and federal grants to states. To successfully compete for funds, it is necessary to understand the state budget process and how to prepare a competitive budget request (see Chapter 17). To maintain a viable level of nutrition services during times of state budget fluctuations, it is useful to form partnerships with nongovernmental agencies for additional funds and in-kind services. For example, in Idaho, Montana, and Wyoming, state and private funds were used to fund *WIN the Rockies* (Wellness IN the Rockies). The *WIN the Rockies* program seeks to stem the rising tide of obesity in the three states by focusing proactively on prevention and positively on health (rather than weight) at the individual and community levels.

State Health and Nutrition Policy

The administrative structure for state nutrition and health policy varies from state to state. A variety of organizational structures and leadership models are used within state governments. Nutrition and health policy may be administered from various agencies within state governments including freestanding health departments or state divisions of human service. Understanding the structure of nutrition services within the state health agency is the first step to changing or formulating state nutrition policy. The Association of State and Territorial Health Officials (www.astho.org) is a useful resource for gathering information on state government organizational structures.

The secretary of the state human service department, the director of the state health agency, or the designated state health official is the chief public health advisor to the governor. It is usually the role of the state public health nutrition director or chief nutrition consultant to advise this state health official on nutrition policy. Nutritionists working in the local and state health agencies can provide input into state nutrition policy through their state public health nutrition director or their lead public health nutritionist.

Nutrition policy should reflect the food and nutrition needs of the public based on (1) results of formal and informal community needs and assets assessments and market research, (2) consensus recommendations of the public and of health and nutrition professionals throughout the state, and (3) national published nutrition objectives and model standards for nutrition services. Several documents are useful in developing state nutrition objectives: *Healthy People 2010*, the American Public Health Association's *Model Standards: Guidelines for Community Attainment of the Year 2000 Objectives*, and the Association of State and Territorial Public Health Nutrition Director's guidebook, *Moving to the Future*, and their Model State Nutrition Objectives.

POLICY-MAKING STRATEGIES

In-depth knowledge of the community based on the subjective and statistical database from the community assessment (see Chapter 3) is essential to develop policy. This requires effective study of the community and considers political, social, economic, and geographic implications as well as health and scientific concerns.

Policy makers, whether they are state legislators, county commissioners or supervisors, members of boards of health, or state or local health officials—elected or appointed—are necessarily political. Even policy recommendations strongly buttressed by scientific rationale and evidence of program effectiveness yield to budgetary constraints and special interests.

In recent years there have been major cuts in the federal grants-in-aid to states for health and social programs. As a result, competition for available state and local revenues has intensified. State and local advocates who have identified needs close to home have generated public support for policies not tenable at a national level. Local initiatives can often succeed with less funding and more cooperative voluntary efforts.

Well-documented community assessments, feasible recommendations, local community support, and persuasive presentations influence policy makers. For example, in Montana a group of dietitians organized and founded a state nutrition advisory council, representing State Cooperative Extension Agencies, WIC nutritionists, hunger advocates, food industry specialists, commodity groups, and clinical dietitians. The group became formally known as the Montana State Advisory Council on Food and Nutrition. One of the group's major initiatives is to produce an annual report entitled, "The State of Food and Nutrition in Montana." After providing this report to policymakers, the Governor mandated the establishment of WIC Programs in all Montana counties. This annual report has also been instrumental in increasing coordination and information sharing between nutrition agencies within the state. This is just one example of how a coalition of concerned dietitians can bring about needed changes in state-level nutrition policy.[1]

Policies that respond to documented community needs and that affect the lives of a large constituency are more likely to gain support and be adopted. Success is more likely to come to those who advocate broad innovative programs than to those who plead for more money, staff, or resources to maintain the status quo.

Formulate Policy

At the agency, local, state, or national level the general steps to develop policy are as follows:

- Document needs through community assessments, direct observations, and communications from consumers, scientific studies, and government reports.
- Draft a preliminary policy statement, using past and existing policies as models.
- Seek and gain support from key administrators and policy makers.
- Mobilize a broad grassroots constituency.
- Invite public and professional comments, and refine the statement to reflect this input.
- Implement the policy, and monitor its community application effectiveness to ensure that programs operate according to their intent and achieve the desired outcomes.

Frame a Policy to Win

The more simple, relevant, and immediate the issue, the more likely it is to succeed. Both the public and the policy makers must agree on the benefits. The many paradoxes and controversies in nutrition science need clarification. As policy makers confront questions regarding nutrition services, nutrition education, food labeling, food assistance, and nutrition research, the cost effectiveness and public benefits of each nutrition intervention must be clearly communicated.

A winning policy capitalizes on the policy makers' agenda. Most policy makers have several paramount concerns. They seek job advancement, either in an agency or in the legislature. They intend to be reappointed or reelected. If an agency administrator seeks reappointment, then it is important to accentuate successful programs conducted by the agency to make the official "look good." If a legislator seeks a leadership position, then consensus building on a successful campaign issue counts. Issues they support must enjoy general popularity among a wide group of constituents. Policy makers like to be perceived as serving their constituents. Arguments that demonstrate the human and health benefits, as well as the cost benefits, of a nutrition program boost its chances of gaining support.

The specific purpose of a winning policy must be clear to the audience. For example, the specific purpose of state bills to license dietetic practitioners can be to control the quality of nutrition services available to the public. The consistency in quality of care achieved by licensed nurses and physicians attests to the fulfillment of their purpose. Improvement of the public's health is an expected consequence of licensing bills. Policy makers want tangible proof that harm to the public will be minimized when nonqualified individuals are prohibited from practicing and that good to the public will result when only qualified nutrition professionals serve the public.

Secure Approval of Policy

Successfully promoting policies does not depend on luck. It depends on choosing the right strategies.

Strategy 1: Prepare a Scientific Base

Begin with a comprehensive study of the issue, the target audience, and the environment, and prepare clear answers to these questions: Is there a need for this policy or legislation? What studies have been conducted on this issue? By whom? What were the findings? Does any similar policy exist? Who sponsored it? Who opposed it? What were the arguments for or against it? Nutritionists and health colleagues in key administrative or legislative positions or on university faculties can often answer these questions. Information might come from state or local nutritionists, the state dietetic or public health association, nutrition educators, published research in peer-reviewed journals, or other professional organizations. Careful research provides data to buttress arguments and strategic assumptions.

Strategy 2: Develop and Mobilize Broad Support

Building broad organizational coalitions and grassroots support requires a far-reaching educational campaign. Forming active coalitions among diverse groups such as researchers, health professionals, educators, farmers, consumers, religious groups, women's groups, and environmentalists brings nutrition issues to public attention. Nutrition networks should include not only nutrition experts, but also influential citizens in the community; friends of decision makers; respected community groups with political power, including the League of Women Voters, chamber of commerce, parent and teachers associations; local affiliates of such voluntary health agencies as the American Heart Association, the American Diabetes Association, the American Dietetic Association, and the March of Dimes; and lead media personalities. Networking mobilizes multiple voices to move legislators to action (see Chapter 22). Policy makers need to understand that past reductions in funding for nutrition programs may not indicate a failure of programs to meet goals, but rather an unorganized constituency. Policy makers need to recognize that immediate savings may mean much larger costs for health care in the future. Finding that cuts in federal health expenditures reversed the previous decline in infant mortality rates has motivated legislators in several states to increase health care coverage for pregnant women and to provide state monies to supplement the federal WIC and Medicaid funds.

If uninformed or confused, colleagues, organization members, and agency staff who could be potential allies may engender skepticism or even launch an opposition campaign. Wide dissemination of concise and informative fact sheets and press releases on the policy should mobilize the greatest number of potential supporters in the widest geographical area.

Strategy 3: Analyze the Opposition Policy Makers

To have successful interactions with policy makers, knowledge of their priorities, personal relationships, and prior political history is essential. For example, if a policy maker has a university in his or her district, it may be beneficial to gain the endorsement of the university for the proposed policy as a first step in the policy-making process. Or if a policy maker has school-aged children and the proposed policy change would impact this group, it may be helpful to speak to the policy-maker as a parent and appeal to their sensitivity to children's issues.

Strategy 4: Anticipate Problem Opposition, and Develop Alternative Approaches or Compromise Positions

A successful campaign responds constructively to the opposition's arguments and contributes to their defeat. Because policy makers must weigh all views, they need to hear strong factual arguments that refute the opponent's position. If a strong scientific base has been prepared (Strategy 1), it will facilitate responses to opposing arguments. It is important to also mentally prepare several compromise positions, but be careful of compromising too early and relinquishing the goals of the original policy.

For example, the desire to decrease infant mortality might compel policy makers to increase state Medicaid benefits, thus creating a potential risk of high-government costs and subsequent taxpayers' revolts. An alternative solution might be to provide tax advantages to private health care providers serving low-income women so that they can significantly reduce their fees to low-income women who need prenatal care. When no clear solution can be found, policy makers may elect to study several alternatives.

Strategy 5: Estimate Needed Resources and Time

The resources and time that must be devoted to an issue differ depending on whether the issue can be resolved within agency policy or whether it requires legislation. Costs for carrying out a legislative campaign must be paid, and it takes time to identify resources or in-kind contributions. Before the campaign begins, significant resources must be in place. Media coverage must be arranged, key contributors identified, and individuals who will maintain contact with policy makers secured.

Strategy 6: Adopt Successful Strategies from Others

Learning from the successful experiences and strategies of other professionals or other interest groups provides a competitive edge. The drive for dietetic licensure legislation illustrates how dietitians have learned from experiences in the states that initiated the movement.

Strategy 7: Set a Clear Direction Before Starting

Points for possible compromise must be decided and points for "bailout" established. Being readily accessible to policy makers during the process is essential to staying on track and being able to negotiate as necessary.

Strategy 8: Stay on Course

Successful promotion of policy changes requires more than just getting the ball rolling. Promoting policy change is a dynamic process that necessitates persistent monitoring, reacting, regrouping, and remobilizing. Promoting change effectively requires engagement from all parties involved in the process.

Communicate the Message

Charismatic messages are concise, consistent, creative, and sensitive to the community. Successful persuaders communicate precisely what they want their audience to remember. The persuasive message focuses on a single critical point and leaves the details to the fine print. Effective communicators establish credibility over time by being consistent and by avoiding tangential statements that detract from their central message. When rallying support for their viewpoint, they rarely confront the opposition. Good communicators interpret the science simply and clearly. Popular nutrition issues must offer direct, positive solutions to public concerns, while representing the consensus of the scientific and professional community. Popularizing a nutrition issue requires skillful use of the media to assure clear community understanding.

The memorable message is creative. It must be heard and seen repeatedly. The central idea is personalized for the specific audience—whether they are health professionals, the public, consumers, administrators, or legislators. To trigger legislative or administrative action, catchy phrases have been launched in the media to capture public attention:

- SMART—Stop Marketing Alcohol on Radio and TV
- Steps to a Healthier US
- Eat Smart, Play Hard
- Strong Bones, Strong Girls
- America on the Move
- Healthy Mothers, Healthy Babies
- Hunger Watch
- Best Start

The message must focus policy makers on community needs, successful programs using public funds, and the negative impact of budget cuts on the lives of the people in their own communities. Elected officials are especially interested in the views of their constituents, including nutritionists, but more importantly, those the nutritionists serve.

LEADERSHIP ROLES FOR PUBLIC HEALTH NUTRITIONISTS

Policy development has often begun in the offices of professionals. The process of planting and nurturing the seed until it becomes policy utilizes a network of persons who serve in a variety of influential roles.

- Advisors to state or local health officials
- Staff of key boards or committees
- Educators and researchers on university faculties
- Members of key advisory committees, commissions, or expert panels
- Members of one or more health and nutrition professional societies
- Members of consumer, citizen, or service clubs
- Constituents of legislators
- Speakers or writers appearing in the media

In their capacity of advising officials on food and nutrition policy, nutritionists function as organizers, network builders, and resource persons. As staff to policy makers, they analyze and interpret findings of research, another possible channel to influence their administrators. Nutritionists are also often asked to write speeches for key health or elected officials, to communicate with the press, and to conduct public relations.

Another natural and most persuasive role is that of constituent of an elected official. From that perspective, too, a nutritionist may advise as an expert. Nutritionists have served in advisory positions to elected or appointed officials and as professional staff on boards or committees.

Officials and legislators often ask nutrition experts to provide relevant research or to evaluate a food program or an educational campaign. As part of an evaluation team, nutritionists have helped to answer policy questions directly or indirectly, for example: Was the intended target audience reached? What was accomplished? Were the costs justified? What other alternatives exist? At what cost?

Representatives of professional societies educate policy makers through written and oral communications that address current critical food and nutrition issues. A nutritionist may serve as an expert witness at the public hearing of an appointed or elected panel. When their own staff is limited, policy makers may use the expertise of interested and available professionals to suggest witnesses for hearings or even to draft policy statements or legislation.

The most powerful and influential position in the policy process is that of decision maker. This may be a member of an advisory committee, commission, or expert panel or a person to be appointed as a health agency administrator.

Learn by Example

Three brief case studies illustrate how nutritionists have participated in developing state policy by advocating for school breakfast programs in Vermont, establishing a nutrition-monitoring system for those at highest nutritional risk in California, and by securing state supplemental funding for federal nutrition programs in New York.

Vermont Campaign to End Childhood Hunger

In Vermont, a group of concerned nutritionists and health professionals founded the Vermont Campaign to End Childhood Hunger (VTECH) out of a shared concern with escalating emergency food bank use and the small number of Vermont schools participating in the federal funded School Breakfast Program. VTECH began its efforts by contacting individual schools to identify barriers to School Breakfast Program participation and working to overcome those barriers by providing minigrants and educating school administrators on how to enroll in the school meal programs. To strengthen their efforts, VTECH worked with legislators to introduce a bill requiring every Vermont school district without both a school breakfast and school lunch program to put school meals on the ballot to let voters decide if the programs were needed. As a result of this legislation, Vermont has increased the percentage of schools participating in the School Breakfast Program from 20% to more than 90% over the past 10 years.[2]

California Redefines Government's Role

California's Nutrition Monitoring Act, passed in 1986, places the complementary responsibility for nutrition among several levels of government and demonstrates how nutrition monitoring fits into a contemporary redefinition of government's proper role in society.[7] Findings from hunger surveys and a surveillance system spurred nutritionists and other staff of the Northern California Anti-Hunger Coalition (NCAHC) to draft and seek passage of the Monitoring Act.[4] NCAHC included the California Dietetic Association, the California Church Council, and the California Legal Assistance Foundation. Analysis by the coalition showed that policy makers favored legislation that (1) links diet and disease, (2) demonstrates how electronic data systems can economically target existing resources, and (3) shows that nutrition interventions are cost effective.[5] Active participation of local public health nutrition groups and NCAHC's quick response to legislative and administrative requests for data brought success. The 1989 report to the governor and legislature on nutrition monitoring for California identifies the gaps in data collection and makes eight policy recommendations for the computer-based coordinated system of nutrition data management to improve program planning, management, and accountability.[6]

New York Hunger Watch

New York's governor authorized Hunger Watch to direct future public health policies and intervention programs. Program goals were to determine the scope and distribution of undernutrition among high-risk populations in order to evaluate contributing causes and to ascertain whether reduced socioeconomic status adversely affected the nutritional status of certain populations. Health professionals and medical students conducted two studies: a descriptive survey of populations at nutritional risk and a case-control study of observed differences in the growth of preschool children. Data from these studies prompted the New York State Assembly to establish the Supplemental Nutrition Assistance Program (SNAP), which adds state dollars to the federal funding for WIC, senior meal programs, and emergency feeding. Out of the studies were developed methods to estimate the seriousness of hunger, determine reasons for hunger, identify undernourished children, and analyze associated risk factors.[7]

Policy development begins with identifying problems, collecting data, and establishing networks. After a policy is adopted and implemented, it must be monitored and evaluated. Opportunities to influence policy making are unlimited for those who are assertive, energetic, and creative.

POINTS TO PONDER

- As priorities for public health dollars shift to new concerns (e.g., AIDS and emergency care for the homeless), how can nutritionists link nutrition to quality of care, preventive interventions, or sustained independence for high-risk individuals?
- Which coalitions should public health nutritionists join that will provide opportunities to anticipate legislative actions, shifts in funding, and revisions of health improvement plans?
- How can public health nutritionists make time in their overcrowded schedules to participate in formal and informal policy making in their agency, city, county, or state?

HELPFUL WEB SITES

Association of State and Territorial Health Officials: www.ashto.org

NOTES

1. The State of Food and Nutrition in Montana. Report of the Montana State Advisory Council on Food and Nutrition. Accessed at www.dphhs.state.mt.us/hpsd/pubheal/disese/cardio/pdf/annual_report_2002.pdf-8/31/04.

2. Vermont Campaign to End Childhood Hunger. Accessed at http://www.vtnohunger.org/-7/12/04. Personal communication with Dorigan Keeny. 7/12/04.

3. Neuhauser L. Northern California hunger surveys: 1948–85. *National Nutrition Monitor.* 1985;11:2–6.

4. Cohenour SH. Monitoring legislation in California. *National Nutrition Monitor.* 1985;11:4–6.

5. California Department of Health Services. *Report to the Governor and the Legislature on Nutrition Monitoring in California.* Sacramento, Calif: California Department of Health Services; 1989.

6. California Department of Health Services. *Report to the Governor and the Legislature on Nutrition Monitoring in California.* Sacramento, Calif: California Department of Health Services; 1989.

7. Lamphere J-A. Hunger Watch—New York State. *National Nutrition Monitor.* 1984; 11:2–4.

CHAPTER 6

Advocate for National Health and Nutrition Policies

Nancy Chapman

Reader Objectives

- List the interacting private- and public-sector influences on national nutrition policy.
- Discuss the important roles of public health officials and nutritionists in shaping national nutrition policy.
- Know how federal nutrition policy evolves and the operational steps of policy making.
- Review the history of national nutrition policy as background for revising existing policies or formulating new policies.
- Examine the current climate in which nutrition emerges as a national focus.

IDENTIFY PRIVATE-SECTOR AND PUBLIC-SECTOR POLICIES AND INFLUENCES

Food and nutrition policies grow out of the needs, problems, and solutions identified by both public and private sectors at the local and national level. Public health nutritionists express their voices directly to their elected officials or through various groups with which they are affiliated or work. Figure 6–1 shows the wide range of converging forces that influence food and nutrition policy development. The role of elected or appointed public officials is to balance the myriad of often competing policy ideas and construct public policies that benefit the majority and harm the fewest constituents.

The influence each entity exerts varies with the issue and the profile of that entity's leadership, stature, and relationship with the policy makers. Public policy

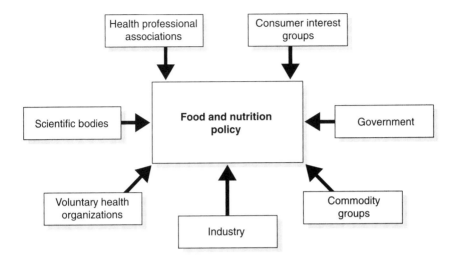

Figure 6–1 Influences on Food and Nutrition Policy Development

ideas may emanate from scientific bodies, such as the Food and Nutrition Board of the Institute of Medicine; nutrition and health professional associations, such as the American Public Health Association and the American Dietetic Association; and voluntary health organizations, such as the American Heart Association and the American Cancer Society. Nutritionists working with consumer groups and public interest groups, such as Food Research and Action Center and the Center for Science in the Public Interest, bring forward many issues that evolve into policies. Food industry trade associations and commodity groups help shape the positions on nutrition policies affecting food producers. Although nutritionists working for government agencies must use formal routes of policy development and approval, their policy ideas and programs often lay the foundation for broader public health nutrition policy initiatives.

Numerous policies emerging from the private sector as well as the public sector affect the public's health. Guiding principles adopted by farmers, producers, food processors, food retailers, and food service operations all along the food system affect consumer food choices initially and public health eventually. Producer and distributor policies guide pricing, marketing, production, distribution, safety, sanitation, and product promotion decisions. In turn, what food consumers can obtain and at what price they pay profoundly influences the public's health and nutritional status.

Other private groups, including nutrition professional associations, voluntary health organizations, and consumer interest groups adopt policies that affect the public. These organizations' policy statements guide their legislative initiatives, public awareness campaigns, and standards of practice, continuing education requirements, and the content of their publications. Likewise, quasi-governmental scientific bodies such as the National Academy of Sciences (NAS) issue publications with important policy implications. The Food and Nutrition Board of the Institute of Medicine has published a wide range of reports that influence health policy, nutrition labeling, military rations, and nutrition assistance programs, including *Preventing Childhood Obesity: Health in the Balance*[1]; the series of Dietary Reference Intakes for major nutrients, vitamins, and minerals; the Guiding Principles in Nutrition Labeling[2]; High-energy, nutrient-dense emergency relief food product,[3] and Proposed Criteria for Selecting the WIC Food Packages.[4]

UNDERSTAND THE ROLES OF BRANCHES OF GOVERNMENT

In the public sector, federal food, nutrition, and health programs and policies are usually based upon laws enacted by the legislative branch or Congress, but others begin as administrative initiatives in the executive branch. The executive branch agencies then develop rules and formal regulations to implement the programs and policies. Lastly, the courts or judicial branch may step forward to ensure that the executive branch carries out the intent of Congress when writing the rules and implementing the programs. The judicial branch also assesses whether citizens' rights granted under the Constitution are violated by any rules or laws. Figure 6–2 portrays the three branches of the federal government—the

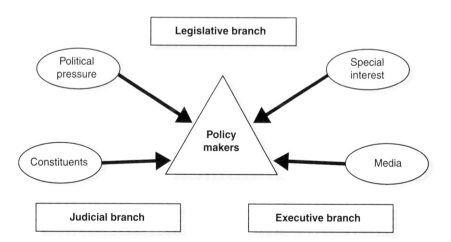

Figure 6–2   The Three Branches of the Federal Government Determine Food and Nutrition Policy.

legislative, executive, and judicial—that develop, implement, and uphold the laws, respectively. More details about these roles appear in Chapter 7. Policy makers are at the center in all three branches. The sources of influence on policy decisions may differ slightly depending on the branch, but scientific or legal evidence, special interests or political bias, and media reports are universal factors in policy making.

Food, nutrition, and health issues fall under the jurisdiction of numerous committees of Congress and numerous agencies in the cabinet-level departments. Committee structure and the legal jurisdictions in the House of Representatives and the Senate differ substantially. Making contact and building a relationship with a representative or senator who cares about nutrition issues or represents a concerned public health institution or nutrition constituent is often the place to begin. In the executive branch, a number of agencies take responsibility for various aspects of food, nutrition, and health. The Department of Health and Human Services (DHHS) and the Department of Agriculture (USDA), however, dominate federal nutrition activities. (Chapter 7 further discusses some specific programs within these departments.)

Key congressional committees and their counterpart executive agency offices are responsible for nutrition education, food assistance, nutrition research and monitoring, and food safety. Most of the federal agencies have staff that offer consultation; administer grants, contracts, or cooperative agreements; conduct training: sponsor continuing education; and prepare and distribute publications appropriate to their respective nutrition program areas. These activities influence, implement, and disseminate policies. Evaluations of the federal food programs, for example, have been widely cited when new policies or changes in existing policies are being considered.

Formulate National Policy

Attention to nutrition policy ebbs and flows depending on the philosophies of the majority of elected officials and the level of media attention on nutrition issues. Compelling scientific evidence, grassroots focus, and a high level of advocacy for nutrition also strengthen the resolve of legislators and agency administrators to revise existing nutrition policies and introduce new ones. A nutritionist may help formulate national policy in different roles—constituent, advisor, staff, family, or public witness. By understanding the steps to formulating policy and knowing the policy makers, nutritionists can contribute effectively to the legislative and administrative process of policy development.

A sequence of steps is shown in Table 6–1 in a logical order, but in reality, policy making may be truncated or accelerated at any time. The astute nutritionist tracks the progress closely through newsletters or news alerts from various organizations and then inserts comments on the policy at critical points.

The eight policy-making steps summarized in Table 6–1 are described below:

1. Policy makers (e.g., members of Congress or heads of federal agencies) *identify needs* from reported scientific assessments or direct communications from constituents, scientific studies, or governmental reports. The media often amplify these needs by focusing broader and more dramatic attention on the problem. Legislative and administrative staffs also attempt to forecast future needs by studying trends. Besides federal policy and evaluation shops, including the White House Office of Science and Technology Policy, several private groups, such as the Institute of Medicine and the Life Sciences Research Organization, are charged with generating reports that make policy recommendations.

2. Staff from a member of Congress, committee, or agency *draft preliminary policy statements* (e.g., legislation or regulations). In drafting these statements, staff review past and current policies and actions and address concerns related to identified needs.

3. Policymakers *generate strong support* for a new policy or a policy change. Staff assesses likely sources of support or opposition as they develop the purpose, scope, and rationale for the policy. Thus, successful policy statements are worded to maximize support and minimize opposition. Support is sought from scientists, educators, professionals, industry representatives, concerned constituents, and other policy makers who will commit time and resources to manage a policy initiative through the steps required to make it law.

4. Policymakers *hear public testimony* to determine if revisions in the policy are necessary.

5. Staff *refines the policy document* to reflect and balance public sentiment.

6. Policymakers *approve (or reject) the policy* statement and appropriations, if authorized.

7. Agency staff translates approved policy statements or legislation into programs to be implemented in communities across the nation. Regulations are written to guide *program implementation*.

8. Program staff and the public *monitor implementation to ensure program compliance* with the new policy. In some cases, the court system or the legislators intervene to enforce compliance with the law or rules.

Table 6–1 Operational Steps of Policy Making

1. Identify needs.
2. Draft preliminary policy statements.
3. Generate strong support.
4. Hear public testimony.
5. Refine policy document.
6. Reject or approve policy statements.
7. Implement approved policy.
8. Monitor implementation to ensure compliance.

Nutritionists need to understand each step in the development of food, nutrition, and health policies. They should be ready and willing to provide data from their needs assessments, recommend policies, participate in drafting statements, mobilize support, testify, and refine policy statements. They should also know how to translate policies into funding priorities, regulations, standards, and implemented programs.

Evolution of the Nation's Nutrition Policy

Public health legislation and administrative policies embrace the broad concern of preventing disease and protecting and promoting the public well-being. The medical model attempts to cure or control disease. Nutrition interventions are paramount in public health policy because so many diseases are diet related, that is associated with over- or underconsumption of nutrients, energy, and other components of food. Besides public health issues, nutrition has also taken a central role in policies on food safety, food security, consumer protection, national security, antipoverty reforms, and international relations. Table 6–2 lists selected federal domestic nutrition policy initiatives from 1862–1988.

Early Developments in National Nutrition Policy

In the early 1900s, concerns about food safety provided the impetus for strong legislation on pure food and drugs, milk inspection, and better sewage disposal. The Federal Pure Food and Drug Act of 1906 prohibited interstate commerce of misbranded and adulterated food, beverages, and drugs.

Also during the early 1900s, researchers such as E. V. McCollum isolated vitamins A, B, and D and strongly advocated eating a proper diet to prevent deficiency diseases and perhaps to guard against the more or less constant, but unperceived causes that undermine health.[5] In 1917, the USDA published its first dietary guidance plan, Five Food Groups, to help consumers select nutritionally balanced diets.

Continuing the prevention movement in a different direction, the state of Michigan began the first iodine fortification campaign in 1924 to prevent the endemic problem of goiters caused by iodine deficiency.[5,7] George Rosen, in his History of Public Health,[6] described the attention to nutrition as an elixir in America: "By the third decade of this century, scientific nutrition had become in the United States not only an important medicine, but an important component of industry and commerce as well as a major instrument of social policy."

The early pioneers in community nutrition—Lucy Gillet in New York, Frances Stern in Boston, and Lydia Roberts in Chicago—worked with pediatricians to advance nutrition as essential to child growth and development.[7] The high percentage of Selective Service rejectees in World War I suggested that poor nutrition

Table 6–2 Selected Federal Domestic Nutrition Policy Initiatives, 1862–1988

1862	US Department of Agriculture (USDA) created. Morrill Act establishes land grant colleges.
1867	Office of Education established with responsibilities for nutrition education within public schools.
1887	Hatch Act establishes agricultural experiment stations. Federal Research Laboratory established at Staten Island. (Name is changed to the National Institute of Health in 1930.)
1889	US Public Health Service Commissioned Corps authorized for duty on communicable, nutritional, and other diseases.
1893	USDA authorized by Congress to conduct research on agriculture and human nutrition.
1906	The Pure Food and Drug (Wiley) Act prohibits interstate commerce in misbranded and adulterated foods, drinks, and drugs. Federal Meat Inspection Act passed.
1914	Cooperative Extension Service created as part of USDA.
1916	USDA publishes *Food for Young Children*, first dietary guidance pamphlet.
1917	US Food Administration established to supervise World War I food supply. First dietary recommendations issued by USDA—*Five Food Groups*.
1921–29	Maternity and Infancy Act enabled state health departments to employ nutritionists.
1924	Addition of iodine to salt to prevent goiter is first US food fortification program.
1927	Food, Drug, and Insecticide Administration established. Name is changed to Food and Drug Administration (FDA) in 1932.
1930	USDA and Federal Emergency Relief Administration buy and distribute surplus agricultural commodities as food relief. Public Health Service Hygienic Laboratory designated as National Institute of Health (later changes to National Institutes of Health).
1933	Agricultural Act amendments permit purchase of surplus commodities for donation to child nutrition and school lunch programs.
1935	Food Distribution Program established. Social Security Act authorizes grants to states for nutrition services to mothers and children.
1936–37	USDA conducts first *Nationwide Food Consumption Survey* (NFCS).
1938	The Food, Drug, and Cosmetic (FD&C) Act includes provisions for food standards. FDA nutrition research program established. Social Security Act provides support for role of nutrition in health.
1939	Federal Surplus Commodities Corporation initiates experimental Food Stamp Program.
1940	National Defense Advisory Commission draws attention to malnutrition in the United States.
1941	President Roosevelt calls National Nutrition Conference, with announcement of first Recommended Dietary Allowances by the Food and Nutrition Board. FDA promulgates standards for enrichment of flour and bread with vitamins B complex and iron.
1946	National School Lunch Program established.
1947	Laboratories of Nutrition, Chemistry, and Pathology of the National Institutes of Health incorporated into Experimental Biology and Medicine Institute.
1954	Special Milk Program established.
1955	Interdepartmental Committee on Nutrition for National Defense established (discontinued 1967).

(continues)

Table 6–2 continued

1956	Title VII of the Public Health Service Act authorizes funds to support graduate training in public health nutrition.
1958	Food Additives Amendment to FD&C Act prohibits use of a food additive until safety established by manufacturer. Delaney Clause prohibits carcinogenic additives. GRAS (Generally Recognized as Safe) List established.
1961	President Kennedy expands the use of surplus food for needy people at home and abroad and announces a new pilot Food Stamp Program.
1963	Maternal and Child Health and Mental Retardation Planning Amendments to the Social Security Act allow for an expanded number of nutritionists in health care programs.
1965	Food Stamp Act passed by Congress. Nationwide Food Consumption Survey collects first data on dietary intake of individuals.
1966	Child Nutrition Act passed. School Breakfast program established. President Johnson outlines Food for Freedom Program, the "war on hunger." Allied Health Professions Personnel Training Act includes support for training of dietitians.
1966–70	The Department of Health, Education, and Welfare (DHEW), which later becomes the Department of Health and Human Services (DHHS), sponsors a National Academy of Sciences study, Maternal Nutrition and the Course of Pregnancy, which makes major recommendations related to the role of nutrition in human reproduction.
1968	US Senate Select Committee on Nutrition and Human Needs established.
1968–70	DHEW sponsors Preschool and Ten-State Nutrition Surveys that report evidence of hunger and malnutrition in poverty groups in the United States.
1969	President Nixon calls White House Conference on Food, Nutrition, and Health. Secretary of Agriculture establishes the Food and Nutrition Service to administer federal food assistance programs.
1971–74	The National Center for Health Statistics conducts the first *National Health and Nutrition Examination Survey* (NHANES) to measure the nutritional status of the US population. This is followed by NHANES II in 1976–1980, Hispanic HANES in 1982–1984, and NHANES III in 1988.
1972	USDA establishes Special Supplemental Food Program for Women, Infants, and Children (WIC). Agriculture and Consumer Protection Act provides price supports to farmers.
1974	US Senate Select Committee on Nutrition and Human Needs issues *Guidelines for a National Nutrition Policy*, prepared by the National Nutrition Consortium. Safe Drinking Water Act passed.
1975	National Institutes of Health establish Nutrition Coordinating Committee.
1977	US Senate Select Committee on Nutrition and Human needs issues two editions of *Dietary Goals for the United States*. Food and Agricultural Act and Child Nutrition and National School Lunch Amendments passed.
1978	Joint Subcommittee on Human Nutrition Research established in Office of Science and Technology Policy (in 1983 becomes Interagency Committee on Human Nutrition Research under joint direction of USDA and DHHS). DHEW and USDA submit proposal to Congress for national nutrition monitoring system.
1979	DHEW established department-wide Nutrition Policy Board and issues *Healthy People: The Surgeon General's Report on Health Promotion and Disease Prevention*.

Table 6–2 continued

1980	USDA and DHHS jointly issue *Nutrition and Your Health: Dietary Guidelines for Americans*. A second edition follows in 1985. DHHS issues *Promoting Health/Preventing Disease: Objectives for the Nation*, which contains 17 nutrition objectives to be achieved by the year 1990. The Surgeon General's Workshop on Maternal and Infant Health makes recommendations about improving nutrition for these vulnerable groups.
1981	DHHS and USDA issued *Joint Implementation Plan for a Comprehensive National Nutrition Monitoring System*, revised in 1987 as the *Operational Plan for the National Nutrition Monitoring System*. The Select Panel for the Promotion of Child Health, created by Public Law 95-626, submits to Congress and the Secretary of DHHS its report, which includes recommendations on nutrition.
1984	The Surgeon General's Workshop on Breast-feeding and Human Lactation develops strategies for promoting breast-feeding.
1985	USDA initiates Continuing Survey of Food Intakes by Individuals, repeated in 1986.
1986	DHSS and USDA issue *Nutrition Monitoring in the United States*, the report of the Joint Nutrition Monitoring Evaluation Committee.
1988	DHHS publishes the *Surgeon General's Report on Nutrition and Health*.

Source: Reprinted from *Surgeon General's Report on Nutrition and Health*, pp. 29–33, U.S. Government Printing Office, Washington, D.C., 1988.

delayed physical development of the nation's youth. To reverse this trend, several public policy initiatives were launched, among them (1) the 1918 Children's Year Campaign that included weighing and measuring infants and preschool children, (2) federal publications that emphasized giving children priority milk allocations, and (3) volunteer community feeding programs that supplemented the food of the poor.[8]

Nutrition services as part of public health were first suggested at the White House Conference on Children in 1910. Services began about 1915 in the Children's Bureau, part of the Department of Labor, with efforts to educate health and welfare workers and teachers who worked with children and families.[9] During this time, a bureau survey found malnutrition to be prevalent in children of low-income families in the Appalachian area of Kentucky.

During the 1920s, federal funds provided under the Shepherd Towner Maternity and Infancy Act enabled nine states to employ the first nutritionists as consultants to other health workers. Passage of Title V in the Social Security Act of 1935 expanded public health nutrition services in state and local health agencies. With the 1963 and 1965 amendments to Title V of the Social Security Act, nutrition services were further expanded in direct health care programs such as the Maternal and Infant (M&I) and Children and Youth (C&Y) projects and in diagnostic and treatment programs for children who are mentally retarded or have developmental disabilities.

Federal food assistance programs began in 1930 when the USDA and the Federal Emergency Relief Administration bought and distributed surplus agricultural commodities as food relief. Distribution of surplus commodities marked the beginning of child nutrition, school lunch, and food stamp programs during the

1930s, and until recently provided the political engine for authorizing the programs. The National School Lunch Program and the Special Milk Program were established in 1946 and 1954, respectively.

National Nutrition Policy from the 1960s to the 1990s

The 1969 White House Conference on Food, Nutrition, and Health positioned food and nutrition on the national agenda in its own right.[10] Conference participants made recommendations to:

- Enhance nutrition in health services throughout the life span.
- Improve nutrition education in schools, in the training of health care providers, and for the public.
- Improve food assistance to low-income families.
- Expand and coordinate basic and applied nutrition research.
- Establish a nutrition monitoring and surveillance system for the entire population and for targeted high-risk groups.
- Strengthen food safety and inspection activities.

These concepts laid the groundwork for today's array of national nutrition policies.

NUTRITION SERVICES AND EDUCATION

Policy makers in the 1970s continued to view nutrition as an integral part of many public health and food programs. The Special Supplemental Food Program for Women, Infants, and Children (WIC) passed in 1972 as part of child nutrition legislation. Though primarily designed as a food assistance program, it strengthened the food–nutrition–health connection.

State and locally funded primary health care programs began requiring nutrition services. Nutrition became a component of community health education programs that reached persons with diabetes, hypertension, and other chronic diseases. More state and local nutritionist positions were funded as grants from such federal programs as WIC, maternal and child health, health promotion, home health services, congregate meals for the elderly, and the Head Start Program.

Nutrition policy shifted from defining nutrition problems as arising from too little food to recognizing the risks of overconsumption of certain dietary factors. This concept ushered in federal dietary guidance on health promotion and disease prevention. The Senate Select Committee on Nutrition and Human Needs examined the evidence linking diet and the major killing and crippling chronic diseases, and in 1977 issued the *Dietary Goals for the United States*.[11]

After much debate, in 1980 the USDA and DHHS jointly published nonquantitative recommendations in the first edition of the *Nutrition and Your Health:*

Dietary Guidelines for Americans.[12] The debate about the issuance of the *Dietary Guidelines for Americans* in 1980 led to a US Senate Committee on Appropriations report directing DHHS and USDA to convene a Dietary Guidelines Advisory Committee of outside scientists that would assess the scientific need for updates and revise the guidelines every five years, if necessary. The nine-member Dietary Guidelines Advisory Committee established in 1983 helped in the development of the second edition, the *1985 Dietary Guidelines*[13] that closely followed the earlier publication with minor clarifying changes. The second edition received wide acceptance and served as the basis for several consumer brochures.

Congress wanted to ensure that the guidelines would be updated regularly and formalized the requirement in language in the 1987 *Conference Report of the House Committee on Appropriations*[14] stating that USDA, in conjunction with the DHHS, "shall reestablish a Dietary Guidelines Advisory Group on a periodic basis. This Advisory Group will review the scientific data relevant to nutritional guidance and make recommendations on appropriate changes to the Secretaries of the Departments of Agriculture and Health and Human Services." In 1989, a third panel of nutrition experts was convened to consider revisions to the 1985 dietary guidelines.

As is evident in the 1988 *Surgeon General's Report on Nutrition and Health*,[15] the current nonquantitative recommendations remained the federal policy on dietary advice for Americans. The National Research Council's report *Diet and Health*[16] signaled a shift to quantifying dietary guidelines for the intake of fat, cholesterol, saturated fat, sodium, fruits, vegetables, and grain products. For adults at risk of chronic diseases, the National Cancer Institute and the National Heart, Lung, and Blood Institute launched their own national nutrition education campaigns.

The 1979 Surgeon General's report *Healthy People*[17] focused significant attention on nutrition, as did a follow-up DHHS publication, *Promoting Health/ Preventing Disease: Objectives for the Nation 1990.*[18] This latter report devoted 1 of the 15 chapters to nutrition and identified 17 objectives to reduce nutritional risk factors, compared to 24 nutrition objectives for the year 2000.[19]

To monitor progress toward meeting the objectives, DHHS conducted midcourse reviews every five years.[20] This 1986 midyear analysis found that the lack of baseline data and data collection systems hindered assessing progress. Some evidence suggested gains in the number of women breast-feeding and in the number of persons adopting weight control regimens; however, the prevalence of overweight and high blood cholesterol remained critical. To achieve national nutrition objectives, a more comprehensive approach to nutrition programming, more resources, and more extensive nutrition monitoring systems are needed based on state and federal data.[21]

In the 1970s, use of the food label as a nutrition education tool added to the listing of ingredients information on the nutrient content of foods. The Food and Drug Administration (FDA) implemented the voluntary Nutritional Labeling

Program, permitting food product labels to present the nutrient content based on US Recommended Dietary Allowances (RDAs). The US RDAs were the nutrient standards set for nutrition labeling and reflect the highest of the RDAs for all sex–age categories for most nutrients as published in 1968.

As nutrition policy embraced health promotion, the FDA issued regulations that extended voluntary nutrition labeling to include sodium.[22] Proposed regulations and legislation would later extend labeling to cholesterol and several of the individual fatty acids.[23] Food companies, viewing nutrient labeling as an opportunity, made claims about the potential health benefits associated with a product. The cacophony of labels confused the consumer, and eventually propelled Congress to set criteria for formal nutrition labeling.

The 1980s saw a policy climate of consolidation and fiscal constraint. In passing the Omnibus Budget Reconciliation Act of 1981, Congress combined a large number of categorical public health programs under several federal block grants and reduced levels of funding. With block grants, more responsibility for public health policy was delegated to state and local health agencies.

After three years of reduced health expenditures, studies by the National Academy of Sciences,[24] the National Commission to Prevent Infant Mortality,[25] and Congress documented negative effects on low-income populations and a leveling off in the infant mortality rate decline. In response, Congress began to reinstate modest increases in funds to the Maternal and Child Health block grant, Medicaid, and other public health programs.

Reduced government regulation has also been a policy thrust of the 1980s. For example, in 1987, the Health Care Financing Administration (HCFA) issued a proposed rule that, among other things, dropped the requirement for dietary services staffing and professional qualifications from Medicare and Medicaid regulations. Using its legislative network and joining a coalition, The American Dietetic Association (ADA) successfully mobilized forces to stop this HCFA proposal and maintained the standards for dietary services. The ADA continued to advocate for appropriate dietary services for Medicare and Medicaid patients as well as adequate reimbursements.

Food Assistance

In the 1970s, congressional representatives responded to identified problems of poverty by improving food assistance to needy families. They expanded the Food Stamp Program and the National School Lunch Program. They created the National School Breakfast Program and the Special Supplemental Food Program for Women, Infants, and Children (WIC). Faced with rising budget deficits in the early 1980s, Congress reduced expenditures for food assistance programs by one third. Tightened program eligibility criteria, coupled with reduced or frozen benefits, substantially decreased the number of recipients. Ironically, as program reductions were being enacted, evidence from several program evaluations confirmed the effectiveness of programs and recommended areas for program improvement.

By 1983, hunger emerged again as a powerful social and public health issue and Congress gathered information.[26,27,28] Nutritionists and others[29] reported expanding lists of eligible WIC applicants. Soup kitchens were serving increasing numbers of families with children, and there was heavy demand for emergency food packages. Staff of hospital emergency rooms reported observing children and adults suffering from malnutrition.[30]

Responding to the paradox of reports of increased hunger at the time that agricultural surpluses were swelling in warehouses, Congress enacted the Temporary Emergency Food Assistance Program (TEFAP) of 1984. TEFAP distributed surplus commodities to families at nutritional risk. In further response, Congress began to reverse earlier legislative actions that had reduced benefits and eligibility for the Food Stamp, National School Lunch, National School Breakfast, Commodity Food Distribution, and WIC programs.

By gathering relevant data and communicating their observations to policy makers, nutritionists have influenced the direction of legislation. Their findings provided part of the justification for strengthening food assistance programs. For example, based on the national evaluation,[31] lawmakers secured additional appropriations for WIC from 1984 through 1989. This evaluation showed that infants participating in WIC had larger head circumferences, fetal death rates were reduced, and intakes of key nutrients were improved in the diets of women, infants, and children. The recommendation from the USDA national evaluation of school breakfasts[32] that breakfast include more iron and vitamins A and B_6 led to the authorization of increased reimbursements for breakfasts in the 1986 School Lunch and Child Nutrition Program amendments.

Nutrition Research

Several legislative and administrative actions served to expand and coordinate inter- and intra-agency nutrition research. The Food and Agriculture Act of 1977 designated the USDA as the lead agency for investigations in human nutrition. A structure to coordinate research and dietary guidance was then created under one director in the Department of Agriculture. The Department of Health and Human Services (DHHS) was authorized to study the causes, diagnosis, treatment, control, and prevention of physical and mental diseases of man. A nutrition coordinating office was set up to oversee research at the National Institutes of Health. The Office of Science and Technology Policy under the executive office of the President formed a Joint Subcommittee on Human Nutrition Research, raising nutrition to unprecedented status. The congressional Office of Technology Assessment reviewed federal nutrition research activities and published reports that contributed to enhanced coordination.

Although some of the formal organizational structures have disappeared, some efforts to coordinate federal nutrition research continue. The report *Human Nutrition Research: The Federal Five-Year Plan*[33] identifies current and proposed areas for government-wide nutrition research. The *Surgeon General's Report on Nutrition and Health*[34] reviewed current scientific literature and suggested future directions for nutrition research.

Nutrition Monitoring and Surveillance

Because policy development depends in part on scientific data, lack of quality data has often translated into inaction or inappropriate policy. The USDA has surveyed household food consumption since 1936; however, the system has not tracked individual dietary intakes or nutritional status.

In 1968, Congress sought information on the nutritional health of the nation and mandated the *Ten-State Nutrition Survey*. Between 1968 and 1970, nutrition status indicators of populations in five low-income and five high-income states were surveyed and reported by DHHS. This survey spearheaded implementation of the DHHS *National Health and Nutrition Examination Survey* (NHANES) as a periodic survey beginning in 1971. The *USDA National Food Consumption Survey* added an individual interview component in 1977 and the *Continuing Survey of Intakes by Individuals* in 1985. The Centers for Disease Control and Prevention began tracking nutrition indicators for children and women through the pediatric and pregnancy nutrition surveillance systems developed in collaboration with state public health agencies. These surveys are discussed in detail in Chapter 16.

Evidence from national nutrition surveys has often guided policy decisions on nutrition education initiatives, food assistance, health programs, and food fortification. At the request of Congress, joint reports of the national nutrition-monitoring activities conducted by the USDA and DHHS were published in 1986 and 1989, reporting the dietary and nutritional status of the U.S. population as shown by the available survey data. Nutrition, health, and antihunger advocacy groups questioned the timeliness and completeness of the data and lobbied Congress to pass the 1988 National Nutrition Monitoring and Related Research Act that called for improvements in federal monitoring activities. Congress passed the bill in 1988, and President Reagan vetoed it. A coalition of nutrition professional societies, private health organizations, commodity groups, and advocacy groups continued to lobby for the nutrition-monitoring bill, with eventual enactment in 1990.

FOOD SAFETY AND QUALITY

In the late 1970s and early 1980s, food safety debates expanded from concerns about food contamination because of poor sanitation and inspection practices to concerns about birth defects, cancer, and health problems associated with pesticides, drugs, and such additives as nitrates, saccharin, and cyclamates in foods. The 1958 Delaney Clause was enacted to prevent food processors from adding any substance to food that has been shown to induce cancer in humans or in laboratory animals. Subsequently, animal drugs were covered by this prohibition. Drugs found to be carcinogens could be used if no residues were found in the food analyzed by acceptable methods.

Exemptions to absolute prohibition under the anticancer clause were created for numerous substances. In the absence of an acceptable substitute for the artificial sweetener saccharin or the curing agent nitrite, the public and hence policy makers found ways to place a moratorium on a ban of saccharin and to postpone action on nitrites.[35] The 1977 saccharin debate and the 1978 nitrite case tested the concept of absolute abolition and initiated an examination of food safety policy.[36]

In 1981, some scientists, regulators, consumers, policy makers, and the food industry attempted to reform food safety laws to redefine acceptable levels of risk associated with food additives. Current and more sensitive analytical techniques for risk assessment had rendered the legal definitions of "safe" (the zero standard of the Delaney Clause) obsolete. To correct the perceived problem, some members of Congress sought changes in the Food, Drug, and Cosmetic Act that would substitute risk–benefit appraisals for the hazard-free approach of the Delaney Clause. Strong opposition from consumer groups stalled the reform initiative in Congress, although administrative and congressional actions have permitted exceptions to the Delaney Clause to remain.

Reports of serious outbreaks of food-borne illnesses and media attention to pesticides in food continued to raise questions about food safety and the need to examine meat and poultry inspection policies,[37] the cleanliness of water and fish products, the use of antibiotics in livestock, and the amount of pesticide residues on plants.[38] As biotechnology changes the methods of food production, preservation, and protection and manipulates the composition of the food supply, public health professionals must raise more questions and sharpen their understanding of the trade-offs (see Chapter 13).

TURN-OF-THE-CENTURY NUTRITION POLICY (1990–2005)

If the 1980s was the decade of consolidation and fiscal constraint, the 1990s to present represent a time of lessened government regulation and intervention and more attention to constitutional rights, personal accountability, and national security, as shown in Table 6–3. Initially nutrition labeling laws and rules governing school nutrition programs emphasized rigorous science-based policy, but over the decade, these rules changed with pressure from industry, and the federal nutrition education and public health efforts waned with lack of funding. Attention to bioterrorism, homeland security, and the Iraq war drained funds from all the discretionary programs and staff from health-oriented tasks at FDA and DHHS.

Table 6–3   Selected Federal Domestic Nutrition Policy Initiatives, 1990–2005

1990	The National Nutrition Monitoring and Related Research Act was enacted requiring review of the *Dietary Guidelines for Americans* every 5 years and joint USDA and HHS review of Federal nutrition publications.
	Congress passed the Nutrition labeling and Education Act that mandated nutrition information on the food label and permitted nutrient and health claims.
	HHS and USDA jointly released the third edition of the *Dieatry Guidelines for Americans* including numerical recommendations for intakes of dietary fat and saturated fat and specific food selections to achieve the dietary goals.
	IOM released reports *Nutrition During Lacatation* and *Nutrition during Pregnancy: Part I: Weight Gain, Part II: Nutrient Supplements*, which changed the guidelines for these population groups.
1991	FDA publishes the rules for labeling fresh fruits and vegetables, fish, and meat and begins an educational campaign, "Read the label, Set a Better Table."
1992	USDA issued the Food Guide Pyramid as the new food guidance system that visually represents the number of servings from each food grouping.
	Enactment of the WIC Farmers Market and Nutrition Act of 1992, increased access of WIC participants to fresh fruits and vegetables.
1993	FDA issues regulations permitting health claims and ingredient declarations, including percent juice, based on NLEA.
	USDA published *School Nutrition Dietary Assessment* showing that school lunches are too high in fat but overall provide essential nutrients for children.
1994	The Better Nutrition and Health for Children Act of 1994 made a number of changes primarily emphasizing the need to improve the nutritional quality of school meals and required school lunches to conform to the *Dietary Guidelines* by 1996.
	USDA established Team Nutrition and launched the Healthy School Meals Initiative to support improvements in school lunches and increased nutrition education for children.
	Congress enacted the Dietary Supplement Health and Education Act (DSHEA), which requires FDA to establish special regulatory procedures for dietary supplement labels describing the nutrient and dietary supplement effect on the structure and function in humans.
	Institute of Medicine released *How Should the Recommended Dietary Allowances Be Revised?*, a report of the Food and Nutrition Board.
1995	USDA and HHS jointly released the fourth edition of the *Nutrition and Your Health: Dietary Guidelines for American* including the Food Guide Pyramid, Nutrition Facts labels, boxes highlighting good food sources of key nutrients, and a chart illustrating three weight ranges.
	USDA published *The Healthy Eating Index*, an analytic tool to assess dietary quality of individuals and groups.
1996	The Food Quality Protection Act (FQPA) of 1996 amended the Federal Insecticide, Fungicide, and Rodenticide Act (FIFRA) and the Federal Food Drug, and

Table 6–3 continued

Cosmetic Act (FFDCA) that fundamentally changed the way EPA regulates pesticides and set a new safety standard—reasonable certainty of no harm—that must be applied to all pesticides used on foods.

1997 The USDA charter established the 2000 Dietary Guidelines Advisory Committee. DHHS issues the midcourse review assessing progress toward the Healthy People 2000 objectives.

IOM released report, *Dietary Reference Intakes for Calcium, Phosphorus, Magnesium, Vitamin D, and Fluoride*.

1998 Congress passed the FDA Modernization Act of 1997 allowing health claims or nutrient claims based on authoritative statements of scientific body.

IOM released the report *Vitamin C Fortification of Food Aid Commodities: Final Report*.

1999 USDA released the Food Guide Pyramid for Young Children 2 to 6 years old.

Congress passed the Child Nutrition and WIC Reauthorization Amendments of 1998 that reauthorized the School Food Service programs and the WIC program and increased access by expanding eligibility, reducing stigma, and streamlining the participation process for participants and providers.

2000 USDA and HHS jointly issued the fifth edition of the *Nutrition and Your Health: Dietary Guidelines for Americans* that made 10 recommendations by separating physical activity from the weight guideline, emphasizing the grains and fruits/vegetables as separate groups, and adding a safe food handling guideline.

DHHS and USDA sponsored the National Nutrition Summit in Washington, DC, to highlight accomplishments since the 1969 White House Conference on Food and Nutrition with a focus toward the epidemic of overweight and obesity.

IOM released two reports *Dietary Reference Intakes for Vitamin C, Vitamin E, Selenium, and Carotenoids* and the *Dietary Reference Intakes for Thiamin, Riboflavin, Niacin, Vitamin B_6, Folate, Vitamin B_{12}, Pantothenic Acid, Biotin, and Choline*.

2001 DHHS and USDA began to integrate the CDC/NCHS National Health and Nutrition Examination Survey and the ARA Continuing Survey of Food Intakes of Individuals to connect health indices with average dietary intakes of a nationally representative sample of Americans.

IOM released the report on *Dietary Reference Intakes for Vitamin A, Vitamin K, Arsenic, Boron, Chromium, Copper, Iodine, Iron, Manganese, Molybdenum, Nickel, Silicon, Vanadium, and Zinc*.

2002 IOM released the report, *Dietary Reference Intakes for Energy, Carbohydrate, Fiber, Fat, Fatty Acids, Cholesterol, Protein, and Amino Acids* that served as the basis for the updates of the 2005 *Dietary Guidelines*.

Passage of the Benefits Improvement and Protection Act that permitted reimbursement for nutritional services.

Passage of the 2002 Farm Bill permitting seniors to use coupons at farmers' markets from 2003 to 2007.

(continues)

Table 6–3   continued

2003	FDA launched the Consumer Health Information for Better Nutrition Initiative that included new requirements for qualified health claims for dietary supplements and conventional foods.
	FDA issued final rule requiring labeling of trans fatty acid with cholesterol and saturated fats in nutrition labeling, nutrient content claims, and health claims.
	IOM released the report, *Dietary Reference Intake: Guiding Principles for Nutrition Labeling and Fortification* intended for FDA to use as a basis for updating the Nutrition Facts Panel.
2004	Congress passed the Child Nutrition and WIC Reauthorization Act of 2004 that made a number of changes to the child nutrition programs: National School Lunch program, School Breakfast Program, Special Milk Program, Child and Adult Care Food Care Program, and Summer Food Service Program, including a mandatory School Wellness Policy Plan.
	IOM issued two reports, *Preventing Childhood Obesity: Health in the Balance, Proposed Criteria for Selecting the WIC Food Package*, and *Dietary Reference Intakes: Water, Potassium, Sodium, Chloride, and Sulfate.*
2005	DHHS and USDA jointly issue the sixth edition of the *Dietary Guidelines for Americans* that serves as the basis of federal nutrition policy and for the first time a consumer brochure to provide advice to consumers about food choices that promote health and decrease the risk of chronic disease.

Public Health Nutrition Goals

The decade began with the DHHS release of *Healthy People 2000: National Health Promotion and Disease Prevention Objectives*[39] that reviewed the current state of public health and set forth guideposts for the 1990s to increase the span of healthy life for all Americans, reduce health disparities, and increase access to preventive services. Nutrition was elevated to the second priority area with 24 nutrition objectives.[20] For the first time, the report estimated the economic impact of diet-related diseases at a cost of $200 billion, and noted that the increasing prevalence of obesity carried a cost of $99 billion related to comorbidities of hypertension, diabetes, coronary heart disease, sleep apnea, cancer, strokes, gall bladder disease, and osteoarthritis.[40]

At the beginning of the 1990s, there had been advances in reducing cholesterol as Americans chose lower fat, saturated fat, and cholesterol but not necessarily lower-calorie foods. Fewer individuals used diet, controlled portion sizes, or engaged in physical activity to lose weight, while the prevalence of diabetes rose among those at highest risk of obesity and with lowest access to preventive services—Native Americans, Mexican-Americans, and African-Americans. By 1996, when the *Healthy People 2000 Mid Course Review*[41] was completed, the trend continued toward a higher prevalence of obesity among all ages and an increase in diabetes in adults. Individuals were eating a lower percentage of calories from fat, but consumed more calories.

By January 2001 when DHHS issued the *Healthy People 2010*,[42] obesity had become a leading health indicator. Charter 19 titled Nutrition and Overweight states 18 measurable objectives and refers readers to related objectives in 13 of the other focus areas. The proportion of children, adolescents, and adults who are overweight grew, with two in three adults and one in five children being overweight or obese. The links to chronic disease became stronger and the disparity of prevalence among certain ethnic groups became clear. The 2010 goals included increasing the quality as well as years of life and eliminating, not just reducing, health disparities. Despite the abundance of food and calories, food security among US households also grew, and the 2010 report included an objective for food security for the first time.

Nutrition Education and Nutrition Labeling

The beginning of the 1990s found a flurry of Congressional and executive branch actions on nutrition issues to improve public health. Congress passed the 1990 Nutrition Labeling and Education Act, then the 1994 Dietary Supplement Health and Education Act, and lastly the FDA Modernization Act of 1997, all of which has resulted in a decade of laborious FDA rule making. In 1990, Congress also enacted the National Nutrition Monitoring and Related Research Act that directed the DHHS and USDA to integrate the collection of health and nutrition data on a national representative sample of Americans. Urged by an alliance of nutrition, consumer, and industry groups, Congress funded nutrition and health monitoring activities to identify causes of the obesity epidemic and blunt the related health problems and rising health care costs. In addition, every five years the DHHS and USDA updated the *Dietary Guidelines for Americans*, making them more specific but increasing the number of recommendations.

Over 15 years, FDA issued rules implementing the provisions of the Nutrition Labeling and Education Act of 1990 (NLEA)[43] that initially set forth the criteria for the new Nutrition Facts panel for most foods (except meat and poultry) and authorized the use of nutrient content claims and appropriate FDA-approved health claims. The passage of DSHEA[44] brought generally less burdensome rules for labeling dietary supplements. Over time, the FDA rules for nutrition labeling of food and dietary supplements have become more consistent and less stringent overall, including FDA's 2003 *Consumer Health Information for Better Nutrition Initiative*[45] that allowed use of qualified health claims when there is emerging evidence, but not significant scientific consensus for a relationship between a food, food component, or dietary supplement and reduced risk of a disease or health-related condition. In 1991 the Food and Drug Administration (FDA) (Department of Health and Human Services) and Food Safety and Inspection Service (FSIS)

(US Department of Agriculture) initiated a multiyear food labeling education campaign, called *Read the Label, Set a Healthy Table* to help consumers make healthy food choices in accordance with the *Dietary Guidelines for Americans.* Fourteen years after NLEA and evidence that Americans read the labels, FDA and other federal agencies shifted the focus to obesity and issued an *Action Plan on Obesity*[46] report calling for increased prominence of calories on the label and changing the portion sizes for larger single-serve packages, among other things. FDA began a "Calories Count" campaign.

Also from 1990 to 2005, nutrition research findings catalyzed a change in the nutrient standards used for nutrition labeling, school meals, military rations, and dietary guidance. In the mid 1990s, the Food and Nutrition Board of the Institute of Medicine (IOM) contemplated a change in setting nutrient requirements[47] and adopted an alternative framework, *Dietary Reference Intakes* (DRIs) that replaced the single sets of nutrient specific values (i.e., Recommended Dietary Allowances), with multiple sets of values (Estimated Average Requirements (EAR), Recommended Dietary Allowances (RDA), Adequate Intakes (AI), and Tolerable Upper Intake Levels, (UL)) for designated age groups, physiologic states, and sexes.[48] From 1997 through 2004, the IOM issued DRIs for various categories of nutrients and a guide to reforming the nutrition label using the DRIs (see Chapter 2).

During this time, the USDA conducted several important evaluations of federal nutrition programs. The findings of the 1993 School Nutrition and Dietary Assessment[49] provided the impetus for Congress a year later to require that meals served under the National School Lunch and Breakfast Programs conform to the *Dietary Guidelines* by 1996. The 5-year periodic congressional reauthorizations of the Child Nutrition Programs continued to bring more attention to improving the nutritional quality of the programs with each subsequent law through the Child Nutrition and WIC authorization Act of 2004 that required all schools to have School Wellness Policy Plans.[50] Actual funding for nutrition education and training declined, and Team Nutrition replaced the National Nutrition Education and Training Program, limiting the previous national scope to a portion of the states. An emphasis on nutrition was a significant departure from the initial basis in surplus commodity distribution of these programs.

Passage of the Nutrition Monitoring and Related Research Act of 1990 (P.L. 101-445)[51] formally directed the two departments to convene a scientific panel to review the dietary guidelines and revise the text every five years, if necessary. Although there has been a tremendous amount of consistency throughout the guidelines, there have also been some notable changes throughout the years that reflect the emerging science. The 1990 *Dietary Guidelines for Americans*[52] offered more positive guidance and numerical recommendations for dietary fat and saturated fat and specific food choice suggestions. In 1991, the National Cancer Institute initiated a campaign, 5 a Day for Better Health to promote the consumption of fruits and vegetables, and it is now one of the most widely recognized campaigns around the world.[53]

Shortly after release of the third edition, USDA issued the 1992 Food Guide Pyramid[54] as the new guidance system, but not without controversy. Commodity groups disapproved of the lessened position of animal-based food groups compared to fruits, vegetables, and grain products in the new graphic. The graphic was rescinded temporarily for a review of the research, but eventually republished without any changes. The fourth edition (1995) of the *Nutrition and Your Health: Dietary Guidelines for Americans*[55] included this Food Guide Pyramid, the FDA Nutrition Facts Panel, boxes suggesting good food sources of key nutrients, and a chart illustrating three weight ranges. To assess how well individual diets met the *Dietary Guidelines* and Food Guide Pyramid, USDA published *The Healthy Eating Index*[56] as an analytic tool in 1995.

Like the pyramid, the fifth edition of the *Nutrition and Your Health: Dietary Guidelines for Americans*[57] gave more prominence to fruits and vegetables, separating them from whole grains; it also separated physical activity from the weight guideline, and added a safe food handling guideline, increasing recommendations to 10. This document also recognized dietary supplements as a source of calcium, sodium, iron, and other nutrients. In the 1990s, besides schools and health care settings, community settings and worksite food services were identified as places to implement the *Dietary Guidelines* and to offer nutrition counseling and weight management classes.

Reimbursement for nutrition counseling languished in the Medicare and Medicaid program until passage of the 2002 Benefits Improvement and Protection Act, which included reimbursement for diet counseling for diabetes and kidney disease. DHHS changed the name from Health Care Finance Administration to Center for Medicare and Medicaid Services to ensure better understanding of the agency's role. The American Dietetic Association has worked closely with CMMA to assure that the rules permit appropriate and adequate funding for nutrition counseling.

FUTURE DIRECTIONS FOR NATIONAL NUTRITION POLICY

To anticipate the future of national nutrition policy requires learning lessons from past and present policy priorities. It also requires attempting to forecast population dynamics, budget realities, technological capabilities, and the expansion of the science base through research. As the Centers for Disease Control and Prevention forecasts escalating and uncontrollable costs related to obesity,[58] Congress and multiple federal agencies have rushed to propose and undertake new research, intervention, and educational program initiatives but without substantial funds to ensure comprehensive, sustained interventions. With discretionary funds for research and education unavailable this decade thus far, public health initiatives will depend more on partnerships with the private sector.

What will be funded will depend in large measure on strong scientific evidence of need and/or a link to bioterrorism, homeland security, or other high priorities of Congressional leaders and the president. In the future, public health nutritionists can help (1) document and publish changes in nutrition knowledge, dietary behavior, and nutrition-related health outcomes resulting from education and intervention programs, (2) develop new systems to collect and analyze program data, (3) create new methodology to gather data from hard-to-reach populations (e.g., the homeless, deaf, elderly, institutionalized, migrant, Native American, and non-English-speaking populations), and (4) advocate at local, state, and national levels for adequate funding for successful programs, promotion of the dietary guidelines, and nutrition research.

POINTS TO PONDER

- What will be the effect on public health and public health nutrition services in the future if today's public health policy continues to focus on "putting out fires" by using most of the available funds to respond to the crisis of the moment?
- What are the best approaches to prevention of weight gain and treatment of obesity at local, community, and federal levels? Should communities have more autonomy to structure programs and environments that help overweight individuals adopt lifestyle habits that support a healthier weight? How should these programs be evaluated to assure effective and efficient use of public and private funding?
- If universal health insurance becomes a reality, what nutrition services and education programs should be covered? What steps should be implemented now to assure collection of data to justify the inclusion of nutrition services as promoting health and reducing health care costs?
- Does the food label remain a credible source of health and nutrition information for consumers? If not, what can be done to assure consumers find the nutrition label informative, understandable, and applicable to their daily diets?
- Will today's advances in food technology and food marketing deliver a food supply that fosters food choices that benefit the nation's long-term health?
- What role should the federal government undertake to promote a healthier food supply at schools, workplaces, government buildings, airlines, entertainment centers, and other public places? What standards for food safety and nutritional adequacy are needed? How can nutritionists work with agribusiness and food processors to assure that corporate policies consider public health implications?

NOTES

1. Koplan JP, Liverman CT, Kraak VA. *Preventing Childhood Obesity: Health in the Balance*. Washington, DC: National Academies Press; 2005.

2. Subcommittee on Use of Dietary Reference Intakes in Nutrition Labeling, Food and Nutrition Board. *Dietary Reference Intakes: Guiding Principles in Nutrition Labeling.* Washington, DC: National Academy of Sciences; 2003.

3. Subcommittee on Use of Dietary Reference Intakes in Nutrition Labeling, Food and Nutrition Board. *Dietary Reference Intakes: Guiding Principles in Nutrition Labeling.* Washington, DC: National Academy of Sciences; 2003.

4. Committee to Review the WIC Food Package. *Preliminary Report on Proposed Criteria for Selecting the WIC Food Packages.* Washington, DC: National Academy of Sciences; 2004.

5. Markel H, Cowie DM. "When It Rains It Pours": Endemic goiter, iodized salt, and David Murray Cowie, MD. *Am J Pub Health.* 1987;77:219–229.

6. Rosen G. *History of Public Health.* New York, NY: M.D. Publications; 1958:404–419.

7. Egan M. Public health nutrition services: issues today and tomorrow. *J Am Diet Assoc.* 1980;77:423–433.

8. Egan M. Public health nutrition services: issues today and tomorrow. *J Am Diet Assoc.* 1980;77:423–433.

9. Egan M. Federal nutrition support programs for children. *Pediatr Clin North Am.* 1977;24:229–239.

10. White House Conference on Food, Nutrition, and Health. *Summary of Actions on Food, Nutrition, and Health.* Washington, DC: Government Printing Office; 1970.

11. Senate Select Committee on Nutrition and Human Needs. *Eating in America: Dietary Goals for the United States.* Cambridge, Mass: MIT Press; 1977:12–51.

12. US Department of Agriculture (USDA), US Department of Health and Human Services (DHHS). *Nutrition and Your Health: Dietary Guidelines for Americans.* Washington, DC: USDA, DHHS; 1980. Home and Garden Bulletin 232.

13. US Department of Agriculture (USDA), US Department of Health and Human Services (DHHS). *Nutrition and Your Health: Dietary Guideline for Americans.* 2nd ed. Washington, DC: USDA, DHHS; 1985. Home and Garden Bulletin 232.

14. House of Representatives Conference Committee, 100th Cong, 1st Sess (1987) (H. Rep. 498).

15. Department of Health and Human Services, Public Health Service. *The Surgeon General's Report on Nutrition and Health.* Washington, DC: Government Printing Office; 1988. DHES (PHS) Publication No. 88-50215.

16. National Academy of Sciences, National Research Council, Food and Nutrition Board. *Diet and Health: Implications for Reducing Chronic Disease Risk.* Washington, DC: National Academies Press; 1989.

17. Department of Health, Education, and Welfare. *Healthy People: The Surgeon General's Report on Health Promotion and Disease Prevention.* Washington, DC: Government Printing Office; 1979.

18. Department of Health and Human Services. *Promoting Health/Preventing Disease: Objectives for the Nation.* Washington, DC: Government Printing Office; 1980.

19. Department of Health and Human Services. *Promoting Health/Preventing Disease: Year 2000 Objectives for the Nation.* Washington, DC: Government Printing Office; 1989:1–24. Available at: http://odphp.osophs.dhhs.gov/pubs/hp2000/hppub97.htm.

20. Department of Health and Human Services. *The 1990 Health Objectives for the Nation: A Midcourse Review.* Washington, DC: Government Printing Office; 1986.

21. Kaufman M, Heimendinger J, Foerster S, Caroll MA. Progress toward meeting the 1990 nutrition objectives for the nation: nutrition services and data collection in state/territorial health agencies. *Am J Pub Health.* 1987;77:299–303.

22. House Subcommittee on Investigations and Oversight, Committee on Science and Technology, 97th Cong, (1981) (*Sodium in food and high blood pressure*).

23. Food and Drug Administration, Department of Health and Human Services. Food labeling: declaration of sodium content of foods and label claims for foods on the basis of sodium content: OMB approval and effective date. 49 *Federal Register* 126 (1984).

24. Institute of Medicine. *Preventing Low Birth Weight.* Washington, DC: National Academies Press; 1985.

25. National Commission to Prevent Infant Mortality. *Death before Life.* Washington, DC: National Commission to Prevent Infant Mortality; 1988.

26. House Select Committee on Hunger, 98th Cong, (1984) (Serial no. 98-2, *Alleviating Hunger: Progress and Prospects*).

27. Subcommittee on Domestic Marketing, Consumer Relations, and Nutrition, Committee on Agriculture, 98th Cong, (1984) (Serial no. 98-63, *Hunger in the United States and Related Issues*).

28. Senate Subcommittee on Nutrition, Committee on Agriculture, Nutrition, and Forestry, 98th Cong, (1983) (*Oversight on nutritional status of low-income Americans in the 1980s*).

29. Food Research and Action Center. *Hunger in the Eighties: A Primer.* Washington, DC: Food Research and Action Center Inc; 1984.

30. *Report of the President's Task Force on Food Assistance.* Washington, DC: President's Task Force on Food Assistance; 1984.

31. Rush D. *The National WIC Evaluation.* Washington, DC: USDA Food and Nutrition Service, Office of Analysis and Evaluation; 1985.

32. Systems Development Corporation. *National Evaluation of School Nutrition Programs: Overview and Presentation of Findings,* Final Report. Vol 1. 1983.

33. Interagency Committee on Human Nutrition Research. *Human Nutrition Research: The Federal Five-Year Plan.* Washington, DC: Government Printing Office; 1986.

34. Department of Health and Human Service, Public Health Service. *The Surgeon General's Report on Nutrition and Health.* DHES (PHS) publication 88-50215, 1988.

35. Porter DV. *The Delaney Clause: Current Application and Proposed Changes.* Washington, DC: Congressional Research Service; 1984.

36. Senate Committee on Agriculture, Nutrition, and Forestry. *Food Safety: Where Are We?* Washington, DC: Government Printing Office; 1979.

37. National Research Council, National Academy of Sciences. *Meat and Poultry Inspection.* Washington, DC: National Academies Press; 1985.

38. National Research Council, and National Academy of Sciences. *Regulating Pesticides in Food.* Washington, DC: National Academies Press; 1987.

39. Department of Health and Human Services (DHHS). *Promoting Health/Preventing Disease: Year 2000 Objectives for the Nation.* Washington, DC: DHHS; 1989:1–24. Available at: http://odphp.osophs.dhhs.gov/pubs/hp2000/hp2kfact.htm.

40. Wolf AM, Colditz GA. Current estimates of the economic rate of obesity in US. *Obesity Research.* 1998;6:97–106.

41. Centers for Disease Control and Prevention, National Center for Health Statistics. *Healthy People 2000 Midcourse Review.* Washington, DC: National Center for Health Statistics; 1997. Available at: http://www.cdc.gov/nchs/data/hp2000/hp2k97.pdf.

42. Department of Health and Human Services, Office of Disease Prevention and Health Promotion. *Healthy People 2010.* Washington, DC: DHHS; 2000. Available at: http://www.healthypeople.gov/document. Accessed December, 2005.

43. Center for Food Safety and Applied Nutrition Web site. Nutrition Labeling and Education Act of 1990. Available at: http://www.cfsan.fda.gov/label.html. Accessed December 5, 2005.

44. Center for Food Safety and Applied Nutrition Web site. Dietary Supplement Health and Education Act of 1994. Available at: http://www.cfsan.fda.gov/~dms/dietsupp.html. Accessed December 5, 2005.

45. Center for Food Safety and Applied Nutrition Web site. Consumer Health Information for Better Nutrition Initiative. July 2003. Available at: http://www.cfsan.fda.gov/~dms/nuttftoc.html#oview. Accessed December 5, 2005.

46. US Food and Drug Administration (FDA). FDA report of the Obesity Working Group, 2002. Available at: http://www.fda.gov/oc/initiatives/obesity/. Accessed December 5, 2005.

47. Institute of Medicine. *How Should the Recommended Dietary Allowances Be Revised? A Report of the Food and Nutrition Board.* Washington, DC: National Academies Press; 1994.

48. Garza B. Moving beyond the RDAs to Dietary Reference Intakes (DRIs). *Cornell University Food and Nutrition.* July 2002.

49. USDA, Food and Nutrition Service. *School nutrition dietary assessment study, summary of findings.* 1993. Available at: http://www.fns.usda.gov/oane/MENU/Published/CNP/FILES/SNDA-Sum.pdf.

50. Child Nutrition and WIC Reauthorization Act Pub L No. 108-265, (2004). Available at: http://www.fns.usda.gov/cnd/Governance/Legislation/PL_108-265.pdf.

51. House of Representatives, Committee on Agriculture. *Report on National Nutrition Monitoring and Related Research Act of 1990.* Washington, DC: Government Printing Office; 1990. Report Number 101-788.

52. USDA, US Department of Health and Human Services (DHHS). *Nutrition and Your Health: Dietary Guidelines for Americans.* 3rd ed. Washington, DC: USDA, DHHS; 1990. Home and Garden Bulletin 232.

53. National Cancer Institute. Available at: http://www.5aday.gov/index-about.shtml#background.

54. USDA, Center for Nutrition Policy and Promotion. *The Food Guide Pyramid.* Washington, DC: USDA; 1996. Garden Bulletin 252. Available at: http://www.usda.gov/cnpp/pyrabklt.pdf.

55. USDA, US Department of Health and Human Services (DHHS). *Nutrition and Your Health: Dietary Guidelines for Americans.* 4th ed. Washington, DC: USDA, DHHS; 1995. Garden Bulletin 232.

56. Variyam JN, Blaylock J, Smallwood D. *USDA's Healthy Eating Index and Nutrition Information.* Washington, DC: USDA; 1998. Publication TB1866.

57. USDA, US Department of Health and Human Services (DHHS). *Nutrition and Your Health: Dietary Guidelines for Americans.* 5th ed. Washington, DC: USDA, DHHS; 2000. Garden Bulletin 232.

58. Finkelstein EA, Fiebelkorn IC, Wang G. National medical spending attributable to overweight and obesity: How much, and who's paying? *Health Affairs.* 2003;W3; 219–226.

Chapter 7

Speak Out on Health and Nutrition Legislation and Regulations

Robert Earl

Reader Objectives

- Compare and contrast the functions of the legislative, executive, and judicial branches of the United States government.
- Describe the major federal agencies that administer programs relating to public health and public health nutrition.
- Discuss how nutritionists and dietitians can influence federal legislation and regulations.
- List the strategies to use to advocate for public health nutrition programs and services.
- Discuss acceptable strategies that public health agency staff, who may be prohibited by law to engage in legislative activities, can use to promote public policies to benefit their communities.

WHY SPEAK OUT FOR PUBLIC HEALTH NUTRITION?

Shaping public health nutrition programs requires not only excellence in professional practice, but also contributing time and energy to the political and regulatory processes that govern these programs. Public health personnel are employed to carry out programs and services established by federal, state, and local laws and regulations. Most public health programs receive their support from federal, state, and local revenue. These positions in public health were envisioned and then established to carry out programs and services enabled by federal or state legislation or city or county ordinances. In that context, public health nutrition personnel ensure that their services meet the legislation's intent, are cost effective, and that there is no waste, fraud, or abuse in their operation. When operational problems arise because of the "red tape" of the legislation or regulations, or when the community assessment identifies unmet or insufficiently met needs in the community, public health nutrition personnel are challenged to advocate for the changes needed.

In the democratic society of the United States, all power is vested in the people. The U.S. Constitution begins with "We the people. ..." Representatives elected by the people enact laws to serve the interests of their constituents. Elected officials, whether they are city or county commissioners, state legislators, or federal representatives or senators, should represent the prevailing values and will of the majority of their constituents. They should be accessible to their constituents and responsive to their concerns and their needs. However, public health nutritionists should be sophisticated enough to understand that in the political process there is an ongoing power play between conflicting values, vested interests, and ambitious personalities. The public and their elected officials can be fickle, constantly changing their views, and subject to multiple pressures. Willingness to negotiate and make trade-offs is central to success in the political and regulatory arena. This chapter provides background on the structure and function of American government and describes the workings of the legislative and regulatory process. It suggests how the public health nutritionist can participate actively, effectively, and ethically to advocate for policies and programs to protect and promote the public's nutritional health.

To influence the governing process requires understanding how it works and where the power lies. The government of the United States has evolved over 200 years, based on a Constitution that provides an interlocking system with checks and balances that distribute the decision making and the power between the legislative, judicial, and executive branches.

UNDERSTAND HOW THE FEDERAL GOVERNMENT WORKS

Legislative Branch Responsibilities

The legislative branch enacts laws to initiate, modify, authorize, and fund all the programs and services administered by the federal government. In the United States, Congress, composed of the House of Representatives and the Senate, is the legislative branch.

In the Congress most of the action occurs at the committee or subcommittee level. There are several types of committees that consider food, nutrition, and health issues. A standing committee is permanently established to develop and approve legislation to authorize programs. Standing committees that have jurisdiction over programs related to food, nutrition, and health are:

Senate Standing Committees

The five Senate standing committees are listed below:

- Committee on Agriculture, Nutrition, and Forestry (child nutrition and other food programs)
- Committee on Appropriations (program funding for all federal food, nutrition, and health programs)
- Committee on Finance (Medicare and Medicaid programs)
- Committee on Foreign Relations (international hunger)
- Committee on Health, Education, Labor, and Pensions (Department of Health and Human Services programs: elderly nutrition, maternal and child health, and food labeling)

House of Representatives Standing Committees

The six House standing committees are listed below:

- Committee on Agriculture (food programs)
- Committee on Appropriations (program funding)
- Committee on Education and the Work force (child and elderly nutrition programs)
- Committee on Energy and Commerce (public health, food, and drugs)
- Committee on Science (environment, EPA)
- Committee on Ways and Means (Medicare and Medicaid programs, Aid to Families with Dependent Children)

Select or special committees are established for a specified time or for a specific purpose, such as monitoring issues applicable to several committees. Select or special committees do not have the authority to authorize or to appropriate funds for programs. The Senate Special Committee on Aging, established in 1961 to study issues, conduct oversight of programs, and investigate reports of fraud and waste, serves as the focal point in the Senate for discussion and debate on matters relating to older Americans (see Chapter 10).

Conference committees represent members of relevant House and Senate committees appointed to reconcile differences between legislative proposals approved by the House and Senate. They are appointed for a brief period to negotiate compromise so that commonly supported legislation can move forward for a final vote by both chambers.

The Legislative Process—How a Bill Becomes a Law

The enactment of legislation by Congress occurs through a specified system of development, review, debate, and approval. Ideas for new legislation may be conceived by members of Congress based on problems and concerns of their constituents; they may be ideas generated by consumer, health, or industry groups; or ideas for new legislation may be issues resulting from needs evidenced in the implementation of federal programs.

Participation by public health nutrition professionals in the legislative process requires a clear understanding of the steps in the development of legislation. Knowing the steps, the key decision makers at each step and the responsibilities of these decision makers suggests the appropriate actions for the concerned professional to take. Timing and contacting the key decision makers is critical to success in the legislative process. Figure 7–1 graphically represents the steps in how a bill becomes a law from introduction to enactment by the president. It describes when grassroots advocacy efforts can influence a legislative outcome. Public health nutritionists should study this sequence to determine the contact points and

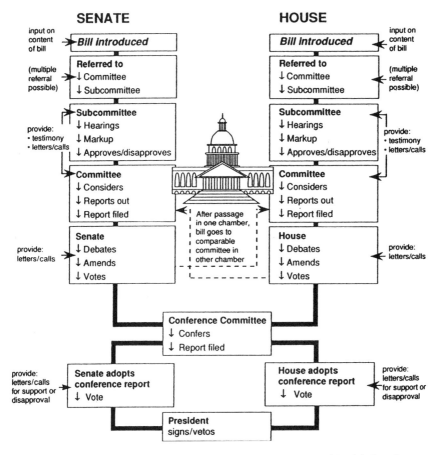

Figure 7–1 How a Bill Becomes Law—Typical Path to Passage of Legislation. Source: Prepared by Robert Earl, contributing Chapter 7 author.

consider who and when to call when a piece of critical health or nutrition legislation is being considered.

FEDERAL BUDGET DEVELOPMENT AND CONTROL

The federal budget system provides the framework to make decisions about the allocation of funds for federal programs. This framework allows budgetary decisions to be made in relation to the requirements of the nation, the available resources, and the rules for accountability of federal funds. The president and the Congress develop the federal budget simultaneously. The nation's budget is shaped in three main phases: executive branch development, Congressional action, and budget execution. These three processes interface with each other. Table 7–1 describes the timetable for federal budget development from the Congressional perspective. In practice in recent years, competing priorities for limited federal resources has caused delays in meeting the standard timetable— from budget development to finalizing appropriations bills.

Table 7–1   Congressional Budget Process Timetable

Date	Action to be completed
First Monday in February	President submits budget to Congress.
February 15	Congressional Budget Office submits economic and budget outlook report to Budget Committees.
Six weeks after president submits budget	Committees submit views and estimates to Budget Committees.
April 1	Senate Budget Committee reports budget resolution.
April 15	Congress completes action on budget resolution.
May 15	Annual appropriations bills may be considered in the House, even if action on budget resolution has not been completed.
June 10	House Appropriations Committee reports last annual appropriations bill.
June 15	House completes action on reconciliation legislation (if required by budget resolution).
June 30	House completes action on annual appropriations bills.
July 15	President submits mid-session review of his budget to Congress.
October 1	Fiscal year begins.

Source: Congressional Research Service. *The Congressional Budget Process Timetable.* Washington, DC: Library of Congress. Order Code 98-472 GOV.

In passing legislation, Congress authorizes a maximum level of funding for a program. It separately appropriates the actual amount to be spent, which may be less than the authorized amount. Authorization legislation can create programs or agencies for a specific time period or indefinitely.

Congressional Action on the Federal Budget

When Congress receives the president's budget request, it acts through legislation to approve, modify, or disapprove it. Congress can change the level of program funding, eliminate programs, or add programs not requested by the president. It can also enact legislation to raise or lower taxes or generate other sources or revenue.

The Congressional Budget Act of 1974 requires that current service estimates be transmitted to Congress with the budget to provide a basis for reviewing the president's budget recommendations. The current services estimates of budget authority and outlays are the funds required to continue federal programs and activities at their present level during the fiscal year in progress. For example, in relation to public health nutrition programs, current services estimates have been very important in efforts to maintain funding for the WIC Program.

Appropriations legislation establishes the specific funding level to support federal programs and agencies for a given fiscal year. Appropriation legislation generally follows the enactment of authorization legislation. Congress does not vote on the level of outlays directly, but rather on budget authority to incur obligations for immediate or future outlays of federal funds to federal departments and agencies.

When action on appropriations has not been completed by the beginning of the fiscal year, Congress must enact a continuing resolution to provide authority for the affected agencies to continue operations up to a specified date or until their regular appropriations are enacted. In recent years, continuing resolutions have become more of a reality in the congressional budget and appropriations cycle. This creates a substantial level of uncertainty for federal agencies to operate and manage programs effectively. Congress has relied on enacting continuing resolutions to keep the federal government operating. These bills are commonly known as omnibus budget reconciliation acts (OBRA).

Executive Branch Budget Development and Control

Federal agencies begin budget development approximately 18 months in advance of a fiscal year (October 1 to September 30). Agency requests are reviewed and budget decisions made based on the president's fiscal policy, the resources needed to carry out the programs, Congressional budget authority, total outlays, current receipts, and anticipated economic conditions.

During the formation of the budget, there is a continual exchange of information, proposals, evaluations, and policy decisions between the president, Office of Management and Budget (OMB), federal departments, and their agencies. Budget decisions are based upon and influenced by the results of previous budgets, including those currently in use by federal agencies and the previous year's budget being considered by Congress. Final decisions on budget requests are generally completed by the end of the calendar year that precedes the upcoming fiscal year (December for the fiscal year that begins the following October).

The president's proposed financial plan indicates administration priorities for the federal government. This budget process operates in the context of a multi-year planning system that covers several years into the future as a long-range plan to accomplish the fiscal and programmatic goals of the president's administration. By law, the president is to submit the budget to Congress on or before the Monday that follows January 3 of each year.

Following congressional action on the budget and approval of annual appropriations bills, the president signs the budget into law. The budget serves as the basis for financing operations of the agencies of the federal government. The OMB distributes appropriations to each agency by time periods and activities (line items) to ensure effective use of resources and guard against the need for additional program funding.

Regulatory Responsibilities

When the House and Senate have passed legislation, it is sent to the president to be signed into law. Writing to the president to urge him to sign a piece of desirable legislation or to veto legislation that is opposed is another important responsibility in advocacy. When the president vetoes a piece of legislation it is sent back to Congress. The House and Senate must act with a two thirds majority vote to override a presidential veto.

After legislation is passed and signed by the president, or a veto overridden, implementation and enforcement of laws becomes the responsibility of the executive branch department and agency to which it is assigned. In the federal agencies, appointed and career civil servants (or bureaucrats) prepare regulations or rules to more specifically define the requirements to implement a law. Regulations are designed to carry out the "intent of Congress" and have the power of laws. This may or may not include establishment of fines or other punitive measures for non-compliance. Whether or not regulations precisely carry out the legislative intent may depend on how well the philosophy and policies of Congress and the administering agencies agree. When the president and the majority of the members of both houses of Congress are the same political party, there is usually some degree of unanimity. When they are of opposing parties there may be some discrepancies noted in the proposed rules and guidance materials.

Regulations for federal programs are compiled in the *Code of Federal Regulations* (CFR), which is revised and published each year. Interim regulatory activity is proposed in the *Federal Register*. The CFR and the *Federal Register* generally are readily accessible on the Internet at www.gpoaccess.gov/cfr/index.html (CFR) and www.gpoaccess.gov/fr/index.html (*Federal Register*).

Understand the *Federal Register*

The *Federal Register* is the source for meeting announcements, requests for proposals for special program funding and federal grants, and notices for advanced rulemaking, proposed rules, and final rules for federal programs. The *Federal Register* is published daily. Items in the *Federal Register* fall into categories relative to the action to be taken. A notice generally announces meetings or other items under agency review. An advanced notice of proposed rulemaking (ANPR) announces an action that an agency is considering. Such notices precede the issuance of a proposed rule, and the response to an ANPR can affect the form and substance of a proposed rule. A proposed rule declares an agency's intention to issue new regulations or to revise existing regulations. Both ANPR and proposed rules invite public comment on the content of the proposal. Comment periods range from 30 to 90 days, at the discretion of the agency. Usually, the more complex the proposal, the longer the comment period.

When proposed program regulations are revised and approved by the agency and administration, a final rule is published. A final rule carries an effective date that can range from its time of publication to up to several years into the future. For example, federal food labeling regulations are implemented on a "uniform effective date," which is generally at the end of 2-year cycle following the year in which the final rule became effective (time from publication of final rule to effective date could be from 25 months up to 47 months). Alternatively, implementation dates can align with the beginning of a fiscal or calendar year.

Petitions are also published in the *Federal Register*. A petition is a formal request by an individual, organization, or firm to a department or agency that a certain action be taken or not taken, or that a regulation or order be established, revoked, or revised. In the public health arena, most petitions are submitted to the Food and Drug Administration for regulation of food ingredients, food labeling policy, and nutrient content and health claims.

Respond to Proposed Rules

Because regulations promulgated by federal agencies have the force of law, commenting on proposals or other items in the *Federal Register* is equally important as communicating views to Congress about specific pieces of legislation. Involvement in the federal regulatory development process is essential to speak out for public health nutrition.

Public health nutritionists must develop an ongoing process to monitor activity of administrative agencies related to food and nutrition programs. First, it is necessary to identify the agencies involved. At the federal level, the primary agencies are the Department of Health and Human Services (DHHS) and the Department of Agriculture (USDA). Public health professionals should establish a network of contacts to ensure that they are aware of current and upcoming administrative proposals. Establishing relationships involves networking at the federal level.

When responding to a regulatory proposal, it is critical to accurately identify it. Profession and interest in the proposal should identify the respondent. Comments should be indexed to specific regulatory citations and should be concise, targeted, and when possible, referenced. Because regulations may influence program plans and content, staff qualifications, services provided, budget use, and reporting requirements, proposed rules should be carefully studied and analyzed for cost effectiveness and potential overload of red tape and paperwork.

FEDERAL AGENCIES AND PROGRAMS

To speak out effectively, the public health nutritionist should understand the role of the agency or department assigned responsibility for administering food, nutrition, and health legislation. In carrying out their responsibilities, agencies usually offer consultation, training, and guidance materials that are useful in understanding how to implement the laws and regulations. Becoming acquainted with agency responsibilities and staff, particularly at the federal level, facilitates program implementation and helps resolve misunderstandings about laws and regulations.

Department of Health and Human Services

The Department of Health and Human Services (DHHS) is the United States government's principal agency for protecting the health of all Americans and providing essential human services, especially for those who are least able to help themselves. The department oversees more than 300 programs, covering a wide spectrum of activities ranging from research to food and drug regulation and health care (Medicare and Medicaid). DHHS receives approximately 25% of federal budget outlays. The Social Security Administration was made an independent federal agency in 1995. Before that time, DHHS was the second largest federal department behind the Department of Defense.

Public Health Service (PHS)

The chief Public Health Service (PHS) officer is the Surgeon General of the United States (www.surgeongeneral.gov). The Surgeon General reports directly to the Secretary of the Department of Health and Human Services. Numerous agencies and units compose the PHS. The Office of Disease Prevention and Health Promotion (ODPHP; www.odphp.osophs.dhhs.gov) provides management and oversight to many federal health promotion and disease prevention programs. Key projects include coordination of development of the *Dietary Guidelines for Americans* (along with the U.S. Department of Agriculture; www.health.gov/dietaryguide lines/), updated every five years. Other projects include the *Healthy People* project, currently working on the *2010 Health Objectives for the Nation*. The Food and Drug Administration (FDA; www.fda.gov) is responsible for the regulation of food, drugs, cosmetics, biologics, veterinary medicines, medical devices, and other products. FDA regulates food labeling, including nutrition labeling on food products and nutrient content and health claims on food labels (www.cfsan.fda.gov/label.html).

Several of the National Institutes of Health (NIH; www.nih.gov) have responsibilities for nutrition research and education programs.

The National Cholesterol Education Program (NCEP) and the National High Blood Pressure Education Program are administered by the National Heart, Lung, and Blood Institute (www.nhlbi.nih.gov). The National Cancer Institute (NCI; www.nci.nih.gov) is developing its leadership in research on innovative nutrition education interventions for cancer prevention. NCI also supports the "5 a Day for Better Health Program" encouraging Americans to increase consumption of fruits and vegetables (www.5aday.gov/homepage/index_content.html).

The NIH Office of Dietary Supplements (www.dietary-supplements.info.nih.gov/) explores the role of dietary supplements in maintaining health and preventing chronic diseases. It also supports and coordinates government research on dietary supplements and advises all DHHS agencies about dietary supplements.

The Centers for Disease Control and Prevention (CDC; www.cdc.gov) administers national prevention programs, nutrition monitoring, and other nutrition surveillance activities of DHHS. In 1987, the National Center for Health Statistics (NCHS; www.cdc.gov/nchs/) became a center within CDC. NCHS administers the continuous *National Health and Nutrition Examination Survey* (NHANES; www.cdc.gov/nchs/nhanes.htm) and publication and dissemination of the data (jointly with USDA). In 1988, the Centers for Chronic Disease and Health Promotion and Education were combined to form the Center for Chronic Disease Prevention and Health Promotion (CCDPHP; www.cdc.gov/nccdphp/). The preventive health services block grant, which covers screening and referral for many chronic diseases, is administered by CCDPHP. In 1988, Congress proposed the addition of cholesterol screening to the items currently covered in the preventive health services block grant. The Division of Nutrition and Physical Activity (www.cdc.govnccdphp/bb_nutrition/index.htm) has responsibility for pediatric and maternity surveillance programs, the nutrition content of the *Behavioral Risk Factor Survey* (BRFS), and support of national and state programs for obesity prevention and promotion of physical activity.

The Health Resources and Services Administration (HRSA; www.hrsa.gov) serves to improve and expand access to quality health care by assuring the availability of quality health care to low-income, uninsured, isolated, vulnerable, and special needs populations and that the care meets their unique health care needs. HRSA programs implement strategies to eliminate health disparities and barriers to care, to assure quality care, and to improve public health and health care. HRSA's maternal and child health services and training programs are administered through the Maternal and Child Health Bureau (MCHB; www.mchb.hrsa.gov) governed by Title V of the Social Security Act. Traditionally this agency has funded public health nutrition programs at the state and local level. MCHB provides expert consultation, training materials, and funding for continuing education and graduate training of public health nutritionists. HRSA also administers community health centers, migrant health, allied health professions training programs, and HIV/AIDS services under the Ryan White Preventive Care Act (www.hab.hrsa.gov).

Administration on Aging

The Administration on Aging (AoA; www.aoa.gov) administers programs authorized by the Older Americans Act (OAA). For over 35 years, the AoA has provided home and community-based services to millions of older Americans. The AoA administers congregate and home-delivered meals programs under Title III of the OAA. In addition to meals, many programs provide nutrition education and counseling for older Americans (see Chapter 10).

Administration for Children and Families

The Administration for Children and Families (ACF; www.acf.dhhs.gov) administers the Head Start program (www.acf.hhs.gov/programs/hsb/about/index.htm) that provides food and nutrition education for young children. The health component of Head Start, including nutrition, is administered through a cooperative agreement between HRSA and PHS of DHHS.

Centers for Medicare and Medicaid Services (CMS)

The Centers for Medicare and Medicaid Services (CMS; formerly the Health Care Financing Administration; www.cms.hhs.gov) administers the Medicare (Title XVIII, Social Security Act) and Medicaid (Title XIX, Social Security Act) programs. The Medicare program provides coverage for health services for older Americans and individuals on disability. Medicare regulations cover nutrition and dietetic services in hospitals, nursing homes, home health agencies, hospices, and other facilities. The Medicaid program, administered through state agencies, provides health services for economically disadvantaged individuals and the disabled. Medicaid regulates the Early Periodic Screening, Diagnosis, and Treatment Program (EPSDT), providing comprehensive and preventive child health services up to 21 years of age (www.cms.hhs.gov/medicaid/epsdt/default.asp).

Coverage of nutrition services under Medicare by qualified personnel became a reality in 2000. The Medicare program added medical nutrition therapy (MNT) for individuals with diabetes and kidney disease. This program expansion was championed by the American Dietetic Association and efforts continue to expand Medicare MNT coverage for cardiovascular disease and other conditions for which nutrition services and intervention has been determined to improve health outcomes and be cost effective. The Medicare prescription drug law, passed in 2003, sets the stage for coordinated disease management services that could include evidence-based MNT for a variety of nutrition-related conditions.

U.S. Department of Agriculture

The U.S. Department of Agriculture (USDA; www.usda.gov) has responsibility for food assistance and agriculture promotion and support programs. The primary USDA agency that covers most food, nutrition, and public health programs is the Food and Nutrition Services (FNS; www.fns.usda.gov/fns/). Other human nutrition activities with a public health focus or relevance are located within the Agriculture Research Service's human nutrition research group (www.ars.usda.gov/News/docs.htm?docid=1276). ARS food and nutrition programs cover research, food, and nutrient databases (www.barc.usda.gov/bhnrc/foodsurvey/home.htm), and nutrition monitoring surveys (along with DHHS' NCHS). Regulation, safety, and labeling of meat and poultry products are led by the Food Safety Inspection Service (FSIS; www.fsis.usda.gov).

Food and Nutrition Service (FNS)

FNS administers the National School Lunch Program (www.fns.usda.gov/cnd/Lunch/default.htm), National School Breakfast Program (www.fns.usda.gov/cnd/Breakfast/Default.htm), Summer Food Service Program (www.fns.usda.gov/cnd/Summer/Default.htm), Child and Adult Care Food Program (www.fns.usda.gov/cnd/Care/CACFP/cacfphome.htm), Special Supplemental Nutrition Program for Women Infants and Children (WIC; www.fns.usda.gov/wic/), Commodity Supplemental Food Program (www.fns.usda.gov/fdd/), and the Nutrition Education and Training Program (NETP). These programs provide a critical food security safety net that offers both food and nutrition education and information to low-income individuals. The WIC Program is the nation's largest public health nutrition program delivering supplemental food, nutrition education, and health care.

The Center for Nutrition Policy and Promotion (www.cnpp.usda.gov) supports USDA's role in development of the *Dietary Guidelines for Americans* and the Food Guidance System (currently the Food Guide Pyramid; www.usda.gov/cnpp/pyramid.html) and the Healthy Eating Index (www.usda.gov/cnpp/healthyeating.html). These programs and educational tools are the cornerstone for national nutrition education efforts and nutrition policy across the federal government.

Department of Education

The Department of Education (www.ed.gov) has responsibility for educational programs for children with special needs. Public Law 99-457, Education of the Handicapped Amendments of 1986, integrates health services into early intervention programs for infants and children with special needs. Nutrition services are listed as a required health service, and dietitians and nutritionists are designated as part of the early intervention team.

Department of the Treasury

The Bureau of Alcohol, Tobacco and Firearms (www.atf.gov) regulates the sale and labeling of alcoholic beverages (e.g., "lite" beer labeling). The Federal Trade Commission (FTC; www.ftc.gov) regulates the content of food and dietary supplement advertising and truth in labeling laws.

JUDICIAL BRANCH

Involvement with the judicial branch generally occurs only when legislative and regulatory options have been exhausted and legal authority or procedures have been violated. Utilizing the judicial system should never be attempted without first obtaining legal counsel and thoroughly weighing financial and time commitments against the outcome of the process.

Over the years, judicial activity in federal courts and the Supreme Court related to nutrition and public health programs has been related to class action lawsuits to force the release of program funding impounded by the president (e.g., WIC funding).

SPEAK OUT TO ADVOCATE FOR
PUBLIC HEALTH NUTRITION

Many agencies support their professional staff in advocating policies, legislation, and regulations that promote and protect the public health. Such activities should always be conducted in compliance with agency policy. Speaking out on food, nutrition, and public health issues should also conform with professional and ethical standards of conduct, be nonpartisan, and without personal conflict of interest.

As responsible citizens, public health nutrition professionals should study, discuss, and speak on current issues related to the public's health, particularly those related to food and nutrition policy. This can be accomplished by participating in coalitions, public forums, town meetings, field hearings, and other legislative and regulatory inquiries at the local level.

Public health personnel should study the qualifications and interests of candidates running for local, state, and federal public office. Informed voters in all primary and general elections can help to put into office those candidates whose views support public health. As a concerned citizen, it is important to write, telephone, e-mail, or make personal contacts with candidates and elected officials to present expert views.

When managing federally funded programs, public health nutritionists, with their administrator's approval, might invite their congressman (or staff) or local elected officials to visit and observe nutrition programs in action. This provides elected officials with firsthand information on the benefits of the program to their constituents and lets the officials observe the needs and problems that exist. Media coverage adds to the interest and visibility of the official's visit.

Agency policy may dictate whether advocacy activities can be undertaken as an agency representative on official time, or whether they must be done as an informed citizen on personal time, using a home address on correspondence. If agency policy discourages active advocacy efforts, it is possible to work "behind the scenes" through the legislative efforts of professional organizations, church groups, and issue-oriented citizen lobbies. For example, The American Dietetic Association has established a grassroots network and provides training at its annual public policy workshops. The American Public Health Association issues "action alerts" to members regarding national public health legislation and regulation. The Society for Nutrition Education develops members' skills in advocacy at the national and grassroots level through forums at their annual conference and their advisory committee for public policy.

Lobbying

The process by which individuals or groups advocate for passage or to block passage of legislation is popularly called "lobbying." In many ways, it is similar to the way in which nutritionists attempt to influence others through education, promote a program in the community, or secure support for budget from agency administration.

In the democratic process, shaping policy decisions through lobbying is a privilege and a right. Many people think that one voice makes no difference in the legislative halls. The reality is that it is the process or strategy by which that one voice presents an issue that makes the difference between success and failure.

Effective lobbying correctly targets appropriate information. Each issue must be approached differently, and no one strategy always works. The degree to which lobbying is effective depends as much upon the method of communication as the content of the proposal. Effective communication with busy officials is concise, convincing, consistent, and cordial. Communication with members of Congress and other elected officials can be through personal contacts, letters, e-mail, or by telephone. Communication with elected officials can express a viewpoint on an issue or obtain information about the official's stand on an issue or voting record. Care should be taken to accurately present evidence-based analysis and science to support each issue under discussion.

Visiting an elected official's office benefits both the official and the constituent. In Washington, visits are generally handled by congressional staff, but may occur with the member of Congress. When Congress is in recess, visits can also be scheduled when members of Congress are in their home state or district. Meetings are usually brief because of the busy schedules of members of Congress and their staff. An appointment should always be made in advance by phone or in writing. The time of the meeting should be confirmed shortly before it is scheduled.

The meeting begins with an introduction, stating one's name, profession, and professional affiliation. Conversation should clearly and concisely state the purpose of the meeting and its content. It is wise to speak from notes that highlight the pertinent points. Leaving additional supporting material with the member or staff is recommended. After the meeting, there should always be a follow-up letter summarizing the discussion and thanking the member or staff for taking the time to discuss an issue.

Corresponding with congressmen and other elected officials helps establish ongoing dialogue to promote nutrition issues. In congressional offices, correspondence is entered on a tracking system by issue. Frequent letters related to legislative proposals provides a record of the opinions of constituents. Letters should be limited to one page. The letter should open by identifying the issue and the writer's professional affiliation. The body should identify the writer's position on the issue and include brief statements in support or opposition. When in opposition, an alternative proposal should always be offered. The writer should close the letter by offering to provide additional information about the topic.

When time is critical, telephone calls and e-mail are effective strategies. These are especially useful when an immediate vote is expected on a piece of legislation. Phone calls can be made to the legislator's Washington or home office.

Brevity is critical when communicating by telephone or e-mail. The caller should identify the legislation, the position, then make one or two points that may explain the issue and its relevance to the constituency. Phone numbers of Congressional offices can be obtained by calling the capitol switchboard at (202) 224-3121. E-mail addresses for congressional offices are found on both the House and Senate Web sites (www.house.gov and www.senate.gov).

Establishing an open line of communication through a variety of channels will establish the public health nutritionist as an interested constituent and as a nutrition expert in public health issues. By taking the time to communicate with officials, the nutritionist's message will be heard. Over time, effective presentations positively affect food, nutrition, and public health policy.

Testify at Hearings, Town Meetings, and Other Forums

Getting to know legislators and other elected officials by frequent contact will promote invitations to testify at hearings. Testifying at hearings before Congressional committees or regulatory bodies provide public health nutritionists with the opportunity for expert input that can influence the outcome as well as authorization or appropriations levels of legislation. Congressional hearings are generally conducted in Washington, but field hearings may be held at sites where there may be a particular problem or concern to members of Congress.

Testifying generally means presenting information in both oral and written form. While both oral and written remarks become part of a hearing report, oral remarks should highlight the written testimony. Testimony on legislation is generally conceptual in nature. A 5-minute time limit is usually provided for each individual testifying. One page of double-spaced typewritten text can usually be delivered in one minute. Oral and written testimony must be well researched and adhere to the rules of communication with elected officials. Both content and style of presentation are equally important. Testimony should include the following:

- Introduction—Identification of the speaker, group represented, and proposal being addressed.
- Position on the issue—Clear statements supporting the proposal, supporting the proposal with modification, or opposing the proposal.
- Explanation of proposal—Elaboration of position and issues within the proposal in nontechnical language. References to written testimony or supporting documents are appropriate.
- Summary—Restatement of position and recommendations. If testimony partially supports or opposes a proposal, an alternative is suggested.

To conclude the testimony, the official conducting the hearing should be thanked and an offer made to answer questions and provide additional information. The record for congressional hearings is open for 10 working days. During that time additional supporting documents can be provided to the committee conducting the hearing. Following the hearing, the person testifying usually will be provided with a copy of transcribed remarks to edit for accuracy.

Sometimes organizations or agencies will be asked to supply testimony on a specific subject. It is important that the most knowledgeable person be selected so that questions can be handled with ease. This may not always be the organization's leader or agency director. The public health nutritionist needs to maintain a file of experts on specific topics to suggest at such times.

Cultivate Elected Officials

Becoming involved in political campaigns is another effective way to influence nutrition policy decisions. Campaign involvement may not lead directly to favorable outcomes for public health nutrition programs, but it creates a favorable impression on public officials. Involvement in campaigns provides an opportunity to meet and talk with the elected officials and provides for improved accessibility.

Working with political action committees, (PACs), provides another way to become involved in political campaigns. PACs represent a group of volunteers who join to support candidates of their choice. By collecting funds from individuals and pooling them, PACs contribute directly to candidates or political fundraisers. They sponsor events or finance printing and/or mailing of campaign materials. Although PACs frequently are criticized for "buying" votes or promoting single issues, they remain an important part of the political process of accessing and generating interest in nutrition issues.

Public health nutrition professionals can seek appointments to federal, state, and local boards and commissions. Public health nutritionists should seek appointments to boards of health, special committees of legislatures, and local and national commissions.

Build Coalitions to Promote Nutrition Programs

Coalitions supplement involvement in the legislative and regulatory process. When building a coalition to achieve a public policy goal, it is critical to not only work with those who wholeheartedly support the same issues but also with groups that have differing views. In conferring with colleagues interested in the public policy proposal, the following questions might be asked.

- Who are the key players?
- What groups are allied with similar views?
- What groups are expressing opposing views?
- What expertise is necessary to ensure a balanced discussion of issues?

A coalition can be established for a single issue or be established permanently to address issues over time. Coalitions are effective because advocacy work can be shared among several members of the coalition according to expertise, contacts, and time commitment. By joining forces in coalitions, an impressive number of diverse constituents can work together demonstrating strength and unity to policy makers.

POINTS TO PONDER

- Faced with drastic budget cuts in public programs, what rationales and explanations can be proposed to influence congressional budget assumptions and program appropriations?
- What types of coalitions could be joined to promote public health and nutrition programs?
- How can clients who benefit from a federally funded program be mobilized to work for its continuation or expansion?

HELPFUL WEB SITES

Administration for Children and Families: www.acf.dhhs.gov
Bureau of Alcohol, Tobacco, Firearms, and Explosives: www.atf.gov
Center for Food Safety and Applied Nutrition:
   www.cfsan.fda.gov/label.html
CDC: www.cdc.gov
CDC Chronic Disease Prevention: www.cdc.gov/nccdphp
CDC National Center for Health Statistics: www.cdc.gov/nchs
CDC National Health and Nutrition Examination Survey:
   www.cdc.gov/nchs/nhanes.htm
Code of Federal Regulations (CFR): www.gpoaccess.gov/cfr/index.html
Dietary Guidelines for Americans: www.health.gov/dietaryguidelines
Eat 5 to 9 A Day: www.5aday.gov/homepage/index_content.html
Federal Register (FR): www.gpoaccess.gov/fr/index.htm
Federal Trade Commission: www.ftc.gov
Food and Drug Administration: www.fda.gov
National Institutes of Health: www.nih.gov
National Heart, Lung, and Blood Institute: www.nhlbi.nih.gov
National Cancer Institute: www.nci.nih.gov (www.cancer.gov)
Office of Disease Prevention and Health Promotion:
   www.odphp.osophs.dhhs.gov
Office of Dietary Supplements: dietary-supplements.info.nih.gov
U.S. Administration on Aging (AoA): www.aoa.gov
      Head Start Bureau: www.acf.hhs.gov/programs/hsb/about/index.htm
U.S. Department of Agriculture: www.usda.gov

U.S. Department of Agriculture — Agricultural Research Service:
www.arrs.usda.gov
  Human Nutrition Reseach: www.ars.usda.gov/News/docs.htm?docid=1276
  Food Surveys: www.barc.usda.gov/bhnrc/foodsurvey/home.htm
U.S. Department of Agriculture – Food Safety and Inspection Service:
www.fsis.usda.gov
U.S. Department of Agriculture — Food and Nutrition Service:
www.fns.usda.gov
  National School Lunch Program:
  www.fns.usda.gov/cnd/Lunch/default.htm
  School Breakfast Program:
  www.fns.usda.gov/cnd/Breakfast/default.htm
  Summer Food Service Program:
  www.fns.usda.gov/cnd/Summer/default.htm
  Child and Adult Care Food Program:
  www.fns.usda.gov/cnd/Care/CACFP/cacfphome.htm
  Women, Infants, and Children: www.fns.usda.gov/wic
  Food Distribution Programs: www.fns.usda.gov/fdd
**U.S. Department of Agriculture – Center for Nutrition Policy and
Promotion:** www.usda.gov/cnpp
  The Original Food Guide Pyramid: www.usda.gov/cnpp/pyramid.html
  USDA Healthy Eating Index: www.usda.gov/cnpp/healthyeating.html
U.S. Department of Education: www.ed.gov
**U.S. Department of Health and Human Services —Health Resources
and Services Administration:** www.hrsa.gov
  Maternal and Child Health Bureau: www.mchb.hrsa.gov
**U.S. Department of Health and Human Services — Centers for
Medicare & Medicaid Services:** www.cms.hhs.gov
  EPSDT Dental Coverage: www.cms.hhs.gov/EPSDTDentalCoverage
U.S. House of Representatives: www.house.gov
U.S. Senate: www.senate.gov

BIBLIOGRAPHY

Earl R. In Kaufman M, ed. *Nutrition in Public Health, A Handbook for Developing Programs and Resources.* "Influencing Federal Health and Nutrition Legislation and Regulations." Rockville, MD: Aspen Publishers Inc; 1990:7–136.

Chapter 8

Nurture Women, Infants, and Children

Alice J. Lenihan and Diane R. Wilson

Reader Objectives

- List the federal laws enacted to provide health care services to women and children.
- Describe why nutrition services are essential in maternal and child health (MCH) programs.
- Discuss nutrition issues for women, infants, and children.
- Discuss current issues in and the nutritional support of breast-feeding women.
- List and describe services meeting nutritional needs of the MCH population.
- Describe the roles of public health nutrition MCH service personnel.
- Identify opportunities for nutrition services in organizations offering MCH services.

MATERNAL AND CHILD HEALTH PROGRAMS— A HISTORICAL PERSPECTIVE

A nation's health is often judged by the health status of its mothers and children. Maternal and infant health has been improving in the United States as reflected by a decreasing trend in both the country's infant mortality and adolescent pregnancy rates. Decreases reflect the efforts of a number of public health and educational programs, improved access to health care, early identification of risks, and improved technology and health care enhancements.

The infant mortality rate in 1990 was 8.9 per 1000 live births. In 2001, the rate was at an all time low of 6.8. In 2002 it increased to 7.9 and was attributed to an

163

increase in the number of infants born weighing less than 750 grams (1 lb., 10.5 oz.) to women ages 10 to 34 years of age.[1,2] The overall US adolescent pregnancy rate declined 17% between 1990 and 1996.[3,4] Despite these declines in infant mortality and teenage pregnancies within the past 10 years, the US rate is still higher than other industrialized countries.[5] As a result, maternal and child health continues to be a national priority.

The high rates of maternal and infant morbidity and mortality in the early 1900s led Congress to pass the Maternity and Infancy Act. This act was in effect from 1920 to 1929. Beginning in 1935, Title V of the Social Security Act provided formula grants to states for maternal and child health as well as crippled children's services. Initially legislation was administered by the Children's Bureau of the Department of Labor. In the 1960s, however, the Department of Health and Human Services took over the administration and began to promote and improve maternal and child health services across the nation.

Over the years, Title V has supported MCH services including the development and provision of guidance materials, technical assistance to local and state programs, and special projects targeted to specific MCH population group needs. Research, and professional training, also included training for public health nutritionists. Now, over 70 years later, Title V remains the main federal program that targets the improvement of health for the nation's mothers and children.

In 2000, *Healthy People 2010: Objectives for Improving Health*, the nation's health plan, was published.[6] Several of the plan's key objectives for the MCH population are included and discussed later in this chapter. Each objective in this national plan offers opportunities for public health nutritionists in program planning and development, nutrition education, and policy development.

Specific objectives include:

- Increase the proportion of pregnant women who receive early and adequate prenatal care.
- Increase the proportion of pregnant women who attend a series of prepared childbirth classes.
- Reduce low birth weight and very low birth weight.
- Reduce preterm births.
- Increase the proportion of mothers who achieve a recommended weight gain during their pregnancies.
- Reduce the occurrence of spina bifida and other neural tube defects.
- Increase the proportion of women who begin their pregnancy with an optimum folic acid level.
- Increase the proportion of mothers who breast-feed.[7]

Each of these objectives relates to a woman's optimal nutritional health. Providing nutrition services to women in the childbearing years is critical to improving pregnancy outcome and preventing low birth weight, disabilities, and birth defects. Public health nutritionists need to seek opportunities to reach women in their childbearing years and promote good preconception nutritional status. Family planning programs, exercise and health programs for young adults, and other community-based programs and organizations are sites where women in the childbearing years may be found.

Education for women should emphasize the following:

- Prepregnancy weight recommendations
- Appropriate weight gain during pregnancy
- Eating a variety of foods following the *Dietary Guidelines for Americans 2005*
- Vitamin and mineral supplementation
- Avoidance of alcohol, tobacco, and use of harmful substances

To learn more, go to www.healthypeople.gov/Document/HTML/Volume2/16MICH.htm.

Maternal and Child Health Bureau

The nation's lead agency for promoting and improving the health of mothers and children is the Maternal and Child Health Bureau (MCHB) located within the Health Resource Service Administration of the US Department of Health and Human Services. MCHB administers Title V funds, provides national leadership, and works with public and private partners to strengthen the MCH infrastructure. Partners include state and local health departments, community health centers, professional organizations, academic institutions, and other groups and organizations to assure the availability and use of health care services to the MCH population.

MCHB uses a pyramid to describe core public health services for the MCH population. Figure 8–1 illustrates the framework for MCH services.[8] To learn more, go to www.mchb.hrsa.gov.

MCHB administers seven major programs:

- Maternal and Child Health Services Block Grant Program
- Healthy Start Initiative
- Emergency Medical Services for Children Program
- Abstinence Education Program
- Traumatic Brain Injury Program
- Universal Newborn Hearing Screening Program
- Poison Control Centers Program

The two key programs where public health nutrition personnel are involved as integral members of the health care planning and service delivery teams are the Maternal and Child Health Services block grants and the Healthy Start Initiative.

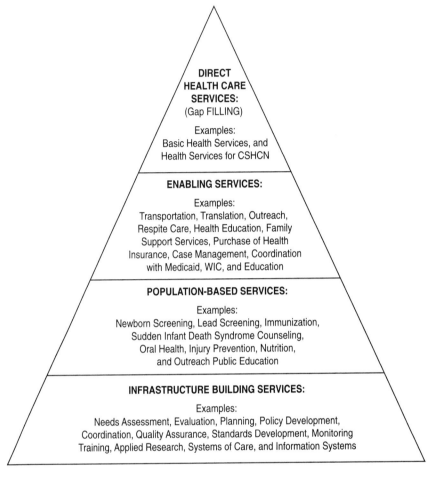

Figure 8–1 Core Public Health Services for MCH Population. Source: Maternal and Child Health Bureau. Rockville, MD: U.S. Department of Health and Human Services, Health Resources and Services Administration, Maternal and Child Health Bureau.

MCH Block Grants

In 1981, changes in Title V resulted in the discontinuation of MCH formula grants to states and the creation of the MCH Services Block Grant Program. This program consolidated former categorical MCH programs into a single grant to enable states to more effectively meet the needs of mothers, children, and their families.

The MCH Block Grant Program funds are also available for projects of regional and national significance (SPRANS), community-integrated service systems (CISS) projects, and professional training and research.

SPRANS

SPRANS grants support innovative MCH research, training, genetic services, and maternal and child health improvement projects. One example of a SPRANS grant initiative involved in nutrition care is Partners in Program Planning for Adolescent Health (PIPPAH). The American Dietetic Association is the lead organization for PIPPAH. The American Medical Association, the American Bar Association, the American Psychological Association, the American Nursing Association, and other organizations are partners with the American Dietetic Association working to fulfill PIPPAH's primary objective of improving adolescent health.

The goals of this partnership are to accomplish the following:

- Develop strategies among the partners to improve adolescent health.
- Develop strategies to create and improve the systems that serve adolescents and their families.
- Strengthen organizational commitment to focus on adolescent health.
- Enhance communication among disciplines and training needs in the area of adolescent health.
- Encourage coordination and collaboration across disciplines and professional organizations.[9]

CISS

The Community Integrated Service Systems (CISS) grant program funds projects to develop and expand integrated health, education, and social services for mothers and children at the community level. An example of a CISS project is the Washington State Department of Health's Children with Special Health Care Needs Program (CSHCN). This project promotes integrated systems of care to assure that children with special health care needs have the opportunity to achieve the healthiest lives possible and develop to their full potential. Children served by CSHCN have physical, behavioral, or emotional conditions that require health and related services beyond those required for the general child population.

The program has developed state level leadership in three key areas:

- Identifying and addressing health system issues that impact the CSHCN population
- Working with families and other leaders to influence planning, priority setting, and policy development
- Supporting community efforts in assuring the health and well-being of children with special health care needs and their families[10]

Nutrition for Children with Special Health Care Needs in Washington state is a partnership between the Special Health Care Needs Program in the state's Department of Health and the University of Washington in Seattle. Information is available through this program on current nutrition issues for the pediatric special needs population, available programs and services, resources, publications, education and training, and links to related Web sites. To learn more, go to www.depts.washington.edu/cshcnnut/.

Healthy Start Initiative

The Healthy Start Initiative was authorized under the Public Health Services Act in 1991 and reauthorized by Congress as part of the Children's Health Act of 2000. The premise of this program is that communities can best develop and implement the necessary steps needed to eliminate those factors contributing to infant mortality, low birth weight, and racial disparities in perinatal outcomes. Over 96 Healthy Start projects are currently funded.

These are the common principles for every Healthy Start project:

- Innovations in service delivery
- Community commitment and involvement
- Personal responsibility demonstrated by expectant parents
- Integration of health and social services
- Multiagency participation
- Increased access to care
- Public education[11]

Each Healthy Start project is mandated to form a coalition of women, their families, neighborhood residents, health care providers, social service agencies, faith-based representatives, and the business community to work together to address local perinatal health issues. These issues include the following:

- Providing adequate prenatal care
- Promoting positive prenatal health behaviors
- Meeting basic health needs (nutrition, housing, psychosocial support)
- Enabling client empowerment[12]

The Healthy Start projects offer opportunities for public health nutritionists to collaborate in planning community-based services and the provision of education and referrals. To learn more, go to www.healthystartassoc.org.

MCH Training Program

The MCHB, through its MCH Training Program, funds public and private nonprofit colleges and universities to provide leadership training in maternal and child health. The aim of these training programs is to improve the knowledge of health needs and needed services and to improve the effectiveness of MCH services. Training grants are available to promote public health nutrition services for children, adolescents, women, and families. Funded programs also support graduate training for public health nutritionists and dietitians, fellowships, and short-term training focused on public health and clinical issues in maternal and child nutrition. Focused areas for education and training include maternal and pediatric nutrition, neonatal nutrition, MCH leadership training, and nutrition services for children with special health care needs. To learn more, go to www.mchb.hrsa.gov/training/.

National Center for Education in Maternal and Child Health

In 1982, Georgetown University established the National Center for Education in Maternal and Child Health (NCEMCH). The center provides national leadership in the following efforts:

- Launch national initiatives involving multiple partners.
- Develop and disseminate culturally competent child health and development materials for families and professionals.
- Provide a virtual MCH library of state-of-the-art knowledge and information for health professionals, educators, researchers, policy makers, service providers, business leaders, families, and the public.[13]

The center offers numerous resources for public health nutrition personnel. For example, the center's library contains a knowledge path of current and high-quality resources on the identification, prevention, management, and treatment of overweight and obesity in children and adolescents.

To learn more, go to www.mchlibrary.info/KnowledgePaths/kp_overweight. html.

Children with Special Health Care Needs

Children with special health care needs (CSHCN) are defined as those who have or are at increased risk for a chronic physical, developmental, behavioral, or emotional condition and who also require health and related services of a type or amount beyond that required by children generally.[14] These groups comprise nearly 20% of all children but accounts for 45% of the total expenditures for all children's health care.[15]

State health agencies have been providing services to children with special health care needs through Title V funding since 1935. Until the 1970s, most state programs were called crippled children's services (CCS) and focused on identifying and providing diagnosis, treatment, and ongoing care to children with orthopedic problems.[16] A gradual expansion of CCS state programs since then has resulted in the provision of health and related services to children with other chronic health conditions, developmental disabilities, sensory impairments, and other special health care needs. The term *crippled children* was replaced by the more appropriate term *children with special health care needs.*

In addition to providing direct health care services to eligible children, state CSHCN programs have the responsibility to improve the quality and responsiveness of the overall health care system for these children. In 1989, Congress amended Title V to require state CSHCN programs to provide and promote family-centered, community-based, coordinated care and to facilitate development of community-based systems of services for children with special health care needs and their families.[17]

Each state has its own financial eligibility criteria, list of services for different populations of children with special health care needs, and funding provisions for health care and related services. The federal Maternal and Child Health Bureau has supported the development of a publication to assist families and health care providers in determining what each state CSHCN program requires and offers. The publication is titled *Directory of State Title V CSHCN Programs: Eligibility Criteria and Scope of Services* and is available online at www.ichp.edu.

To further assist families in understanding and making use of state CSHCN programs, the Families in Title V project, supported through MCHB, provides opportunities for families to contribute to the planning of programs and use of Title V block grants. Materials are available for presentations and workshops to encourage and support family participation.[18] To learn more, go to www.familyvoices.org/.

Department of Agriculture Food and Nutrition Service

The Food and Nutrition Service (FNS) administers the nutrition assistance programs of the US Department of Agriculture. In this role, FNS is responsible for providing children and low-income families with access to foods through its nutrition assistance programs and nutrition education. FNS works in partnership with state and local governments, Indian tribal organizations, nonprofit organizations, and faith-based organizations to fulfill its mission.

Programs administered by FNS include the following:

- National School Lunch Program (see Chapter 4)
- School Breakfast Program (see Chapter 4)
- Special Milk Program
- Special Supplemental Nutrition Program for Women, Infants, and Children (WIC)
- Child and Adult Care Food Program (see Chapter 4)
- Summer Food Service Program (see Chapter 4)
- Team Nutrition

To learn more, go to www.fns.usda.gov/fns/.

Each of the preceding programs is authorized by the Child Nutrition Act of 1966. This legislation recognized:

the demonstrated relationship between food and good nutrition and the capacity of children to develop and learn, based on the years of cumulative successful experience under the National School Lunch Program with its significant contributions in the field of applied nutrition research. It is hereby declared to be the policy of Congress that these efforts shall be extended, expanded, and strengthened under the authority of the Secretary of Agriculture as a measure to safeguard the health and well-being of the Nation's children, and to encourage the domestic consumption of agricultural and other foods, by assisting States, through grants-in-aid and other means, to meet more effectively the nutritional needs of our children.[19]

The most recent reauthorization of this law, PL 108-265, in June of 2004 mandated a number of changes to promote health and nutrition through these FNS-administered programs. A most significant change is the requirement for local school districts to develop local wellness policies, which address nutrition standards and education and physical activity goals.

Opportunities exist for the active participation of public health nutritionists in all Child Nutrition Act programs. This can include policy development, program planning, training of program personnel, direct nutrition intervention services, community resource development, and consultation.

Special Milk Program

The Special Milk Program provides milk to children in schools, child care institutions, and eligible camps that do not participate in other federal child nutrition meal service programs, such as the school lunch or school breakfast programs. This program provides reimbursement to the participating institutions for the milk they serve.

Special Supplemental Nutrition Program for Women, Infants, and Children (WIC Program)

Established in 1972, the Special Supplemental Nutrition Program for Women, Infants, and Children (WIC Program) has grown to be the nation's largest public health nutrition program providing nutrition education and specific supplemental foods to low-income, nutritionally at-risk pregnant and lactating women, infants and children up to five years of age. The WIC Program also provides breast-feeding promotion and referrals to health and social service agencies and programs. It is designed to improve the nutritional status, health, and birth outcomes in low-income populations.

In the Child Nutrition Amendments of 1975, Congress stated that "the purpose of the WIC Program was to provide supplemental nutritious food as an adjunct to good health care during such critical times of growth and development in order to prevent the occurrence of health problems."[20]

The WIC Program operates in all 50 states, the District of Columbia, Puerto Rico, Guam, American Samoa, American Virgin Islands, and 33 Indian tribal organizations. This involves more than 2000 local agencies and over 10,000 clinic sites.[21] In federal fiscal year 2004, the WIC Program served over 7.9 million women, infants, and children.[22]

The WIC Program applicants must meet income, residence, categorical (pregnant or lactating woman, infant, or child up to 5 years of age) eligibility criteria and must have a nutrition risk. Nutrition risk categories include anthropometrical, biochemical, medical, and dietary factors affecting health status and/or predisposing health conditions. Income eligibility is a gross family income of less than 185% of the federal poverty level (see Chapter 4) or participation in the Food Stamp Program, Medicaid, or the Temporary Assistance for Needy Families Program. The categorically eligible woman, infant, or child must reside within the service area of the local WIC agency.

Nutritionists and other health professionals in local agencies certify WIC applicants for eligibility and prescribe the supplemental foods. WIC supplemental foods are selected to meet specific nutrient requirements needed during the critical times of growth and development for the targeted population. Key nutrients in the WIC food package include iron, vitamins A and C, protein, and calcium. WIC supplemental foods include iron-fortified infant and adult cereals, vitamin C-enriched fruit or vegetable juices, eggs, milk, cheese, peanut butter, dried beans and peas, tuna fish, and carrots. If an infant is not breast-fed, iron-fortified infant formula is provided. Program participants receive special WIC checks that are redeemed at participating grocery stores for the authorized foods.

WIC participants receive a minimum of two nutrition education contacts within each 6-month certification period. The purpose of nutrition education is to address the nutritional risk of the participant and to provide information on nutrition, health, and physical activity targeted to the participant's needs. The education is provided in a variety of ways, including classes, one-on-one sessions, computer-assisted nutrition education, Web-based education, and other teaching methods. The WIC Works Resource System contains a number of federal and state nutrition education methods and materials. Resources include WIC Learning Online, Databases, Sharing Center, Learning Center, Topics A-Z, and WIC Talk, a list serve for nutrition and health care professionals providing nutrition services and maternal and child health services. To learn more, go to www.nal.usda.gov/wicworks/.

Within the Sharing Center of the WIC Works Resource Center is information on FIT WIC, a 5-state obesity prevention program. Training manuals and educational materials along with background information about the program are included. The states of California, Kentucky, Vermont, Virginia, and the Inter-Tribal Council of Ari___a developed resources to utilize in the WIC Program to target obesity preve_____ learn more, go to www.nal.usda.gov/wicworks/.

The legislativ_____nt for the WIC Program remains the same today as it did in 19_____m's success has been shown through numerous studies den_____lth outcomes and cost benefits.[23,24,25,26,27] Maternal pa_____nancy improves birth outcomes, infant birth weight_____lted in reduced rates of low and very low birth w_____associated with increased use of preventive c_____ervices.

Integrati_____d child health services as well as othe_____rtunity to enhance services for pr_____anding of the varied programs ar_____egration may mean that progra_____ne time of the WIC or MCH clinic_____ional services, and referrals can be s_____message and services in an integrated v

In additi_____ervices, the Head Start Program also offers _____r service integration. Both the WIC Program an_____re nutrition assessment and offer nutrition educati_____children. There is potential for both programs to shar_____ssessment data, joint referrals for preventive health care, nutri_____.nd staff.

Team Nutrition

Team Nutrition is an integrated, behavior-based, comprehensive system to promote the nutritional health of children in the United States. Team Nutrition includes the following:

- Training and technical assistance for personnel involved in Child Nutrition Act programs to assist in offering meals that look good, taste good, and meet nutrition standards
- Provision of multifaceted, integrated nutrition education for children and their parents to help build skills and behaviors for children to make healthy food and physical activity choices within a healthy lifestyle
- Support for healthy eating and physical activity by including school administrators and other school and community personnel in the Team Nutrition effort

A number of print and electronic resources are available to public health nutrition staff at the Team Nutrition Web site. One example is the Changing the Scene

Action Kit. In collaboration with 16 education and nutrition organizations, Team Nutrition developed this action kit to provide local staff with materials to assist in promoting healthy school environments and allow students to learn and participate in healthy eating and physical activity. To learn more, go to www.fns.usda.gov/tn/.

Team Nutrition also provides grants to states to develop and implement innovative approaches to healthy school environments. A menu of options for creating healthful school nutrition environments in North Carolina was funded by Team Nutrition in 2002. This project was a partnership between the state health department, state department of public instruction, the North Carolina Cooperative Extension Service, and local partners. The following training modules targeting school nutrition were developed:

- Soft Drinks and School-age Children
- Portion Sizes and School-age Children
- 5-a-Day and School-age Children
- Food for Thought
- Winner's Circle—Healthy Dining Program
- Walk to School

The modules focus on trends, effects, and solutions. Implementation training was provided to 50 local teams of school and community partners. Twelve demonstration projects implementing the modules were funded. To learn more, go to www.nutritionnc.com/.

SIGNIFICANT MCH-RELATED FEDERAL LEGISLATION

Education of the Handicapped Act Amendments of 1986

The Education of the Handicapped (EHA) Act Amendments of 1986, PL 99-457, is aimed at children with handicaps and their families. The IDEA 97 Part C (formerly Part H 99-457) program assists states to develop a comprehensive, multidisciplinary, statewide system of early intervention services for infants and toddlers (birth to age 3).

Early intervention services to meet a handicapped infant's or toddler's development needs can include the following services:

- Physical development
- Cognitive development
- Language and speech development
- Psychosocial development
- Self-help skills

An individualized family service plan (IFSP) is prepared for each child and family emphasizing case management and community-based support.

Public health nutritionists are among the qualified personnel named in the legislation to serve children and their families in this program.

Individuals with Disabilities Education Act

In 1990, PL 99-457 was reauthorized and became the Individuals with Disabilities Education Act (IDEA), PL 101-476. IDEA guarantees all children with disabilities access to a free and appropriate public education. Nutrition services for children birth to three years of age are listed as a reimbursable service in Part C of this legislation.

Title XIX of the Social Security Act

Title XIX of the Social Security Act also plays a significant role in the health of women and children through three programs: Medicaid; the Early Periodic Screening, Diagnosis, and Treatment Program (EPSDT); and the State Children's Health Insurance Program (SCHIP).

Medicaid

Medicaid is a program that provides reimbursement for medical assistance for certain individuals and families with low incomes and resources. Established by Congress in 1965, it is jointly funded by the federal government and by each state. Medicaid is the largest source of funding for medical and health-related services for people with limited incomes. Each state's legislature sets its state's eligibility guidelines, reimbursement services, and policies.

Since the 1980s, Congress has enacted numerous laws concerning Medicaid eligibility for children and pregnant women. Federal law requires that state Medicaid programs cover pregnant women, infants, and children from ages one to eight whose family income is less than 133% of the federal poverty level. Many states have expanded beyond the federal levels. Some states have increased the limit to 300% of the poverty level for pregnant women and children. A list of state income eligibility tables is available at www.cbpp.org/shsh/tables.htm.

Early Periodic Screening, Diagnosis, and Treatment Program

The Early Periodic Screening, Diagnosis, and Treatment Program (EPSDT) was established in 1969 through an amendment to Title XIX of the Social Security Act. It serves as Medicaid's comprehensive and preventive child health program for children under the age of 21. The EPSDT program consists of two mutually supportive and operational components:

1. Assuring the availability and accessibility of required health care resources
2. Assisting Medicaid recipients and their parents or guardians in effectively using these resources

In conjunction with medical and health professionals, states develop a periodicity schedule for screening, vision, and hearing services.

EPSDT services include the following:

- Comprehensive health and developmental history
- Comprehensive unclothed physical exam
- Appropriate immunizations
- Laboratory tests (including lead toxicity)
- Health education (expectations in child's development, leading healthy lifestyles, and injury prevention)
- Vision services
- Dental services
- Hearing services
- Other necessary health services

To learn more, go to www.cms.hhs.gov/medicaid/epsdt/default.asp.

State Children's Health Insurance Program

The Balanced Budget Act of 1997 created a new children's health insurance program called the State Children's Health Insurance Program (SCHIP). It is a state-administered program. Each state determines the level of income eligibility and the scope of services available for children up to age 19 who are not already insured.

Opportunities for Nutrition Services in Title XIX Programs

The Medicaid, EPSDT, and SCHIP programs offer opportunities for medical nutrition therapy (MNT). Selected states include MNT for individuals with specific risk conditions and chronic diseases. Nutrition services may be required based on findings from an EPSDT screening. Participants with conditions such as growth retardation, iron deficiency anemia, obesity, or lead toxicity all benefit from nutrition counseling. The nutritionist should plan referral arrangements with clinicians involved in these programs.

WEIGHT

The serious public health epidemic of overweight and obesity cannot be ignored. Although public health professionals have been working to call attention to the problem and provide a number of preventive actions, the 2001 Surgeon General's *Call to Action to Prevent and Decrease Overweight and Obesity* brought the issue to significant media attention and became the focus of several public policy forums.[28] To learn more, go to www.surgeongeneral.gov.

The *Healthy People 2010* objectives related to overweight and obesity are aimed at increasing the proportion of adults who are at a healthy weight and reducing the proportion of children and adolescents who are overweight or obese.[29]

The challenge of obesity prevention and weight management crosses all of the segments of the maternal and child health population. Obesity and overweight are caused by many factors including genetics, metabolic, behavioral, environmental, cultural, and socioeconomic factors.

A woman's preconception weight should be in a healthy range with a body mass index (BMI) of 18.9 to 26.[30] BMI is a mathematical formula used to state the ratio of weight to height calculated as [Weight in Pounds/(Height in Inches)^2] $\times$ 703. Individuals with a BMI of 25 to 29.9 are considered overweight, while individuals with a BMI of 30 or more are considered obese. BMIs at a high level (greater than 25) have been associated with greater risk for a number of chronic diseases and early mortality.[31] Women who are overweight and obese are at increased risk for hypertension, gestational diabetes, and other pregnancy complications when compared to women of a normal weight. Children born to obese women are at greater risk of childhood obesity. To learn more, go to www.cdc.gov/nccdphp/dnpa/bmi/bmi-for-age.htm.

Although there is not an overall national plan for the public health response to the prevention and treatment of overweight and obesity, the majority of federal health agencies, state governments, and professional health organizations have taken up the issue.

An example of a federal initiative is the Centers for Disease Control and Prevention's state-based nutrition and physical activity grants to prevent obesity and other chronic diseases. Twenty-three states in 2004 received as much as $1.5 million to develop and implement science-based nutrition and physical activity interventions. To learn more, go to www.cdc.gov/nccdphp/dnap/obesity/state_programs.

A national initiative of the Weight-control Information Network (WIN) funded by the National Institutes of Health, National Institute of Diabetes and Digestive and Kidney Diseases is the Sisters Together: Move More, Eat Better Program. It is designed to encourage African-American women 18 years of age and older to maintain a healthy weight by becoming more physically active and eating healthier foods. To learn more, go to www.win.niddk.nih.gov/sisters/index.htm.

Prenatal Weight Gain

Recommendations for weight gain during pregnancy should be individualized according to prepregnancy body mass index. Table 8–1 below illustrates the recommendations based on individual BMI status.[32]

The Colorado Department of Health provides guidelines and resource recommendations for public health nutritionists in evaluating and providing services to a woman who has inadequate weight gain during pregnancy. To learn more, go to www.dcphe.state.co.us/ps/bestpractices/topicsubpages/inadequateweightgain.html.

The Texas Department of Health's fact sheet on gestational weight gain provides comprehensive information on assessment of prenatal weight gain and recommendations for nutrition intervention for varied weight gain, inadequate weight gain, and twin birth. For more detailed information, go to www.dshs.state.tx.us/wichd/nut/pdf/fac6%2Ds.pdf.

The Missouri Department of Health and Senior Services provides a chart and guidance for tracking prenatal weight gain. The chart includes graphic illustrations for the varied weight gain recommendations based on a woman's BMI status. To see this chart and other useful information, go to www.dhss.mo.gov/npe_pdfs/PrenatalWtGainChart.pdf. Although not specific to pregnancy, the *Dietary Guidelines for Americans 2005* provide useful messages and guidance for women throughout the lifecycle. For a complete review of the *Dietary Guidelines for Americans 2005*, see Appendix A.

VITAMIN AND MINERAL SUPPLEMENTATION

Iron and folic acid status are of key concern during pregnancy to assure maternal health and a successful pregnancy outcome. During pregnancy, a diet high in iron and a daily iron supplement of 30 milligrams per day is recommended to prevent iron deficiency anemia.[33]

In 1992, the US Public Health Service recommended that all women of childbearing years should take 400 micrograms of folic acid daily to prevent neural tube defects (NTD).[34] The Food and Nutrition Board, National Academy of

Table 8–1   Recommendations for Total Weight Gain for Pregnant Women

		Weight Gain	
Status	BMI	lb	kg
Underweight	< 19.8	28–40	12.5–18.0
Normal	19.8–26.0	25–35	11.5–16.0
Overweight	> 26.0–29.0	15–25	7.0–11.5
Obese	> 29	≥ 15	≥ 7.0

Sciences, and Institute of Medicine recommend that women take 400 micrograms of synthetic folic acid daily from fortified foods or supplements or a combination of the two in addition to consuming foods from a varied diet.[35] In 1998, the fortification of cereal grain products went into effect. Since 1995, the number of infants born with neural tube related birth defects has declined by approximately 26%.[36]

The American Medical Association has stated the following with regard to folic acid and women's health:

> One of the most exciting medical findings of the last part of the 20th century is that folic acid, a simple, widely available water-soluble vitamin, can prevent spina bifida and anencephaly. Not since the rubella vaccine became available 30 years ago have we had an opportunity for primary prevention of such common and serious birth defects.[37]

The Centers for Disease Control and Prevention in collaboration with the March of Dimes, the National Council on Folic Acid, and partner organizations communicate new and emerging science on the promotion of folic acid and the reduction of NTD-related birth defects.[38]

Many state health departments have an ongoing folic acid education campaign. Public health nutritionists have an important role in the leadership and dissemination of information on the benefits of and need for folic acid.

To learn more, go to any of the following:

- www.folicacidinfo.org/
- www.cdc.gov/doc.do/id/0900f3eec8000e2e0
- www.marchofdimes.com/
- www.cfsan.fda.gov/~dms/wh-preg.html
- www.folicacidnow.net/Resources/Resources1.html
- www.getfolic.com/

AVOIDANCE OF HARMFUL SUBSTANCES

Although moderate alcohol consumption has been advised for the US population, the recommendation for women who are pregnant or who are planning pregnancy is to avoid alcohol to prevent fetal alcohol syndrome, alcohol-related neurodevelopment disorders, and alcohol-related birth defects in newborns.[39,40]

Tobacco use, specifically cigarette smoking, is to be avoided by the general US population. This is especially true during pregnancy because of the relationship of smoking to low birth weight and the increased risk for mental retardation.[41,42]

The use of prescription and over-the-counter drugs during pregnancy should be reviewed with a medical professional because of possible effects on fetal development. Any harmful and/or illicit substance should be avoided especially during pregnancy to prevent neonatal morbidity and mortality.

BREAST-FEEDING

There is no question that breast-feeding is the optimal choice for infant nutrition. It is the gold standard for infant feeding. The *Healthy People 2010* objectives for breast-feeding are to achieve levels of 75% who initiate breast-feeding and 50% who maintain breast-feeding for at least six months.[43] Current *Healthy People 2010* data indicate that the breast-feeding objectives are far from being met. In the United States, less than 54% of mothers breast-feed their infants for a brief period with fewer than 22% of infants receiving breast milk by six months of age.[44]

A number of medical and health organizations including the American College of Obstetricians and Gynecologists, American Academy of Pediatrics Section on Breastfeeding, American Academy of Family Physicians, The American Dietetic Association, Academy of Breastfeeding Medicine, World Health Organization, United Nation's Children's Fund and others recommend exclusive breast-feeding for the first six months of life. These organizations along with many others participate in the United States Breastfeeding Committee formed in 1998 to protect, promote, and support breast-feeding. To learn more, go to www. usbreast feeding.org/.

The Office on Women's Health and the Advertising Council have developed the National Breastfeeding Awareness Campaign to highlight the importance of breast-feeding and to encourage more mothers to breast-feed exclusively for six months. Exclusive breast-feeding is defined as an infant's consumption of human milk and no other supplements of any type except for vitamins, minerals, and medications.[45] To learn more, go to www.4woman/.

The benefits of breast-feeding are significant for both the mother and her infant. A number of relationships between breast-feeding and health outcomes has been documented. For the infant, these include decrease in the incidence of selected infectious diseases, sudden infant death syndrome, insulin-dependent (type 1) and non-insulin-dependent (type 2) diabetes mellitus, overweight and obesity, and asthma. The breast-feeding mother can benefit from decreased postpartum bleeding, earlier return to prepregnancy weight, decreased risk of breast and ovarian cancer, and possible decreased risk of osteoporosis and hip fractures in the postmenopausal period.[46]

There are few situations where infants should not be breast-fed. These include the following:

- Infant with diagnosed galactosemia
- Mother's use of illegal drugs during pregnancy
- Mother with active tuberculosis
- Mother infected with HIV or acquired immunodeficiency system or other diseases in which the immune system is compromised[47]

In these situations or when breast-feeding is not chosen or is discontinued before the infant's first birthday, iron-fortified formula is recommended for the first year of life.[48] The standard of choice infant formula is a cow milk-based formula. Soy formulas and other alternative formulas are available for infants with gastrointestinal problems or metabolic diseases.

To achieve the nation's objectives for breast-feeding, public health nutritionists and other health care professionals must commit to the promotion of breast-feeding and understand how to effectively manage lactation to assist breast-feeding mothers.

In 2004, Congress appropriated approximately $15 million to expand WIC breast-feeding support services through peer counseling. These funds enable state WIC agencies to begin implementation of an effective and comprehensive peer-counseling program and/or to enhance existing breast-feeding peer-counseling programs. States will follow the Loving Support Makes Breastfeeding Work model developed in 1996.

Loving Support Makes Breastfeeding Work is the name of the USDA National WIC Breastfeeding Promotion Campaign. The goals of the campaign are listed below:

- Encourage WIC participants to initiate and continue breast-feeding.
- Increase referrals to WIC for breast-feeding support.
- Increase general public acceptance and support of breast-feeding.
- Provide technical assistance to WIC state and local agency professionals in the promotion of breast-feeding.

For a more complete listing, refer to www.fns.usda.gov/wic/Breastfeeding/lovingsupport.htm.

To promote and support breast-feeding, women participants in WIC are provided with counseling and breast-feeding educational materials during the prenatal period. Women who choose to breast-feed receive an enhanced WIC food package (carrots and tuna), follow-up support through peer counselors, ongoing counseling and education to continue breast-feeding, and are eligible for a 1 year breast-feeding certification period. The WIC program provides breast pumps, breast shells, and other items to help support and sustain breast-feeding.

The San Diego Breastfeeding Coalition is a nonprofit organization of health professionals devoted to the promotion and support of breast-feeding through education and outreach in the community. Coalition activities include the distribution of a breast-feeding resources guide to parents in the San Diego community, community education programs, community outreach to promote breast-feeding, and recognition of breast-feeding-friendly businesses. To learn more, go to www.breastfeeding.org/.

WOMEN'S HEALTH

Traditionally, women's health has addressed reproductive issues. More recently, women's health has evolved to address health issues across the lifespan.[49] A new program to promote preventive health care for women is the Bright Futures for Women's Health and Wellness Initiative (BFWHW) sponsored by the US Department of Health and Human Services' Office of Women's Health in partnership with other federal agencies, private organizations, professional associations, and consumer groups. The objectives of BFWHW are the following:

- Provide information to women on recommended preventive health services so that they seek care based on their individual needs and share in the decision making about their health services.
- Provide tools for practitioners to use in making all health care visits an opportunity to offer preventive care.
- Provide materials for community organizations to use in promoting women's health.
- Support health professions curricula for students and continuing education modules for practitioners on women's preventive health.
- Stimulate a research and data collection agenda that recognizes relevant differences across preventive health behavior and practice.

Physical activity and healthy eating guides are available for women and practitioners. To learn more, go to www.hrsa.gov/womenshealth/bfwhw.htm.

Along with this initiative, the Office of Women's Health is also sponsoring a public education campaign, Pick Your Path to Health, to help women take simple, active steps to wellness. To learn more, go to www.4woman.gov.

Two of the top priority health issues for women today are cardiovascular disease and osteoporosis.[50] Both have nutrition care implications.

Heart Disease

Cardiovascular disease is the leading cause of death for women in the United States.[51] The current recommendation to identify women with cardiovascular risks is routine lipid screening and treatment of abnormal lipid levels in women aged 45 years and older. Screening and treatment for women 20 to 45 years of age is recommended if they have other risk factors for heart disease.[52]

The National Heart, Lung, and Blood Institute along with a number of partners have initiated a national campaign, The Heart Truth, to make women aware of the danger of heart disease. Although the campaign is aimed at women ages 40 to 60, its messages are of importance to younger women because heart disease can start even in adolescence. To learn more, go to www.nhlbi.nih.gov/health/hearttruth/index.htm.

Osteoporosis

Osteoporosis is a major public health disease in the United States today. Of the 10 million Americans estimated to have osteoporosis, 80% are women, and one in two women over the age of 50 will have an osteoporosis-related fracture in her remaining lifetime.[53] Osteoporosis is a "silent disease" because bone loss occurs without symptoms and is unknown to a person until a fracture occurs.

Some of the risk factors for developing osteoporosis include the following:

- Personal history of fracture after age 50
- Current low bone mass
- Being female
- Being thin and/or having a small frame
- Advanced age
- Family history of osteoporosis
- Estrogen deficiency as a result of menopause, especially early or surgically induced
- Abnormal absence of menstrual periods
- Anorexia nervosa
- Low lifetime calcium intake
- Vitamin D deficiency
- Inactive lifestyle
- Current cigarette smoking
- Excessive use of alcohol
- Being Caucasian or Asian

Because the average woman has acquired 98% of bone mass by about the age of 20, building strong bones during childhood and adolescence is a key to osteoporosis prevention.[54] The following steps are recommended to optimize bone health and prevent osteoporosis:

- Consume a balanced diet rich in calcium and vitamin D.
- Perform weight-bearing exercise.
- Live a healthy lifestyle with no smoking or excessive alcohol intake.
- Test bone density and take medication, when appropriate.[55]

Daily calcium intake should be at least 1000 milligrams in premenopausal women and 1500 milligrams in postmenopausal women who do not take estrogen. When adequate calcium intake cannot be achieved through diet, calcium supplementation is required.[56]

A daily intake of 800 International Units (IU) of vitamin D is recommended. Vitamin D supplementation may be needed and is recommended for women with osteoporosis whose dietary intake of vitamin D is below 400 IU per day.[57]

Bone density should be measured in all women under age 65 who have one or more risk factors (in addition to menopause) for osteoporosis-related fracture.[58] To learn more the following sites are helpful:

- www.nof.org/
- www.healthywomen.org/

Nutrition Care Planning for Women

A nutrition assessment should be completed at an individual's initial visit for nutrition counseling. The assessment should consist of the following elements:

- Medical, obstetric, and psychosocial history
- Diet assessment
- Anthropometrical determinations (height, weight, BMI)
- Laboratory assessment (hematocrit/hemoglobin)
- Economic status

The information gathered assists the public health nutrition staff to develop an appropriate plan of care including referrals for nutrition assistance and social services if needed. Women who have preexisting risk factors such as diabetes, cardiovascular problems, renal disease, hypertension, or inborn errors of metabolism should be referred to a registered dietitian for medical nutrition therapy (MNT).

INFANT AND CHILD HEALTH

In the United States, access to child health care is a national priority and is being addressed by numerous federal, state, and local agencies, organizations, associations, and consumer groups. Many of the laws, initiatives, and programs affecting infant and child health and access to care have previously been reviewed in this chapter. Other programs of importance to public health nutritionists include newborn screening and the Bright Futures project.

Newborn Screening

All states and territories provide newborn screening for a variety of inherited metabolic conditions and hemoglobinopathies. Disorders identified through such screening can include the following:

- Phenylketonuria (PKU)
- Maple syrup urine disease (MSUD)
- Homocystinuria
- Tyrosinemia
- Galactosemia
- Some disorders of organic metabolism

Each state and territory mandates specific tests to be done on an infant following birth. These tests can be paid by the state or territory or by a mix between state or territory and MCHB funds. Each state or territorial health department can provide information on mandated tests and referral sources. For information on tests mandated by each state or territory, go to www.genes-r-us.uthscsa.edu/nbsdisorders.pdf.

Public health nutritionists need to be aware of their state's requirements for newborn screening and should be familiar with resources available to assist families in nutrition care for infants and children with these genetic disorders. Failure to initiate appropriate medical nutrition therapy shortly after birth in diagnosed infants can result in mental retardation or death.

Bright Futures

The Bright Futures project was initiated in 1990 by the Maternal and Child Health Bureau with support from the Medicaid Bureau. Partnerships were formed with many associations and organizations including The American Dietetic Association and the American Academy of Pediatrics. The principle of Bright Futures is that every child deserves to be healthy and that optimal health involves a trusting relationship between the health professional, the child, the family, and the community as partners in practice.[59]

Major objectives include the following:

- Develop materials and practical tools for health professionals, families, and communities.
- Disseminate Bright Futures philosophy and materials.
- Train health professionals, families, and communities to work in partnership on behalf of children's health.
- Develop and maintain public-private partnerships.

In working towards the first objective, Bright Futures has developed a series of health supervision guidelines:

- *Bright Futures: Guidelines for Health and Supervision of Infants, Children, and Adolescents*
- *Bright Futures in Practice: Mental Health*
- *Bright Futures in Practice: Nutrition*
- *Bright Futures in Practice: Oral Health*
- *Bright Futures in Practice: Physical Activity*

These publications can be viewed online by going to the Bright Futures Web site at www.brightfutures.org/.

These Bright Future publications provide specific information on health supervision visits specific to infancy, early childhood, middle childhood, and adolescence. They review the following:

- A snapshot of the developmental period
- A developmental chart

- Information on how a family can prepare for health supervision visits
- A periodicity schedule for health supervision visits
- A table of strengths and issues that emerge during each development period[60]

Public health nutrition personnel can access and use these materials to guide parents and caretakers in planning and meeting nutrition care standards specific to age and developmental stages.

Infant and Child Growth

Public health nutrition staff working in child health clinics, the WIC program, programs for children, or community agencies are often the primary monitors of a child's growth. This is done through use of clinical growth charts developed by the Centers for Disease Control and Prevention. Although these charts are not intended to be used as a sole diagnostic tool, they contribute to an overall impression of a child's health status. The charts are gender specific and include the following:

- Infants, birth to 36 months
  - Length-for-age and weight-for-age
  - Head circumference-for-age and weight-for-length
- Children and adolescents, 2 to 20 years
  - Stature-for-age and weight-for-age
  - BMI-for-age
- Preschoolers, 2 to 5 years
  - Weight-for-stature[61]

The BMI-for-age charts were introduced in 2000. They are recommended for use beginning at 2 years of age when an accurate stature can be obtained to screen for overweight children.[62]

These clinical growth charts can be viewed, printed, and reproduced by going to www.cdc.gov/growthcharts.

Using the same data as was used to develop the clinical growth charts, the Centers for Disease Control and Prevention created weight-for-age and stature-for-age growth charts for 2- to 5-year olds.

Overweight and Obesity Prevention

Childhood obesity is a growing epidemic. Nearly 9 million children in the United States aged 6 through 19 are overweight.[63] Among children ages 2 to 5, more that 10% are overweight.[64] Early prevention and identification of at-risk children is the key to stopping this epidemic.

Overweight and obesity prevention recommendations include the following:

- Identify and track patients at risk through family history, birth weight, or socioeconomic, cultural, or environmental factors.
- Calculate and plot BMI once a year in all children and adolescents.
- Use change in BMI to identify rate of excessive weight gain relative to linear growth.
- Encourage, support, and protect breast-feeding.
- Encourage parents and caregivers to promote healthy eating patterns by offering nutritious foods, encouraging self-regulation of food intake, setting appropriate limits on choices, and promoting healthy food choices.
- Routinely promote physical activity, including unstructured play at home, in school, in child care settings, and throughout the community.
- Recommend limiting television and video time to a maximum of 2 hours per day.
- Recognize and monitor changes in obesity-associated risk factors for adult chronic disease, such as hypertension, dyslipidemia, hyperinsulinemia, impaired glucose tolerance, and symptoms of obstructive sleep apnea syndrome.[65]

The American Dietetic Association Foundation (ADAF) has established the Healthy Weight for Kids Initiative. In conjunction with the Centers for Disease Control and Prevention, the US Department of Agriculture, the National Institutes of Health, and the International Life Science Institute, ADAF is developing screening and counseling tools and techniques for the detection, prevention, and treatment of obesity among children and adolescents.[66]

The US Department of Health and Human Services in conjunction with Discovery Networks, US, has developed two innovative DVD programs to help prevent and treat childhood obesity and overweight. *Max's Magical Delivery: Fit for Kids* is an interactive DVD aimed at children ages 5 through 9 and their families. For health care providers, *Childhood Obesity: Combating the Epidemic* addresses both prevention and treatment and also contains educational materials eligible for continuing medical education. Both DVDs are available at no cost by going online to www.ahrq.gov/child/dvdobesity.htm.

Physical activity in conjunction with good nutrition is essential in preventing and treating overweight and obesity. Figure 8–2 shows the Children's Activity Pyramid, which is a tool to be used along with the Kid's Food Pyramid.[67]

Vitamin and Mineral Supplements

In light of the growing concerns with skin cancer, sun exposure as a source of vitamin D is not recommended for infants and children. To prevent rickets and vitamin D deficiency, the recommendation is that all breast-fed infants receive

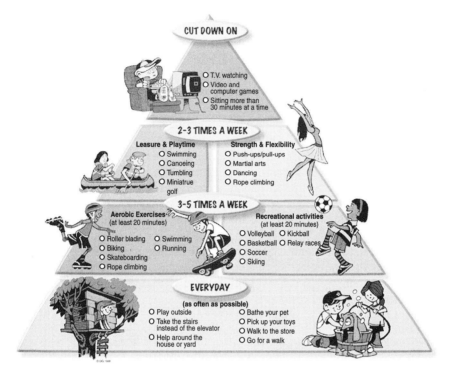

Figure 8–2   Children's Activity Period. *Source:* Prepared by University of Missouri Extension.

200 IU of vitamin D daily starting during the first two months of life. The supplementation should continue until the infant or child either receives more than 500 ml a day of vitamin D fortified formula or milk daily.[68]

Fluoride supplements can be prescribed by physicians and dentists when appropriate. Fluoride supplementation may be needed in situations where fluoridated drinking water is unavailable or is not consumed because of the growing trend in use of unfluoridated bottled drinking water. Parents should check with their child's physician to determine if fluoride supplementation is required.

Other vitamin and mineral supplementation is normally not required if a child is consuming the appropriate quantity and quality of foods for age and developmental stage.

Young girls need at least 1300 milligrams of calcium daily. They also need to participate in weight-bearing activities. These simple steps help to prevent osteoporosis. A number of state health departments and nonprofit organizations are leading efforts in osteoporosis prevention through public education, particularly targeting young girls. Adequate consumption of calcium through a combination of foods along with weight-bearing activities all contribute to the prevention of osteoporosis. Calcium supplementation may be required when needed calcium intake from foods is not achievable such as in children with lactose intolerance.

The US Department of Health and Human Services' Centers for Disease Control and Prevention in partnership with Office of Women's Health and the National Osteoporosis Foundation has developed a multiyear campaign to promote optimal bone health for girls ages 9 to 12. This Web-based campaign, *Powerful Bones, Powerful Girls*, offers a number of activities, incentive items, and guidance on calcium rich foods and physical exercise. An accompanying parent's Web site offers advice and information to parents. To learn more, go to www.cdc.gov/powerfulbones/parents/index.html.

ADOLESCENT HEALTH

The adolescent years are characterized by dramatic growth and development beginning with the onset of puberty and continuing throughout the teen years. Significant health and nutritional risks occur during adolescence as a result of the following:

- Increased need for energy and nutrients
- Increasing financial independence
- Increasing need for autonomy
- Immature cognitive abilities
- Peer pressure[69]

The Centers for Disease Control and Prevention through the Division of Adolescent and School Health (DASH) has initiated the *Healthy Youth!* project to address six critical types of preventable adolescent health behaviors:

- Alcohol and drug use
- Injury and violence
- Tobacco use
- Nutrition
- Physical activity
- Sexual behaviors, including teenage pregnancy[70]

These behaviors are usually established in childhood and persist into adulthood if not addressed early.

Resources for public health nutrition personnel are available through the project to address adolescent nutrition, health, and safety. To learn more, go to www.cdc.gov/HealthyYouth/NationalInitiative/guide.htm.

The mission of the 4GirlsHealth project, developed by the Office on Women's Health in the US Department of Health and Human Services, is to promote healthy, positive behaviors in girls between the ages of 10 and 16. The site gives female adolescents reliable, useful information on the health issues they will face as they become young women, and tips on handling relationships with family and friends, at school and at home.[71] The nutrition section of the Web site provides useful messages addressing the following:

- Eating well everyday
- Vitamins, nutrients, and other essentials
- Weight
- Vegetarian eating
- Bone health

ROLE AND RESPONSIBILITIES OF NUTRITIONISTS IN CHILD AND ADOLESCENT HEALTH

The position of the American Dietetic Association on the role and responsibilities of dietetic professionals in child and adolescent food and nutrition programs serves as the basis for the role and responsibilities of public health nutritionists.[72] Public health nutritionists are the health care practitioners most qualified to administer programs that help ensure that all women, infants, and children obtain safe, nutritious, and adequate diets for optimal nutrition and health. Public health nutritionists are preeminently qualified to provide nutrition screening and assessment, education, and counseling in accordance with national health recommendations. They also plan, administer, and monitor food and nutrition programs for the nation's women and children.

The responsibilities they carry out include the following:

- Advocating for continued and adequate funding of food assistance and nutrition education programs at the local, state, and national levels
- Facilitating the application of evidence-based research on nutrition for women and children to the development, provision, and evaluation of food and nutrition programs
- Serving as a resource to health and education disciplines, agencies, and organizations that provide nutrition-related services to women and children through the provision of technical assistance and training
- Participating in and advocating for adequate and continued funding for nutrition surveillance efforts to document the need for publicly funded food and nutrition programs for women, infants, children, and their families
- Advocating for healthy prenatal care, child care, school environments, and community services that include comprehensive nutrition education
- Supporting the development of universal health care reimbursement for comprehensive nutrition services, including screening and assessment, education and counseling, and developmentally appropriate anticipatory guidance

- Developing advocacy, program planning, evaluation, and media skills through education, including continuing professional education, that enhance the ability to support and administer food and nutrition programs
- Advocate for adequate and sustained support for a strong infrastructure for nutrition education in child care facilities, schools, and health care sites.

POINTS TO PONDER

- How can public health nutritionists obtain a share of available resources to develop nutrition services for women in the childbearing years?
- How can public health nutritionists assure that health care team members (physicians, nurses, health educators, social workers and other professionals) provide credible and realistic nutrition information to MCH clients?
- What can public health nutritionists do to combat the misconception that weight gain during pregnancy for overweight and obese women is unhealthy?
- How can public health nutritionists promote the coordination of nutrition services among public health services, day care centers, schools, and special health care needs services?
- What MCH public policy issues are of concern today and how can public health nutritionists affect these issues?

HELPFUL WEB SITES

Bright Futures at Georgetown University: www.brightfutures.org
Calculating Body Mass Index:
  www.dhss.mov.gov/npe_pdfs/PrenatalWtGainChart.pdf
CDC: www.cdc.gov
CDC 2000 United States Growth Charts: www.cdc.gov/growthcharts
CDC National Initiative to Improve Adolescent Health:
  www.cdc.gov/powerfulbones/parents/index.html
CDC Powerful Bones. Powerful Girls:
  www.cdc.gov/HealthyYouth/AdolescentHealth/NationalInitiative/index.htm
Centers for Medicare and Medicaid Services – EPSDT Dental Coverage:
  www.cms.hhs.gov/EPSDTDentalCoverage
Family Voices: www.familyvoices.org
Institute for Child Health Policy: www.ichp.edu
List of DVDs to Help Prevent Childhood Obesity:
  www.ahrq.gov/child/dvdobesity.htm
March of Dimes: www.marchofdimes.com
Maternal and Child Health Bureau: www.mchb.hrsa.gov

Maternal and Child Health Library — Knowledge Path: Overweight in Children and Adolescents:
www.mchlibrary.info/KnowledgePaths/kp_ overweight.html

Maternal, Infant, and Child Health:
www.healthypeople.gov/Document/ HTML/Volume2/16MICH.htm

National Council on Folic Acid: www.folicacidinfo.org

National Healthy Start Association: www.healthystartassoc.org

National Osteoporosis Foundation: www.nof.org

National Women's Health Information Center: www.4woman.gov

National Women's Health Resource Center: www.healthywomen.org

North Carolina Folic Acid Council: www.getfolic.com

Nutrition Fact Sheet – Maternal Nutrition: Gestational Weight Gain:
www.dshs.state.tx.us/wichd/nut/pdf/fac6%2Ds.pdf

Nutrition Services: www.nutritionnc.com

Office of the Surgeon General: www.surgeongeneral.org

San Diego County Breastfeeding Coalition: www.breastfeeding.org

Start Healthy, Stay Healthy – Tables: www.cbpp.org/shsh/tables.htm

The Heart Truth: A Campaign About Heart Disease in Women:
www.nhlbi.nih.gov/health/hearttruth

U.S. Department of Agriculture – Food and Nutrition Services:
www.fns. usda.gov/fns

U.S. FDA – Information for Pregnant Women:
www.cfsan.fda.gov/~dms/ wh-preg.html

United States Breastfeeding Council: www.usbreastfeeding.org

Weight-Control Information Network – Sisters Together:
www.win.niddk. nih.gov/sisters/index.htm

WIC Works Resource System: www.nal.usda.gov/wicworks

NOTES

1. National Center for Health Statistics. Infant Mortality. Available at: http://www. cdc.gov/nchs/fastats/infmort.htm. Accessed May 7, 2005.

2. National Center for Health Statistics. Health, United States 2004, with chartbook on trends in the health of America. Available at: http://www.cdc.gov/nchs/data/hus/ hus04trend.pdf#022. Accessed May 7, 2005.

3. Alan Guttmacher Institute. *Teenage Pregnancy: Overall Trends and State-By-State Information.* New York, NY: Alan Guttmacher Institute; 1999:Table 1.

4. Henshaw SK. *Teenage Pregnancy Statistics with Comparative Statistics for Women Aged 20–24.* New York, NY: Alan Guttmacher Institute; 1999:5.

5. UNICEF. Statistical tables. Available at: http://unicef.org/sowc05/english/statistics. html. Accessed May 7, 2005.

6. US Dept of Health and Human Services. *Healthy People 2010: Objectives for Improving Health*. Washington, DC: US Dept of Health and Human Services; 2000.

7. US Dept of Health and Human Services. *Healthy People 2010: Objectives for Improving Health*. Washington, DC: US Dept of Health and Human Services; 2000.

8. Maternal and Child Health Bureau. Maternal and child health strategic plan. Available at: http://mchb.hrsa.gov/about/stratplan03-07.htm. Accessed May 1, 2005.

9. VanDyke PC. Introduction, PIPPAH supplement. *J Am Diet Assoc.* year?;102:5.

10. Washington State Dept of Health, Maternal and Child Health Programs. Children with special health care needs. Available at: http://www.doh.wa.gov/cfh/mch/CSHCNhome2.htm. Accessed May 25, 2005.

11. National Healthy Start Association. The Healthy Start Program. Available at: http://www.healthystartassoc.org. Accessed May 7, 2005.

12. National Healthy Start Association. The Healthy Start Program. Available at: http://www.healthystartassoc.org. Accessed May 7, 2005.

13. National Center for Education in Maternal and Child Health. About NCEMCH. Available at: http://www.ncemch.org/about/default.html. Accessed May 27, 2005.

14. US Dept of Health and Human Services. *The National Survey of Children with Special Health Care Needs*. Available at: http://www.mchb.hrsa.gov/cshcn/pages/intro.htm. Accessed June 4, 2005.

15. Agency for Healthcare Research and Quality. Access to medical care among children under 18 years of age with special health care needs. *MEPS Statistical Brief.* 2002;75.

16. Reiss J. Introduction to state Title V programs for children with special health care needs. Available at: http://www.ichp.edu. Accessed June 4, 2005.

17. Reiss J. Introduction to state Title V programs for children with special health care needs. Available at: http://www.ichp.edu. Accessed June 4, 2005.

18. Family Voices. Project: families in Title V. Available at: http://www.familyvoices.org/. Accessed June 4, 2005.

19. Child Nutrition Act of 1966, Pub L 108-498.

20. Child Nutrition Amendments of 1975, Pub L 94-105.

21. USDA Food and Nutrition Service. About WIC. Available at: http://www.fns.usda.gov/wic/aboutwic/wicataglance.htm. Accessed May 25, 2005.

22. USDA Food and Nutrition Service. WIC Program: total participation. Available at: http://www.fns.usda.gov/pd/wifypart.htm. Accessed May 25, 2005.

23. Buescher PA, Larson LC, Nelson MD, Lenihan AJ. Prenatal WIC participation can reduce low birth weight and newborn medical costs: a cost-benefit analysis of WIC participation in North Carolina. *J Am Diet Assoc.* 1993;93:163.

24. US General Accounting Office. *Early Intervention: Federal Investments Like WIC Can Produce Savings*. Washington, DC: US General Accounting Office; 1992. Publication No. GAO/HRD-92-18.

25. Devaney BL, Bilheimer L, Schore J. Medicaid costs and birth outcomes: the effects of early prenatal WIC participation and prenatal care. *J Policy Analysis Manage.* 1992;11:573.

26. Buescher PA, Horton SJ, Devaney BL, et al. Child participation in WIC: Medicaid costs and use of the health care services. *Am J Pub Health.* 2003;93:145.

27. Owen AL, Owen GM. Twenty years of WIC: a review of some effects of the program. *J Am Diet Assoc.* 1997;97:777.

28. US Dept of Health and Human Services. *The Surgeon General's Call to Action to Prevent and Decrease Overweight and Obesity.* Rockville, Md: DHHS, Office of the Surgeon General; 2001.

29. US Dept of Health and Human Services. *Healthy People 2010: Objectives for Improving Health.* Washington, DC: US Dept of Health and Human Services; 2000.

30. Institute of Medicine. *Nutrition During Pregnancy Part I: Weight Gain Part II: Supplements.* Washington, DC: National Academies Press; 1990.

31. National Heart, Lung, and Blood Institute. Clinical guidelines on the identification, evaluation, and treatment of overweight and obesity in adults. Available at: http://www.nhlbi.nih.gov/guidelines/obesity/ob_home.htm.

32. Institute of Medicine. *Nutrition During Pregnancy Part I: Weight Gain Part II: Supplements.* Washington, DC: National Academies Press; 1990.

33. Centers for Disease Control and Prevention. Recommendations to prevent and control iron deficiency in the United States. *MMWR.* 1998;47:1.

34. Centers for Disease Control and Prevention. Recommendations for the use of folic acid to reduce the number of cases of spina bifida and other neural tube defects. *MMWR.* 1991;41:2.

35. Food and Nutrition Board, Institute of Medicine. *Dietary Reference Intakes for Thiamine, Riboflavin, Niacin, Vitamin B6, Folate, Vitamin B12, Pantothenic Acid, Biotin, and Choline.* Washington, DC: National Academies Press; 1998.

36. Centers for Disease Control and Prevention. Spina bifida and anencephaly before and after folic acid mandate—United States, 1995–1996 and 1999–2000. *MMWR.* 1992;41:No. RR-14.

37. Oakley G. Folic acid-preventable spina bifida and anencephaly. *JAMA.* March 1993; 1292.

38. Centers for Disease Control and Prevention. Recommendations for the use of folic acid to reduce the number of cases of spina bifida and other neural tube defects. *MMWR.* 1992;41:No. RR-14.

39. Surgeon General. Surgeon General's advisory on alcohol use in pregnancy. Available at: http://www.hhs.gov/surgeongeneral/pressrelease/sg02222005.html. Accessed May 1, 2005.

40. Committee on Substance Abuse and Committee on Children with Disabilities. Fetal alcohol syndrome and alcohol-related neurodevelopment disorder. *Pediatrics.* 2000; 106:358.

41. Centers for Disease Control and Prevention. Smoking during pregnancy—United States 1990–2002. *MMWR.* 2004;53:No. 39.

42. Centers for Disease Control and Prevention. Tobacco information and prevention source. Available at: http://www.cdc.gov/tobacco/research_data/health_consequences/matsmkg.htm. Accessed May 30, 2005.

43. US Dept of Health and Human Services. *Healthy People 2010: Objectives for Improving Health*. Washington, DC: US Dept of Health and Human Services; 2000.

44. Centers for Disease Control and Prevention. Pediatric and pregnancy nutrition surveillance reports. Available at: http://www.cdc.gov/pednss_tables/pdf/national_table3. pdf. Accessed June 4, 2005.

45. American Academy of Pediatrics. Breastfeeding and the use of human milk. American Academy of Pediatrics Policy statement, February 2005. *Pediatrics*. 2005;115:496.

46. American Academy of Pediatrics. Breastfeeding and the use of human milk. American Academy of Pediatrics Policy statement, February 2005. *Pediatrics*. 2005;115:496.

47. American Dietetic Association. Position of the American Dietetic Association: promoting and supporting breastfeeding. *J Am Diet Assoc*. 2005;105:810.

48. Academy of Pediatrics, Committee on Nutrition. Iron fortification of infant formula. *Pediatrics*. 1999;104:119.

49. Weisman CS. Changing the definition of women's health: implications for health and health care policy. *Maternal and Child Health Journal*. 1997;1:179.

50. Weisman CS. Measuring quality in women's health care: issues and recent developments. *Quality Managed Health Care*. 2000;8:14.

51. National Heart, Lung, and Blood Institute. What is the Heart Truth? Available at: http://www.nhlbi.nih.gov/health/hearttruth/whatis/index.htm. Accessed May 30, 2005.

52. US Preventive Services Task Force. Screening for lipid disorders in adults. Available at: http://www.ahrq.gov/clinic/uspstf/uspschol.htm. Accessed May 30, 2005.

53. National Institutes of Health. Osteoporosis and related bone disease – National Resource Center, fast facts on osteoporosis. Available at: http://www.osteo.org/ newfile.asp?doc=fast&doctitle=Fast+Facts+One+Osteoporosis&doctyp. Accessed June 3, 2005.

54. National Institutes of Health. Osteoporosis and related bone disease – National Resource Center, fast facts on osteoporosis. Available at: http://www.osteo.org/ newfile.asp?doc=fast&doctitle=Fast+Facts+One+Osteoporosis&doctyp. Accessed June 3, 2005.

55. National Institutes of Health. Osteoporosis and related bone disease – National Resource Center, fast facts on osteoporosis. Available at: http://www.osteo.org/ newfile.asp?doc=fast&doctitle=Fast+Facts+One+Osteoporosis&doctyp. Accessed June 3, 2005.

56. Rosen HN. Patient information: prevention and treatment of osteoporosis. Up-To-Date: Patient information site. Available at: http://patients.uptodate.com/print.asp?print= true&file=endo_hor/10905. Accessed June 3, 2005.

57. Rosen HN. Patient information: prevention and treatment of osteoporosis. Up-To-Date: Patient information site. Available at: http://patients.uptodate.com/print.asp?print= true&file=endo_hor/10905. Accessed June 3, 2005.

58. Rosen HN. Patient information: prevention and treatment of osteoporosis. Up-To-Date: Patient information site. Available at: http://patients.uptodate.com/print.asp?print= true&file=endo_hor/10905. Accessed June 3, 2005.

59. Bright Futures. About Bright Futures. Available at: http://www.brightfutures.org/ about/index.html. Accessed June 3, 2005.

60. Bright Futures. About Bright Futures. Available at: http://www.brightfutures.org/about/index.html. Accessed June 3, 2005.

61. Centers for Disease Control and Prevention. Clinical growth charts. Available at: http://www.cdc.gov/nchs/about/major/nhanes/growthcharts/clinical_chart.htm.

62. Centers for Disease Control and Prevention. Clinical growth charts. Available at: http://www.cdc.gov/nchs/about/major/nhanes/growthcharts/clinical_chart.htm.

63. National Center for Chronic Disease Prevention and Health Promotion. Healthy Youth! health topics. Available at: http://www.cdc.gov/HealthyYouth/healthtopics/index.htm.

64. Ogden CL, Flegal KM, Carroll MD, Johnson CL. Prevalence and trends in overweight among US children and adolescents. *JAMA*. 2002;288:1728.

65. American Academy of Pediatrics, Committee on Nutrition. Prevention of pediatric overweight and obesity. *Pediatrics*. 2003;112:424.

66. Myers EF, Shelke K, Johnson GH. Healthy Weight for Kids: Hertzler Fund kicks off the Family Nutrition and Physical Activity Screening Initiative. *J Am Diet Assoc.* May 2002;102:727.

67. University of Missouri Extension. Children's activity pyramid. Available at: http://muextension.missouri.edu/xplor/hesguide/foodnut/gh1800.htm. Accessed May 30, 2005.

68. Gartner LM, Greer FR, the Section on Breastfeeding and Committee on Nutrition. Prevention of rickets and vitamin D deficiency: new guidelines for vitamin D intake. American Academy of Pediatrics Clinical Report. *Pediatrics*. 2003;111:908.

69. Stang J, Story M, eds. Guidelines for adolescent nutrition services. Available at: http://www.epi.umn.edu/let/pubs/adol_book.htm. Accessed June 4, 2005.

70. National Center for Chronic Disease Prevention and Health Promotion. Healthy Youth! Available at: http://www.cdc.gov/HealtyYouth/healthtopics/index.htm.

71. 4GirlsHealth. 4Girls—about us. Available at: http://www.4girls.gov/about/mission.htm. Accessed June 4, 2005.

72. American Dietetic Association. Position of the American Dietetic Association: child and adolescent food and nutrition programs. *J Am Diet Assoc*. 2003;103:887.

CHAPTER 9

Shape Up the Adults

Margaret Tate, Nicole Olmstead, and Marie Tymrak

Reader Objectives

- Discuss the leading and actual causes of death in the United States.
- Identify the leading causes of disability in the United States.
- Understand the economic burden caused by chronic disease in the United States.
- Learn how to select the evidence-based nutrition interventions for public health programs.
- Specify the differences between primary, secondary, and tertiary interventions for the leading causes of death and disability in the United States.
- Understand the importance of expanding partnerships and collaborations in public health programming.

LEADING VS ACTUAL CAUSES OF DEATH IN THE UNITED STATES

Chronic diseases are now the leading causes of death and disability in the United States. A chronic disease is defined as a disease which has one or more of the following characteristics: (1) is permanent and leaves residual disability; (2) is caused by nonreversible pathological alteration; and (3) requires educating the patient for self-care as an essential part of rehabilitation, and usually requires continuing supervision, observation, and care.[1] Chronic diseases account for 7 of every 10 deaths in the United States and effect the quality of life for over 90 million Americans. The leading causes of death, as shown in Figure 9–1, are diseases of the heart, cancer, stroke, chronic obstructive pulmonary disease, and diabetes.[2] Not only are these diseases some of the most costly and long-term illnesses, but

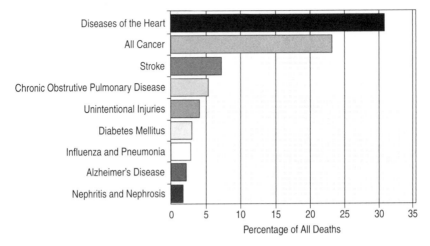

Figure 9–1 Leading Causes of Death in the United States. Source: CDC National Center for Chronic Disease Prevention and Health Promotion, 2000.

they also can be prevented through lifestyle changes. When observing the leading causes of death, it is necessary to look at the "real" causes. The actual causes of death for the United States according to the Centers for Disease Control and Prevention (CDC) are shown in Figure 9–2. Use of tobacco, poor diet, lack of exercise, and alcohol abuse are the most common actual causes of death, all of which are modifiable behaviors.[3]

A diagnosis of a chronic disease does not have to be perceived as a death sentence. Many chronic diseases can be managed by exercising, physical activity,

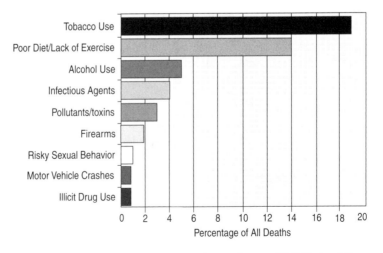

Figure 9–2 Actual Causes of Death in the United States. Source: CDC National Center for Chronic Disease Prevention and Health Promotion, 2000.

smoking cessation, and improved nutrition, thus limiting the death and disability. The most disturbing chronic disease of our time is the increasing obesity epidemic. In 1991, only four states reported obesity rates of 15–19% in their populations, and no states reported that 20% or more of their population was obese or overweight. In 2002, the CDC *Behavioral Risk Factor Surveillance Survey* (BRFSS) reported that 18 states had an obesity prevalence of 15–19%, 29 states had an obesity prevalence of 20–24%, and 3 states had a prevalence rate of over 25%.[4] Three primary factors contribute to overweight and obesity:

- Overweight and obesity result from an energy imbalance: eating too many calories and too little physical activity.
- Body weight is the result of genes, metabolism, behavior, environment, culture, and socioeconomic status.
- Both the social environment and an individual's behavior play a large role in causing people to become overweight and obese.

Modifying the individual's environment affects two out of three of these factors. Diet and physical inactivity play the greatest role in contributing to the obesity epidemic. In the United States, the food choices in markets, restaurants, popular fast-food outlets, cafeterias, and vending machines have greatly expanded. A variety of packaged convenience foods, soft drinks, pastries, and confections are readily accessible. These types of foods, while quick and easy to eat, are generally high in "empty" calories from saturated and trans fats and refined sugars. In addition to the prevalent convenience foods, portion sizes have become larger. People consume more calories at meals or snacks than in the past. For most adults, this results in a higher intake of calories than their bodies can burn off. Without enough physical activity, the extra calories are stored as fat.[5] Diet is not the only factor contributing to the obesity epidemic. In the 2000 *Behavioral Risk Factor Surveillance Survey* (BRFSS), more than one quarter of the population of the United States reported that they had engaged in no leisure time physical activity. Increasingly, Americans are becoming more sedentary, and the obesity problem continues to grow which in turn contributes to other chronic diseases. By addressing the growing obesity and overweight issues, diabetes, cardiovascular disease, stroke, arthritis, and other chronic diseases can be greatly reduced.

ECONOMIC BURDEN OF CHRONIC DISEASES

In the United States, health care costs are exploding. On average, this nation spent $5035 per American in 2001, more than any other country in the world.[6] According to the federal Centers for Disease Control and Prevention (CDC), chronic diseases account for approximately 75% of all health care costs each year.[7] The CDC cites the following impact of chronic diseases on the health care system[8,9]:

- More than 90 million Americans live with chronic illnesses.
- Chronic diseases account for 70% of all deaths in the United States.

- Medical care for people with chronic diseases account for more than 75% of the nation's $1.4 trillion medical care costs.
- Chronic diseases account for one third of the years of potential life lost before age 65.
- In 2001, approximately $300 billion was spent on all cardiovascular diseases. Of this amount, over $129 billion in lost productivity was due to cardiovascular diseases.
- In 2002, the overall cost for cancer was $171.6 billion; this includes $60.9 billion for direct medical expenses, $15.5 billion for lost worker productivity due to illness, and $95.2 billion for lost worker productivity due to premature death.
- The direct and indirect costs of diabetes are nearly $132 billion a year.
- Each year, arthritis results in estimated medical care costs of more than $22 billion, and estimated total costs (medical care and lost productivity) of almost $82 billion.
- Estimated direct and indirect costs associated with smoking exceed $75 billion annually.
- Direct medical care costs associated with physical inactivity were nearly $76.6 billion in 2000.
- Yearly, approximately $68 billion is spent on dental services.

Health disparities must also be examined in relation to these escalating health care costs. The National Institutes of Health (NIH) defines health disparities as the differences in the incidence, prevalence, mortality, and burden of diseases and other adverse health conditions that exist among specific population groups in the United States. Populations currently experiencing poor health status are increasing, while those experiencing good health status are decreasing.[10] Because of technological advances and environmental improvements, the average life expectancy in this nation has increased from 59 years in 1950 to 77 years today. Despite these improvements, health disparities occur that affect longevity, disease rates, and access to care. Some examples of these health disparities include the following:

- African-American women are more likely to die of breast cancer than are women of any other racial or ethnic group. The incidence of cervical cancer, a 100% preventable cancer, is more than five times greater among Vietnamese women than among Caucasian women in the United States.
- In 1998, rates of death from cardiovascular disease were about 30% higher among African-American adults than among Caucasian adults.
- Prevalence of diabetes is 70% higher among African-Americans and nearly 100% higher among Hispanics than among Caucasians. The prevalence of diabetes among American Indians and Alaska Natives is more than twice that of the total population, and the Pima Indians of Arizona have the highest known prevalence of diabetes in the world.[11]

EVIDENCE-BASED PUBLIC HEALTH PRACTICE

When considering any public health intervention, especially a nutrition intervention, it is important to document the following:

- The research evidence supports the application of basic nutrition science findings to practice.
- There is published evidence of credible studies documenting that the intervention will result in population-wide as well as individual behavior change.

Both government agencies and private foundations are no longer willing to fund "feel-good" interventions, projects that have no scientific basis to prove that they will work. Interventions must be designed and implemented with built-in evaluation to document their achievement. Evidence-based interventions should demonstrate their effectiveness in reducing the burden of chronic disease in targeted populations. Evidence-based public health is the development, implementation, and evaluation of effective programs and policies in public health. It means applying scientific reasoning, using systematic data and information systems, and appropriate behavioral science theory and program planning models.[12] Key characteristics of evidence-based public health interventions include the following:

- Approaches based on the best available published scientific research findings are used.
- Use a multidisciplinary team for planning and problem solving.
- Theory and systematic planning approaches are followed.
- Sound evaluation principles are built-in.
- Results are widely disseminated to others who need to know.

Successfully implementing evidence-based public health interventions requires the use of several tools, including, but not limited to, performing systematic reviews that address key questions before making decisions, addressing health status outcomes and not just intermediate process outcomes, and all the while considering the potential harms as well as the benefits of the interventions being considered.[13]

PREVENT AND MANAGE CHRONIC DISEASES IN ADULTS

Most chronic diseases in adults can be prevented. Regretfully our current health care system is designed to treat diseases that have already developed, not to prevent them from occurring in the first place. Federal and local governments have consistently underfunded prevention interventions. Investing in a system that prevents disease and stops it from taking a toll on the population's health could substantially reduce the enormous costs to society, taxpayers, and medical care organizations.

As discussed in Chapter 1, there are three stages of prevention. Primary prevention refers to the complete prevention of the disease, often through methods that inhibit exposure to risk factors.[14] Secondary prevention activities detect disease early and, thereby, limits the adverse effects after diagnosis. Tertiary prevention strives to prevent further disability and restores a higher level of functioning to patients with a diagnosed disease.[15]

The primary function of public health programs and services is to prevent disease and disability. Prevention is "a proactive process that empowers individuals and systems to meet the challenges of life events and transitions by creating and reinforcing conditions that promote healthy behaviors and lifestyles."[16] More focus needs to be on primary prevention, which targets "generally healthy individuals to decrease the probability that they will develop a disease or disability."[17]

In adults, primary prevention activities include educating individuals and population groups to reduce risk factors by implementing evidence-based interventions to help modify their behavior. With increasing obesity rates in the population, many of the interventions currently being implemented focus on dietary intake and physical activity.

Obesity

The prevention of obesity and overweight has become the primary focus of many public health programs at the national, state, and local levels. Every state is reporting at least a 15% obesity rate, with Mississippi, Alabama, and West Virginia reporting obesity rates of greater than 25%, according to the 2002 BRFSS.[18] The health consequences of overweight or obesity include high blood pressure, high blood cholesterol, type 2 diabetes, insulin resistance, glucose intolerance, coronary heart disease, stroke, gallstones, gout, osteoarthritis, some types of cancer (breast, prostate and colon cancer), and poor female reproductive health. According to the *Healthy People 2010* objectives, about 75% of Americans do not eat enough fruit, more than half do not eat enough vegetables, and about 64% consume too much saturated fat.[19] Poor diet and physical inactivity have been attributed to 310,000 to 580,000 deaths per year and linked to 23% of chronic disease–related deaths in the United States.

To curb the rising obesity prevalence, the Association of State and Territorial Public Health Nutrition Directors (ASTPHND) developed *Guidelines for Comprehensive Programs to Promote Healthy Eating and Physical Activity*, a document designed to help state and local health advocates create comprehensive nutrition, physical activity and obesity control programs.[20] For more information, go to: www. astdhpphe.org.

This document makes seven recommendations that obesity programs should focus on:

1. Leadership in planning, management, and coordination
2. Environmental, systems, and policy change

3. Mass communications
4. Community programs and community development
5. Programs for children and adolescents
6. Health care delivery
7. Surveillance, epidemiology, and research

Secondary interventions focus on losing weight by reducing calorie intake and participating in more physical activities. These interventions often need to start small and grow, as the target population tends to be sedentary and may have multiple health problems as a result of their overweight or obesity. Interventions need to be tailored specifically to the participants and build in a social support network as well as goal setting and problem-solving skills.[21]

Diabetes

The goal of primary prevention in diabetes is to delay or prevent the development of the disease entirely.[22] To reach the largest number of people who might be affected with this disease later in life, public health organizations generally focus primary prevention on persons who have an impaired glucose tolerance, and therefore, the highest risk for developing diabetes. Most primary interventions urge participants to maintain a diet that includes fruits, vegetables, whole grains, reduced fat dairy products, and lean meats. These programs suggest reducing or eliminating foods high in "empty" calories from saturated fats and sweets and incorporating exercise into daily activities. The National Diabetes Education Program, a collaboration between the CDC, the National Institutes of Health, and more than 200 other partners, developed a program called "Prevengamos la Diabetes Tipo 2: Paso a Paso" (Let's Prevent Type 2 Diabetes: Step by Step). Participation in this primary prevention program is aimed at Hispanic and Latino Americans to prevent the development of type 2 diabetes.[23] They received recipe cards utilizing the recommended foods and free products to encourage them to eat better. They were encouraged to be physically active for at least 30 minutes a day. Most of the participants chose brisk walking as their activity. They were also encouraged to maintain a desirable body weight. Most participants lost 5–7% of their body weight.[24] Through this program, two out of every three of the 500 participants were able to prevent or delay the onset of diabetes. This program showed that by making modest lifestyle changes, it is possible to delay or prevent the onset of type 2 diabetes.

Secondary and tertiary interventions focus on people with diagnosed diabetes and aim to prevent (secondary) or control (tertiary) the devastating complications of the disease.[25] For example, maintaining medically recommended blood glucose levels, blood pressure, and cholesterol levels have been repeatedly shown to reduce the common complications of diabetes. Foot screening, frequent hemoglobin A1C screening, and eye examinations are well-established components of any quality diabetes management program.[26] Most secondary and tertiary interventions encourage persons with diagnosed diabetes to become physically active, maintain desirable body weight, and adhere to a physician-prescribed diet and meal plan as counseled by a nutritionist or registered dietitian in order to avoid further complications of diabetes such as renal failure, limb amputations, blindness, and death.

Type 1 diabetes is a disease that develops when the body's autoimmune system destroys the pancreatic beta cells, rendering the body incapable of producing the necessary insulin.[27] The risk factors for type 1 diabetes include autoimmune, genetic, and environmental factors. Type 1 diabetes can affect adults as they move through their lives, but generally, this type of diabetes sets in prior to adulthood. Many of the diet and exercise recommendations for this population are the same as for adults with type 2 diabetes.

Gestational diabetes is a form of glucose intolerance diagnosed during a pregnancy. As this condition is related to the state of being pregnant, the only primary prevention for it is to not get pregnant. Many of the interventions focus on secondary prevention. It is recommended that the pregnant women monitor sugar intake and increase exercise.[28] In many cases, this form of diabetes can be controlled with diet and exercise, but in severe cases, the patient may require daily insulin therapy. Gestational diabetes usually disappears when the baby is born. Babies born to women who were affected with gestational or any other type of diabetes tend to be larger than those born to mothers without any form of diabetes. Women who are diagnosed with gestational diabetes have a 20–50% chance of developing one of the other forms of diabetes within 5 to 10 years after their diagnosis during pregnancy.[29]

Cardiovascular Disease

Primary prevention in cardiovascular disease (CVD) is targeted toward people who are at risk for a first CVD event because they have one or more of the CVD risk factors.[30] These primary risk factors are high blood pressure, high cholesterol, tobacco use, physically inactive, and poor diets, usually evidenced as overweight or obesity and possibly diabetes. An example of a program with both primary and secondary prevention components is the *New York Healthy Heart Program*. Most of the worksites participating in this program have made blood pressure screening available for employees on a regular basis. They have placed healthier low-fat food choices in vending machines; instituted smoke-free workplace policies, and are now providing physical activity breaks for employees during the day. Through this program, participants in businesses and worksites are evaluated by the New York Department of Health Services Cardiovascular Health Program and followed over a 3-year period to determine if the recommended changes were made and maintained.[31] Some of the dietary guidelines that are used for those with CVD risk factors are to eat a diet that is moderate in salt, with an intake of no more than 2400 mg per day.[32] New guidelines recently released by the National Cholesterol Education Program Expert Panel lowered the recommended LDL level from < 130 mg/dL to 100 mg/dL.[33] New blood pressure guidelines released by the Joint National Committee on Prevention, Detection, Evaluation, and Treatment of High Blood Pressure indicated that the goal blood pressure is < 140/90 mm HG.[34]

Secondary prevention targets people diagnosed with established CVD to prevent recurrent events.[35] In addition to reducing risk factors for cardiovascular disease through lifestyle changes such as weight loss and smoking cessation, secondary intervention programs present information regarding the use of aspirin, beta-blockers, ACE inhibitors, anticoagulants, and other antiplatelet agents. Frequently, the American Heart Association's *Get with the Guidelines* program is used as a secondary and tertiary intervention. This program is aimed at patients being discharged from the hospital after a cardiac event. The hospital setting has been identified as a "teachable moment" because patients can relate the intervention strategies to the event they have just experienced. Patients are counseled on medications as well as diet and lifestyle changes. If they smoke, they are advised to quit. They are advised to maintain a desirable weight with a body mass index (BMI) between 18.5 and 24.9. Finally, they are counseled to increase their physical activity to at least 30 minutes three to four times per week, ideally every day.[36]

For more information, go to the American Heart Association www.americanheart.org.

Cancer

In the past, cancer prevention has focused on site-specific interventions. The current trend is to look at cancer in a more comprehensive fashion. Cancer is another chronic disease in which 50–70% of cancer deaths are attributable to preventable risk behaviors,[37] with more than 30% of those specifically attributable to poor eating habits.[38]

Primary cancer prevention refers to the complete prevention of the disease by reducing or eliminating exposure to risk factors. The four primary risk factors for cancers are tobacco use, lack of physical activity, exposure to ultraviolet light, and poor diet. Some important interventions in prevention and early detection of cancer focus on reducing smoking; reducing consumption of saturated fats while increasing the consumption of fiber, minerals, and antioxidants from fruits, vegetables, and whole grains; increasing physical activity; increasing the number of cancer screenings that are done on a regular basis; and decreasing the level of ultraviolet light exposure a person receives. As with other chronic diseases, the diet and physical activity recommendations are very similar. According to the American Cancer Society recommendations for cancer prevention, a person should do the following:

- Eat a variety of healthful foods, with an emphasis on plant sources.
  - Eat five or more servings of a variety of vegetables and fruits each day.

- ○ Choose whole grains instead of processed grains and sugars.
- ○ Limit consumption of red meats, especially those that are processed and are high in fat.
- ○ Choose a diet to maintain a desirable weight and BMI.
- Adopt a physically active lifestyle.
  - ○ Adults should engage in at 30 minutes of moderate activity on five or more days of the week; 45 minutes or more of moderate to vigorous activity on five or more days of the week may further enhance reductions in the risk of breast and colon cancer.
  - ○ Children and adolescents should engage in at least 60 minutes per day of moderate-to-vigorous physical activity at least five days per week.
- Maintain a desirable weight throughout life.
  - ○ Balance caloric intake with physical activity.
  - ○ Lose weight if currently overweight.
- Limit consumption of alcoholic beverages.[39]

Secondary cancer prevention activities use screening programs to detect the disease in its early stages and attempt to limit the negative effects after diagnosis. Early detection is the key as outcomes can be dramatically improved if the cancer is caught before it has spread throughout the body. Secondary interventions are mainly concerned with early detection. Programs such as the National Breast and Cervical Cancer Early Detection Program play a key role in secondary intervention. Through yearly screening of women who are at risk of developing cervical and breast cancer, this program detects cancers before they become advanced. It encourages women to get yearly Pap tests, conduct regular self-breast exams, and go for yearly mammograms when they reach the recommended age.[40]

Tertiary prevention involves two very different concerns. One is to prevent further disability and prevent the cancer from returning or metastasizing. The other concern is to limit pain from the cancer and to rehabilitate the cancer patient. Usually, tertiary intervention methods are not handled by the public health system, but it is important for public health professionals to work with medical professionals to ensure a comprehensive cancer control program.[40]

Arthritis

Arthritis is the leading cause of disability in the United States.[41] Nearly 70 million Americans have arthritis, about one in every three adults. With the increasing population of aging Americans, this number will continue to rise. Untreated, arthritis can lead to severe joint pain, physical disfiguration, loss of mobility, and increase the risk of developing other chronic diseases. In addition to the physical effects that arthritis has on individuals, the cost of arthritis was more than $82 billion in 1995. This includes both direct and indirect costs and lost productivity. These costs will continue to rise as the aging population increases.

There are few primary prevention strategies to prevent arthritis. Many of the different types of arthritis are linked to genetics, and usually prevention does not begin until a diagnosis has been made. Interventions for arthritis are secondary and tertiary in nature. The focus of many arthritis programs is to reduce the impact that arthritis has on a person's life after they have been diagnosed and to prevent pain and the loss of mobility. The CDC awards grants to 36 states across the United States to conduct arthritis programs. One of the requirements is that the interventions must be evidence based. Currently, there is only one evidence based intervention for those with arthritis, the Arthritis Self-Help Course (ASHC). The ASHC, developed by Dr. Kate Lorig at Stanford University, is the most widely tested and accepted intervention for those with arthritis. It is a 6-week course designed to help patients with arthritis increase their mobility and maintain their quality of life. Participants are encouraged to implement problem-solving skills into their daily lives. The course also emphasizes maintaining a physically active life, and modifying activities as necessary in order to do so. Research has shown that physical activity decreases pain, improves function, and delays disabilities associated with arthritis. It helps if the person afflicted with arthritis maintains a desirable body weight or reduces the amount of weight on the joints.[42] Research has shown that even a 5-pound weight loss can decrease pain in joints when excess wear and tear on the joints is decreased. In addition to traditional treatments for arthritis, many alternative treatments can also be tried. However, they have not been tested to the extent that physical activity has been, and should be recommended with caution. What works for one patient may not necessarily work for another. It is important to strongly recommend that persons with arthritis continue to exercise on a regular basis and remain mobile.

Osteoporosis

Osteoporosis is another chronic disease that can result in serious disability. Osteoporosis is a disease of the skeletal system and is characterized by low bone mass and deterioration of the bone tissue. This disease is estimated to affect nearly 10 million individuals, and almost 24 million more are estimated to have low bone mass, placing them at increased risk of developing the condition.[43]

Each person's potential bone mass is genetically determined. By age 20, most people have acquired the majority of the bone mass they will have during their lifetime; this is especially true for women. Preventing osteoporosis involves attaining peak bone mass early in life to maintain bone health throughout life. The group most affected by osteoporosis is postmenopausal women, especially of Caucasian decent. However, an increasing number of women of other ethnicities, as well as men, are being diagnosed with the condition.

Osteoporosis prevention can be primary, secondary, or tertiary. Primary prevention ensures that everyone has an adequate calcium intake and encourages participation in weight-bearing activities early in life to reduce the risk of developing osteoporosis later. Because the body cannot produce calcium, it must be obtained from food. The recommended daily calcium intake for adults is:

- 19–50 years—1000 mg/day
- 51 and older—1200 mg/day
- Pregnant and lactating women—1000 mg/day[43]

Recommended food sources of calcium are reduced-fat and nonfat dairy products, dark green leafy vegetables, calcium-fortified foods such as orange juice, and nuts, especially almonds. With high intake of these foods, combined with weight-bearing physical activities, such as walking, jogging, running, dancing, hiking, or basketball, osteoporosis can be avoided.[44]

Once osteoporosis has been diagnosed, there are some secondary and tertiary interventions that can still be effective. Many of the recommendations are the same as those in primary prevention. People diagnosed with osteoporosis should get an adequate intake of calcium every day. As the body can only absorb 500 mg of calcium at a time, calcium intake should be spaced throughout the day with food.[51] It is also important to participate in weight-bearing activities to maintain a desirable weight and maximum bone mass. Individuals with osteoporosis should consult their medical practitioner to learn about the safest types of exercises to effectively strengthen their back and hips. Regular screening should also be done for those younger age groups that are at highest risk of developing osteoporosis later in life. It is often referred to as the "silent disease" because it develops without symptoms. The symptoms may present themselves as a hip, wrist, or spinal fracture. Although osteoporosis cannot be cured, it can be prevented, and in those who have already developed the disease, its progression can be slowed with proper interventions.[43]

Acquired Immune Deficiency Syndrome (AIDS/HIV)

AIDS is not a chronic disease like the others discussed in this chapter, but it has great public health significance. The primary risk factors for AIDS are risky sexual behavior, injection drug use with contaminated needles, and transmission from HIV-infected women to their babies before or during birth or breast feeding after birth.[30] Primary prevention focuses on reducing risky sexual behavior and increasing condom use among those that are infected, decreasing the sharing of contaminated needles, and educating pregnant women infected with HIV on the risk to their child.

Once contracted, there is no cure for the virus, but the survival rate has increased dramatically. The major cause of the extended survival period has been the use of pharmaceutical treatments. Between 1995 and 1997, the mortality from AIDS declined 75%.[30]

The American Dietetic Association (ADA) published medical nutrition therapy protocols for both adult and pediatric patients with HIV/AIDS. These guidelines help dietitians to standardize practices in ambulatory care settings, representing the best evidence-based care. Secondary prevention would be considered the following: (1) optimization of nutrition status, immunity, and well-being; (2) prevention of the development of nutritional deficiencies; (3) prevention of the loss of weight and/or lean body mass; (4) reducing the onset and complications of comorbid conditions; and (5) maximizing the effectiveness of medical and pharmacological treatment. Additionally, food insecurity has been a problem for many people with AIDS. The largest and fastest growing numbers of infected individuals in the United States and other developed countries are in the poor segments of the population who may have the least access to both medical care and food.[31]

Consuming adequate calories from safe food sources and having clean drinking water is often a major need for immune-compromised individuals. They are the most likely to suffer from food-borne and waterborne illnesses. One public health measure that addresses this concern are the public warnings posted in restaurants about consuming raw or undercooked foods in restaurants. There are several waterborne parasites that are not destroyed by the chlorine-based water treatments in most counties. HIV-positive and other immune-compromised individuals should use only water which has come to a rolling boil for one minute or been processed through a filtration system that can document filtrations for *Cryptosporidium* organisms. Monitoring total body weight and lean body mass should be a part of regular care. A regular physical activity program that includes resistance training is important to the maintenance of the lean body mass, endurance, and muscle function.[31]

In addition to the HIV infection, there may be nutrition status changes caused by both short- and long-term side effects from medications. Alterations in appetite, taste, smell, and diarrhea are common changes that may be managed with individualized diet counseling.

Lipodystrophy, dyslipidemia, diabetes, hypertension, heart disease, osteoporosis, and renal disease are increasingly common in HIV-infected individuals. The causes may be genetic, lifestyle, from treatment with certain types of HIV medications, long-term chronic inflammatory disease, and longer-term HIV infection. Recommended medical nutrition therapy may be complicated and dependent on a team of providers that includes family and peer support as well as physicians, a nutritionist, and a social worker. Use of caloric supplements, individualized vitamin and mineral supplements, appropriate dental care, and special foods by supportive caregivers are examples of secondary and tertiary nutrition interventions that can be used with this population.

COLLABORATIONS AND PARTNERSHIPS

Public health professionals are beginning to recognize that by working together they can maximize already scarce resources and broaden their impact. With obesity and overweight as the primary causes of many chronic diseases, health promotion and chronic disease programs are beginning to incorporate weight loss strategies into their interventions. Programs of public and private agencies and foundations are beginning to look to each other to determine how they can collaborate to make biggest impact. Public health nutritionists offer a unique contribution in this collaboration. They offer their extensive knowledge of food and nutrition science and can aid in the design of interventions to ensure they are effective and based on the most current dietary knowledge.

Two examples of successful collaboration are the Steps to a Healthier US program and a partnership between the American Diabetes Association (ADA), American Heart Association (AHA), and American Cancer Society (ACS).[13]

The Steps to a Healthier US Initiative from the US Department of Health and Human Services (DHHS) is designed to help Americans live longer, better, and healthier lives. To kick off this initiative in 2003, a national health summit was convened to call on Americans to take actions that will lead to a healthier nation. Over 1000 community leaders including policymakers, health officials, and other interested stakeholders, attended the summit, entitled Steps to a Healthier US: Putting Prevention First. The summit focused on the importance of prevention and highlighted promising approaches for promoting healthy environments.[13] One of the primary programs put forth by this initiative is the Steps to a Healthier US program. Eleven communities were awarded grants from the CDC to fight obesity, diabetes, and asthma. The programs are to be community driven with members of the participating communities making decisions as to what needs to be done and what evidence-based interventions should be implemented in their communities. Public health nutritionists play a significant role in the design and implementation of the interventions that will take place in the participating communities. In this program, the primary diseases being addressed all have a dietary risk factor. By including public health nutritionists, the dietary component can truly be examined and interventions can be designed to effectively reduce diabetes, asthma, and obesity.

Another unique collaboration is between the ACS, AHA, and ADA. These three health organizations collectively recognized that cardiovascular disease, cancer, and diabetes account for approximately two thirds of all deaths in the United States and about $700 billion in direct and indirect costs each year.[44] To address these diseases and the suffering and death they cause, the ACS, the ADA, and the AHA made a national commitment to prevention and early detection of cancer, cardiovascular disease, and diabetes. Their goal is to bring about substantial improvements in primary prevention and early detection strategies through collaborative efforts; creating public awareness about healthy lifestyles; lobbying for legislative action that results in more funding for and access to primary prevention programs and research; and reconsidering the periodic health checkup as an effective platform for prevention, early detection, and treatment.[44] The screening guidelines developed by this collaboration include the following:

- Use the body mass index (BMI) as part of each regular health care visit for persons 20 years of age or older.

- Blood pressure: Test with each regular health care visit, or at least once every two years.
- Lipid profile: Test every five years at 20 years of age and older.
- Blood glucose test: Test every year for persons at age 45 and older.
- Clinical breast exam: Test every three years at age 20 years of age and older.
- Mammography: Test every year at age 40 and older.
- Pap test: Test every year at age 20 and every one to three years at age 30, depending on type of test and past results.
- Colorectal screening: Test at age 50; frequency depends on preferred test.
- Prostate specific antigen and digital rectal exam: Test yearly at age 50, and assist with informed decision.

The collaboration of these three national health organizations offers new opportunities to advance a collective cause for prevention and early detection of cancer, cardiovascular disease, and diabetes.[45] Because of the reach of this group, they will be able to educate more people and achieve significant progress in health promotion and disease prevention. There will be fewer mixed messages presented to consumers. Multiple messages from different organizations about the same health issue tend to confuse consumers and can be heard as inconsistent. This collaboration provides the opportunity to stimulate new initiatives that could improve health care delivery, such as taking better histories to identify familial disease patterns.[45] By uniting in a common goal with common themes and messages, the ACS, ADA, and AHA may be able to move forward to combat these diseases that cause disability, decrease quality of life, and result in death for millions of Americans.

Role of Public Health Nutritionists

There are key roles that public health nutritionists can play in preventing chronic diseases in adults, although these roles are not limited to just the adult population. These roles can be universally applied to all age ranges. There are seven public health competency areas to be developed by any professional working in the public health area.[22]

Visionary Leadership/Empowerment

This competency is concerned with collaborative leadership to help the organization reach a shared vision. A public health professional competent in visionary leadership and empowerment is capable of promoting self-worth in the client they are serving, of facilitating the process of empowerment for clients through knowledge of risk factors, is supportive in choosing health-promoting lifestyles, and is receptive to new ideas and innovative solutions.

Communication

This competency is focused on listening to others in an unbiased manner and having respect for diverse ideas and opinions. The public health professional that is competent in this area can demonstrate respect for the unique characteristics of the client. Such public health professionals also listen to the client and assist in identifying his or her needs. Demonstrating cultural sensitivity towards the client and teaching or counseling at the client's level of understanding are also important skills in communication with the public.

Information Management

Information management focuses on using technology to manage the transfer of information to end users or clients. Information can be in the form of quantitative or qualitative data, facts, news, knowledge, and ideas. The skills required in this area is the ability to stay up to date on current health services treatments and case management plans, the ability to organize data and give the appropriate information to clients regarding public health and other community resources, and the ability to facilitate the sharing of information between providers, within legal and ethical boundaries.

Assessment, Planning, and Evaluation

Assessment, planning, and evaluation are the competencies that epitomize the continuous quality improvement cycle. The individual with these skills can assess the client needs based on risk factor profiles, medical history, and current systems. Such professionals also plan treatments with the client in order to promote compliance instead of dictating what needs to be done and expecting the client to comply. Individuals with these skills evaluate treatments based on outcomes, expected compliance, and status of high-risk behaviors. Finally, they follow up after the treatment to identify unmet needs and ways to improve the health service delivery system, continually striving to improve treatment options and compliance rates.

Partnership and Collaboration

Through partnerships and collaboration, resources within the public health system can be shared and responsibilities can be spread among several public health professionals instead of relying solely on one individual. To be competent in this area, the public health nutritionist must be able to increase treatment compliance of high-risk individuals through interaction with families and other sources of support. Public health nutritionists also need to function as a member of the case management team and facilitate interaction among groups of clients and providers to communicate the needs of the client and identify effective solutions to health problems.

Systems Thinking

Individuals with a "systems thinking" perspective are concerned with solving problems through future oriented methods and decision making. It is important for the public health nutritionist to be competent in this area in order to optimize the opportunities to improve the health status of the community. To be competent in the area, the professional needs to be able to look at problems from the client's perspective as well as involve the client and support network in solving the problem. The professional also needs to show outcome and benefits of prevention in order to enable the client to take responsibility for his or her own health. This skill also requires that the public health nutritionist be receptive to new ideas and innovative solutions and be able to modify their behavior accordingly if necessary.

Promoting Health and Prevention Disease

Promoting health and preventing disease is the competency that is concerned with putting the science and art of public health into practice. The role of the public health nutritionist in this area is extremely important. Not only is it necessary to understand the disease process, but the professional also needs to understand the determinants of disease and the appropriate primary or secondary interventions. Public health nutritionists who are competent in the area have the abilities to develop and revise protocols for preventive and primary care based on the latest scientific information. They also provide disease prevention and clinical care services in a manner consistent with the mission, priorities, and resources of the organization they work for. Finally, the public health nutritionist who is competent in this area can use every patient encounter as a prevention opportunity.

The public health competencies are not only applicable to public health nutritionists. These principals can be applied to all professionals who work in the public health arena and across the age spectrum. It is important to be skillful in all of these areas in order to achieve the mission and vision of the public health organization and ensure that those individuals who need health information are receiving the most up-to-date information available.

POINTS TO PONDER

- Should public health agencies conduct screening programs for chronic diseases even if there is no money for follow-up treatment?
- How much responsibility should a public health agency take for the obesity epidemic, and how much should the obese individuals take?
- How should public funds be reallocated for primary prevention? How can it be documented that "an ounce of prevention is better than a pound of cure?"
- How can and should public health nutritionists and their professional organizations move into leadership positions in adult health promotion?

HELPFUL WEB SITES

Arthritis

Administration on Aging: www.aoa.gov
American College of Rheumatology: www.rheumatology.org

American Society on Aging: www.asaging.org
Arthritis Foundation: www.arthritis.org
National Council on Aging: www.ncoa.org

Cancer

American Cancer Society: www.cancer.org
Improving Chronic Illness Care: www.improvingchroniccare.org
Susan G. Komen: www.komen.org

Cardiovascular Disease

American Heart Association: www.americanheart.org
American Public Health Association: www.apha.org
Association of State and Territorial Health Officials: www.astho.org/
Centerwatch Clinical Trials Listing Service:
   www.centerwatch.com/patient/index.html
CDC Cardiovascular health: www.cdc.gov/cvh/index.htm
CDC Prevention Chronic Disease Journal: www.cdc.gov/pcd
Chronic Disease Directors, Cardiovascular Health Council:
   www.chronicdisease.org/cvh_council/cvh-index.htm
Healthfinder: healthfinder.gov
Eat Smart Move More—North Carolina: www.eatsmartmovemorenc.com
National Association of County and City Health Workers:
   www.naccho.org/general927.cfm
National Conference of State Legislatures:
   www.ncsl.org/programs/health/phchronic.htm
National Heart, Lung, and Blood Institute: www.nhlbi.nih.gov/index.htm
Partners in information access for public health workers:
   phpartners.org/hp/evidence.html
Public Health Foundation: www.phf.org/index.htm
Public Health Infrastructure Resource Center:
   www.phf.org/infrastructure/index.php
Women's Cardiovascular Health Network: www.hsc.wvu.edu/womens-cvh

Diabetes

American Diabetes Association: www.diabetes.org/homepage.jsp
Arizona Diabetes Prevention and Control Program:
   www.hs.state.az.us/phs/oncdps/diabetes/index.htm
CDC State-based Diabetes Programs:
   www.cdc.gov/diabetes/states/index.htm

CDC Division of Diabetes Translation Web site:
  www.cdc.gov/health/diabetes.html
Diabetes at Work: www.diabetesatwork.org
Health Disparities Collaborative:
  www.healthdisparities.net/training_manuals_and_tools.html
Institute for Healthcare Improvement: www.ihi.org
National Diabetes Education Program: www.ndep.nih.gov
Pan American Health Organization: www.fep.paho.org

Nutrition and Physical Activity

Arizona Action for Healthy Kids: www.ActionForHealthyKids.org
Arizona Department of Health Services: www.hs.state.az.us
Arizona Department of Health Services P.L.A.Y. Program:
  www.maricopa.gov/publichealth/play/about.asp
Arizona Nutrition Network: www.eatwellbewell.org
Arizona's Governor's Council on Health, Physical Fitness, and Sports:
  www.getactivestayactive.org
American Academy of Pediatrics: www.aap.org
**American Alliance for Health, Physical Education, Recreation, and
  Dance:** www.aahperd.org
American Council on Exercise: www.acefitness.org
American Dietetic Association: www.eatright.org
American Obesity Association: www.obesity.org
American Public Health Association, Food & Nutrition Section:
  www.aphafoodandnutrition.org
Association for Worksite Health Promotion: www.uwsp.edu/hphd/awhp
Association of State and Territorial Public Health Nutrition Directors:
  www.astdhpphe.org
CDC Division of Adolescent and School Health:
  www.cdc.gov/nccdpdp/dash/index
CDC 5 A Day: www.5aday.org
CDC Nutrition, Physical Activity, and Obesity Program:
  www.cdc.gov/prgrams.health9
National Association of State Boards of Education:
  www.nasbe.rog/HealthySchools/SamplePolicies/healthyeating
National Center for Chronic Disease Prevention and Health Promotion:
  www.cdc.gov/nccdphp
National Coalition for Promoting Physical Activity: www.ncppa.org
North American Association for the Study of Obesity: www.naaso.org
Partnership for Prevention: www.prevent.org
President's Council on Physical Fitness and Sports: www.fitness.gov
Shaping America's Youth Initiative: www.shapingamericasyouth.com

USDA Center for Center for Nutrition Policy and Promotion:
www.cnpp.usda.gov
USDA Food and Nutrition Service: www.fns.usda.gov

NOTES

1. Delaware Healthcare Association Glossary of Health Care Terms and Acronyms. Available at: http://www.deha.org/Glossary/GlossaryC.htm. Accessed July 29, 2004.

2. National Center for Chronic Disease Prevention and Health Promotion (NCCDPHP). Chronic Disease Overview. Available at: http://www.cdc.gov/nccdphp/overview.htm. Accessed July 29, 2004.

3. National Center for Chronic Disease Prevention and Health Promotion (NCCDPHP). Available at: http://www.cdc.gov/nccdphp/overview_longdesc.htm. Accessed July 29, 2004.

4. National Center for Chronic Disease Prevention and Health Promotion (NCCDPHP). Arthritis Web pages. Available at: http://www.cdc.gov/nccdphp/arthritis/index.htm Background Accessed July 29, 2004.

5. National Center for Chronic Disease Prevention and Health Promotion (NCCDPHP). Available at: http://www.cdc.gov/nccdphp/dnpa/bonehealth/bonehealth.htm. Accessed July 29, 2004.

6. National Osteoporosis Foundation Web site. Available at: http://www.nof.org/osteoporosis/stats.htm.. Accessed July 29, 2004 .

7. National Center for Chronic Disease Prevention and Health Promotion (NCCDPHP). Available at: http://www.cdc.gov/nccdphp/dmpa/obesity/contributing_factors.htm. Accessed July 29, 2004.

8. National Center for Chronic Disease Prevention and Health Promotion (NCCDPHP). Available at: http://www.cdc.gov/nccdphp/power_prevention/pdf/power_of_prevention. pdf. Accessed July 29, 2004.

9. National Center for Chronic Disease Prevention and Health Promotion (NCCDPHP). Chronic disease prevention Web site. Available at: http://www.cdc.gov/nccdphp. Accessed July 29, 2004.

10. www.preventions.org. Accessed July 29, 2004.

11. Brownson RC, Baker EA, Leet TL, Gillespie KN. *Evidence-Based Public Health.* New York, NY: Oxford University Press; 2003:4.

12. Available at: http://www.cdc.gov/ncbddd/cg/day1/Helfand_files/frame.htm#slide 0100.htm. Accessed July 29, 2004.

13. US Dept of Health and Human Services, Steps to a Healthier US. Primary, secondary, and tertiary prevention. Available at: http://www.healthierus.gov/steps/summit/prevportfolio/strategies/reducing/cancer/opportunities.htm#primary. Accessed July 29, 2004.

14. US Dept of Health and Human Services. Partners for Substance Abuse Prevention Web site. Available at: http://preventionpartners.samhsa.gov/resources_glossary_p2. asp. Accessed March 21, 2005.

15. Kaufman M. *Nutrition in Public Health: A Handbook for Developing Programs and Services*. Rockland, Md: Aspen Publishers; 1990.

16. CDC. Overweight and obesity: obesity trends: US obesity trends 1985-2004. Available at: http://www.cdc.gov/nccdphp/dnpa/obesity/trend/maps/index.htm. Accessed July 29, 2004.

17. National Diabetes Education program. Prevengamos la Diabetes tipo 2. Paso a paso. Available at: http://www.ndep.nih.gov/campaigns/Tipo2/Tipo2_overview.htm. Accessed July 29, 2004.

18. National Diabetes Education program. Prevengamos la Diabetes tipo 2. Paso a paso. Available at: http://www.ndep.nih.gov/campaigns/Tipo2/Tipo2_overview.htm. Accessed July 29, 2004.

19. USDA. Choose a diet moderate in salt and sodium. Available at: http://www.nal.usda.gov/fnic/dga/dga95/sodium.html. Accessed July 29, 2004.

20. Association of State and Territorial Public Health Nutrition Directors (ASTPHND) Guidelines of Comprehensive Program to Promote Healthy Eating and Physical Activity. http://www.lastdhpphe.org. Accessed, July 29, 2004.

21. US Dept of Health and Human Services, National High Blood Pressure Education Program. 7th Report of Joint National Committee on Prevention, Detection, Evaluation, and Treatment of High Blood Pressure. Available at: http://www.nhlbi.nih.gov/guidelines/hypertension/express.pdf. Accessed July 29, 2004.

22. US Dept of Health and Human Services, Centers for Disease Control and Prevention. *Promising Practices in Chronic Disease Prevention and Control: A Public Health Framework*. Atlanta, Ga: Department of Health and Human Services; 2003.

23. Available at: http://www.cdc.gov/nccdphp/bb_heartdisease/index.htm. Accessed July 29, 2004.

24. American Heart Association. What Is "Get With the Guidelines"? Available at: http://www.americanheart.org/presenter.jhtml?identifier=1106. Accessed July 29, 2004.

25. University of Pittsburgh. AHA/ACC secondary prevention for patients with coronary and other vascular disease: 2001 update. Available at: http://www.pitt.edu/~super1/lecture/lec5201/pic2.htm. Accessed July 29, 2004.

26. American Cancer Society. Prevention and early detection. Available at: http://www.cancer.org/docroot/PED/content/PED_3_2X_Recommendations.asp?sitearea=PED. Accessed July 29, 2004.

27. Available at: http:/www.cdc.gov/nccdphp/arthritis/index.htm. Accessed July 29, 2004.

28. University of Arizona, College of Agriculture and Life Sciences. Building Strong Bones for a Lifetime. Available at: http://ag.arizona.edu/maricopa/fcs/bb/nutrition.html. Accessed July 29, 2004.

29. CDC. How is HIV passed from one person to another? Available at: http://www.cdc.gov/hiv/pubs/faq/faq16.htm. Accessed July 29, 2004.

30. Palella F Jr, Delaney K, Moorman A, et al. Declining morbidity and mortality among patients with advanced human immunodeficiency virus infection. *N Engl J Med.* 1998;338:853-860.

31. American Dietetic Association and Dietitians of Canada. Nutrition intervention in the care of persons with human immunodeficiency virus infection. *J Am Diet Assoc.* 2004; 104(9):1425-1441.

32. Nelson J, Essien J, Loudermilk R, Cohen D. *The Public Health Competency Handbook: Optimizing Individual and Organizational Performance for The Public's Health.* Atlanta, Ga: Center for Public Health Practice of the Rollins School of Public Health; 2002.

33. Karon J, Fleming P, Steketee R, DeCock K. HIV in the United States at the turn of the century: an epidemic in transition. *Am J Public Health.* 2001;91:1060-1068.

34. Available at: http://www.cdc.gov/ncidod/diseases/crypto/hivaids.htm. Accessed March 21, 2005.

35. US Dept of Health and Human Services. Steps to a Healthier US Initiative. Available at: http://www.healthierus.gov/steps/index.html. Accessed July 29, 2004.

36. Eyre H, Kahn R, Robertson RM. Preventing cancer, cardiovascular disease, and diabetes: a common agenda for the American Cancer Society, the American Diabetes Association, and the American Heart Association. *CA: A Cancer Journal for Clinicians* July 14, 2004.

37. National Cancer Institute, National Institutes of Health. *Cancer Progress Report 2001.* Washington, D.C.: Department of Health and Human Services, 2001.

38. Doll R, Peto R. *The Causes of Cancer: Quantitative Estimates of Avoidable Risks of Cancer in the United States Today.* New York: Oxford University Press, 1981.

39. http://www.cancer.org/docroot/PED/content/PED_3_2X_Recommendations.asp?sitearea=MH. Accessed May 5, 2006.

40. http://www.cdc.gov/cancer/nbccedp/about2004.htm#future, Accessed May 5, 2006.

41. Targeting Arthritis: Reducing Disability for 16 Million Americans and Arthritis: The Nation's Leading Cause of Disability. http://www.cdc.gov/nccdphp/publications/aag/arthritis.htm. Accessed May 9, 2006.

42. http://patienteducation.stanford.edu/internet/arthritisol.html. Accessed May 5, 2006.

43. http://www.cdc.gov/nccdphp/dnpa/nutrition/nutrition_for_everyone/bonehealth/index.htm. Accessed May 5, 2006.

44. ACS/ADA/AHA Scientific Statement. Preventing Cancer, Cardiovascular Disease, and Diabetes: A Common Agenda for the American Cancer Society, the American Diabetes Association, and the American Heart Association. 2004;109:3244–3255. http://www.everydaychoices.org/downloadables/pdf/scientific_stat_acs_ada_aha.pdf. Accessed May 5, 2006.

45. ACS/ADA/AHA Scientific Statement. Preventing Cancer, Cardiovascular Disease, and Diabetes: A Common Agenda for the American Cancer Society, the American Diabetes Association, and the American Heart Association. 2004;109:3244–3255. http://www.everydaychoices.org/downloadables/pdf/scientific_stat_acs_ada_aha.pdf. Accessed May 9, 2006.

BIBLIOGRAPHY

Willett, WC. *Eat Drink and Be Healthy: The Harvard Medical School Guide to Healthy Eating.* New York, NY: Free Press; 2001.

CHAPTER 10

Add Life to Years

Nancy S. Wellman and Barbara Friedberg Kamp

Reader Objectives

- Appreciate the new aging reality and how aging is being redefined.
- Gain sensitivity to ageism stereotypes and avoid their use.
- Learn how nutrition, physical activity, and primary, secondary, and tertiary disease prevention contribute to a life-affirming view of aging.
- Understand the basis for specific nutrient requirements and dietary recommendations for healthy aging and evidence-based disease management.
- Understand the aging services network and opportunities to collaborate with state and local public health agencies.
- Compare and contrast federally funded food assistance and nutrition education programs for older adults as well as Medicare and Medicaid reimbursement available for some prescribed medical nutrition therapy (MNT).
- Utilize expanded opportunities for nutritionists who understand the new aging reality to fill gaps in nutrition services for older adults.

UNDERSTAND THE NEW AGING REALITY

The new reality of aging is that older adults now live longer, healthier, more functionally fit, and more independent lives. Termed *successful* aging,[1] it is also called *active* aging, *productive* aging, *positive* aging, and *healthy* aging. Maintaining optimal nutritional health is vital to successful aging, and contributes to primary, secondary, and tertiary disease prevention. Optimal nutrition helps prevent and reduce the risk or progression of disease and disability. Along with physical activity, optimal nutrition helps older adults maintain high cognitive and physical functioning. A health-promoting diet not only helps *add years to life*, but more importantly it *adds life to years*.

Nutrition fits into the two aging domains of gerontology and geriatrics, although the traditional emphasis has focused on nutrition-related chronic diseases. Gerontology, the study of normal aging, derives from sciences including biology, psychology, and sociology. Public health nutrition, or gerontological nutrition, focuses on health promotion and disease prevention for older adult populations. Health promotion programs are offered to these populations in their communities.

Geriatrics is the study of the chronic diseases frequently associated with aging, including their diagnosis and treatment. Medical nutrition therapy for older adults is often called geriatric nutrition. Although medical nutrition therapy has commonly been practiced in hospitals, this distinction is blurring as nutrition therapy services move out of hospitals and into home and community services. A broader focus on nutrition in all aspects of aging is evolving, as is the focus on healthy lifestyles and disease prevention. Without increasing the emphasis on disease prevention, health care expenditures will increase exorbitantly as the United States' population ages.

Define Ageism

The term *ageism* is defined as any prejudice or discrimination against or in favor of an age group.[2] Despite the new aging reality of vim and vigor, ageism abounds in the United States, a country characterized as one of the most death-denying in the world. Ageism is likely to affect all people at some point in their lifetimes. Even those who believe they are not ageist probably have some ageist attitudes based on myths, stereotypes, and misinformation. Common misconceptions are that most older adults live in nursing homes, are in very poor health, have some degree of mental decline ranging from occasional forgetfulness to severe dementia, are unable to work due to illness or mental decline, are depressed, and live alone. Another misconception is that older people are a homogeneous group, yet they are no more alike than a younger cohort. They encompass several generations and differ considerably based on culture, race, ethnicity, religion, language, gender, sexual orientation, income, education, employment, life experiences, marital status, living arrangement, cognitive capacity, health, and functional status.

In popular American culture, "over the hill" birthday cards poke fun at those who are no longer young. Images in advertisements and on TV programs are often negative when older adults are depicted. There is widespread use of demeaning ageist language, including colloquialisms such as *geezer*, *old fogey*, *old biddy*, *old coot*, *old timer*, and *old goat*. Some nutrition textbooks, as well as other texts, have been found to contain ageist language. Style manuals for writers now include age among the biases to avoid. The American Psychological Association[3] states *elderly* is not acceptable as a noun and is considered by some to be pejorative as an adjective. The term *senior* is considered passé by most, especially today's 78 million *baby boomers*. To sharpen sensitivity to *ageism*, consider the typical classification of words used to refer to people 65 years and older in Table 10–1.

Since aging in the United States' language and culture equates with deterioration and impairment, facts about aging surprise many.[4,5] Only about 5% of adults age 65 years and older are institutionalized, with most nursing home residents being age 85 years and older. Among the 95% residing in communities, over half (54%) live with a spouse. Although many older people have at least one or more chronic health condition, about four in five are healthy enough to engage in their normal activities. The most commonly diagnosed conditions are hypertension (49%), arthritic symptoms (36%), all types of heart disease (31%), any type of cancer (20%), sinusitis (15%), and diabetes (15%). Older adults suffer from fewer acute illnesses and accidents than younger adults. Poor health is not an inevitable consequence of aging. Measures are now available that can improve health, reduce the effects of disease, delay disability and the need for placement in a long-term care facility. Mental decline or mental illness is not inevitable with age. Most older adults maintain normal mental abilities including the ability to learn and remember. Reaction time may become slower with age, and it may take longer to learn something new. Older adults are particularly motivated to maintain their independence and avoid nursing home placement.

Palmore, a (grand) parent of anti-ageism cautions that the consequences of ageism are similar to any discrimination. People subjected to prejudice and discrimination tend to adopt the dominant group's negative image and to behave in

Table 10–1   Typical Categorization of Words Used to Refer to People 65+ Years

Positive	Neutral	Negative
active	adaptable	antiquated, archaic
experienced	aged, aging	cantankerous, crotchety
independent	dementia	difficult, rigid
mature	eccentric	dying, terminal
quick-witted	older adult, older person	feeble, slow, impaired
useful	retired	grouchy, grumpy, peevish
veteran	self-sufficient	old, child-like
vigorous	seasoned	senile, senescent
wise	warm	withered, wizened
youthful	vulnerable	helpless, frail

Source: Excerpted from Palmore EB. *Ageism: Negative and Positive.* 2nd ed. New York, NY: Springer Publishing Co Inc; 1999.

ways that conform to it.[2] In the case of ageism, older adults may give up their freedom to be sexually active, creative, productive, effective, and engaged. Some older adults fail to seek medical treatment for chronic health problems that they believe are a normal part of the aging process and cannot be reversed. Ultimately, these ailments tend to worsen and multiply until it may be too late for treatment.[2] Ageism itself can directly affect longevity. Unlike racism or sexism, ageism's damage is caused by the internalization of the negative images individuals have about older adults. People with positive views of aging, formed before they become older adults, live seven years longer than those who held negatives views of aging.[6]

Government entitlement programs reinforce ageism when they apply a higher federal poverty standard for older adults and target job training to younger age groups. Health care systems in the United States reinforce ageism by focusing on acute care and cures rather than on health promotion and disease prevention throughout the lifespan. Because of the cost of the current obesity epidemic and resulting chronic diseases, federal, state and local public health programs are now beginning to emphasize health promotion and disease prevention. This is an opportune time to advocate for universal access to food and nutrition services in public health, with special attention to needs of older adults (see Chapters 5, 6, and 7).

Understand the Changing Demographics and Trends

Life expectancy in the United States is at an all time high of 77.2 years compared to 47 years a century ago. Women who reach age 65 can expect to live an additional 19.4 years; men, 16.4 years. By year 2030, the population over age 65 will double in number from 36 to 72 million, increasing from 12.5% to 20% of the population. The 85 years and older age group is the fastest growing, from the current 4.6 to 9.6 million in 2030. Members of minority groups will also increase from 17% to 26.4% of the older population. Eligibility for Social Security and other retirement benefits many years ago established age 65 as the cutoff point to classify individuals as older adults. Now, the Census Bureau and other demographers categorize those over 65 years of age as young old (65–74), old (75–84), and oldest old (85+). Some consider today's new old to be those in their nineties. Centenarians now number 50,000 and are no longer considered unique as many of them live independently.[4,5,7]

The gender ratio of three older women to two older men shows up in marital and financial status statistics. While almost 50% of older women are widows, 73% of older men are married. Half of women age 75 years and older live alone. The educational level of older adults is rising; 70% have high school diplomas, and 17% have college degrees.

Median annual income in 2002 was $11,406 for older women and $19,436 for older men. Sources of income of these older people include about 38% from Social Security benefits; 23% from earnings; 18% from assets, and 17% from pensions. Almost 4 million (10.4%) of older adults are classified as poor with another 2.2 million (6.4%) classified as near poor, living on incomes between the poverty level and 125% of the poverty level. Among the poorest are minorities, women, central city and rural residents, Southerners, and those who live alone. Older Hispanic women who live alone had the highest poverty rate, 47%.[4] The adage "Men die married, and women die alone" is even truer if amended to ". . . and women die alone and poor."

As the proportion of the United States population living to older ages grows, it increases demands on the public health system, health care, and social services, including various types of food and nutrition services. Although most (72%) older adults rate their own health as excellent, very good, or good, hospitalization rates for older adults are triple those for people aged 45–64.[4,5] While lengths of stay have decreased overall since 1980 when diagnostic-related groups (DRGs) were established, lengths of stay, office visits to physicians, and out-of-pocket health care expenditures are greater for older people. Health care expenditures for older adults average $3586 compared to $2350 per year for the population as a whole. Many older Americans spend almost 13% of their incomes on health care, more than double that of all consumers (6%). In 2001, health care costs paid by older people averaged $1886 (53%) for supplemental health insurance, $955 (27%) for drugs, $582 (16%) for medical services, and $163 (5%) for medical supplies.[4] Even with the recent addition of a modest prescription drug benefit to Medicare, many older adults who live on low and fixed incomes must choose between paying for their prescribed medicines, food, utilities, or housing. The case study (Table 10–3) later in this chapter illustrates the difficult financial situation common to many older adults.

Functionality and *functional status* are terms used to describe physical abilities and/or limitations in, for example, ambulation.[8,9] Functionality, as does health status, correlates with independence and quality of life. Disability rates among older adults are declining, but the actual number considered disabled is increasing as the size of the aging population grows. Limitations in activities of daily living (ADLs), instrumental activities of daily living (IADLs), and other measures are used to monitor physical function. ADLs include eating independently, and IADLs include shopping and food preparation. Regardless of the measure used, older Americans are aging more successfully in terms of functionality. There are myriad connections between nutrition-related chronic conditions, diets, and functionality.[8–12] For example, diabetes-related amputations impair ambulation, and osteoporosis-weakened bones fracture more easily. Nutrient relationships are now recognized in age-related hearing loss, age-related macular degeneration, cognition, infections, and wound healing. Dehydration impairs cognition, and inadequate or excessive calories affect mobility, stamina, quality of life, and depression. A new curriculum jointly developed by the American Society on Aging and the Centers for Disease Control and Prevention (CDC) emphasizes the connection between older adults' ability to drive and their health.[13] Those who seek to improve their driving longevity are encouraged to increase their physical activity, improve the nutrient quality of their diets, engage in mental exercise, manage their medications, and engage in safe driving practices. For more, see www.asaging.org/cdc/index.cfm.

COMPARE AND CONTRAST THE PUBLIC HEALTH AND AGING SERVICES NETWORKS

In addition to the United States personal health care provider systems, two distinct tax-supported networks—public health and aging services—address the needs of older adults. Although these two service networks share responsibilities for ensuring optimal health in the nation's rapidly aging society, each reaches the older population through different state and local service delivery systems with their priorities driven by their funding sources.

The DHHS Administration on Aging (AoA) is the federal agency responsible for policy development, planning, and funding the delivery of supportive home and community-based services to older people and their caregivers. The AoA works through its national aging services network established when the Older Americans Act (OAA) was legislated in 1972. State leadership of the networks may be administratively placed in the state health department (SHD), in a separate state unit on aging (SUA), or as a separate entity as a part of another state agency such as the governor's office.

This national network, shown in Figure 10–1, consists of 56 state units on aging that provide services through 655 area agencies on aging, 241 tribal and Native American organizations representing 300 American Indian and Alaska Native tribal organizations and two organizations serving Native Hawaiians. This aging network is made up of thousands of service providers, which include adult care centers, caregivers, and volunteers. The estimated 12,000 senior centers nationwide serve 10 million older adults annually.

Over 4400 local OAA funded nutrition programs serve 250 million congregate and home-delivered meals to about 3 million older adults each year. These nutrition programs also provide nutrition screening, education, and counseling, and some provide supportive and health services including transportation, health screening, wellness and fitness programs, and in-home services. The AoA works in partnership with constituent agencies in the USDHHS or DHHS, such as the Centers for Medicare and Medicaid Services (CMS), Centers for Disease Control and Prevention (CDC), and the National Institute on Aging (NIA). About two thirds of the state units on aging employ a nutritionist. Some, but not all, area agencies on aging employ a full-time nutritionist or consultant, as do some of the larger

National Aging Services Network

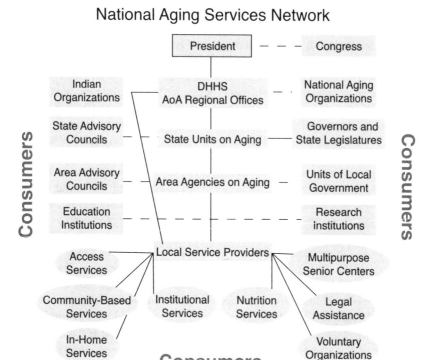

Figure 10–1 National Aging Services Network. *Source:* Administration on Aging. Washington, DC: U.S. Department of Health and Human Services, Administration on Aging.

local Older Americans Nutrition Program providers. Qualified nutrition expertise is limited throughout the aging network, while almost half of the OAA annual budget funds Older Americans' Nutrition programs.

State health departments are part of the public health network supported by state general revenue, as well as by health block grants from several of the constituent agencies of the DHHS. To protect and promote the health and well-being of all Americans, the public health network has developed a system to provide services to prevent diseases, promote health to specified high-risk populations and collect health statistics. Using population-based data, the public health network prioritizes the most urgent health problems and develops policies and programs to address the assessed needs (see Chapter 3). The network includes state public health departments, city and county health departments, as well as university-based schools of public health, and other community-based health agencies. Depending on size of the population and their assessed nutrition-related health needs, state health departments employ a staff of qualified nutritionists (see Chapters 19, 20). If the state unit on aging is part of the state health department, its public health nutrition staff may be responsible for aging services. In recent years, however, public health nutritionist positions in state and local public health departments have been largely employed to work with clients enrolled in the Special Supplemental Nutrition Program for Women, Infants, and Children (WIC) with funds from the US Department of Agriculture (see Chapter 8). With this funding earmarked to serve high-risk, low-income pregnant/breast-feeding women, infants and preschool children, most public health nutritionists have limited opportunities to offer related community nutrition services to older adults.

Resulting from the need to strengthen collaboration and cooperation between these two essential networks, the Association of State and Territorial Chronic Disease Program Directors and the National Association of State Units on Aging with support from AoA and CDC initiated an Aging States Project in 2001.[14] Information was compiled about health needs, activities, and partnerships related to health promotion and disease prevention for older adults served by SUAs and SHDs and to identify opportunities for collaboration. Chronic diseases, especially heart disease, and prescription drug coverage were the greatest shared concerns, but both agencies acknowledged limited involvement in these top aging health issues and perceived multiple barriers. SUAs cited individual lifestyle barriers, and SDH cited systems barriers. The aging services network grows out of the social service model of providing one-on-one services to each client with an addressed need and referral. The public health network, on the other hand, is built on an assessment of community population needs to develop programs and services to promote health and prevent disease through organized programs. Since the agencies collaborate minimally, each was generally unaware of the other's strengths. Each used different data sources to plan and evaluate their programs. The Aging States Project found that the quality and quantity of health promotion programs for older adults could be enhanced without requiring substantial additional funding. In each state, a lead coordinator might be assigned to mobilize the chronic disease prevention expertise of health professionals employed by state and local health departments and build on the community outreach capacity of state units on aging. Nutrition and physical activity were the topics most frequently noted in best practice models for risk reduction through behavior change. This presents an opportunity to increase the amount of nutrition expertise as public health and aging networks collaborate to help older adults live healthier, more independent, and satisfying lives.

NUTRITION STATUS AND DIETS OF OLDER AMERICANS

There are many gaps in knowledge about nutrition and aging. The needs for specialized anthropometric, biochemical, clinical, and dietary assessment methods and standards for older populations are beginning to be developed. Although a number of longitudinal studies on aging populations are underway, data are lacking to clarify changes in nutritional status with advancing age to 100 years and beyond.[15]

Characteristics to consider when assessing the nutritional status of older adults include their physical activity level, dentition, and any difficulties in absorption, transport, metabolism, and/or excretion of essential nutrients. Chronic diseases, drug/nutrient, and drug/drug interactions due to multiple prescriptions and self-prescribed medications such as vitamins, minerals, and herbs must be assessed. Functional fitness, mental health, recent weight loss or gain, alcohol intake, and social isolation must also be assessed. The older adult's socioeconomic status and participation in food or nutrition assistance programs and other community services must be part of the assessment.

Preventive health services recommended for adults age 65 years and older include an annual nutrition screening followed by a comprehensive assessment. Care planning should include nutrition therapy and physical activity counseling as needed.

Interpretation of nutrition assessment data should differentiate characteristics of the normal aging process from those attributable to degenerative chronic diseases. More specific nutritional assessment data on older adults, particularly those aged 75 years and older are needed both for those who live independently in their own homes, and also those in institutional care, for whom there is virtually no national data. Memory lapses and impaired hearing and/or vision might limit accuracy of food and nutrient intake data using traditional dietary interview methods. The Automated Multiple Pass Method (AMPM) is a new US Department of Agriculture (USDA) computer-assisted interviewing tool to help people remember and report actual foods they have eaten over a 24-hour period.[16] Because it more precisely captures food consumption data and achieves almost total 24-hour recall, it holds promise for use with older age groups. Changes in body composition and stature should also be considered when taking anthropometric measurements of older adults. Body mass index (BMI) should be interpreted with caution due to differing correlations than those found with younger adults.

For more, go to www.ars.usda.gov/is/AR/archive/jun04/recall0604.htm.

Poor nutrition is a serious problem for many older adults, especially minorities with health disparities.[11,17] Although most older adults do not display clinical evidences of overt nutrient deficiencies, surveys show that many consume inadequate diets and are at increased risk of malnutrition and subclinical nutrient deficiencies that may affect function and quality of life.[11,17,18] Since micronutrient needs may increase as calorie needs decline with age, older adults must be advised to choose more nutrient-dense foods.

A recent 12-year European study, the Hale Project, investigated the combined effect of a Mediterranean diet, physical activity, moderate alcohol use, and non-smoking on older adults aged 70–90 years. The study found 50% lower mortality rates, all-cause and cause specific, in those older adults who followed a Mediterranean style diet and made healthful lifestyle choices including regular physical activity and not smoking.[19]

Protein-Energy Undernutrition (PEU)

Protein-energy undernutrition (PEU) is diagnosed in many older adults. It is defined as the presence of clinical signs that include wasting or involuntary weight loss, low BMI, and biochemical evidence such as low serum albumin and insufficient nutrient intake.[20] Because those people 85 years and older are at greatly increased risk of being hospitalized and/or institutionalized, they are the most likely to develop severe undernutrition. As many as 40–85% of nursing home residents are malnourished, making PEU the most serious long-term care problem. Upon admission, 40% to 60% of hospitalized older patients are malnourished or at risk of malnutrition. Complications and mortality are two to three times more common, and hospital care costs are 35–75% higher. Hospital stays are longer and home care needs are greater for older patients who are malnourished. PEU is also observed in 20% to 60% of homebound older adults and is predictive of mortality.[20–22]

Several syndromes associated with undernutrition that may occur singly or in combination have been recently diagnosed in older adults.[20] Sacropenia, the age-related loss of skeletal muscle mass, affects strength and accelerates functional decline. At the other end of the weight spectrum, morbidly obese older people may have sarcopenic obesity as their muscle mass loss may be greater due to immobility in addition to increased age.[23] Cachexia is the cytokine-mediated inflammatory injury response, and wasting is semistarvation with inadequate food intake that results in weight loss. Neither cachexia nor wasting are a normal part of the aging process. These terms have often been used interchangeably to describe loss of body cell mass. Newer evidence separates these two conditions, which are particularly challenging to treat when increased extracellular fluids mask the weight loss of cachexia. Another age-related catchall term, *failure to thrive*, is being replaced by its four treatable components: impaired physical functioning, malnutrition, depression, and cognitive impairment.

Factors that contribute to poor food intake, less nutrient-dense food choices, overeating or undereating, include loneliness and grief as spouse, relatives, and friends pass away; fear of illness and disability; forgetfulness; vision and hearing loss; tooth loss or poor dentition; or moving out of the home of a lifetime. Side effects of medications can cause many older people to lose their appetites and interest in eating. Declining income, living in substandard housing, lack of transportation, limited education, and purposeful self-starvation contribute to poor health and nutritional status. Ability to shop for, safely store, prepare, and consume a nutritionally adequate diet may decrease with age, depending upon the individual's functional and health status. The cost to the community of providing a homebound older adult with a nutritious home-delivered midday meal for one year is the same as the cost of one day of hospital care. Not surprisingly, Older Americans Act Nutrition programs often have waiting lists. The small number of qualified nutritionists employed in the aging network and in home health care programs has delayed establishment of risk-based criteria to prioritize people on these waiting lists. Comprehensive care planning should include nutrition therapy, ongoing monitoring of the homebound who receive meals, and some nutrition services.[17]

Overweight and Obesity

Overweight tendancies and obesity, the most common nutrition-related health risks in the United States, are problems for older adults too. Overweight risks generally increase through age 55, then stabilize in women, and decline in men.[20] Between ages 65 to 74, 34% of women and 24% of men are overweight, and an additional 27% of women and 24% of men are obese. Older African-Americans and women living on poverty-level incomes have the highest obesity rates. In 1999, 37% of older adults were overweight, and nearly 18% were obese.[24] Although being overweight is associated with increased risk for many chronic diseases including heart disease, high blood pressure, diabetes, arthritis-related disabilities, and some cancers, this association is not as clear in older adults. Many epidemiological studies suggest that the relationship between body mass index (BMI) and mortality lessens as age increases, especially among people aged 75 and older. BMI is not a predictor of mortality or hospitalization for most individuals aged 75 and older.[25,26] Several factors have been proposed. Older adults are more likely than younger adults to have diseases that both increase mortality and cause weight loss leading to lower body weight.

Treatment for overweight and obese older adults should be based on an individual benefit versus risk analysis. Obesity not only affects the health of older adults, it also affects their day-to-day lives. Older people who are obese report more limitations of activity and more feelings of sadness and hopelessness than those who are not obese. Differences between the obese and nonobese populations are particularly striking for people ages 51 to 69. Some data support the association of obesity and premature mortality in older people and, therefore, life expectancy may have peaked in the United States.

Chronic Diseases

Four out of five older adults have one chronic condition and half have two or more chronic conditions.[4,20] Minorities and people age 85 and older are at greatest risk for chronic disease. In 2003, of Medicare's annual $300 billion budget, 99% was spent on chronic disease management, with about $71 billion for medical care costs associated with diseases attributable to poor diet.[27] Many physicians acknowledge the importance of nutrition, but seldom incorporate nutrition screening and intervention into their care plans for older adults. Every dollar spent on nutrition screening and intervention saved one health care system $5.63.[27] Disease-specific nutrition screening and interventions are crucial to management of many chronic diseases. In general, medical nutrition therapy identifies and addresses calorie and nutrient intakes that are excessive or inadequate, body weight, and fitness.

Coronary Heart Disease

Coronary heart disease (CHD) causes one in five deaths in the United States. Of those who die from coronary heart disease, 85% are age 65 years or older. Evidenced-based nutrition therapy to lower blood lipid levels and improve drug effectiveness includes diet counseling to reduce intake of saturated fats, trans-fatty acids, and cholesterol. Patients are advised to increase their daily intake of fruits, vegetables, whole grains, nuts, legumes, fiber, and to reduce their body weight, when appropriate. Dietary restrictions may be contraindicated for frail older people, especially those in nursing homes or those assessed to be appropriate for nursing home placement and who receive home and community services through the Medicaid-waiver program.[21]

Hypertension

Hypertension (HTN) is a manageable risk factor for CHD, occurring in one in three American adults, with many unaware that they have it.[28,29] It is more prevalent in people over age 60. Prevalence in African-Americans is double that of white Americans between ages 55 and 64. Among African-Americans, hypertension occurs at an earlier age and with higher average blood pressure readings. African-Americans have a greater rate of nonfatal stroke and heart disease death. Hypertension is a leading risk factor for stroke, congestive heart failure, and end-stage renal disease. Stroke is the leading cause of long-term disability in the United States. Evidenced-based medical nutrition therapy is cost effective even when drugs are prescribed. Nutrition therapy includes reduced salt/sodium intake, weight reduction for those who are overweight, and the *Dietary Approaches to Stop Hypertension* diet, commonly called the DASH diet, with more fruits, vegetables, low-fat milk products, and unsalted nuts.[30]

Congestive Heart Failure

Congestive heart failure is the most common diagnosis in hospitalized patients over age 65, and occurs in even greater numbers for African-Americans. Evidence-based medical nutrition therapy focuses primarily on reducing salt/sodium intake, limiting fluid intake when edema is present, and weighing the patient daily to detect rapid weight gain from fluids. Noncompliance with prescribed diet and/or medication results in hospital readmissions of about half of older patients. This is another chronic disease where patient compliance to prescribed medical nutrition therapy contributes to reducing health care costs.

Diabetes

Diabetes mellitus affects one in five older adults. In descending order, incidence is higher in Native Americans and Alaskan Natives, Hispanic Americans, and African-Americans. As obesity rates climb, the incidence in all populations is increasing. In older adults, atypical symptoms can delay diagnosis and treatment. Diabetes mellitus is the leading cause of heart disease, stroke, blindness, end-stage renal disease, and lower-limb infections and amputations. Gum disease and tooth loss are also common. Diabetes is the costliest chronic disease, because of comorbidities and the detrimental effects on quality of life. Individually prescribed evidence-based medical nutrition therapy normalizes blood sugar levels by limiting calorie intake and encouraging daily exercise to attain a healthier body weight. Costly complications caused by elevated blood glucose can be reduced by managing diabetes with individually prescribed diets and prescription drugs. Data documents that every dollar spent on outpatient diet counseling and education can save $2–3 in hospital costs.

Osteoporosis

Osteoporosis is a bone-thinning disease that increases the risk of fractures with age.[31] Among the almost 30 million affected, four in five are women, especially white women with low body mass indices (BMI). The 1.5 million osteoporosis-related fractures each year are costly both to individuals and to tax payers. Evidence-based medical nutrition therapy emphasizes increased dietary intake of calcium and Vitamin D, and/or supplements along with encouraging weight-bearing activities and advising the older patient on strategies to prevent falls.

An Institute of Medicine Committee on Nutrition Services for Medicare Beneficiaries concluded that evidence strongly supports reimbursement for medical nutrition therapy for Medicare beneficiaries diagnosed with dyslipidemia, hypertension, diabetes, and osteoporosis. Evidence also supports medical nutrition therapy for patients diagnosed with heart failure, predialysis kidney failure, and undernutrition.[20]

NUTRITION SCREENING INITIATIVE

The Nutrition Screening Initiative (NSI), a national coalition of health and social service organizations under the direction of the American Dietetic Association and the American Academy of Family Physicians, promotes routine nutrition screening and intervention for older adults as a cost-effective strategy to improve the health of older Americans and manage their chronic diseases.[22,27] Nutrition Screening Initiative members conclude that effective nutrition intervention can help keep older adults at home and in their communities, reduce costs of prescription drugs, hospital, and nursing home care. A brief review of nutrition-related chronic diseases excerpted from NSI's *Nutrition Statement of Principle* and *A Physician's Guide to Nutrition in Chronic Disease Management for Older Adults* documents the contributions of optimal nutrition to healthy aging for all racial, ethnic, and income groups.[22,27] These guides recommend physicians refer patients to registered dietitians for prescribed medical nutrition therapy. *A Nutrition Guide for Older Adults* provides some food tips specific to diagnosed chronic diseases.

Based on the USDA *Healthy Eating Index (HEI),* most diets of older Americans need improvement.[18] Only 9% of those who live on incomes at or below the poverty level and 21% of those who live on incomes above poverty level had diets rated as *good.* People aged 65 years and older, 77% living on incomes at or below poverty level and 65% living on incomes above the poverty level, have poor diets. Diets rated as poor included insufficient calories, protein, and vitamins, and excessive calorie and fat intakes contributing to obesity and related conditions. Data from the *National Health and Nutrition Examination Survey III* (NHANES III) found many older adults' diets to be low in calories, total fat, fiber, calcium, magnesium, zinc, copper, folate, and vitamins B_6, C, and E. The Institute of Medicine committee studying the need to reimburse for nutrition services for Medicare beneficiaries found strong evidence that older adults are at high risk for vitamin D deficiency, given the limited food sources of vitamin D. Contributing factors included their insufficient sunlight exposure in winter especially among those who live in long-term care facilities, having reduced subcutaneous production of vitamin D_3, and increased use of sunscreen and protective clothing.[32]

Only one in three older adults consume the recommended five or more servings of fruits and vegetables each day. Three servings of whole grains are recommended, but intakes averaged only one serving. Daily dietary calcium intake is less than 800 mg compared to the 1200 mg recommended. Vitamin D intake averages 4–6 µg daily, while the recommendation is the highest for older adults, 10 µg (400 IU) for those aged 51 to 70 years, and 15 µg (600 IU) for those 70 years or older.[31] Unless older adults drink about four 8-ounce glasses of milk daily, they need to use calcium-fortified foods (e.g., calcium fortified fruit juices or milk, breakfast cereals, soy foods), a multivitamin, and a calcium supplement with vitamin D to meet the recommended requirements.[28]

Vitamin B_{12} deficiency increases with age, because the decreased ability to digest the forms of Vitamin B_{12} found in meat, poultry, fish and dairy foods.[20]

Vitamin B_{12} is necessary for cognition, nervous system function, vascular health, and formation of red blood cells. Consequently, older adults need to consume most of their vitamin B_{12} in the easier-to-absorb crystalline form found in many, but not all, fortified breakfast cereals as well as in multivitamin supplements.

DIETARY RECOMMENDATIONS FOR HEALTHY OLDER AMERICANS

Many older adults have special nutrient requirements because aging effects absorption, utilization, and excretion.[33] The Dietary Reference Intakes (DRIs) groups recommendations for those age 51 to 70 years and for those over age 70 years. Previously published recommendations combined both in a 50+ age category.[34,35] Dietary studies suggest that older people consume low intakes of calories, total fat, fiber, calcium, magnesium, zinc, copper, folate, and vitamins B_6, C, E, and D.[18,28,31]

The *Dietary Guidelines for Americans* translate the nutrient-based DRIs into food-based *Guidelines*. The year 2000 edition was the first to address the specific needs of healthy older people. Updated every five years, the 2005 *Dietary Guidelines* emphasize eating a variety of foods while staying within energy needs and controlling calories to manage body weight.[36] Because of newer scientific information, the 2005 *Dietary Guidelines* emphasize being physically active 30 minutes per day, staying hydrated by drinking fluids, eating more whole grains, potassium-rich fruits and vegetables, and non-fat or low-fat dairy products, decreasing sodium (salt) intake, and, for older adults, getting some vitamin B_{12} and vitamin D from fortified foods and/or supplements. The *Guidelines* recommend selecting fiber-rich foods for their digestive, intestinal, cholesterol lowering, and other health benefits, including relief from constipation, a common complaint of Americans young and old. There is no specific guideline about sugars, which include table and other sugars added during food processing. However, older adults who are overweight should limit added sugars to lower total calories.

The Food Guide Pyramid is an illustration of the *Dietary Guidelines*. It helps one visualize the types and amounts of foods to eat each day in various food groups.

Healthy People 2010, a comprehensive set of health promotion and disease prevention objectives for the nation, has two overarching goals, both relevant to older adults.[11] These are to increase quality and years of healthy life and to eliminate health disparities. While aging is not addressed in a separate chapter as it was in *Healthy People 2000*, a topic search for aging found 67 relevant objectives in 19 of the focus areas. Almost two thirds of these age-related objectives address chronic conditions associated with obesity, overweight, or specific nutrient excesses or deficiencies. Data can be used to convince administrators, colleagues, funders, health planners, and policymakers that funding community nutrition programs, which include both nutrition education to promote health and medical nutrition therapy to manage diagnosed chronic diseases, are cost effective. *Healthy People 2010* challenges people throughout their lives to practice health promotion and chronic disease prevention through healthy food choices and regular physical activities (see Chapter 9). This publication endorses self-management and personal responsibility.

The National Institute on Aging (NIA) established by Congress in 1974, conducts and supports biomedical, social, behavioral research and training related to the aging process, as well as degenerative diseases, and other special problems and needs of older people. The Gerontology Research Center in Baltimore, Maryland, the USDA Human Nutrition Research Center on Aging at Tufts University in Boston, and the National Resource Center on Nutrition, Physical Activity, and Aging at Florida International University in Miami focus on nutrition and aging from the cellular to the food and people programmatic levels. Of the many university-based gerontology centers, few others study the nutritional aspects of aging.

Several simplified tools have been developed to encourage nutrition screening of older adults, including the Nutrition Screening Initiative Nutrition Checklist[37] and the Mini Nutritional Assessment shown in Figure 10–2.

Both recognize the multiple factors that may contribute to poor nutritional status in older adults. These tools flag those individuals most likely to be at increased risk of malnutrition. Use of these tools alerts health professionals of the need to refer at-risk clients to a registered dietitian (RD) for a complete nutrition assessment and comprehensive care planning as appropriate.

RECOMMEND MORE PHYSICAL ACTIVITY FOR OLDER AMERICANS

The American College of Sports Medicine Position Stand: Exercise & Physical Activity for Older Adults is resoundingly reassuring in the following excerpt and throughout the text:[39]

> In the past, exercise generally has been considered inappropriate for *frail* or very aged older individuals. The past decade has seen an accumulation of data that dispels the myths of frailty and provides reassurance of the safety of exercise.

Connections between regular physical activity for disease prevention, weight control, and overall good health are necessary for people of all ages. For older adults, especially for those who are frail, physical activity lessens the consequences of chronic diseases such as hypertension and diabetes; it can also improve mobility and functionality.[8–10] Despite overwhelming evidence of benefits, few older adults engage in the recommended 30 minutes or more of moderate physical activity on most days of the week. Moderate physical activity can be defined as activities that cause light to moderate sweating and may increase the heart and breathing rate. The CDC's *Behavioral Risk Factor Surveillance Survey* (BRFSS) in 2000 found that 28% to 34% of adults ages 65 to 75 years are physically inactive, increasing to 35% to 44% of adults age 75 years and older who

Mini Nutritional Assessment
MNA

Last name:	First name:	Sex:	Date:
Age:	Weight, kg:	Height, cm:	I.D. Number:

Complete the screen by filling in the boxes with the appropriate numbers.
Add the numbers for the screen. If score is 11 or less, continue with the assessment to gain a Malnutrition Indicator Score.

Screening

A Has food intake declined over the past 3 months due to loss of appetite, digestive problems, chewing or swallowing difficulties?
0 = severe loss of appetite
1 = moderate loss of appetite
2 = no loss of appetite ☐

B Weight loss during last months
0 = weight loss greater than 3 kg (6.6 obs)
1 = does not know
2 = weight loss between 1 and 3 kg (2.2 and 6.6 lbs)
3 = no weight loss ☐

C Mobility
0 = bed or chair bound
1 = able to get out of bed/chair but does not go out
2 = goes out ☐

D Has suffered psychological stress or acute disease in the past 3 months
0 = yes   2 = no ☐

E Neuropsychological problems
0 = severe dementia or depression
1 = mild dementia
2 = no psychological problems ☐

F Body Mass Index (BMI) (weight in kg)/(height in m)^2
0 = BMI less than 19
1 = BMI 19 to less than 21
2 = BMI 21 to less than 23
3 = BMI 23 or greater ☐

Screening score (subtotal max. 14 points) ☐☐

12 points or greater Normal–not at risk– no need to complete assessment

11 points or below Possible malnutrition–continue assessment

Assessment

G Lives independently (not in a nursing home or hospital)
0 = no   1 = yes ☐

H Takes more than 3 prescription drugs per day
0 = no   1 = yes ☐

I Pressure sores or skin ulcers
0 = no   1 = yes ☐

Ref.: Guigoz Y, Vellas B and Garry PJ. 1994. Mini Nutritional Assessment: A practical assessment tool for grading the nutritional state of elderly patients. *Facts and Research in Gerontology.* Supplement #2:15–59. Rubenstein, LZ, Harker J, Guigoz Y and Vellas B. Comprehensive Geriatric Assessment (CGA) and the MNA: An Overview of CGA, Nutritional Assessment, and Development of a Shortened Version of the MNA. In: "Mini Nutritional Assessment (MNA): Research and Practice in the Elderly". Vellas B, Garry PJ and Guigoz Y, editors. Nestlé Nutrition Workshop Series. Clinical & Performance Programme, vol. 1. Karger, Bâle, in press.
© Société des Produita Nestlé S.A., Vevey, Switzerland, Trademark Owners

J How many full meals does the patient eat daily?
0 = 1 meal
1 = 2 meals
2 = 3 meals ☐

K Selected consumption markers for protein intake
• At least one serving of dairy products (milk, cheese, yogurt) per day?   yes ☐ no ☐
• Two or more serving of legumes or eggs per week?   yes ☐ no ☐
• Meat, fish or poultry every day   yes ☐ no ☐
0.0 = if 0 or 1 yes
0.5 = if 2 yes
1.0 = if 3 yes ☐.☐

L Consumes two or more servings of fruits or vegetables per day?
0 = no   1 = yes ☐

M How much fluid (water, juice, coffee, tea, milk . . .) is consumed per day?
0.0 = less than 3 cups
0.5 = 3 to 5 cups
1.0 = more than 5 cups ☐.☐

N Mode of feeding
0 = unable to eat without assistance
1 = self-fed with some difficulty
2 = self-fe3d without any problem ☐

O Self view of nutritional status
0 = view self as being malnourished
1 = is uncertain of nutritional state
2 = views self as having not nutritional problem ☐

P In comparison with other people of the same age, how do they consider their health status?
0.0 = not as good
0.5 = does not know
1.0 = as good
2.0 = beetter ☐.☐

Q Mid-arm circumference (MAC) in cm
0.0 = MAC less than 21
0.5 = MAC 21 to 22
1.0 = MAC 22 or greater ☐.☐

R Calf circumference (CC) in cm
0 = CC less than 31   1 = CC 31 or greater ☐

Assessment (max. 16 points) ☐☐.☐

Screening score ☐☐

Total Assessment (max. 30 points) ☐☐.☐

Malnutrition Indicator Score
17 to 23.5 points   at risk of malnutrition ☐
Less than 17 points   malnourished ☐

08. 95 USA

Figure 10–2   Mini Nutritional Assessment MNA. Copyright (2005), Nestle Nutrition Services USA.

are inactive.[40] Most older women are less physically active than men, and African-American older adults are less active than white older adults.[41,42]

Sedentary lifestyle has been correlated to increased morbidity and mortality. Those who engage in regular physical activity usually are found to live longer than those who are sedentary. Sedentary lifestyles pose both a physical and financial threat to all Americans. The health care system bears these increased costs. Medicaid and Medicare spend billions of dollars each year to pay for medical care for the five most commonly diagnosed chronic conditions—diabetes, heart disease, cancer, depression, arthritis—all of which can be moderated by regular physical activity. The word *exercise* is less acceptable to older adults than *physical activity* or *physical fitness*.

HealthierUS, a DHHS initiative, encourages Americans to live longer, better lives by being physically active, eating health-promoting foods, getting periodic preventive screenings, and making healthy choices, like not smoking.[43] As part of this initiative, the Administration on Aging designed the *You Can! Steps to Healthier Aging* to increase the number of older adults who are active and healthy.[44] *You Can!* is built on partnerships that mobilize communities, create public awareness, and make programs more available to help older Americans improve their food choices and increase their physical activity. For more go to: www.aoa.gov/youcan.

Nutritionists understand the relationship between calorie intake and expenditure. They are the logical leaders to implement national initiatives in local communities that encourage older adults to be more physically active and improve the nutrient density of their diets. To link food and fitness for older adults, the National Resource Center on Nutrition, Physical Activity, and Aging has prepared *Eat Better & Move More: A Guidebook for Community Programs*.[45] This ready-to-use program has plans for 12 weekly sessions including minitalks, group activities, and take-home "Tips & Tasks" sheets. Simple food checklists are used to encourage healthier food choices, and step counters motivate participants to walk more. This program is designed to fit the interests and needs of older adults who need encouragement to maintain their quality of life and independence. It is successful, because small changes in diet and physical activity can make a difference at any age.

FOOD INSECURITY

For many older adults, food insecurity is a broader concern than limited or uncertain food affordability, accessibility, and availability due to lack of resources. For many older adults, food insecurity also includes their inability to prepare, shop for, or eat healthy food due to functional limitations.[46] Food insecurity rates vary in households with older adults by household composition, income, race, ethnicity, and location of residence. Over 7% of older adults live alone. Between 1998 and 2000, this older population group experienced the only increase in food insecurity or hunger.[47]

Food insecurity results in a less varied diet and lower intakes of essential nutrients and calories. Consequences for older adults include a higher risk of underweight and/or reporting fair or poor health. Known linkages between poverty and obesity are attributed to poor-quality diets with an excess of high-calorie, low nutrient–dense foods, including some fast foods and snack foods. Food insecurity makes it difficult for many older adults to follow physician-prescribed diets to manage their diagnosed chronic diseases. This can have life-threatening and costly consequences, such as insulin shock in people with diabetes.

Many older Americans who live on poverty-level incomes are food-insecure, even hungry, and need both food and financial assistance. Inadequate nutrient intake affects nearly 40% of individuals 65 years of age and older. In 2000, 1.5 million households with older adults reported that they did not have enough of the right types of food they needed to maintain their health. Some reported that they simply did not have enough food to eat. Federally funded programs are available to combat food insecurity and poor-quality diets, as well as to address special dietary needs and other functional limitations that compromise the health of older Americans who must live on low fixed incomes.

Federally Funded Food and Nutrition Programs That Serve Older Adults

About $1 billion is appropriated annually for *all* food and nutrition programs that serve older adults. The largest are funded through the Older Americans Act.

Nutrition programs funded by the Older American Act focus on social service aspects with limited input from qualified nutritionists. There is less emphasis on documented health risk eligibility criteria or on nutrition standards. The assumption is that five midday meals weekly are sufficient for all older adults. Federally funded food assistance and nutrition programs that serve older adults are summarized in Table 10–2.

DEPARTMENT OF HEALTH AND HUMAN SERVICES (DHHS)

The Administration on Aging (AoA) administers funding to qualifying local agencies to provide food and nutrition services under the Older Americans Act of 1965. There are six core service areas. Aside from **Title IIIC**, not all are dedicated to support food and nutrition services, but many states use these to fund such services for older adults.

Title IIIB, Supportive Services provides local agencies with funds to provide transportation to medical appointments, grocery, and drug stores. It provides handyman, chore, and personal care services. Additional services that can be funded include: housing subsidies, long-term care, legal assistance, services to encourage employment of older workers, and crime prevention. Title IIIB funds

Table 10–2 Federal Programs Providing Food Assistance to Older Adults

Program	Purpose	Federal Appropriation	Target Populations	Services	Number Served
US Department of Health & Human Services (USDHHS) Administration on Aging (AoA)					
Older Americans Act Titles I–VII	Grants to state, tribal, community programs on aging; research, demonstration projects, etc.[1]	$1.37B Total FY2004[2]	Age 60+ in greatest economic need and/or social need, with particular attention to low-income minorities and those in rural areas	See below	7.5M older adults FY2003
"	Title III Nutrition services to older adults[1]	$714M FY2004	See above	Congregate and home-delivered meals; nutrition screening, education, counseling; array of other supportive and health services	2.9M older adults 250M meals FY2002
"	Title VI Tribal and native organizations for aging programs & services[1]	$26M FY2004	Age requirement determined by tribal organizations or Native Hawaiian program	Congregate and home-delivered meals; nutrition screening, education, counseling; array of other supportive and health services	67,000 older adults 3M meals FY2003

Program	Purpose	Federal Appropriation	Target Populations	Services	Number Served
US Department of Health & Human Services (USDHHS) Administration on Aging (AoA)					
Nutrition Services Incentive Program[3] (NSIP)	Provides proportional share to states and tribes of annual appropriation based on number of meals served in prior yr.	$148M FY2004	Age 60+, < 60 yrs, and disabled who live in elderly housing, disabled living at home and eat at congregate sites w/ older adults	Cash and/or commodities to supplement meals	2.9M older adults ~252M meals FY2001
USDHHS		**Indian Health Service (IHS)**			
Indian Health Service[4]	Nutrition and Dietetics Program	No line item funded; funded through clinical services	American Indians and Alaska Natives	Array of nutrition services including clinical nutrition counseling, home and community-based nutrition services, such as diabetes self management and nutrition education	$87,000 older adults FY1998

(continues)

239

Table 10-2 continued

Program	Purpose	Federal Appropriation	Target Populations	Services	Number Served
USDHHS					
			Centers for Medicare & Medicaid Services (CMS)		
Medicaid Waiver Program[5]	Reimbursements to states for Medicaid recipient services	No data available	Older adults with physical and developmental disabilities; those who qualify for Medicaid	Array of home and community-based services as an alternative to long-term care in institutional settings	No data available
Medical nutrition therapy (MNT)	Reimbursements to providers of nutrition services	Medicare covers 80% of approved amount for MNT after individual pays $100 deductible for Part B services[6]	Medicare beneficiaries with diabetes and predialysis renal disease[7]	Diabetes self-management training; predialysis nutrition therapy by registered dietitians (RDs)	No data available
United States Department of Agriculture (USDA) Food & Nutrition Service (FNS)					
Food Stamp Program	Assists low-income families to buy food that is nutritionally adequate[8]	$30.9 B FY2004[9]	US citizens and legal residents who are most in need, gross income ≤ 130% federal poverty level; up to $2000 countable resources, $3000 if age 60+ or disabled	Coupons or electronic benefits to purchase breads and cereals, fruits and vegetables, meats, fish, poultry; dairy products, seeds and plants that produce food for households	21 M 51% Children 40% Adults 9% Age 60↑ FY2002

Program	Purpose	Federal Appropriation	Target Populations	Services	Number Served
United States Department of Agriculture (USDA) Food & Nutrition Service (FNS)					
Food Stamp Nutrition Education Program[10]	Nutrition education	$192 M FY2003	Low-income individuals receiving or eligible for food stamps	Programs focusing on healthy food choices and active lifestyles	19 M FY2002 Age groups not defined
Food Distribution Program on Indian Reservations[11]	Provides commodity foods to low-income households living on or nearby Indian reservations	$86.2 M FY2004	Low-income American Indians and non-Indians that reside on a reservation or those on approved areas near reservations or in Oklahoma that contain at least one person who is a member of a federally and recognized tribe	Supplemental foods for a nutritionally balanced diet Receives a box of commodities once a month Nutritional information for healthy food choices	1.3 M FY2003 Age groups not defined
Commodity Supplemental Food Program	Food and administrative funds to states and tribes to supplement diets Available in 33 states and 2 tribes[12]	$98 M FY2004[13]	Pregnant and breast-feeding women, mothers up to 1 year postpartum, infants, children up to age 6 with incomes ≤ 185% federal poverty Adults 60+ with incomes ≤ 130% federal poverty guideline	Supplemental foods to complete the diet of recipient. Participants receive a free box of commodities up to once a month	5.5 M 85% older adults FY2003

(continues)

241

Table 10-2 continued

United States Department of Agriculture (USDA) Food & Nutrition Service (FNS)

Program	Purpose	Federal Appropriation	Target Populations	Services	Number Served
Seniors' Farmers Market Nutrition Program[14]	Grants to state and tribes to provide fresh foods and nutrition services while providing the opportunity for farmers to enhance their business	$15 M FY2002–2007	Low-income older adults: at least 60 years old and who have household incomes of not more than 185% federal poverty	Coupons or vouchers to be exchanged for fresh fruits and vegetables at local farmers markets	47 agencies FY2004; 700,000 older adults FY2003
The Emergency Food Assistance Program (TEFAP)[15]	Provides food to local agencies that directly serve the public	$190 M FY2003; $172 M worth of food FY2002	Adults aged 60+ who meet state criteria based on income, including homeless, low-income older adults	Emergency food for low-income needy persons, including older adults. States provide food to local agencies, usually food banks, which in turn, distribute food to soup kitchens and food pantries that directly serve the public	No data available
Child and Adult Care Food Program[16]	Healthy, nutritious meals for children and adults in day care centers	$1.8 B FY2003	Children < 12 yrs, homeless children, migrant children < 15 yrs. Disabled citizens regardless of age. Age 60+; functionally impaired; reside with family members	Nutritious meals and snacks	86,000 adults FY2003; Age groups not defined

Sources:

1. US Dept. of Health & Human Svcs., Administration on Aging: www.aoa.gov

2. US Dept. of H&HS, FY 2005 Budget in Brief: www.dhhs.gov/budget/05budget/aoa.html#ao

3. US Dept. of H&HS, Admin. on Aging, Nutrition Services Incentive Program: www.aoa.gov/eldfam/Nutrition/Nutrition_services_incentive.asp

4. DHHS, HIS Trends in Indian Health, 1998–1999. US Dept. of Health & Human Svcs.

5. US Dept. of H&HS, Medicaid, Medicare Coverage: www.cms.hhs.gov/medicaid/waiver1.asp

6. US Dept. of H&HS, Medicare, Medicare Answers: MNT Benefit, www.medicare.gov

7. Centers for Medicare & Medicaid Services, *Medicare News*, March 1, 2002, "Medicare Revises Medical Nutrition Therapy Policy," www.cms.hhs.gov/media/press/release.asp?Counter=425

8. USDA Food & Nutrition Svcs., "Applicants & Recipients: Introduction," www.fns.usda.gov/fsp/applicant_recipients/about_fsp.htm FSP Services

9. "USDA Food Stamp Program Participation and Costs" (Data as of 2005–12/21), "USDA FY2005 Budget Summary," www.fns.usda.gov/pd/fssummar.htm FSP Federal Appropriation (www.usda.gov/agency/obpa/Budget-Summary/2005/FYbudsum.pdf)

10. USDA Food & Nutrition Svcs., Governments/Nutrition Education Information, "Nutrition Program Facts: Food Service Program Nutrition Education," www.fns.usda.gov/fsp/nutrition_education/factsheet.htm FSNEP

11. USDA Food & Nutrition Svcs., Food Distribution Fact Sheet, March 2005, "Food Distribution Program on Indian Reservations," www.fns.usda.gov/fdd/programs/fdpir/pfs-fdpir.pdf FDPIR

12. USDA Food & Nutrition Svcs., Food Distribution Pgms., "About CSFP: Commodity Supplemental Food Program," www.fns.usda.gov/fdd/programs/csfp/about-csfp.htm CSFP Services offered

13. USDA Food & Nutrition Svcs., "Senior Farmers' Market Nutrition Program," www.fns.usda.gov/wic/SeniorFMNP/SFMNPmenu.htm

14. USDA Food & Nutrition Svcs., Food Dist. Programs, www.fns.usda.gov/fdd/programs/csf/pfs-csfp.pdf CSFP Number Served, Service Units, Federal Appropriation

15. USDA Food & Nutrition Svcs. Pgm., Food Distribution Programs, "About TEFAP," USDA Food & Nutrition Svcs., "Child and Adult Care Food Program," www.fns.usda.gov/fdd/programs/tefap/about-tefap.htm

243

can be extended to cover community adult day care and information referral and assistance.

Title IIIC, Nutrition Services funding supports local agencies that provide nutritious meals in congregate settings and home-delivered meals. The OAA targets those in greatest economic or social need with particular attention to low-income minorities and rural individuals. Although this is the only federally funded nutrition assistance program that is not means tested, 84% of home-delivered and 65% of congregate meal participants are considered to be poor or near poor. All meals served must meet one third of the most recently published *Dietary Reference Intakes* for older adults, as published by the Food and Nutrition Board of the National Academy of Sciences (See Chapter 2, Table 2–1). These nutrition programs must also provide nutrition education, counseling, and health screening, and often are the gateway to many other services. Since it was enacted, the nutrition programs funded by Older American Act have served nearly 6 billion meals to at-risk older people. Each day in communities throughout the United States, older adults come together in groups to share a meal and companionship. Homebound people can have meals delivered, sometimes by an older volunteer who may be their only regular visitor. The Older Americans Act Nutrition Program has been shown to improve the nutritional status and decrease the social isolation of its participants.[48,49]

Congregate meals are offered at community centers such as senior centers, faith-based settings, schools, and adult day centers. These nutrition programs serve 3 million participants annually. The meal provides an estimated 40–50% of recommendations for daily nutrients and calories. Most older adults who participate say that this single meal provides half or more of their total food intake for the day. Many eat more food at congregate sites than they would eat at home. In addition to providing a hot meal, the congregate sites provide seniors with social interaction and stimulation, and an opportunity to feel more involved in their community. Almost all participants like to visit with friends, and 60% say that their social opportunities have increased since attending.[47]

Home-delivered meals are provided to frail homebound unable to travel to a congregate meal site. Like the congregate meals, home-delivered meals provide the recipients with more than nutritious food. Volunteers who deliver the meals provide a friendly visitor, especially to the 59% who live alone.[48] Volunteers can help monitor the health of the homebound and make sure that they receive other services they may need. The recipient who becomes able to participate in a congregate meal site is no longer eligible to receive home-delivered meals.

The Nutrition Services Incentive Program (NSIP) provides a cash allotment or commodity foods to states and Indian tribal organizations (ITO) for their Older Americans Act nutrition programs. The amount of funds dispersed is based on the number of meals served in the previous year and averages about 60 cents per meal served. The purpose of the NSIP is to provide incentives to encourage and reward effective performance in the efficient delivery of nutritious meals to older individuals. The funds are received from the government quarterly.[50]

Title IIID, Disease Prevention and Health Promotion Services provides SUAs with funds for health risk assessments, routine health screening, nutrition counseling and education, health promotion programs, exercise and fitness programs, home injury control service, screening for prevention of depression, educational programs, medication management education, counseling regarding social services, and information concerning diagnosis, prevention, treatment and rehabilitation of age-related chronic diseases and conditions. Priority is given to areas of the state that are medically underserved and where there are a large number of older individuals who have the greatest economic need for such services. Since no credentials or qualification are specified in the Older Americans Acts, nutritionists in many states use this title to fund nutrition education and other services as primary prevention.

Title IIIE, National Family Caregiver Support Program funds local community agencies to provide support services to help the primary caregivers of older adults. These may include disseminating information about available services and assistance in accessing services. These may include individual counseling in decision-making and problem-solving, supplemental services to complement caregiver care, and support groups available in the local community. Caregivers also may need help from a registered dietitian to understand the special nutrition and dietary needs of the older person in their care. Caregivers themselves are often at nutritional risk and may need encouragement to make time for themselves and to choose healthy foods. Title IIIE also funds services to meet the needs of grandparents who must care for their grandchildren. States, tribes, and communities across the country are making significant progress in implementing the NFCSP. Communities across the country have reached out to almost 4 million individuals with information about caregiver programs and services, provided assistance in accessing services to approximately 436,000 caregivers, served almost 180,000 caregivers with counseling and training services, provided respite to over 70,000 caregivers, and provided supplemental services to over 50,000 caregivers.[51]

Title IV, Training, Research, and Discretionary Projects and Programs fund competitive grants or cooperative agreements for eligible public or private nonprofit agencies, organizations, and institutions for evidence-based research and interventions with older adults. It supports the National Resource Center on Nutrition, Physical Activity, and Aging at Florida International University. Founded in 1995, the center is the nation's only university-based nutrition source of technical assistance, information dissemination, and applied research directed to assist nutrition programs funded by the Older American Act.

The center's mission is to promote active healthy aging through good nutrition and to increase food and nutrition services in home and community-based social, health, and long-term care systems serving older adults. The center strives to place food and nutrition services in the mainstream of home and community-based care systems serving older adults. The center works with the AoA to provide national leadership for the Older Americans Nutrition Program by providing training and technical assistance to the aging network. The center's Web site, is a digital storehouse of resources, including hundreds of references in its continuously updated bibliography section, many with direct links to journal abstracts. The center's Web site also includes links to relevant nutrition and aging Web sites including federal agencies, national organizations and foundations, educational institutions, and private enterprises.

The center works to reduce nutrition risk among older adults, especially minorities with health disparities. The goals are to support quality of life, improve functionality, promote independence, and decrease early nursing home admissions and hospitalizations through better nutrition and increased physical activity. The center encourages risk-based nutrition screening to identify and serve the most needy, and conducts policy analysis and outcomes research. The center's applied, community-based research has fostered vital links among faculty researchers, local nutrition service providers, older adults, and caregivers.

Title VI funds nutrition and supportive service to organizations that address the unique Native American, Hawaiian, and Inuit cultural and social traditions, especially the tribal elders, as they are among the most disadvantaged groups in the United States. Apparently, the Hawaiian and Inuit nations have separated themselves from continental tribes.

Title VII, Vulnerable Elder Rights Protection Activities allots funds to protect and enhance the basic rights and benefits of vulnerable or abused older people, such as the National Long-Term Care Ombudsman Program. Paid and volunteer ombudsmen advocate for residents of nursing homes, board and care homes, and assisted living facilities (ALFs). Their presence in these facilities monitors care and conditions providing a voice for those unable to speak for themselves. Many nurse and social worker ombudsmen are concerned about food and nutrition issues and are receptive to nutritionist input. Elder abuse includes food deprivation and serving substandard food. Concerned registered dietitians can be effective ombudsmen, and more of them should be trained to become visible Long-term Care Ombudsmen.

Medicaid Waiver Program

Medicaid is a state-federal partnership that pays for health and long-term care services to low-income people who are aged, blind, disabled, or members of families with dependent children, or who meet certain other criteria for need.[52] In 1981, federal legislation established the Home- and Community-based Care Service (HCBS) Waiver program under Section 1915(c) of the Social Security Act.[53] This permits states to provide community-based services by waiving certain Medicaid statutes and regulations. These waivers enable individuals who are at risk of being placed in long-term care facilities to receive care at home, preserving their independence and ties to family and friends. Approved nutrition services include home-delivered meals, nutrition risk reduction counseling, and nutritional supplements as appropriate. Waivers are state-specific so that each state has the flexibility to develop and implement its own benefits package. Only 38 states include meals and/or nutrition services among the specified benefits available through these waivers. Shrinking state budgets and escalating Medicaid/ Medicare expenditures are forcing states to control costs related to health and nursing home care. Older people who are eligible for nursing home placement are not usually able to shop for food, safely store food, plan, and prepare nutritionally appropriate meals. Annual nursing home care now averages $70,000 per year[54]—much more costly than services provided by HCBS waivers. As such, a strong argument can be made to fund all or some meals and nutrition services based on health and nutrition risk criteria. For more detailed information, see www.cms.hhs.gov/medicaid/1915c /default.asp.

Medical Nutrition Therapy Benefit

The Medical Nutrition Therapy (MNT) benefit was added to the Medicare, Medicaid, and State Children's Health Insurance Program (SCHIP) Benefits Improvement and Protection Act of 2000 (BIPA) implemented in 2002.[55] This act authorizes licensed or registered dietitians and nutritionists to be reimbursed directly by Medicare. Only MNT prescribed for diabetes and diabetes self-management training and predialysis renal disease were covered in the 2002 legislation. Continuing advocacy efforts are being made to cover MNT prescribed for cardiovascular disease, end stage renal disease (dialysis), osteoporosis, obesity, and undernutrition. MNT includes comprehensive assessment of the patient's nutrition and health status including food preferences, physical activity level, and lifestyle. Based on this, the credentialed nutrition professional collaborates with the patient and caregiver to develop an individualized care plan that may include diets and meal plans. Recommendations are monitored and adjusted as needed. The benefit does not cover dietary supplements or foods. The American Dietetic Association has detailed information on becoming a provider, Current Procedure Terminology (CPT) codes, Medicare billing, and disease-specific practice guidelines. For more go to: www.eatright. org and www.cms.gov.

US Department of Agriculture (USDA)

Several Department of Agriculture Nutrition Assistance Programs that serve low-income Americans are available to older adults. All are means-tested. To be eligible, recipients must meet stipulated income criteria.

Food Stamp Program

The Food Stamp Program (FSP) is the largest USDA food assistance program. Since 1974, the Food Stamp Program has provided monthly coupons or electronic benefit transfer (EBT) cards to eligible low-income families to purchase food. All 50 states, the District of Columbia, and Puerto Rico are now using some form of EBT system. In most states, FSP administration is a division within departments of health, human services, family services, or economic security. A complete list of state contact agencies can be found at www.fns.usda.gov/fsp/government/ state-contacts.htm.

There is evidence that many older adults are unaccustomed to using these cards or are reluctant to trust others to use them as their surrogate. Only one third of eligible older adults participate in the Food Stamp Program. The 30% of eligible older adults who participate represent less than 10% of food stamp users. Some of the reasons eligible older adults give for not applying for this program include their lack of information, perceived lack of need, low expected benefits, difficult application procedures, and the stigma of receiving public benefits.

Current regulations from USDA's Food and Nutrition Service (FNS) encourages state agencies to provide nutrition education to their food stamp participants and those who are eligible. Specific outreach to older adults however, is limited. The goal of food stamp nutrition education is to encourage food stamp recipients to make healthy food choices within their limited budget consistent with the most recent *Dietary Guidelines for Americans* and the Food Guide Pyramid. Although education is generally provided by the state's cooperative extension service, state nutrition education networks, public health departments, welfare agencies, and university centers may also be sponsors.

Commodity Supplemental Food Program (CSFP)

The Commodity Supplemental Food Program (CSFP) strives to improve the health of low-income Americans by supplementing their diets with nutritious USDA commodity foods. It provides food and administrative funds to states to supplement the diets. Currently, 33 states and two tribal organizations participate. At the state level, CSFP administration is located within one of the following departments: public health, nutrition services, health services, education, family and children, housing, community service, environmental nutrition, WIC services, or agriculture. Eligible populations include adults over age 60 with incomes less than 130% of the federal poverty level. Local agencies responsible for administering CSFP determine eligibility of applicants, distribute the foods, and provide nutrition education. These food packages do not provide a complete diet, but supply good sources of nutrients frequently lacking in diets of low-income populations. This program began to serve older adults in 1982. In 2003, 389,000 older adults participated.[56]

Seniors' Farmers Market Nutrition Program (SFMNP)

The Seniors' Farmers Market Nutrition Program (SFMNP) may be administered by state departments of agriculture, aging and disability services, health and human services, markets, public health, state unit on aging, or state food and nutrition services. SFMNP provides coupons to low-income older individuals to purchase fresh, unprepared foods at farmers' markets, roadside stands, and community-supported agriculture programs. It provides eligible older adults with local seasonal access to fresh fruits, vegetables, and herbs. It is also increases domestic consumption of agricultural commodities, and is specifically designed to help support and create more farmers' markets, roadside stands, and community-supported agriculture programs. Currently, the program is available in 40 states, five Indian Tribal Organizations, the District of Columbia, and Puerto Rico. Annual benefits to older adults range from $15 to $125, averaging $25 annually, are only available during the local harvest season.

Child and Adult Care Food Program (CACFP)

The Child and Adult Care Food Program (CACFP) serves nutritious meals and snacks to eligible children and older adults in participating child care centers, day care homes, and adult day centers. Centers can serve breakfast, lunch, supper, and snacks. Meals are composed of 1-cup milk, 1–2 pieces fruit or vegetable, grain, and meat or meat alternative. Portion sizes vary by age group. Breakfast must include three components; lunch, all four components; supper, three components; and snack, two of the four components. Meals served must meet these minimum requirements to be reimbursable.

Emergency Food Assistance Program (TEFAP)

The Emergency Food Assistance Program (TEFAP) is a commodity food distribution program. The USDA buys food, including processing and packaging, and ships it to the states' distributing agency. The program was designed to help reduce federal food inventories and storage costs while assisting the needy. Each state's allotment depends on the number of its low-income and unemployed population. States provide food to local agencies, usually food banks, which in turn, distribute the food to soup kitchens and food pantries that directly serve those needing food assistance. These organizations distribute the commodities for household consumption or use the foods to prepare and serve meals in a congregate setting. Since TEFAP tracks amounts of food distributed nationally, there are no data regarding number of recipients.

Food Distribution Program on Indian Reservations (FDPIR)

The Food Distribution Program on Indian Reservations (FDPIR) is a commodity food distribution program used instead of food stamps at times, when travel is impossible. USDA purchases and ships commodity foods to Indian tribal organizations and state agencies based on orders from a list of available foods. Administering agencies store and distribute the food, determine applicant eligibility, and provide nutrition education to recipients. USDA provides the administering agencies with funds for program administrative costs. In 2003, FDPIR served 107,000 people; of those, 15% were age 60 years and older.

Table 10–3 illustrates the benefits that an older woman who lives alone might receive from the various assistance programs. Note that the annual benefit amount from each program varies greatly and that expenditures can exceed income when costs of medical care, prescription drugs, housing, and other costs are higher than average.

HOSPICE, A HOME, AND COMMUNITY SERVICE TO MEET END-OF-LIFE NEEDS

Hospice is not a *place*, but a concept of care. Originally used to describe a place of shelter for weary travelers, *hospice* stems from the Latin word *hospitium* meaning *guesthouse*. The modern hospice movement began in England in the 1960s, with a team approach to professional caregiving. It was the first to use modern pain management techniques to compassionately care for the dying. Since 1974, when the first hospice opened in the United States, hospice has grown into a 3100 program network that annually cares for over a half million people, primarily in their own homes. Hospice is an increasingly visible part of communities serving people across the continuum of care.

Hospice care relies on an interdisciplinary team of health professionals that includes physicians, nurses, medical social workers, therapists, counselors, and volunteers. A perfunctory online search of major hospice associations and providers found no mention of nutritionists or dietitians, and little information on food and fluids at the end of life. The American Dietetic Association encourages registered dietitians to become active in hospice care. The American Dietetic Association has self-study continuing professional education (CPE) audio course, *End-of-Life Decisions: Nutrition and Hydration Issues, a Multidisciplinary Management Approach.* It discusses basic legal principles for end-of-life directives; reviews legal cases regarding hydration and nutrition therapy; and explains the role of registered dietitians as team members during ethical decision-making when end-of-life decisions are being deliberated. Medicare Part A covers hospice care and hospital insurance, including physician services, nursing, equipment, drugs, home health aide, physical, occupational and speech therapy, and counseling that may include nutrition. Currently Medicare Part B covers MNT for those with diabetes or kidney disease with a physician's referral.

EXPAND NUTRITION SERVICES FOR OLDER ADULTS

With the growing older population eligible for Medicare and Medicaid benefits and escalating health care costs, urgent priorities for federal and state agencies are to reduce costs for Medicare and Medicaid benefits. Services for more older adults must move from in-patient hospital and long-term care facilities into the home and community. Public health nutritionists and aging network nutritionists can collaborate to establish and expand food assistance, disease prevention, and medical nutrition therapy programs and services to support older adults so they can remain independent in their own homes or with their families. Older adults want to learn about nutrition and physical activity for health promotion, risk reduction, and disease prevention.

Food assistance packages, congregate meal programs, and home-delivered meals must meet the needs of older adults for prescribed medical nutrition therapy to maintain their health and control their many diagnosed chronic diseases. As these programs become more medicalized, public health nutritionists, aging network nutritionists, and community dietitians must present evidence-based data to document that nutrition is essential to maintain healthy active aging. By presenting cost-effectiveness and cost-benefit data, registered dietitians can document that more comprehensive nutrition services in OAA-funded nutrition programs and other home and community-based services programs for older adults, including day service programs, can reduce costly hospital admissions and readmissions and delay the need for nursing home placement.

Nutritionists, registered dietitians, and their professional organizations should work with their state and federal legislators and policy makers to advocate for regulations requiring community food assistance, meal service, and home health agencies to employ credentialed nutrition professionals. Coordinated public policy advocacy should involve state and district dietetic associations, public health nutritionists, aging network nutritionists, and home health care registered dietitians (RDs), along with other health professionals, such as case managers and their respective organizations.

The small numbers of dietitians employed in home and community food assistance and health services for older adults must be expanded to help older Americans successfully maintain optimal health and independence as they age. The campaign for healthy active aging must promote optimal nutrition and physical activity in later years. Because nutrition is prevention, risk reduction, and treatment, nutrition services are essential in planning, positioning, and marketing cost-effective programs to better serve older adults.

POINTS TO PONDER

- If improved nutrition leads to successful aging, should more resources be spent on nutrition services including nutrition education, medical nutrition therapy, and healthy meals for older adults?
- Is it ageist to assume that positive lifestyle changes are ineffective in improving health, nutritional status, functional fitness, and quality of life of older adults?

Table 10-3   Case Study of Typical Low-income Adult

BK, a 79-year-old overweight widow in good health with hypertension, worked part-time after raising children. Her husband, a moderate wage earner, died of a heart attack at age 66. Most of their modest savings went to pay his medical bills and prescriptions. BK receives a monthly Social Security benefit of $875.[1] BK receives $3500 annually ($291 monthly) from her husband's pension. She does not own her home and pays $460 per month on rent (~41% of her income[2]). Monthly, BK spends $155 on food.[3] Utilities expenditures average $115 per month.[4] BK spends $65 per month on transportation, clothing, home maintenance, and toiletries. BK's health care expenses total $3568 annually. This includes monthly out-of-pocket expenses of $157 on insurance, $80 on prescription drugs, $50 on medical services, and $14 on medical supplies.[5] Estimates for out-of-pocket health costs are likely low and are expected to increase over the next few years as health care costs increase. Medicare premiums go up when health care costs rise. After expenses are paid, BK has only $70.

Now consider the importance of federal food and nutrition assistance programs to her. Attending a congregate dining program helps assure that BK has five nutritious meals a week. This is not sufficient as most Americans eat 21 meals and several snacks weekly. According to the USDA's Food and Nutrition Services online food stamp prescreening eligibility tool,[6] BK is eligible for a monthly food stamp benefit of ~$50–80.[7] She can also receive commodity and supplemental foods. Food packages include a variety of foods, such as nonfat dry and evaporated milk, juice, farina, oats, ready-to-eat cereal, rice, pasta, egg mix, peanut butter, dry beans or peas, canned meat or poultry or tuna, and canned fruits and vegetables. The monetary value of food packages is estimated to be $17. She can participate in SFMNP in her state, although this annual benefit totals on average only about $25 during her state's growing season. The table below summarizes her situation.

Description	Monthly Income	Monthly Expense
Social Security	$875	
Widow's pension	$291	
Rent		$460
Food		$155
Utilities		$115
Misc., transportation, clothing, etc.		$65
Health insurance		$157
Drugs/medication		$80
Medical services		$50
Medical supplies		$14
Balance	**$70**	
Federal Nutrition Assistance		
Older Americans Nutrition Program: Value of meals	$100	
Food Stamps	$50	
CSFP actual retail value generally higher	$17	
SFMNP: Note: $25 average annual benefit divided by 12	$2	
Total Value	**$169**	

Sources:

1. Social Security Administration
2. U.S. Dept. of Health & Human Svcs., Administration on Aging site, http://aoa.gov/prof/Statistics/profile/2003/11.asp accessed 1/17/2006, Professionals department, Statistics section, "A Profile of Older Americans 2003" page, "Housing" section. The source cited for this section is noted as

Table 10–3 continued

"American Housing Survey for the United States in 2001, Current Housing Reports" H150/01. www.aoa.gov.

3. U.S. Dept. of Ag., Center for Nutrition Policy and Promotion site, accessed January 17, 2006, Food Plans department, Updates section, report titled, "Official USDA Food Plans: Cost of Food at Home at Four Levels, U.S. Average, July 2004." People can access the report at CNPP's home page: www.cnpp.usda.gov/.

4. U.S. Dept. of Health & Human Svcs., Administration for Children & Families site, www.acf.hhs.gov/programs/liheap/notebook.html, accessed January 17, 2006; U.S. Dept. of Health & Human Svcs. Admin., Admin. for Children & Families home page, Working with ACF section/ACF Programs link; Working with ACF page, ACF Programs section/Low Income Home Energy Assistance link; Low Income Home Energy Assistance Program page, Data/Households section, LIHEAP Home Energy link, "LIHEAP Home Energy Notebook For Fiscal Year 2003" document. (www.acf.hhs.gov/ would be sufficient as a Helpful Web site).

5. U.S. Dept. of Health & Human Svcs., Administration on Aging site, http://www.aoa.gov/, accessed today, January 17, 2006. USAoA home page, Professionals department, Statistics on the Aging Population link; A Profile of Older Americans: 2003 report, Health and Health Care section. www.aoa.gov/prof/Statistics/profile/2003/14.asp

6. & 7. U.S. Dept. of Ag. home page, www.usda.gov/wps/portal/usdahome, accessed January 17, 2006. (Simply using www.usda.gov will bring the reader to the aforementioned URL). Browse by Section sidebar/Food and Nutrition link; Food and Nutrition dept./Related Topics sidebar, Food Assistance link; Food and Nutrition dept./Food Assistance section, Food Stamp Program link; Food Stamp Program page, Featured Areas sidebar/Online Pre-screening Tool; Food Stamps Pre-screening Eligibility Tool page.

- If a virus was found to take seven years off everyone's life expectancy, considerable effort would be devoted to finding the cause and a cure. A likely cause has been identified: societally sanctioned ageism. What curative actions can our country adopt to increase our life expectancy?
- How can public health nutritionists become more involved in home and community-based programs that serve older adults? How can they become more involved in the aging networks?
- Given the cost of health care for treatment of chronic diseases, when are prevention dollars better spent—in early, mid, or later years?
- What are the ethical dilemmas presented by age-based rationing of nutrition services?

HELPFUL WEB SITES

American Dietetic Association: www.eatright.org

CMS (Centers for Medicare & Medicaid Services): www.cms.gov

CMS – Medicaid: www.cms.hhs.gov/home/medicaid.asp

Live Well, Live Long – Health Promotion Modules:
www.asaging.org/cdc/index.cfm

U.S. Administration on Aging – You Can! Steps to Healthier Aging Campaign: www.aoa.gov/youcan/

NOTES

1. Rowe JW, Kahn RL. *Successful Aging*. New York, NY: Pantheon; 1998.

2. Palmore EB. *Ageism: Negative and Positive*. 2nd ed. New York, NY: Springer Publishing Inc; 1999.

3. American Psychological Association. *Publication Manual of the American Psychological Association*. 5th ed. Washington, DC: APA; 2001.

4. Administration on Aging, US Dept of Health and Human Services. *A Profile of Older Americans 2003*. Available at: http://www.aoa.gov/prof/Statistics/profile/2003/profiles2003.asp. Accessed November 12, 2004.

5. National Center for Health Statistics. 1998–2000. Available at: http://www.cdc.gov/aging/health_issues.htm#2. Accessed November 12, 2004.

6. Levy BR, Slade MD, Kunkel SR, Kasl SV. Longevity increased by positive self-perceptions of aging. *J Pers Soc Psycho*. 2002;83:261–270.

7. US Census Bureau. Available at: http://www.census.gov/prod/2001pubs/c2kbr01-10.pdf. Accessed November 12, 2004.

8. US Dept of Health and Human Services. Physical Activity and Health: A Report of *the Surgeon General*. Atlanta, Ga: Centers for Disease Control and Prevention (CDC), National Center for Chronic Disease Prevention and Health Promotion; 1996. Available at: http://www.cdc.gov/nccdphp/sgr/sgr.htm. Accessed November 12, 2004.

9. Physical Activity and Older Americans: Benefits and Strategies. Available at: http://www.ahrq.gov/ppip/activity.htm. Accessed November 12, 2004.

10. Butler RN, Davis R, Lewis CB, et al. Physical fitness: benefits of exercising for the older patient. *Geriatrics*. 1998;53:46–62.

11. US Dept of Health and Human Services. *Healthy People 2010*. Washington, DC: US Government Printing Office; 2000. Available at: http://www.healthypeople.gov. Accessed November 12, 2004.

12. Sharkey JR, Haines PS. Nutrition risk screening of home-delivered meal participants: relation of individual risk factors to functional status. *J Nutr Elderly*. 2002;22:15–34.

13. American Society on Aging and CDC. Road Map to Driving Wellness. Available at: http://www.asaging.org/cdc/signin.cfm?module=4. Accessed November 12, 2004.

14. Administration on Aging. Collaboration between the public health and aging services networks. Available at: http://www.aoa.gov/prof/agingnet/healthyaging/collaboration/collaboration.asp. Accessed November 12, 2004.

15. National Center for Health Statistics, CDC. *Aging* activities. Available at: http://www.cdc.gov/nchs/agingact.htm. Accessed November 12, 2004.

16. US Dept of Agriculture, Agricultural Research Service, Food Surveys Research Group. Automated Multiple Pass Method Survey Tool. Available at: http://www.ars.usda.gov/is/AR/archive/jun04/recall0604.htm. Accessed November 12, 2004.

17. Mathematica Policy Research Inc. *Serving Elders at Risk, the Older Americans Act Nutrition Programs: National Evaluation of the Elderly Nutrition Program 1993–1995, Executive Summary.* Washington, DC: US Dept of Health and Human Services; 1996. Available at: http://www.aoa.gov/. Accessed November 12, 2004.

18. US Dept of Health and Human Services, Center for Nutrition Policy and Promotion. Quality of diets of older Americans. *Nutrition Insight 29.* June 2004. Available at: http://www.cnpp.usda.gov/insights.html. Accessed November 12, 2004.

19. Knoops, de Groot, et al. *JAMA* 2004;292:1433–39. HALE Study.

20. Institute of Medicine, Committee on Nutrition Services for Medicare Beneficiaries. *The Role of Nutrition in Maintaining Health in the Nation's Elderly: Evaluating Coverage of Nutrition Services for the Medicare Population.* Washington, DC: National Academies Press; 1999. Available at: http://www.nap.edu/category.html?id=fn. Accessed November 12, 2004.

21. American Dietetic Association. Position of the American Dietetic Association: liberalized diets for older adults in long-term care. *J Am Diet Assoc.* 2002;102:1316–1323. Available at: http://www.eatright.org/Public/index_7705.cfm. Accessed November 12, 2004.

22. Nutrition Screening Initiative. *NSI Nutrition Statement of Principle.* Available at: http://www.aafp.org/nsi. Accessed November 12, 2004.

23. Jensen GL, Friedmann JM. Obesity is associated with functional decline in community-dwelling rural older persons. *J Am Geriatr Soc.* 2002;50:918–923.

24. *HealthUS* 2002. Available at: http://www.cdc.gov/nchs/data/hus/tables/2002/02hus070.pdf. Accessed November 12, 2004.

25. Luchsinger JA, Lee WN, Carrasquillo O, Rabinowitz D, Shea S. Body mass index and hospitalization in the elderly. *J Am Geriatr Soc.* 2003;51:1615–1620.

26. Association of body mass index with mortality in older adults. Available at: http://www.nhlbi.nih.gov/guidelines/obesity/e_txtbk/ratnl/2222.htm. Accessed November 12, 2004.

27. Nutrition Screening Initiative. *Nutrition Statement of Principle. Chronic Disease Costs.* 2003. Available at: http://www.eatright.org/Public/Files/nutrition(1).pdf. Accessed November 12, 2004.

28. US Dept of Health and Human Services. *NHANES III.* Available at: http://www.cdc.gov/nchs/nhanes.htm. Accessed November 12, 2004.

29. Fields LE, Burt VL, Cutler JA, Hughes J, Roccella EJ, Sorlie P. The burden of adult hypertension in the United States, 1999 to 2000, A rising tide. *Hypertension.* 2004; 44:1–7.

30. Svetkey LP, Simons-Morton DG, Proschan MA, et al. Effect of the dietary approaches to stop hypertension diet and reduced sodium intake on blood pressure control. *J Clin Hypertens.* 2004;6:373–381.

31. US Dept of Health and Human Services. *The 2004 Surgeon General's Report on Bone Health and Osteoporosis.* Available at: http://www.surgeongeneral.gov/library/bonehealth/docs/Osteo10sep04.pdf. Accessed November 12, 2004.

32. Institute of Medicine, Food and Nutrition Board. *Dietary Reference Intakes for Calcium, Phosphorus, Magnesium, Vitamin D, and Fluoride.* Washington, DC: National Academies Press; 1997. Available at http://www.nap.edu/category.html?id=fn. Accessed November 12, 2004.

33. Weddle DO, Fanelli-Kuczmarski M. Position of the American Dietetic Association: Nutrition, aging, and the continuum of care. *J Am Diet Assoc.* 2000;100:580–95. Available at: http://www.eatright.org/Public/index_7705.cfm. Accessed November 12, 2004.

34. Institute of Medicine. Food and Nutrition Board. *Dietary Reference Intakes for Energy, Carbohydrate, Fiber, Fat, Fatty Acids, Cholesterol, Protein, and Amino Acids.* Washington, DC: National Academies Press; 2004. Available at http://www.nap.edu/category.html?id=fn. Accessed November 12, 2004.

35. Institute of Medicine. DRI table for older adults, as compiled by the National Resource Center on Nutrition, Physical Activity & Aging. Available at: http://www.fiu.edu/~nutreldr. Accessed November 12, 2004.

36. US Dept of Agriculture, US Dept of Health and Human Services. *Dietary Guidelines for Americans 2005.* Available at: http://www.health.gov/dietaryguidelines/dga2005/report/. Accessed November 12, 2004.

37. Nutrition Screening Initiative. *Determine Your Nutritional Health Checklist.* Available at: http://www.aafp.org/x16138.xml?printxml. Accessed November 12, 2004.

38. *Mini Nutritional Assessment.* Revised 1998. Available at: http://www.mna-elderly.com/. Accessed November 12, 2004.

39. American College of Sports Medicine. Position stand: exercise and physical activity for older adults 1998. Available at: http://www.acsm.org. Accessed November 12, 2004.

40. Centers for Disease Control and Prevention, National Center for Chronic Disease Prevention and Health Promotion. *Behavioral Risk Factor Surveillance Survey.* Available at: http://www.cdc.gov/BRFSS/technical_infodata/surveydata/2003.htm. Accessed November 12, 2004.

41. Kamimoto LA, Easton AN, Maurice E, Husten CG, Macera CA. Surveillance for five health risks among older adults: 1993–1997. CDC Surveillance Summaries, Dec 17, 1999. *MMWR* 48(SS08). Available at: http://www.cdc.gov/mmwr/preview/mmwrhtml/ss4808a5.htm. Accessed November 12, 2004.

42. Fried LP, Bandeen-Roche K, Kasper JA, Guralnik JM. Association of comorbidity with disability in older women: the women's health and aging study. *J Clin Epidemiol.* 1999;52:27–37.

43. *Steps to a HealthierUS*; US Dept Health and Human Services. Available at: http://www.healthierus.gov. Accessed November 12, 2004.

44. Administration on Aging. *You Can! Steps to Healthier Aging.* Available at: http://www.aoa.gov/youcan/youcan.asp. Accessed November 12, 2004.

45. Wellman NS, Friedberg B, Weddle DO, et al. *Eat Better & Move More: A Guidebook for Community Programs.* Washington, DC: US Administration on Aging; 2004; Available at http://www.fiu.edu/~nutreldr. Accessed November 12, 2004.

46. Lee JS, Frongillo EA. Factors associated with food insecurity among US elderly persons: importance of functional impairments. *J Gerontol B Soc Sci.* 2001;56B: S94–S99.

47. Nord M. Food security rates are high for elderly households. *FoodReview.* 2002;25:19–24. Available at: http://www.ers.usda.gov/publications/FoodReview/ Sep2002/frvol25i2d.pdf. Accessed November 12, 2004.

48. Wellman NS, Rosenzweig LY, Lloyd JL. Thirty years of the Older Americans Nutrition Program. *J Am Diet Assoc.* 2002;102:348–350. Available at: http://www.fiu. edu/~nutreldr. Accessed November 12, 2004.

49. Performance Outcomes Measures Project. Highlights from the *Pilot Study: First National Survey of Older Americans Act Title III Service Recipients.* Paper No. 2. Available at: http://www.gpra.net/surveys/2ndhighlights.pdf. Accessed November 12, 2004.

50. Food and Nutrition Service. Food Distribution Fact Sheet April 2003. Nutrition Services Incentive Program. Available at: http://www.fns.usda.gov/fdd/programs/nsip/ pfs-nsip.pdf. Accessed November 12, 2004.

51. The Older Americans Act National Family Caregiver Support Program. Executive Summary 2003. Available at: http://www.aoa.gov/prof/aoaprog/caregiver/overview/ NFCSP_Exec_Summary_FULL_03.pdf. Accessed November 12, 2004.

52. US Dept Health and Human Services, Office of the Assistant Secretary for Planning and Evaluation. *Understanding Medicaid Home and Community Services: A Primer.* October 2000. Available at: http://www.aspe.hhs.gov/daltcp/projects.htm#GWo4. Accessed November 12, 2004.

53. Centers for Medicare & Medicaid Services. *Home and Community-Based 1915 (c) Waivers.* Available at: http://www.cms.hhs.gov/medicaid/1915c/default.asp. Accessed November 12, 2004.

54. Nursing home costs average $70,080 per year in U.S. Home care is $18 per hour: 2004 Metlife Mature Market Institute Survey Reports. General News: 2004 and 2003 Press releases. Available at: http://www.metlife.com/Applications/Corporate/WPS/CDA/ PageGenerator/0,1674,P250%257ES589,00.html. Accessed November 12, 2004.

55. *Medicare, Medicaid, and SCHIP Benefits Improvement and Protection Act of 2000* (BIPA). Available at: http://www.cms.gov. Accessed November 12, 2004.

56. USDA Food and Nutrition Service. Food distribution participation, data as of October 2004. Available at: http://www.fns.usda.gov/pd/fdpart.htm. Accessed November 12, 2004.

CHAPTER 11

Ensure Nutrition Services in Primary Health Care for the Underserved

Kathie Westpheling

Reader Objectives

- Define primary care.
- List the lack of access to health care and health care disparities that contribute to the needs for primary care in the community.
- Discuss the contributions of nutrition services to primary care services for the underserved.
- Describe the various local, state, and federal primary care programs and initiatives.
- Discuss the applications of technology in evidence-based practice and the chronic care model.
- Discuss available sources to fund nutrition services in primary care.

DEFINE PRIMARY CARE

Indigent, low-income, and uninsured families are often sicker and diagnosed with a variety of co-occurring diseases. Many speak and read limited English, come from many different cultures, and often are members of working families. They may be at risk for hunger and malnutrition (see Chapter 3) and often need to be treated for more than one diet-related chronic disease (see Chapter 9). Although the Special Supplemental Nutrition Program for Women, Infants, and Children (WIC) has demonstrated its effectiveness when successfully integrated into primary care services for pregnant and breast-feeding women and their children (see

259

Chapter 8), poor diet still contributes to the increased risk of poor outcomes of pregnancy and low birth–weight infants who often have accompanying risks of retarded physical and mental development.

The health care system is also faced with the following:

- Near epidemic levels of obesity and overweight in school-age children and adults, which contribute to increased incidence of type 2 diabetes, hypercholesterolemia, heart disease, and hypertension
- Growing aging populations, including low-income, frail elderly dependent on multiple expensive medications prescribed to manage their chronic diseases (see Chapter 10)
- Widespread untreated periodontal and other dental diseases at all stages of life
- Aggressive treatment regimens for cancer and HIV/AIDS that may have many side effects but can improve survival rates

All have implications for modification of diet and physical activity regimens and require dietary assessment, treatment, monitoring, and follow-up within a comprehensive primary health care system.[1]

The Institute of Medicine defines primary care as "The provision of integrated health care services by clinicians who are accountable for addressing most personal health care needs, developing a sustained partnership with patients, and practicing in the context of family and community."[2] The health care system presents a challenge to many with limited health care literacy and financial resources. Primary care plays a vital role when it reaches out to them.

The Institute of Medicine published six reports written between 2001 and 2004 summarizing the findings of the Committee on the Consequences of Uninsurance.[3] Uninsured children and adults see a physician or dentist less frequently than those insured. Eight out of 10 of these uninsured people are members of working families. Some low-income workers who are offered health insurance coverage by their employers refuse either because of the cost or because they do not perceive the need for personal or family coverage. Annually, approximately 18,000 preventable deaths are attributed to uninsured adults who die before the age of 65.[4] The following lists the committee's recommendations for health care insurance:

- Universal, meaning everyone living in the United States should be covered by health insurance
- Continuous, which allows for the early detection of disease
- Affordable to all individuals and families, with lower-income families offered some financial assistance to participate
- Affordable and sustainable for society
- Enhance health and well-being

The goal is effective, efficient, safe, timely, patient-centered, and equitable health care.[5]

The committee recommends action by legislators, as well as private policy makers, to achieve universal health care coverage by the year 2010. The committee also recommends support of the organizations and health care providers who make up the health care "safety net."[6] Most often, this safety net is provided by community-based primary care clinics and other primary health care providers.

For more, go to www.nap.edu.

Community-Based Primary Care

In 1998, the Institute of Medicine (IOM) convened the Committee on Quality of Health Care in America to study the personal health care delivery system that provides most of the personal, chronic illness, and end-of-life health care. The committee's recommendations, published in *Crossing the Quality Chasm*,[7] provide a blueprint for delivering primary care in the United States. It calls for patient-centered health care with more collaboration and communication among clinicians.

The 2004 IOM report, *Health Literacy: A Prescription to End Confusion*,[8] states that almost half of all Americans are limited in health literacy and are unable to completely benefit from the existing health care system.

Another IOM report, *Unequal Treatment*,[9] cites evidence of racial and ethnic disparities throughout the United States health care system. The rates of obesity, diabetes, heart disease, and cancer are discussed in Chapter 9. Primary care is frequently defined as medical and nursing services. Comprehensive primary health care to prevent and manage chronic diseases can be available within such services and in community settings. All health care professionals and institutions can collaborate in efforts to reduce the burden of illness, injury, and disability, and improve the health and quality of life of the people of the United States. Redesigning the health care system to be more responsive and coordinated to meet the needs of underserved patients will result in more satisfaction for both clinicians and patients. Increased satisfaction is vital to the expansion and vitality of the primary health care workforce.

Some recommendations for changes in primary care services delivery stated by the IOM include:

- Restructure payment systems to ensure availability of services to minority populations.
- Reduce language barriers through reimbursement for services of interpreters.
- Expand the role and responsibilities of community health workers as liaisons between patients, providers, and communities.
- Utilize multidisciplinary teams to optimize patient care.
- Implement education programs to enhance patient-centered health care.[10]

Comprehensive community-based prevention and primary care services include medical, dental, behavioral, and pharmacy services.[11] The Association of Clinicians for the Underserved suggests that patient outcomes will be improved when care is delivered by a transdisciplinary team of health professionals and paraprofessionals educated to work together, with the patient, sharing knowledge and skills across the disciplines with mutual trust and respect.[12] Nutrition services are a part of this comprehensive approach to health care.

The *Future of Primary Care*[13] also recommends that primary care must include a team of clinicians. This team assists the patient with access to information and appropriate care. Seeing the patient as part of this team is necessary for success. The patient must understand the benefits of both having a team delivery of health care and the roles and responsibilities of each team member. The team must become "visible to the patient." A partnership where members share objectives and stated expectations to achieve them is the outcome. The development of the norms, processes, and systems allow the team to function in an integrated primary care setting.[14] Defining nutrition services as more efficient and cost effective when delivered through an organized team approach can be critical to assuring that these services are included.

Primary health care services designed to meet the needs of the underserved can be offered by group practices who may work in community and migrant health centers, hospital outpatient departments, free clinics, health care services for the homeless, mobile medical and dental clinics, health maintenance organizations, school-based health centers, nurse-managed health centers, and public health departments.[15] Physicians, advanced practice nurses (including nurse practitioners and nurse-midwives), and physician assistants are considered the essential primary health care providers in these systems. The physicians may have degrees in medicine (MD) or osteopathic medicine (DO). These clinicians specialize in family medicine, general pediatrics, general internal medicine, or obstetrics/gynecology. Each state practice act defines how advanced practice nurses and physician assistants can work with physicians in their state.

When serving uninsured and underinsured populations, primary care systems seek to offer a comprehensive medical and/or dental home for new and needy members of American society. Offering needy clients more comprehensive health services in the primary care setting is a growing priority. The challenge remains to both add qualified staff and identify sources for reimbursement for many community-based systems.

New immigrant families from many parts of the world encounter an unfamiliar culture and frequently are unable to read or speak fluent English. They often live in poor housing in isolated, rural, and migrant communities or crowded urban dwellings. For them, integration of additional services is essential. Depending on funding and resources available, these services should be provided by nutritionists, dentists, dental hygienists, social workers, psychologists, health educators, pharmacists, medical assistants, and community outreach workers. Enabling services are used to increase the ability of these families to access and participate in primary and preventive health care services.[16] Enabling Services may include transportation; translation and interpreter services; outreach programs, such as promotoras or cultural brokers[17]; and case management to assure and coordinate services.

In community-based primary care, the primary care clinician serves two patients—one is the individual, and the other is the community. Community-oriented primary care[18] includes the best primary care with the support of population-based or public health approaches to address community problems, such as obesity and lack of physical activity. Community-based primary and secondary prevention services can be coordinated within a primary care setting. By increasing collaboration and communication between community agencies and public health nutrition programs, such as school-based nutrition education or church-affiliated chronic disease screening and education programs, services in the primary care clinic are enhanced. The public health nutritionist should take a broad perspective when working to expand nutrition services in primary care.

For more, go to www.health.gov/healthypeople.

ENSURE NUTRITION SERVICES IN PRIMARY CARE

Ensuring nutrition services in primary care is a major responsibility for public health nutritionists, community dietitians, and paraprofessionals. Collaboration with public health nutritionists and existing community nutrition services located at a site other than that of the primary care clinic may be required. Modifying nutrition behaviors, accessing a nutrient-rich food supply, and medical nutrition therapy are part of the self-management of many chronic health conditions seen by primary health care clinicians.

As an essential part of primary and secondary prevention, public health nutritionists demonstrate that nutrition services can be integrated into primary care to meet individual and family needs. Partnerships should be created between the health care providers, the families, and their communities. This presents a challenging opportunity for public health nutritionists to translate evidence-based nutrition and social sciences into realistic personal health behavior plans for those diagnosed with many preventable chronic conditions. The public health nutritionists can assist members of the primary care team to communicate with patients, family caregivers, and the team to determine to what extent the diagnoses and recommended dietary treatment plans are understood. Providing an assessment of the challenges and barriers to patient adherence is a valued service.

To integrate nutrition services in primary care, public health nutritionists need a working knowledge of the several Institute of Medicine reports previously cited.[3,4,7,8,9] Cost-benefit data can document that nutrition services provide patients with health care that is safer, more responsive to their cultural eating patterns, and integrated into their primary health care. Evidence-based clinical nutrition guidelines designed to prevent disease and manage chronic disease conditions such as obesity, heart disease, cancer, and osteoporosis include both medical nutrition therapy and prescription drugs and/or over-the-counter medications.

Crossing the Quality Chasm cites statistics from the 1996 Robert Wood Johnson Report that 40% of people with chronic conditions have more than one condition that requires treatment. Because of this, every health care provider must have access to complete information about the patient, including medical history, summary of services, including the medications prescribed by other clinicians.[19] Nutrition interventions need to make the patient aware of potential nutrient-drug interactions and documented side effects as well as psychological aspects of diet and drug management. These may influence the patient's adherence and willingness to commit to long-term dietary behavioral changes.

New models of primary care recommend shared decision-making. This means new working relationships between patients, their families, and all members of the health care team. The primary care physician is seen as a teacher and coordinator of comprehensive health care services with expanded working relationships with other members of the team,[20] including the public health nutritionist or community dietitian. In this new model of primary care, information technology is used to assist in communicating available resources and assessing health outcomes. It is anticipated that future primary care models will use technology to show evidence of enhanced teamwork, coordinated resources, and documented patient outcomes.

Team Approach to Nutrition Care

Nutrition services require the primary care clinicians, associated outreach, and educational programs to work together. Services still include the fundamental principles of screening and diagnosis, health maintenance, health supervision, and health promotion. To carry out the coordination and integration of these services requires the "buy-in" of administrators and financial officers within health care systems, along with multiple partnerships among nutrition programs in federal, state, and local agencies, and with the various community-based primary health care programs. All members of the health care team must advocate the need for nutrition services. Policy makers, at all levels, seek data of improved health outcomes. Demonstrating improved nutrition outcomes may make a significant contribution to justify expanded nutrition care services in primary care.

Medical nutrition therapy in a primary care clinic should include the following essential components[21]:

- Patient care:
  - Individual screening by the primary health care clinicians to identify patients with nutritional risks who require referrals based on established protocols or evidence-based clinical guidelines

- ° Nutrition assessment using dietary, biochemical, clinical, and anthropometric measures utilizing currently accepted methodology and equipment as required for accreditation by the Joint Commission on Accreditation of Healthcare Organizations (JCAHO)[22]
- ° Nutrition care plans developed by the nutritionist and periodically reviewed and updated in collaboration with the health care team
- ° Culturally competent, documented, individual counseling assisted when needed by interpreters in accordance with the Culturally and Linguistically Appropriate Services (CLAS) guidelines[23]
- ° Appropriate referrals as needed to food assistance programs available in the community (e.g., Food Stamp Program, WIC, food pantries, soup kitchens, congregate meal programs)
- • Program management:
  - ° Coordination with related food and nutrition programs at the local, state, and national levels
  - ° Nutrition action plans, including logic models for evaluation and associated budgets and cost centers, based on needs assessment for specific target areas and populations
  - ° Quality improvement indicators, including nutrition guidelines and a system for peer review
  - ° Written protocols, policies, and procedures for nutrition services and prescribed medical nutrition therapy provided by qualified nutrition personnel and other members of the health care team
  - ° Plans for ongoing continuing education, technical assistance, and case consultation
  - ° Plans for coordinated community outreach and education in nutrition and physical activity to be delivered in the community, including schools, community colleges, work sites, faith-based organizations, and recreation facilities

Role of Public Health Nutritionists and Community Dietitians

To coordinate nutrition services for patients with many nutrition-related health problems, public health nutritionists and community dietitians can be employed by the primary health care center or may contract for services with the primary care organizations. Some may manage a specific program (e.g., WIC), serve a high-risk population group (e.g., mothers and children, the elderly), or be employed to work in a specialty area (e.g., health promotion, chronic disease prevention and management, children's special health care needs). The public health nutritionist can serve as a consultant to write plans for nutrition services for each health program area as required and based on documented needs of the system's consumers and community assessment (see Chapter 3). Nutritionists employed on federal grant funds (e.g., WIC or the Ryan White HIV/AIDS Title III

Prevention and Early Intervention Programs) are required to write periodic nutrition program plans that specify nutrition needs, problems, and resources in relation to the nutrition-related health problems of the whole community.

The public health nutritionist consults and collaborates with other primary health care professionals and administrators to adapt appropriate evidence-based guidelines, policies, and protocols for nutrition services. The lead nutritionist advocates for adequate funding to employ nutrition personnel and may need to seek external funds to expand services through grants, donations, and sliding scale fees for services (see Chapter 17). This public health nutritionist monitors the nutrition services budget and related cost centers. The public health nutritionist also recruits, trains, supervises, and evaluates nutrition personnel and mobilizes and coordinates community resources.[24]

Role of Paraprofessionals

Nutrition services can be expanded through culturally appropriate in-service training of medical or nursing assistants, outreach workers, lay workers or *promotoras* from the community. Lay health workers speak patients' primary languages and know their food preferences, cultural diets, and lifestyles. Continuing in-service training is needed to demonstrate use of patient education resources in the primary language of the clients or in simple English. Paraprofessionals can motivate clients to choose foods and follow meal patterns recommended to promote health and prevent complications of chronic diseases. As relatives, friends, and neighbors, they can help bridge the cultural gap between health professionals and their community.

LOCAL AND STATE PRIMARY CARE INITIATIVES

Local Public Health Departments

Twenty-eight percent of local public health departments are the sole safety net providers in their communities.[25] Denver Health, for example, is an integrated safety net system. It has been recognized nationally as possibly the nation's "most complete medical care system."[26] It is an integrated, seamless delivery system that includes public health services, an acute care hospital in the Denver Health Medical Center, including emergency and trauma services, and an outpatient system, Denver Community Health Services (CHS). The goal of Denver Health is to provide access to quality preventive, acute, and chronic health care for all citizens of Denver regardless of their ability to pay. In addition, Denver Health's mission is to provide for the health education of patients and to participate in educating health care professionals.[27] CHS is the second oldest and largest integrated community health center program in the United States. It includes 9 community health centers and 12 school-based health centers.

The nutrition services within Denver Health are equally integrated. For example, CHS employs community dietitians in programs such as WIC; Kids Care (a service for high-risk children offering traditional one-on-one nutrition counseling); HIV/AIDS ambulatory clinic with diet counseling as part of team case management; Denver's Health Children and Families Program for children with special needs (nutrition case management and resource development); and the community diabetes education program in which a community dietitian participates in monthly education sessions for the community. Medical nutrition therapy, for conditions such as renal disease and diabetes, is available through referrals from the ambulatory clinics to the clinical dietitians at the medical center. With this integrated approach, services are not duplicated and are provided by appropriately trained and funded nutrition and dietetic personnel.[28]

To learn more, go to: www.denverhealth.org.

Free Clinics

According to the National Free Clinic Association, free clinics serve over 3.5 million people and contribute over $3 billion in health care value.[29] The volunteer-based or free clinic is a community and/or faith-based organization that provides medical, dental, prescription drug, and mental health services at little or no cost to low-income, uninsured, and underinsured people. Each free clinic is unique, and services are based on the particular needs and resources of the local community it serves. Funding and support are generally raised locally with little, if any, government assistance. Some free clinics employ a limited number of paid key staff, such as a medical director or clinic manager to assure quality services and coordinate patient care. However, these private, nonprofit free clinics rely upon recruiting volunteer health care professionals and other community volunteers. They also may establish partnerships with community agencies, hospitals, academic health centers, and health care providers, including specialty groups. Free clinics may provide a family practice model of service delivery that sees all family members. Some try to determine the patient's eligibility for Medicaid, Medicare, or the State Children's Insurance Program before establishing the free clinic as a medical or dental home for the patient.

For more, go to www.volunteersinhealthcare.org.

Community-Campus Partnership for Health

The Community-Campus Partnership for Health is a national organization focused on the delivery of community health interventions by students in partnership with a community. This service-learning program provides health professional and paraprofessional students with opportunities to volunteer and collaborate on health programs and services. The involvement of public health nutrition students in this service-learning model provides the opportunity to advocate for nutrition services in primary care settings, share nutrition knowledge, patient counseling skills, and provide nutrition services to the clinic's patients and staff.

To learn more, go to www.depts.washington.edu/ccph.

American Project Access Network

American Project Access Network, a nonprofit organization formed in 2002, assists physicians and clinicians in implementing project access systems for local communities. Public health nutritionists should join other health care colleagues to advocate for free clinics, health systems change, and to include nutrition services as part of this primary care volunteer effort.

For more, go to www.apanonline.org.

STATE AND REGIONAL PRIMARY CARE ASSOCIATIONS

State and regional primary care associations are nonprofit corporations representing the federally qualified health centers in their states or regions.[30] They may recruit and retain the health care workforce, sponsor continuing education courses, establish quality improvement initiatives, collaborate on community-based research, and advocate public policy. Health professional coordinators staff clinical committees and develop clinician support services. The clinical committees of these organizations share best practices in quality improvement and standardize policies and procedures. They promote appropriate applications of information technology including wider use of electronic medical records. They participate in continuing education programs and collaborate on applied research.

Medical and dental directors and clinic nurse managers represent their health centers in state and regional clinical networks to accomplish similar tasks. These associations may work to assure nutrition services in member community health centers. These associations offer opportunities to partner or contract with public health nutritionists employed in state or local official or voluntary public health agencies.

For more, go to www.nachc.com/primcare.

CASE STUDIES ILLUSTRATE NUTRITION INITIATIVES

Connecticut: Reimbursement for Nutrition Services

A large percentage of patients who receive health care in federally qualified health centers in Connecticut have one or more chronic diseases that require prescribed medical nutrition therapy. For this reason, reimbursement for nutrition services is being discussed by the statewide clinical issues committee of the Connecticut Primary Care Association. The major issue is how to make nutrition services self-supporting by billing clients or their health care insurance providers. Credentialing the dietitians/nutritionists who are employed by the managed care organizations in Connecticut appears to be a stumbling block. Working through the Connecticut Women's Health Campaign, the primary care association staff will advocate for access to nutrition services with legislators in upcoming legislative sessions. Advocacy and public policy efforts challenge public health nutrition professionals to partner with clinical affairs departments in their states. Public health nutritionists can provide documented evidence of cost-effective interventions and evidence-based research on improved health outcomes when nutrition services are incorporated into comprehensive chronic disease management.

Culturally Competent Nutrition Workforce

According to the Connecticut Primary Care Association clinical affairs staff, an insufficient number of bilingual nutrition professionals and paraprofessionals is a barrier to expanding nutrition services in the state.[31] Public health nutritionists in state and local official and voluntary health agencies can collaborate with state primary care associations on health workforce agendas to recruit and train culturally competent public health nutritionists, community dietitians, and community health workers. Working with primary care associations offers opportunities for nutrition students, dietetic interns, and dietetic technician students to obtain field experience in working with culturally diverse clients served by community-based primary health centers, including those that are federally qualified. Public health nutrition students benefit by working with the physicians and nurses in state and regional primary care associations on legislative and public policy agendas, such as workforce agendas, to increase access to culturally competent primary care staff members.

New York City: Clinical Research and Education

The Clinical Director's Network (CDN) in New York City is a nonprofit membership organization and practice-based research network founded in 1985 by the medical, dental, and nursing leadership of federally qualified health centers in New York, New Jersey, and Puerto Rico. Most of their research is to document how appropriate behavioral and lifestyle interventions integrated into clinical practice can eliminate health disparities. Citing the influence of vitamin deficiencies on disease progression, the onset of heart disease, diabetes, cancer, and HIV/AIDS, and the limited use of vitamin supplements by low socioeconomic populations, the Clinical Director's Network proposed a project titled VitaGrant: Promotion of Vitamin Supplementation Among Low-Income, Disadvantaged Patients and Their Healthcare Providers.[32] VitaGrant funding came from the Office of the New York State Attorney General, sponsored by the Indirect Vitamin Purchasers Antitrust Litigation Settlement. This settlement provides funding to nonprofit organizations in New York State "for the improvement of the health and/or nutrition of the citizens of New York State and/or the advancement of nutritional, dietary or agricultural science."[33] A nutritionist designed and presented educational programs on the use and benefits of multivitamins to community/migrant health center clinicians and patients. This comprehensive educational program is presented as on-site in-service sessions at some New York State health centers, online as Web casts to health centers in New York State, and is archived online for other interested health professionals. The goal is to increase availability and use of appropriate multivitamin supplements by minority and low-income population subgroups. Educational materials in Spanish, Creole, Chinese, and Russian, at appropriate reading levels, have been developed to use with adult patients.

Using the extensive Internet-based Web cast production service created for the VitaGrant project, nutritionists continue to develop and conduct the nutrition continuing education CME/CEU–approved programs for several health professions through noontime programs. This continuing professional education is made available at no charge to other primary health care professionals in community health centers across the country. E-mails market this service.

Public health nutritionists interested in using Web-based technology to offer continuing education to primary care professionals are encouraged to collaborate on funding proposals with organizations like the Clinical Director's Network to expand professional nutrition education offerings for clinicians.

For more, go to www.cdnetwork.org.

FEDERALLY FUNDED PROGRAMS

Section 330 of the Public Health Service Act—
Consolidated Health Center Funding

The Consolidated Health Center Funding is administered through the Department of Health and Human Services, Health Resources and Services Administration's Bureau of Primary Health Care.[34] Since 1999, access to comprehensive health care services has expanded through this federally funded Health Centers Program. Reauthorized in 2002 by an executive order, a 5-year expansion of this program added six million more people being served by health center programs in 1200 of the most underserved communities. This program serves nearly 15 million people, up from 10 million in 1999.[35] Ninety percent of patients served live on incomes below 200% of the federal poverty level: more than 700,000 are migrant and seasonal farm workers, and 600,000 individuals are currently homeless. In 2003, the health center patient population included 64% from racial and ethnic minorities, and 74% were uninsured or covered by Medicaid.[36] These community-based programs emphasize prevention, early detection, and timely intervention of diagnosed health problems.

For more, go to www.bphc.hrsa.gov.

Community health centers provide primary and preventive health care, outreach, and dental care. Essential ancillary services such as laboratory tests, X-ray, environmental health, and pharmacy services are included, as well as health education, transportation, translation, and prenatal care. Health centers provide links to social services, Medicaid/Medicare, mental health and substance abuse treatment, WIC, and related services. They provide clients with access to a full range of specialty care services as resources are available.

Health care for the homeless programs provide primary care and substance abuse services at locations accessible to people who are homeless, as well as round-the-clock access to emergency health services. Homeless people can be referred for necessary hospital visits, and mental health services unless these services are provided directly at the homeless program site. Outreach informs homeless individuals of the availability of services and also aids them to establish their eligibility for housing assistance and services under entitlement programs.

Migrant health programs support migrant health services using bilingual, bicultural lay outreach workers, health personnel, and culturally sensitive appropriate protocols. Migrant Health Centers are funded to provide preventive and comprehensive adult services, as well as pediatric services, such as immunizations, well-child care, and developmental screenings. Culturally and linguistically appropriate mental health and substance abuse treatment services, environmental and occupational health and safety training, oral health services, and outreach services are offered. These programs increase the capacity of migrant health voucher programs to provide comprehensive primary health care services to seasonal farm workers and their families as they travel in search of work. Migrant health programs increase the visibility of farm worker health issues to leverage additional resources and services unique to farm workers' health and lifestyle needs.

Accreditation of Federally Funded Community Health Centers

A federal executive order in 2001 expanded the number of community and migrant health centers and established a national priority for quality health care measures in these ambulatory health care sites. The Federal Bureau of Primary Health Care encourages health centers to be accredited by an external agency, such as the Joint Commission on Accreditation of Healthcare Organizations

(JCAHO). State primary care associations assist member health centers apply for accreditation. The accreditation standards for ambulatory care sites include evaluation of patient-focused functions, which includes nutrition care.[37] This includes nutrition assessment and screening of the patient at the first primary care visit to an ambulatory clinic or office. Reassessment is needed only as appropriate to the reason the patient is presenting for care or services.

The assessment design standard requires the health care organization to define, in writing, the scope of the assessment, including the data gathered to assess and reassess patient needs. As most health centers do not employ nutrition professionals, public health nutritionists can offer technical assistance to the clinical staff or the primary care associations and local health centers to assure these standards are understood and documentation is in place when on-site evaluations are completed. A comprehensive manual is used to prepare for the accreditation process.

To learn more, go to www.jcrinc.com/publications.

The Health Disparities Collaboratives: Evidence-Based Medicine

The Health Disparities Collaboratives are sponsored by the US Department of Health and Human Services, Health Resources and Service Administration, Bureau of Primary Health Care, in partnership with a number of private and public agencies. These quality improvement projects use the chronic care model to improve chronic illness care.[38] The model was first developed by the Improving Chronic Illness Care Program, supported by the Robert Wood Johnson Foundation with direction and technical assistance by the Group Health Cooperative's MacColl Institute for Healthcare Innovation.

Clinical teams, only from federally qualified health centers, apply for funding to participate in a collaborative. Those served by a collaborative may include urban and rural indigent and low-income patients, the homeless, and migrant or seasonal farm workers.

The Bureau, in cooperation with the Institute for Healthcare Improvement, has developed several prototypes based on the chronic care model. The term used for these collaboratives is "a breakthrough series collaborative." They are short-term (6 to 15 month) learning systems that bring together a large number of teams from federally funded health centers to seek to improve a specific area.[39]

The current work of the Bureau of Primary Health Care focuses on chronic conditions including diabetes, cardiovascular disease, asthma, and depression. General chronic disease prevention, as well as prevention of cancer and diabetes, has also been addressed. A Health Disparities Collaboratives training manual is available to explain the collaborative models and the lessons learned so far to improve the care of people with diabetes, asthma, and depression.

For more, go to www.healthdisparities.net.

Nutrition Services: A Component of the National Health Disparities Collaboratives

Community dietitians play many roles in the collaboratives. They often serve as a team leader for one or more collaboratives, because of their expertise in such areas as the management of diabetes, obesity, and cardiovascular disease.

To be effective in counseling and educating medically underserved clients who receive health care through one of the Health Disparities Collaboratives, dietitians/nutritionists need unique skills and personal sensitivities.[40] Basic counseling skills for individuals require familiarity with a spectrum of special subgroups including the following:

- Substance abusers
- Patients who have multiple health conditions (often referred to as cooccurring conditions) and overlaying (comorbidity) mental health diagnoses, such as depression or schizophrenia
- Patients with low intelligence, some of whom live in group homes or structured living environments
- New and acculturated immigrants
- Migrant and seasonal farm workers, many living in substandard housing without potable drinking water and limited cooking facilities
- Homeless patients, many living on the street or in a shelter who rely on fast foods or soup kitchens
- The elderly living on fixed incomes (see Chapter 10)
- People living in remote areas, inaccessible or greatly affected by geographic barriers where support must be provided by e-mail, phone, and telemedicine

To teach classes on diverse topics to patients who have limited literacy and low health literacy requires knowing and using food and nutrition teaching tools suitable for the target audience. Successful classes use active participant involvement as effective ways to reach low-literacy patients. Collaborating with a state's cooperative extension service provides access to culturally appropriate resources at low reading levels.

Collaboratives using the "group visit" often request dietitians to lead or facilitate group discussions on one of the care aspects of a selected chronic condition. Patients who have the same needs, such as hemoglobin A1c self-management or blood pressure control, participate in the group visit. Patients may also receive individual counseling depending on their condition and self-management objectives. Support groups in collaboratives may focus on the prevention of complications from diabetes and/or obesity with the dietitian utilized as the expert in food and nutrition and lifestyle behaviors. Three core elements required for successful group education and facilitation are empathy, congruence, and positive regard.[41] The goal of education is to empower the patient for self-care.

Other team members, including physicians, physician assistants, and nurse practitioners, may require professional development to learn about new research in nutrition for health promotion and medical nutrition therapy through in-service and other continuing education sessions.

Many centers use community health workers, lay health promoters, or peer educators to extend the work of health professionals in the collaboratives. They are used extensively in nutrition education. They can be trained to present food preparation classes and provide general nutrition information. Practical information presented in easily understood words makes this training most effective and useful to lay learners. Classes for community health workers can be presented to them in a style and format that they can replicate with their client audiences. The dietitian must provide resources that are easily adapted for this purpose.

The National Center for Cultural Competence at Georgetown University and Kaiser Permanente's Institute for Culturally Competent Care have extensive Web-based resources, policy briefs and training materials to develop culturally sensitive health care, as integral component of the work of these collaboratives.

For more, go to www.gucchd.georgetown.edu/nccc/ or www.diver sity.kp.org/.

Computer skills and use of the Internet (see Chapter 22) are important to all health care providers in the collaboratives. Communication in the collaboratives is based on e-mail and on-line discussion lists. The expertise of the dietitian is used by staff and patients for information on accessing appropriate nutrition and general health Web sites. All collaborative staff, including nutritionists and dietitians, participates in computer-based data collection, data analysis, and maintenance of patient registries.

Ryan White Program (Title III)—Primary Care Services for HIV/AIDS Patients

The Ryan White Program was legislated in 1990 to help states, communities, and families cope with the growing effect of the AIDS epidemic. The Title III funds provide grants for comprehensive primary health care services for people living with HIV/AIDS and at-risk populations, including women, the homeless, and substance abusers.

A successful nutrition program as part of a Ryan White Title III Grant has been implemented in Ohio.[42] A local health department provides nutrition services for 14–16 hours each month by contracting with a regional medical center for the services of a registered, licensed dietitian. The dietitian is a member of the prevention and early intervention team, which also includes a physician, registered nurse case manager, mental health counselor, and a peer educator. The dietitian's responsibilities include nutrition assessment, nutrition care planning and implementation, nutrition counseling, and the documentation necessary for nutrition supplements and medication coverage through Medicaid when appropriate. The nutrition care plan is reviewed with the team and tracked on a database to assure that the plan is implemented and updated. A monthly notice sent to patients reminds them of scheduled testing and counseling and provides nutrition tips to focus their attention on their nutrition and diet.

Indian and Alaska Native Health Services

The Indian and Alaska Native Health Service (IHS) currently provides health care to approximately 1.5 million American Indians and Alaska Natives (AI/AN) who belong to more than 557 federally recognized tribes in 35 states.[43] This federal system includes 36 hospitals, 61 health centers, 49 health stations, and 5 residential treatment centers. In addition, 34 urban Indian health projects provide a variety of health and referral services. The IHS is headquartered in Rockville, Maryland. Twelve administrative units, referred to as service area offices, conduct the regional work of the agency.

The IHS clinical staff consists of approximately 900 physicians, 2700 nurses, 350 engineers, 450 pharmacists, 300 dentists, 150 sanitarians, and 83 physician assistants. The IHS also employs various allied health professionals, including nutritionists and dietitians. Approximately 98 public health nutritionists and registered dietitians are employed full- or part-time by IHS, and another 165 dietitians are employed by tribal systems to provide nutrition services on a full- or part-time basis.[44]

The American Indian and Alaska Native populations experience a disproportionate number of health disparities, many of which are nutrition related. Presently, the registered dietitian (RD) is the minimum requirement for hiring professional nutrition personnel. The IHS' nutrition services manual for health and nutrition staff provides guidance regarding nutrition services and staffing. Nutrition services are also coordinated with other specific program areas in the IHS, such as services for the elderly, the Head Start Program, and WIC. Still, resources are insufficient to fully address all of the major nutritional concerns. There remains a great need for dietitians and nutritionists with expertise in obesity, diabetes, and substance abuse, particularly alcoholism. Recovery from alcohol abuse is more likely to be sustained when a client is eating well and has access to nutrition counseling.

The IHS is seeking to identify new strategies, partnerships, and nutrition experts who have the commitment and skills to serve the American Indian and Alaska Native populations. Public health nutrition practitioners are encouraged to assist the IHS nutrition services by promoting IHS as a rewarding career and to refer those interested in working in more rural, culturally diverse communities to IHS job postings at www.his.gov/JobsCareerDevelop/Jobs_index. asp.

Of significance to public health nutrition practitioners is a 2001 *Report to Congress: Obesity Prevention and Control for American Indians and Alaska Natives*.[45] The prevalence of obesity in American Indian and Alaska Native populations has increased dramatically over the past 30 years with preschool and school age children having a rate of up to three times higher than the US population. About 40% of AI children are overweight. Approximately 15% of AI/AN patients, who receive care from the Indian Health Service, have diabetes, an obesity-associated morbidity. AI/AN patients are 2.6 times as likely to have diabetes as non-Hispanic Caucasians of similar age. With more than 500 federally recognized tribes in the United States, data on obesity rates have been difficult to collect. The current epidemics of obesity in children and adults and obesity-associated morbidity, including type 2 diabetes, cardiovascular disease, and some cancers, have profound implications for AI/AN communities.

This report includes a number of recommendations and strategies for partnerships with local tribal governments and other local, state, and federal agencies. It emphasizes developing local initiatives, identifying best practices, and locating community resources. Dietitians participate in evaluation and evidence-based research to document best practices and the impact of nutrition and physical fitness programs on reducing obesity and chronic diseases in AI/AN populations to validate the cost of providing nutrition services. When seeking insurance reimbursement or grant support, outcome evaluation is a critical part of an application.

To access information on primary care and nutrition services of interest to public health nutritionists, go to www.ihs.gov/MedicalPrograms/Medical_index.asp.

The IHS Clinical Support Center offers health professionals a monthly publication, *The IHS Primary Care Provider*, distributed to health care providers working for IHS, urban Indian, and tribal health programs. It is also sent to medical, nursing, and pharmacy schools throughout the country. Articles, letters, commentaries, and editorials of interest to all health care professionals providing services to American Indians and Alaska Natives are welcomed by the editors and can be sent to www.ihs.gov/publicinfo/publications/healthprovider/ provider.asp.

IHS Nutrition and Dietetics Training Program

The IHS Nutrition and Dietetics Training Program is located in Santa Fe, New Mexico, and provides nutrition training to IHS, tribal, and urban health program paraprofessionals and professionals. This includes community health representatives, outreach workers, nutrition coordinators, nutritionists and dietitians, diabetes team members, health educators, registered nurses, substance abuse program staff, as well as food service workers from schools, day care centers, Head Start programs, elderly programs, jails, substance abuse treatment centers, and hospitals.

Protocols for nutrition education in the IHS are found on the Health Education Program page of the US Department of Health and Human Services, Indian Health Service site.

IHS National Diabetes Program

The IHS National Diabetes Program promotes collaborative strategies for the prevention of diabetes and its complications in the 12 IHS service areas through coordination of a network of 19 model diabetes programs and 13 area diabetes consultants.[46] In addition, the program manages the Special Diabetes Program for Indians grant program with 332 grantees in 35 states. The Tribal Leaders Diabetes Committee, established in 1998, partners tribal leaders with IHS.[47] A group of elected tribal officials has voluntarily agreed to form a committee with a special interest in this chronic health condition. They also cooperate with the Centers for Disease Control and Prevention (CDC) National Diabetes Prevention Center to assure the development and dissemination of tools and resources to assist all tribal communities' work in diabetes prevention and care.

The Integrated Diabetes Education Recognition Program for American Indian and Alaska Native Communities manual assists clinics and outpatient departments who seek to have their program recognized and accredited. Evidence-based "best practice" documents are available for nutrition, physical activity, and diabetes care and guide diabetes prevention and management programs. Nutrition professionals can access resources on medical nutrition therapy and diabetes, clinical evidence of program effectiveness, Medicare and Medicaid reimbursement guidelines, and sample forms for referral to, and reimbursement for, nutrition services by contacting the IHS National Diabetes Program.

For more, go to www.ihs.gov/MedicalPrograms/diabetes/nutrition/n_index.asp.

Using 2001 data from the IHS Diabetes Care and Outcomes Audit, the IHS National Diabetes Program has documented evidence of success in its education program for IHS, tribal, and urban Indian health programs participating in the outcomes audit.[48] The study investigated the role of nutrition education and the use of the registered dietitian against a non-registered dietitian counselor on the A1C levels in diabetic patients. Approximately one of three patients received nutrition education from an RD or a team that included an RD. They had greater improvements in their A1C levels when compared to those who received nutrition education from another provider (e.g., physician, nurse, or other nonnutrition professional) or who had no nutrition education. Studies such as this can be used to justify reimbursement for the RD as a member of the diabetes prevention and self-care management health care team.

Food Distribution Program on Indian Reservations

Nutrition practitioners working to reduce obesity and prevent chronic diseases, such as diabetes, cancer, and cardiovascular disease in the AI/AN communities, must think beyond the health care system. Access to a consistent and affordable food supply, including fresh fruits and vegetables, is a challenge to those who live in Indian country. A creative partnership between the IHS and the USDA's

Commodity Food Program has addressed food distribution in remote Indian communities with high poverty and unemployment rates. The Food Distribution Program on Indian Reservations (FDPIR) is administered at the federal level by the Food and Nutrition Service, USDA, and locally by either an Indian tribal organization or a state agency.[49] Currently, there are approximately 243 tribes receiving benefits from this program through 98 Indian tribal organizations and 5 state agencies. Low-income American Indians, non-Indian households residing on a reservation, and households in approved areas near a reservation or in Oklahoma with at least one person who is a member of a federally recognized tribe are eligible to participate. Households are certified based on federal income and resource standards and must be recertified at least every 12 months. Households may not participate in FDPIR and the Food Stamp Program in the same month. Nutrition education is integrated into this commodity food program initiative.

For more, go to www.fns.usda.gov/fdd/programs/fdpir/default.htm.

IHS Maternal and Child Health Program

The IHS Maternal and Child Health Program (MCH) brings together a diverse group of federal, tribal, and urban programs representing geographically over-lapping populations.[50] The MCH population for American Indians and Alaska Natives is extensive with over 70% of the population now living in urban areas. Their needs are broadly distributed beyond the agencies charged to serve the AI/AN population. While IHS is a federal agency of the Department of Health and Human Services that collaborates with other agencies, such as HRSA and CDC, it is a decentralized system of direct health care that must comply with state Medicaid changes, varied reporting systems, and data sharing. Prenatal care may be rendered on-site, privately, or referred to third-party medical centers. Mothers and children, typically a mobile population, require state cooperative agreements to share in providing services, including nutrition services. Local tribal community childhood obesity projects, Head Start programs, and youth initiatives are being coordinated in many communities.

For more, go to www.ihs.gov/Medicalprograms/MCH/MC.asp.

Coordination of breast-feeding programs and services is also a priority of the IHS MCH Program. While all eligible pregnant women may have access to WIC (see Chapter 8), the distances traveled, cultural specific needs, data collection, and local support for breast-feeding may differ. The IHS MCH Program meets with the USDA's ad hoc committee, the Breastfeeding Consortium, the US Breastfeeding Committee, the American College of Obstetricians and Gynecologists, and the American Academy of Pediatrics to address coordination needs for AI/AN mothers and children. For more, go to www.ihs.gov/NonMedicalPrograms/nc4/breastfeed/index. cfm.

NONPROFIT PRIMARY CARE INITIATIVES

Children's Health Fund

The Children's Health Fund is a national network of pediatric programs started in 1987 to provide all children with a stable medical home. There are 16 child health projects across the country operating in urban and rural communities serving homeless and other children who lack access to comprehensive primary care. Care is delivered through mobile medical units, fixed clinic sites, and school-linked programs. Each project is linked to an academic medical program to ensure that all children have access to specialty care. The network has served over 300,000 patients.[51] Services offered include well-child care, anticipatory guidance, preventive care, immunizations, acute care, and chronic illness management.

The Health and Nutrition Action Initiative is a Children's Health Fund project located at the South Bronx Health Center for Children and Families in New York City.[52] It was established in 1995 to promote nutrition services as a component of health care of children. This initiative now provides primary care, nutrition screening, case management, and entitlement assistance to more than 4300 homeless and at-risk children. It also advocates for systemwide improvements, provides public education, and conducts research.

The Children's Health Fund collaborated with the Children's Hospital at Montifiore Medical Center to develop nutrition and food service policies and procedures for homeless family shelters. Nutrition screening tools and selected "best practice" models for improving the nutritional status of children living in shelters are available on the Internet. Starting Right is a nutrition initiative in which children and adolescents at risk for developing type 2 diabetes are identified through pediatric protocols and offered one-on-one nutrition counseling. In addition, Starting Right also informs policy makers and health professionals about the links between obesity and diabetes and the need for culturally appropriate solutions to this public health problem.[53] For more, go to www.childrenshealthfund.org/hfsni.html.

Institute for Healthcare Improvement

The Institute for Healthcare Improvement is a nonprofit organization established to improve health and the quality and value of health care.[54] The Institute's model is based on the recommendations of the Institute of Medicine and incorporates the issues of safety, effectiveness, efficiency, timeliness, and is patient-centered. The patient-centered approach to quality improvement involves patients and their families, and is characterized by shared decision-making and high levels of satisfaction. The proposed outcome is less costly care and a skilled, coordinated, and satisfied health care team. The Institute for Healthcare Improvement is working with many national and international ambulatory health care systems, including the federally funded community health centers through the Health Disparities Collaboratives.

Public health nutrition professionals who seek to enhance their skills in quality improvement and evidence-based practice can find training courses, an electronic newsletter, and other resources through the Institute's Web site. For more, go to www.ihi.org.

e-Health Initiative

Expanded use of technology, such as electronic medical records, enable preventive services, as well as episodic and chronic care services, to be documented and shared throughout the health care system. An evolving e-health initiative advocates for a seamless health care record system that communicates across systems of care to improve the quality, safety, and efficiency of health care. The Health Insurance Portability and Accountability Act (HIPAA) of 1996 is responsible for improving efficiency in health care through the standardization of electronic data. HIPAA guidelines will guide future development of technology and the ability to share patient records and information. Since health professionals must comply with the privacy guidelines of HIPAA, the ability to review components of proposed clinical management information systems, electronic medical records, or other patient electronic computer systems is an evolving skill required by all primary health care providers, including public health nutritionists. For more, go to www.hhs.gov/ocr/hipaa/ or www.ehealthinitiative.org.

SUPPORT FOR NUTRITION SERVICES IN PRIMARY CARE

The greatest challenge for public health nutritionists in primary care is to demonstrate that nutrition services improve the quality of health care delivered, and that patients' health outcomes are enhanced as a result. Whether nutrition services are provided by a nutritionist or dietitian, or by those trained by them, including physicians and other members of the primary care team and community or lay health care workers, the quality and effectiveness of nutrition interventions must be evaluated and documented. A goal of a public health nutritionist is to get nutrition expertise included in the quality improvement teams of the primary care programs in the local community.

Nutrition services in primary care may include direct counseling services for medical nutrition therapy or indirect services through case management and the education and training of other disciplines. An entrepreneurial approach is required to obtain reimbursement for lifestyle behavioral changes, such as weight management, physical activity, and obesity, as a part of chronic disease prevention and management. Nutritionists must work with administrators and case managers of primary care systems to identify state and federal reimbursement resources. The Centers for Medicaid and Medicare Services (CMS) reimburses for some conditions, such as diabetes and chronic kidney disease, and has recently added obesity as a reimbursable medical condition. For more, go to www.cms.hhs.gov/manuals.

Grant funds should be sought to study lifestyle programs that address the nutrition component of chronic disease prevention and management. The Foundation Center and Grantmakers in Health provide information on health grants from state-based private foundations, corporate giving programs, and community foundations. For more, go to www.fdncenter.org or www.gih.org.

A newer source of local funding is the conversion foundation resulting from a nonprofit hospital system converting to a for-profit status.

POINTS TO PONDER

- What are the alternative approaches to serving the medically uninsured and underserved?
- What are the cost-benefit and cost-effectiveness justifications for employing nutritionists on the primary health care team?
- What data can be collected to monitor outcomes of nutrition services in primary care?
- How can assessment of health literacy be completed in the primary care setting to improve nutrition patient care plans and outcomes?
- What coalitions can most successfully advocate for food, clothing, and shelter for the new immigrant families, the homeless, and the hungry?
- What nutrition training should be provided for primary care clinicians, paraprofessionals, and volunteers who serve culturally diverse, vulnerable populations?

HELPFUL WEB SITES

American Project Access Network (APAN): www.apanoline.org
Centers for Medicare & Medicaid Services – Manuals:
   www.cms.hhs.gov/manuals
Children's Health Fund: www.childrenshealthfund.org
Clinical Directors Network (CDN): www.cdnetwork.org/NewCDN/index.aspx
Denver Health: www.denverhealth.org
eHealth Initiative: www.ehealthinitiative.org
Food Distribution Program on Indian Reservations (FDPIR):
   www.fns.usda.gov/fdd/programs/fdpir/default.htm

Foundation Center: www.fdncenter.org

Grantmakers in Health: www.gih.org

Health Disparities Collaboratives:
www.healthdisparities.net/hdc/html/home.aspx

Healthy People 2010: www.health.gov/healthypeople

Indian Health Service (Federal Health Program for American Indians and Alsaka Natives): www.ihs.gov

Chief Clinical Consultant for Obstetrics and Gynecology —
Breastfeeding:
www.ihs.gov/NonMedicalPrograms/nc4/breastfeed/index.cfm

Diabetes National Program:
www.ihs.gov/MedicalPrograms/diabetes/nutrition/n_index.asp

IHS Primary Care Provider:
www.ihs.gov/publicinfo/publications/healthprovider/provider.asp

Jobs and Scholarships:
www.ihs.gov/JobsCareerDevelop/Jobs_index.asp

Maternal Child Health:
www.ihs.gov/Medicalprograms/MCH/index.cfm

Medical and Professional Programs:
www.ihs.gov/MedicalPrograms/Medical_index.asp

National Patient Education Initiative:
www.ihs.gov/NonMedicalPrograms/HealthEd/index.cfm?module=
initiative&option=protocols& newquery=dsp_NatlPatientEd_
Protocols.cfm

Institute for Healthcare Improvement: www.ihi.org/ihi

Joint Commission Resources Publications: www.jcrinc.com/publications

National Academies Press: www.nap.edu

National Association of Community Health Centers, Inc. (Primary Care): www.nachc.com/primcare

National Center for Cultural Competence (NCCC):
www.gucchd.georgetown.edu/nccc

U.S. Department of Health and Human Services – Bureau of Primary Care: www.bphc.hrsa.org

U.S. Department of Health and Human Services – Office for Civil Rights – HIPAA: www.hhs.gov/ocr/hipaa/

Volunteers in Health Care: www.volunteersinhealthcare.org

NOTES

1. Kaufman M, Watkins E. *Promoting Comprehensive Health Care with Emphasis on Nutrition and Social Work Services.* Chapel Hill, NC: School of Public Health, University of North Carolina; 1981:5–7.

2. Shi L, Singh DA. *Delivering Health Care in America. A Systems Approach.* Gaithersburg, Md: Aspen Publishers; 2001:238.

3. Institute of Medicine. *Insuring Health. The Six Reports and Summaries of the Committee on the Consequences of Uninsurance 2001–2004.* Washington, DC: National Academies Press; 2004.

4. Institute of Medicine. *Insuring America's Health: Principles and Recommendations.* Washington, DC: National Academies Press; 2004:8.

5. Institute of Medicine. *Insuring America's Health: Principles and Recommendations.* Washington, DC: National Academies Press; 2004:8–10.

6. Institute of Medicine. *Insuring America's Health: Principles and Recommendations.* Washington, DC: National Academies Press; 2004:14.

7. Institute of Medicine. *Crossing the Quality Chasm. A New Health System for the 21st Century. Executive Summary.* Washington, DC: National Academies Press; 2001: 1–22.

8. Institute of Medicine. *Health Literacy: A Prescription to End Confusion.* Washington, DC: National Academies Press; 2004:1.

9. Institute of Medicine. *Unequal Treatment. Confronting Racial and Ethnic Disparities in Health Care.* Washington, DC: National Academies Press; 2002.

10. Institute of Medicine. *Unequal Treatment. Confronting Racial and Ethnic Disparities in Health Care.* Washington, DC: National Academies Press; 2002:18.

11. DHHS, HRSA, BHPC Fact Sheet. *Community Health Center Program.* Washington, DC: Dept of Health and Human Services; 2001.

12. Association of Clinicians for the Underserved Web site. Available at: http://www.clinicians.org/healthprofessionals/transdisciplinary.shtml. Accessed January 7, 2005.

13. Showstack J, Rothman AA, Hassmiller S, eds. *The Future of Primary Care.* San Francisco, Calif: Jossey-Bass; 2004:31.

14. Showstack J, Rothman AA, Hassmiller S, eds. *The Future of Primary Care.* San Francisco, Calif: Jossey-Bass; 2004:37.

15. Kaufman M. *Nutrition in Public Health,* Rockville, Md: Aspen Publishers; 1990:222.

16. Institute of Medicine. *America's Health Care Safety Net: Intact But Endangered.* Washington, DC: National Academies Press; 2000.

17. National Center for Cultural Competence. *Bridging the Cultural Divide in Health Care Settings. The Essential Role of the Cultural Broker Programs.* Washington, DC: Georgetown University Medical Center; 2004. Available at: http://gucchd.georgetown.edu/nccc/documents/cultural_Broker_Guide_English.pdf. Accessed January 7, 2005.

18. Shi L, Singh DA. *Delivering Health Care in America. A Systems Approach.* Gaithersburg, Md: Aspen Publishers; 2001:239.

19. Institute of Medicine. *Crossing the Quality Chasm. A New Health System for the 21st Century. Executive Summary.* Washington, DC: National Academies Press; 2001:4.

20. Showstack J, Rothman AA, Hassmiller S, eds. *The Future of Primary Care.* San Francisco, Calif: Jossey-Bass; 2004:103.

21. Kaufman M. *Nutrition in Public Health,* Rockville, Md: Aspen Publishers; 1990: 223–224.

22. Joint Commission on Accreditation of Healthcare Organizations. *Joint Commission Resources: 2005–2006 Comprehensive Accreditation Manual for Ambulatory Care.* Oakbrook Terrace, Ill: Joint Commission on Accreditation of Healthcare Organizations; 2005:PC-11–PC-12, PC-17–PC-18.

23. Dept of Health and Human Services, Office of Minority Health. *National Standards for Culturally and Linguistically Appropriate Services (CLAS) in Health Care Final Report.* Washington, DC: Dept of Health and Human Services; 2001.

24. US Department of Health, Education and Welfare. *Guide for Developing Nutrition Services in Community Health Programs.* Washington, DC: US Department of Health, Education, and Welfare; 1978.

25. Keane C, Marx J, Ricci E. *Local Health Departments Changing Role in Provision and Assurance of Safety-Net Services.* Rockville, Md: Health Resources and Services Administration, Center for Health Services Financing and Managed; 2001.

26. Mays GP, Miller CA, Halverson GP. *Public Health Practice: Trends and Models.* Washington, DC: American Public Health Association.

27. Denver Health. Available at: http://www.denverheatlh.org. Accessed January 13, 2005.

28. Personal communication with Bruce Rengers, RD, PhD, Practice manager, Denver Health, Community Health Services, Denver, Colorado.

29. National Free Clinic Association. Available online at http://www.nafclinics.org Accessed January 7, 2005.

30. Lefkowitz B. *Monograph on Clinical Activities on Primary Care Associations and Their Partners Vary in Form and Function.* Washington, DC: National Association of Community Health Centers; August 2003.

31. Personal Communication with Cheryl Hanley Muñoz, MA, Director of State Clinical Program. Connecticut Primary Care Association.

32. Tobin JN, Romanowski A. *Promoting the VitaGrant Project. Community Health Forum.* Washington, DC: National Association of Community Health Centers; 2003: 44–46.

33. New York State, Office of the Attorney General. *Spitzer announces recipients of $18.5 million consumer settlement from vitamin price-fixing case* [Department of Law press release]. March 18, 2002. Available at: http://www.oag.state.NY.US/vita_grant_ update.html.

34. DHHS, HRSA, BPHC. *Fact Sheet. Section 330 of the Public Health Service Act— Consolidated Health Center Funding.* Rockville, Md: Dept of Health and Human Services; 2001.

35. National Association of Community Health Centers. *Policy Brief.* Washington, DC: National Association of Community Health Centers; 2004.

36. US Dept of Health and Human Services, Health Resources and Services Administration, Bureau of Primary Health Care. Uniform Data System; 1999.

37. Joint Commission on Accreditation of Healthcare Organizations. *Joint Commission Resources: 2005–2006 Comprehensive Accreditation Manual for Ambulatory Care.* Oakbrook Terrace, Ill: Joint Commission on Accreditation of Healthcare Organizations; 2005:PC-11–PC-12, PC-17–PC-18.

38. Wagner EH. Chronic disease management: what will it take to improve care for chronic illness? *Effective Clin Pract.* 1998;1:2–4.

39. Institute for Healthcare Improvement. Available at: http://www.ihi.org. Accessed January 7, 2005.

40. Personal Communication with Katherine Breiger, RD, CDE, Hudson River Community Health, Peekskill, New York.

41. Rogers CR. On Becoming a Person. Boston, Mass: Houghton Mifflin; 1961:279–296.

42. Personal Communication with Cathy Castillo, RD, Adena Regional Medical Center, Chillicothe, Ohio.

43. Indian Health Service. *Fact Sheet.* Available at: http://www.ihs.gov. Accessed March 2004.

44. Personal communication from Jean Charles Azure, RD, Chief Nutrition Consultant, IHS, Rockville Maryland.

45. Indian Health Service. *Report to Congress: Obesity Prevention and Control for American Indians and Alaska Natives. Executive Summary.* Washington, DC: Indian Health Service; 2001:6.

46. Indian Health Service. *Overview–IHS National Diabetes Program. Fact Sheet.* Albuquerque, NM: Indian Health Service: 2003.

47. Indian Health Service. *Tribal Leaders Diabetes Committee—Indian Health Service. Fact Sheet.* Albuquerque, NM: Indian Health Service; 2003.

48. Wilson C, Brown T, Gilliland S, Acton K. Effects of clinical nutrition education and educator discipline on glycemic control outcomes in the Indian Health Service. *Diabetes Care.* 2003;26:2500–2504.

49. Food Distribution Program on Indian Reservations. Fact sheet. Available at: http://www.fns.usda.gov/fdd/programs/fdpir/default.htm.

50. Personal communication from Judith Thierry, DO, FACOP, FAAP, Maternal and Child Health, Indian Health Service, Rockville, Maryland.

51. The Children's Health Fund. *Every Child Counts, Every Family Matters. 2003 Annual Report.* New York, NY: 17.

52. *The Children's Health Fund.* Available at: http://www.childrenshealthfund.org/hnai.html. Accessed January 7, 2005.

53. The Children's Health Fund. *Every Child Counts, Every Family Matters.* 26, 28–29.

54. Institute for Healthcare Improvement. Available at: http://www.ihi.org. Accessed January 7, 2005.

CHAPTER 12

Enforce Nutrition and Food Service Standards in Group Care Facilities

Mary C. Maloney

Reader Objectives

- Compare and contrast the types of group care facilities in the community and the clients they serve.
- Identify the food and nutrition services required to meet federal certification, state and/or local licensure requirements, or voluntary accreditation standards for group care facilities.
- Describe the educational needs of group care facility administrators and food service staff and the resources available to provide training.
- Discuss how nutrition consultation can improve health outcomes for populations in group care.

COMMUNITY GROUP CARE FACILITIES

Group care facilities provide day services or room and board to various groups of individuals who require out-of-home care as a result of their educational, custodial, or health care needs. Group care facilities may be operated by federal, state, or local government agencies; voluntary (nonprofit) or faith-based organizations; corporations; or individuals. Facilities may be funded by federal, state, and/or local government tax dollars; sponsored by private philanthropies; or be operated for-profit by corporations or individuals. Educational facilities include child day care, day camps, boarding schools, colleges, universities, and day programs for developmentally disabled individuals. Domiciliary facilities include homeless shelters and domestic violence shelters, which provide basic shelter, meals, and support services. Behavioral treatment facilities include mental health day programs, residential treatment facilities for people who are mentally ill, substance abuse treatment facilities, and psychiatric facilities. Health care facilities include hospitals, nursing homes, rehabilitation facilities, hospices, pediatric extended care facilities, assisted living with limited nursing services, intermediate care facilities for the developmentally disabled, and psychiatric facilities. Health care facilities provide a continuum of health care services, which should include medical nutrition therapy.[1] Table 12–1 presents some of the types of facilities in the community.

ENSURE QUALITY OF FOOD SERVICES IN COMMUNITY GROUP CARE FACILITIES

Most group care facilities are regulated to protect the health and safety of the people they serve, and to ensure they maintain the quality of their services. Federal laws and regulations govern facilities that receive federal funds. Many states and/or local jurisdictions have licensure laws for specified facilities. These and

Table 12–1 Types of Group Care Facilities (not all inclusive)

Nonresidential Facilities	
Child and adult day care centers	Home-delivered meal programs
Day camps	Mental health day programs
Schools	Day programs for developmentally disabled
Soup kitchens	people
Congregate meal programs	

Residential Programs	
Assisted living facilities	Children's homes
— Specialty care assisted living	Overnight children's camps
Independent retirement facilities	Correctional facilities
Residential facilities for developmentally	Homeless shelters
disabled people	Domestic violence shelters
Residential treatment centers for	Colleges, universities, and boarding schools
mentally ill people	Substance abuse rehabilitation facilities

Group Facilities That Provide Health Services	
Hospitals	Rehabilitation centers
Psychiatric facilities	Intermediate care facilities for the
Nursing homes	developmentally disabled
Limited nursing adult assisted living	Pediatric extended care facilities
facilities	
Hospices	

other facilities may elect to become voluntarily accredited to demonstrate their high standards of services. Public health nutritionists employed by the state or local public health agency, as well as the registered/licensed dietitians employed to consult with a staff of group care facilities, must be familiar with the laws and accreditation standards that apply to dietetic services. They are employed to ensure compliance with evidence-based nutrition standards and uphold safe and sanitary food-handling practices.

Licensure

Most types of group care facilities must comply with state and local laws and regulations that establish minimum licensure standards for nutritionally adequate meals and food service sanitation. Facilities must comply with these standards to receive a license to serve the public. Laws vary with each jurisdiction and are enforced by these regulatory agencies through a periodic inspection process. The inspection personnel employed by a state government agency or under contract often include a registered/licensed dietitian as a member of their multidisciplinary team. Some states and local jurisdictions have regulatory enforcement with fines established for facilities that fail to maintain minimum standards. Many state and local laws are now accessible on the Internet through their state or local government Web sites.

Certification

Health care facilities and behavioral treatment facilities that seek reimbursement from the Medicare and/or Medicaid programs must be certified through the federal government. These facilities must meet minimum standards to receive Medicare and/or Medicaid reimbursement. These standards are published in the Code of Federal Regulations (CFR). Federally certified health care facilities may be inspected annually. The Centers for Medicare and Medicaid Services (CMS), formerly the Health Care Financing Administration [HCFA], contracts with state agencies to conduct these inspections or surveys. The CFRs and the survey process for certified health care facilities are available to the public through the Centers for Medicare and Medicaid Services Web site, www.cms.hhs.gov/cop/1.asp.

Of all of the federally certified health care facilities, nursing homes have the most stringent regulatory oversight and enforcement.

Adult day care programs are not certified. These, senior congregate meal programs, and home-delivered meal programs may qualify to receive funding from the Older Americans Act, administered through the DHHS Agency on Aging (see Chapter 10). These programs require some oversight from the designated state and local agencies to ensure that programs provide the quality of food and nutrition services mandated by federal legislation.

Accreditation

Accreditation programs are voluntary. Facilities receive recognition for meeting national and/or international standards of quality established by experts through independent and nonprofit accrediting organizations. Accredited facilities make a commitment to follow the established standards of quality. The most well-known health care accreditation organization is the Joint Commission on Accreditation of Healthcare Organizations (JCAHO), which accredits a variety of health care facilities. These include hospitals, hospices, assisted living facilities, behavioral health care organizations, and long-term care facilities.

The Commission on Accreditation of Rehabilitation Facilities (CARF) is another respected accreditation organization. CARF recognizes physical rehabilitation, substance abuse rehabilitation, mental health services, adult day care, assisted living, and continuing care retirement facilities that meet their quality care standards. The American Osteopathic Association (AOA) also accredits hospitals, particularly those where osteopathic physicians practice.

The JCAHO and AOA are the only two voluntary accreditation programs in the United States authorized by the Centers for Medicare and Medicaid Services (CMS) to survey hospitals for Medicare. When the facility becomes accredited by JCAHO and/or AOA, CMS receives verification that the facility meets or exceeds the federal standards. CMS then deems that the facility meets Medicare and Medicaid certification requirements. Facilities that receive this status may not need to be subjected to a separate certification inspection by CMS.

The major accreditation organization for child care programs is the National Association for the Education of Young Children (NAEYC), which accredits preschool child care centers and after-school child care programs. The National Association for Family Child Care (NAFCC) accredits family-operated child care facilities. Both of these accreditation organizations have established minimum nutritional standards. The American Camping Association (ACA) may accredit day camps, overnight summer camps, and short-term residential camp programs. This accreditation organization sets minimum standards for food service and sanitation. The American Correctional Association (ACA) accredits correctional facilities for adult and juvenile offenders. ACA accreditation standards include food service and sanitation.

To become accredited, the facility completes an application, usually pays a fee, and has an on-site inspection to determine whether the facility meets the accreditor's minimum standards. The accreditation status must be renewed on a specified periodic schedule. More detailed information about these accreditation organizations can be found at their Web sites:

- Joint Commission on Accreditation of Healthcare Organizations (JCAHO)—www.jcaho.org
- Commission on Accreditation of Rehabilitation Facilities (CARF)—www.carf.org
- The American Osteopathic Association (AOA)—www.do-online.osteotech.org
- The National Association for the Education of Young Children (NAEYC)—www.naeyc.org/
- The National Association for Family Child Care (NAFCC)—www.nafcc.org/
- American Camping Association (ACA)—www.acacamp.org
- The American Correctional Association (ACA)—www.aca.org

Public health nutritionists who are registered/licensed dietitians have the knowledge and skills to assist group care facilities to ensure quality food service and nutritional care. Nutritionists ensure that safe and nutritionally adequate food is served in group care settings when they do the following:

- Assist in writing standards for quality food service and client medical nutrition therapy to be incorporated into state licensing laws and regulations, federal requirements for Medicare and Medicaid reimbursement, and/or criteria for accreditation by private nonprofit accreditation organizations.
- Participate as members of the agency team that inspects and recommends licensure, certification, or accreditation of facilities.
- Advise group care facilities on the number of qualified personnel required to provide quality food and nutrition services based on the number and type of clients and the complexity of their nutritional needs.
- Review and approve the layout and equipment for new or renovated food service facilities and provide on-site consultation to group care facilities, administrators, and staff to assist with efficient food service layout and design, food service equipment specifications, and organization of dietetic services.
- Collaborate with environmental and other health care providers to plan and train administrators and food service staff to ensure their compliance with regulations.
- Network with public health and dietetic professionals and consumers to ensure quality nutrition services to meet the needs of the clients in all types of group care facilities/programs.[2]

EDUCATE ADMINISTRATORS AND FOOD SERVICE PERSONNEL

Maintaining licensure and/or federal standards for all aspects of food service and nutritional care requires continual, well-planned in-service education and training for the facility administrators and personnel to enable them to meet the requirements.[3] Depending on the needs, interests, and areas of weakness, the in-service education can be provided by public health nutritionists who are registered/licensed dietitians, dietary managers, and by external specialists, such as environmental health specialists or sanitarians. Nutritionists can collaborate with environmental health specialists or sanitarians to plan and conduct training courses for food service workers on a quarterly, semiannual, or annual schedule.[4] The Consultant Dietitians in Health Care Facilities (CD-HCF), Dietetic Practice Group of the American Dietetic Association has references and materials available to assist in developing in-service education and orientation programs for food service employees. Some teaching styles to make in-service training more interesting and memorable include sharing personal experiences, utilizing humor, quizzes with follow-up discussions, games, demonstrations, and other learner participation activities.[5] Basic food service and nutrition care topics for staff in-service education should include the following:

- Maintain open communications with other departments.
- Respect patient/client/resident rights.
- Meet food safety and sanitation regulations.
- Plan for safety, disasters, and bioterrorism.
- Purchase, receive, and store foods to maintain quality.
- Control food costs and inventory.
- Use standardized recipes to prepare and present foods to preserve nutrients and to appeal to the tastes and needs of clients.
- Meet basic nutritional needs of clients, applying principles of nutrition using the current *Dietary Guidelines* when planning menus.
- Develop and maintain a continuing internal quality improvement system.
- Plan and serve meals that meet the needs of the group.
- Understand medical nutrition therapy that may be prescribed.
- Understand applicable food service regulations and the health agencies' inspection requirements and procedures.[6]

Continuing education programs can be conducted in collaboration with local educational institutions, public health agencies, or with professional organizations to reach the largest numbers of administrators and food service workers from community group care facilities. A study in British Columbia found that adult care facility food service staff who participated in a one-day food service training workshop that included a food service manual was more beneficial than only a manual or no intervention.[7] Computer or Internet-based training reaches large audiences with less expense than conventional classroom training. Training courses might focus on the specific needs of clients served in each type of group care facility, such as child day care or nursing homes, or it might focus on the more generic needs of all types of group care facilities and programs.[8]

Public health programs providing in-service education can be reinforced and extended by selecting, preparing, and mailing or e-mailing guidelines, current manuals, newsletters, and other educational materials to promote and improve the quality of food services and nutritional care in the facilities.[9] Sending informational e-mails or setting up electronic mailing lists for staff can reinforce in-service training. Announcements mailed to qualifying public and nonprofit facilities encourages them to apply for federally subsidized food assistance programs and available donated commodity foods.[10]

The dietitian's consultative report is an excellent tool to educate administrators. The dietitian assesses the food service systems, identifies those areas that need improvement, and makes specific recommendations.

Administrators can keep current on food service trends and newer nutritional care standards through membership in professional organizations such as the American Health Care Association, the American Association of Homes and Services for the Aging, the National Center for Assisted Living, and National Association for Family Child Care. Each of these organizations has a Web site that offers more detailed information.

Registered/licensed dietitians can present or sponsor seminars and conferences to update administrators' knowledge. Many professional organizations and regulatory agencies publish guidelines and "best practices" on the Internet. Two useful Web sites are:

- Agency for Healthcare Research and Quality—www.ahrq.gov
- CD-HCF—www.cdhcf.org

Plan Menus to Meet Client Needs and Tastes

Most food service regulations for group care facilities require nutritionally adequate meals to be served to meet the needs of the population it serves as specified in the Institute of Medicine's *Dietary Reference Intakes: Applications for Dietary Planning.*[11] Written menu plans ensure that adequate nutrients are provided. Group care administrators and staff need and want guidance from the public health nutritionist to assist them in menu development and planning. In addition to basic information on the types, variety, and amounts of food to include, administrators and staff may request guidance to plan menus in a systematic fashion.[12] To ensure that menus meet the unique nutritional needs of their group care population, the menu planner must consider the age, gender, level of physical activity, and health status of the clients they serve. The menu planner should use the up-to-date edition of the *Dietary Guidelines for Americans* for health promotion and disease prevention to ensure the population's recommended needs are met.[13]

The food service managers must understand and respect cultural, religious, and ethnic food preferences of the group care population and the facility's budget.

To achieve well-planned and well-accepted menus in multicultural communities, menu planning must accommodate the variety of cultural and ethnic food preferences of the individuals served or residing in their facility. This may be challenging. Computer software facilitates menu planning and nutrient analysis. Examples of useful menu planning and nutrient analysis software programs include:[14]

- Computrition—www.computrition.com
- Nutritionist Pro—www.nutritionistpro.com
- ESHA Research (food processor)—www.esha.com
- Nutribase nutrition and fitness software—www.nutribase.com
- Gerimenu—www.GeriMenu.com
- USDA Nutrient Data Laboratory, Agricultural Research Service—www.nal.usda.gov/fnic/foodcomp

For maximum variety of foods to minimize monotony, the facility menu planner should consider a seasonal cycle menu. To improve customer satisfaction, limited-choice menus or selective menus may be preferable to consider rather than a "one-size-fits-all" menu. A limited-choice menu offers clients some options, but is not fully selective. A completely selective menu may increase customer satisfaction further. However, offering greater choices of foods and food preparation entails more labor and higher food costs. Hospitals, independent living retirement facilities, nursing homes, intermediate care facilities for the developmentally disabled, behavioral treatment facilities, rehabilitation facilities, as well as school or college cafeterias, are facilities for which selective menus are well suited.

Food service equipment and the skills of the personnel preparing the food must also be considered. Recipes may need to be adjusted to the food preparation skills, reading level, and language of food service employees. To prepare the food items envisioned by the menu planner, the food service staff must clearly understand instructions. They learn best through demonstrations and supervised practice.

The USDA Child Care Food Program has nutritional requirement recommendations based on the number of daytime hours the children spend in the program. Toddlers and preschoolers particularly need to be offered foods to meet recommended needs for calcium, protein, vitamin A, and iron. These are provided by offering a variety of foods. Young children are attracted by interesting shapes and different colors of foods. Most young children prefer plain, unmixed foods that they can easily identify and eat as finger foods. New nutrient-dense foods can be introduced to young children as a surprise "treat" or as a reward for winning a guessing game. Limiting total fat is not recommended for children under two years of age. Limiting total fat, saturated fat, and trans fat intake for children five years and older promotes healthy lifelong food habits. Snacks should be included in menus planned for toddlers, since they can only consume small volumes of food at each meal but require additional energy for growth and physical activity. Snacks should be considered as supplements to the meal, rather than meal replacements, and should be nutrient dense. Menus served can teach young children about their basic nutritional needs and healthy food choices.

Menus for children in group care should include at least the minimum numbers or food portions recommended by the USDA guidelines. Menus should offer five vegetables and fruits each day, with a variety of colors. When planning menus for facilities for school-age children, it is helpful for the menu planner to refer to the current school lunch menu to avoid repeating foods served at school.

Due to their accelerated growth rate, adolescents have high energy needs. Extra calories are best obtained from complex carbohydrates rather than foods high in saturated fats. Adolescent nutrient needs increase from childhood, particularly vitamins A, C, and E, iron, and calcium. Adolescents also need snacks to provide these extra calories and nutrients. A current nutritional concern for children and adolescents that affect menu planning are the increasing numbers of children and adolescents who are overweight or obese. Food allergies, vegetarianism, and fear of weight gain must also be respected.

When planning menus for adults, health promotion and disease prevention issues to consider include obesity and overweight as these may contribute to diabetes, heart disease, and cancer. Osteoporosis and iron-deficiency are issues for women of childbearing age. Menu planning considerations for older adults include their decreased need for calories, while ensuring adequate calcium and fiber. The sense of smell and taste may decrease as part of the aging process. Menus that are flavorful, rather than bland, make foods more appealing. For older adults who have problems with chewing, because of oral or dental problems, it may be necessary to alter the consistency of foods. Due to many of the acute and chronic illnesses diagnosed in the older population, facilities for seniors need to offer a variety of therapeutic diet menus. Carbohydrate-controlled and sodium- and calorie-restricted diets are the most common diet modifications prescribed by physicians. However, there has been a trend in nursing homes to liberalize diets to the greatest extent possible to enhance residents' enjoyment of meals and the quality of their life.[15]

Prepare Appealing, Attractive Food

Many food service workers may have little or no formal training in quantity food preparation, although they may have prepared food for their family, schools, or small restaurants.[16] All food service workers employed in group care facilities benefit from training to ensure quality and consistent food preparation. Training should include use of standardized recipes, portion control, altering food consistencies, foods prepared to be suitable for the various therapeutic diets, and sanitary food handling practices. Dietitians may recommend that the facility purchase a quantity cookbook or standardized recipe file and train food service workers on their use. It may be necessary to demonstrate and supervise cooks, bakers, and others who prepare foods to use the standardized recipes. Food service workers may need training to use portion control utensils, such as scoops, measuring spoons, or cups, to ensure uniform servings. To implement the *Dietary Guidelines*, food service workers may need help to alter popular recipes to reduce amount and type of sugar, fat, and sodium. Although recipes can be modified to make preparation easy, many food service workers may need guidance to use herbs, spices, alternative fats and oils, and artificial sweeteners so that food is still tasty and appealing. Food service workers can be trained to prepare and serve pureed and ground food textures in tasty, eye-appealing combination dishes. Food service workers may need training in principles of food safety. Most state and local health departments require basic and periodic safe food handling training for all food handlers (see Chapter 13).

Serving Meals

People eating in group care look forward to mealtimes as the highlights of their day. Every effort should be made to make the food appealing and the surroundings attractive and comfortable.[17] Depending on the physical and mental abilities of the population, different styles of meal service are used in group care facilities. These include self-service, family-style service, tray service, waited table service, and portable meals. Self-service or cafeteria meal service is common in facilities that serve ambulatory and younger populations, such as schools, colleges, children's summer camps, shelters, and correctional, behavioral treatment, and rehabilitation facilities.

Large hospitals and nursing homes use a centralized distribution system, in which foods are prepared and portioned for individual tray service. Individual meal trays are assembled in the main kitchen, transported, and served to individuals at bedside or in a dining room. Some group care programs, such as senior congregate meal programs, may have a decentralized distribution/service. The food is prepared in a main kitchen and sent in bulk to a satellite location to be served.

Table service is common in independent living retirement facilities and some nursing homes. Portable meal service is used by home-delivered meal programs for seniors. Group care homes for developmentally disabled individuals, mental health facilities, retirement homes, child care facilities, camps, and substance abuse facilities may serve meals in a congregate dining room. They may use tray service, waited table service, or family-style service, in which the individuals are encouraged to serve their own plates.

The style of meal service depends on the functional ability of the individuals served, the dining space and furnishings available, and the number of staff available to supervise or assist with meal service. The trend in dining programs in the community group care over past decades has been to move from the institutional environment to a more homelike environment. This trend is reflected in the dining room decor, furnishings, and tableware. To promote an appealing, aesthetic dining environment, the area should be clean with safe comfortable lighting, temperature, and sound. Space should be adequate for individuals to easily move around tables. Dining room tables with adjustable heights help accommodate individuals in wheelchairs. The tables and chairs should be comfortable, sturdy, and appropriately sized.

A pleasant dining room environment enhances the dining experience for people in group care facilities and programs and makes mealtimes more enjoyable. This is particularly important for populations in which adequate food intake is a challenge, such as in nursing home populations. Another consideration for dining rooms is providing space for trays, carts, soiled dishes, and hand-washing facilities.

Serving attractive meals is important to ensure adequate nutrient intake for people in group care facilities and programs. Meal presentation does not have to be elaborate. One of the basics for attractive meal presentation is to ensure that the food is not overcooked, undercooked, or too dry. Contrasting food colors, textures, temperatures, and methods of food preparation enhances meal attractiveness. Garnishes make the food more attractive. The attractive presentation of meals tells clients and their families that the staff cares for them and takes pride in their work.[18]

Another way to make meal presentation more appealing is to use attractive dishware. However, the type of dishware may depend on the type of washing methods used (manual versus mechanical). It may be more practical for a group care facility or program that serves a high volume of meals, but has little or no mechanical dishwashing equipment available, to consider disposable single-service dishware. However, some elders may have difficulty using single-service items. Expense and storage space are factors to consider when using single-service dishware.

Some individuals may need assistive eating utensils to enhance their ability to eat independently. Administrators should be encouraged to consult with physical or occupational therapists to train staff to assist handicapped clients who have eating disabilities.[19] Many individuals who receive services in group care need assistance with eating, because of developmental level or disability. It is important that there is sufficient trained staff to provide clients assistance with eating. It takes time, patience, and skill to ensure that the patient who needs to be fed consumes enough food to meet nutritional needs.[20] The *CD-HCF Dining Skills Manual* is an available resource to train staff to provide eating assistance to those individuals who require it.[21] CMS has now approved federally certified nursing homes to employ feeding assistants, whose sole function is to feed nursing home residents.[22] This legislation lessens the burden for those nursing homes that have difficulty in maintaining staffing levels needed to provide quality of care and services.

NUTRITIONAL CARE AND MEDICAL NUTRITION THERAPY

Nutritional care in health care facilities usually involves nursing staff or food service workers who can perform the following activities:

- Assist clients with meal service and eating.
- Serve supplements between meals.
- Monitor and record each client's food and fluid consumption.
- Monitor and record each client's weight and body measurements.

Group care workers need to be trained to identify factors that may affect clients' food and fluid intake, such as difficulty in chewing. Training staff to monitor client food preferences and dislikes is also necessary. Staff may need guidance to establish a consistent policy to monitor and document food and fluid intake and refusal. Several tools to record food and fluid intake are available from food companies and nutriceutical companies. For nursing homes, the National Policy & Resource Center on Nutrition & Aging has a validated tool to track food and fluid intake. It is available at www.fiu.edu/nutreldr/.

Group care workers may need to be trained to weigh and take accurate body measurements so that changes in nutritional status may be monitored over time. Nutrition professionals rely on this information to be accurate and use it for nutritional assessment and care planning.

A registered/licensed dietitian is qualified to provide medical nutrition therapy (MNT). This includes individual nutritional assessment, necessary diet modifications, and counseling. The number of clients for whom MNT is prescribed depends on the clinical practice guidelines and regulations. MNT services must be documented in the individual's health record. The evaluation of nutritional status is a core part of MNT and its extent varies in group care facilities. Evaluation of nutritional status may involve basic nutritional screening such as evaluating weight status and food and fluid intake, or it may involve an individualized comprehensive nutritional assessment that evaluates physical condition, laboratory tests results, and medication review, in addition to weight status and nutritional intake. As part of nutritional assessment, it may be necessary for the registered/licensed dietitian to observe the client eating, review food and fluid intake records, collect data such as weight and laboratory values from clinical records, and interview the client, family, or caregiver. In some group care settings, some of these data collection tasks may be delegated to registered/licensed dietetic technicians (DTRs) or certified dietary managers (CDMs). In federally certified nursing homes, the evaluation of nutrition status is part of each resident's comprehensive assessment and requires the use of an accurate, standardized reproducible assessment instrument, called the Minimum Data Set. For more information, go to www.cms.hhs.gov.

The five major components when assessing the nutritional status of children are anthropometric, measures of growth and development; clinical signs, biochemical, dietary patterns, and nutrient intake; and the development of feeding skills in young children.[23] Based on the nutritional assessment, the nutrition professional recommends appropriate nutritional interventions to the physician or health practitioner. Upon approval of the physician or health practitioner, these nutritional interventions are incorporated into the care plan and implemented by the group care staff. The nutrition professional must monitor nutritional interventions for effective outcomes.

A registered/licensed dietitian consultant, who is contracted to make regularly scheduled visits, establishes a referral system to give priority to those who most need nutritional assessment. This referral system assigns priority based on selected nutritional risk criteria. For adult clients, for example, significant weight loss, decreased food and fluid intake, and onset of acute disease are criteria that indicate a high priority for nutritional assessment. A registered/licensed dietitian consultant should establish a tracking system with the food service manager and director of nursing or director of health services to be sure that nutritional recommendations are approved by the physician or health care practitioner. In some settings, nutrition professionals may participate as members of an interdisciplinary health care team.

Facility administrators are ultimately responsible for maintaining the quality of all care and services. The nutrition professional is responsible for overseeing the provision of optimal nutrition and dietary services.[24] This is a part of the facility's quality improvement program. Federally regulated and/or voluntarily accredited group care facilities are mandated to implement a quality assessment and assurance program to demonstrate that they maintain appropriate care and services. Nutrition professionals work with the quality improvement team to collect data, organize results, interpret findings, and develop conclusions, recommendations, initiate actions, and track the results of these actions. Some of the dietary services evaluated in quality improvement include the following:

- Tray accuracy
- Food quality—Attractiveness and temperature
- Meal service satisfaction of clients and families
- Food safety and sanitation
- Nutritional assessment and reassessment
- Nutritional care plans
- Nutrition care communication using client records
- Client and family nutrition education[25]

Counsel Clients and Families

Clients can learn about nutrition, both informally and formally, in group care facilities and programs. Group care clients of all ages can learn about nutritious food choices by observing the meals served to them each day.[26] An education program can teach the principles of basic nutrition through foods served in daily meals that reflect excellence in meal planning and food preparation.[27] Children eating meals and snacks in Head Start programs, day care centers, or residential facilities can be introduced to a wide variety of healthful foods through the menus and food preparation activities planned as part of their daily educational activities.[28]

Family members and caregivers should be involved in nutrition education so they can encourage their child or adult relative to consume an adequate and appropriate amount of food. Family members should participate in nutrition counseling and education with the client, so they understand the reasons why certain foods are selected, prepared, and served in the group care facility or program. Family members and caregivers especially need to understand the underlying principles for any physician-prescribed MNT so that they can serve appropriate meals and snacks at home or bring appropriate food gifts when visiting their relative in the health care or residential facility.[29] Family members may also need guidance in basic food safety to ensure the foods they bring in from outside are safe for the resident to eat.

Those adults who eat only one meal a day in group care or who will be discharged from a group care facility can learn some basic nutrition principles and gain skill in selecting, purchasing, and preparing health-promoting food at home.[30] All residents who will continue to live in group care facilities need to know about the objectives of the food service, the rationale for the menus, and when applicable, the benefits of their physician-prescribed MNT. Client meal satisfaction can be improved by establishing a resident food service and nutrition committee to provide the adult clients the opportunity to make suggestions about menus and meal service. This committee provides valuable feedback to food service staff.

Registered/Licensed Dietitians (RD/LD) in Group Care

Larger facilities employ qualified nutrition personnel who assume the responsibility for maintaining a safe and sanitary food service that meets their clients' nutritional needs.[31] The registered/licensed dietitian and registered dietetic technicians provide each client's medical nutrition therapy and nutrition education. The certified dietary manager (CDM) is a valuable team member and assists with obtaining, monitoring, and documenting data related to nutritional screening and assessment, client food preferences, and food acceptance. These trained personnel are accountable to the administrator for quality improvement, food cost control, supervision and training of the food service staff, and compliance with federal, state, and local regulations.

Smaller group care facilities may share a registered/licensed dietitian or employ a registered/licensed dietitian consultant on contract. Under these circumstances, the registered/licensed dietitian consultant assumes an advisory role, and usually does not have line authority. The consultant dietitian may advise on medical nutritional therapy for patients, residents, or clients, and may advise the administrator, director of health services or director of nursing, and the food service director on the food service operations.

The consultant dietitian's role may have several advantages over other dietetic practice areas. These advantages include a flexible work schedule, opportunity to work with the different types of food services, and facilities. Consultants enjoy the freedom of entrepreneurship, however, consulting offers fewer interactions with other registered/licensed dietitians, lack of fringe benefits, and possible risk of not being reimbursed for all services rendered. The registered/licensed dietitian consultant responsibilities generally include the following:

- Planning and implementing nutritional care for all patients, residents, and clients
- Evaluating the food service delivery system
- Assisting in planning, organizing, implementing, and evaluating staff development programs related to nutritional care
- Documenting these recommendations to the facility administrator[32]

During facility visits, registered/licensed dietitian consultants may conduct required nutritional assessments and counseling; evaluate menus for nutritional adequacy and approve menus; conduct staff in-service education sessions; audit kitchen sanitation; conduct food quality evaluations; review the food budget; and conduct quality improvement activities. In facilities where residents will be returning to their homes or transferred to other types of group care, registered/licensed dietitians should participate in discharge planning, provide appropriate nutrition education and diet counseling, and make referrals for follow-up at home or in the community.[33] By coordinating counseling and referral, registered/licensed dietitians in health care facilities and nutritionists in community agencies collaborate to ensure continuity of nutritional care for clients.[34]

The registered/licensed dietitians who work in group care facilities must be aware of the Occupational Safety and Health Act (OSHA) standards, labor laws, the Health Insurance Portability and Accountability Act (HIPAA), and Medicare provider rules for MNT in addition to federal, state, and local nutrition care standards.

Many consultant dietitians utilize technological devices and software to make some of their tasks more efficient and to better manage their time. Some of these technological devices include handheld personal digital assistants and nutrition assessment software. Dietitians can improve their dietetic practice by using the Internet to obtain disease information, access nutrition and pharmacological industry information, use recipe archives, use online calculators, share information with other dietitians, and connect with clients.

Most consultant dietitians work in nursing homes or long-term care settings, because of the large number of facilities nationally, and because federal regulations require MNT services. Dietitians who consult in health-related group care facilities need to have knowledge and skills in nutrition support and possibly in critical care. Dietitians who consult for group care facilities that serve elders need to know about chronic illness, dysphasia, advance directives, quality of life, and end-of-life issues. Consultants who work in group care facilities that serve children and adolescents must be knowledgeable in weight management and prevention of obesity, vegetarian diets, eating disorders, nutritional needs of persons with HIV, and food allergies.

Public Health Nutritionists as Consultants

Many smaller group care facilities do not employ staff with the training and education necessary to meet the nutritional needs of their clients.[35] Often administrators of small facilities, in addition to administrators of government-sponsored group care, look to the local public health agency for help. They request qualified nutrition consultation to assist them to meet federal Medicare/Medicaid and state licensure requirements. Some local health agencies have the resources and expertise to provide nutrition consultation to group care facilities, particularly those that are nonprofit or public. In the state health agency, specialized nutrition consultants, (also known as institution nutrition consultants, consulting dietitians, or public health dietitians), assume this function.[36] These positions should require education and experience in food service system management, advanced nutrition and dietetics.

The state or local public health agency might charge a cost recovery or sliding scale fee to enable the agency to employ registered/licensed dietitians to provide the requested food service and nutrition care consultation. In some communities, registered/licensed dietitians may be employed as independent contractors to provide the needed services.

When nutritionists from the public health agency work with group care food service operations, they need to clearly define their roles.[37] Many public health agencies are not staffed with sufficient public health nutrition personnel to provide extensive consultation to all group care food services in the community that need such service. The appropriate role should be that of a consultant or educator.[38] The public health nutrition personnel might be able to provide limited consultative services to group care facilities that supplement the services of a regularly scheduled consultant dietitian. Public health agencies would need to plan and develop educational and training programs that reach out to groups of administrators and their food service staff. Public health nutrition personnel are expert resources to develop nutrition education programs that promote health, such as weight management for children, adolescents, and adults in group care facilities. Depending on the nature of the relationship with the facility, it may be appropriate to provide services in cooperation with the monitoring or regulatory agency and follow up to see that recommendations have been implemented.[39]

Public health nutritionists must avoid situations that may be considered a conflict of interest, such as providing consultative services to group care facilities when their health agency's primary role is regulatory. Additionally, public health nutritionists who work in group care facilities, particularly nursing homes, may write litigation related to poor nutritional care. They should protect against legal entanglements by carrying malpractice and liability insurance, provide services and care according to practice standards, and accurately document care and services provided.[40]

Nutritionists can have an important affect on the health of the community by assisting group care facilities develop quality food service and nutrition education. They have the knowledge and skills to demonstrate to group care facility administrators and food services staff the need to promote health and prevent disease through food services. Federal, state, and local governments need to allocate adequate funding to enable the public health agency nutrition staff to provide expert consultation to these community programs.

POINTS TO PONDER

- How should the dietetic practitioner maintain knowledge and skills needed to provide quality services to a variety of group care facilities serving diverse nutritional needs, such as children in group care, homes for people with HIV, and nursing homes?
- How should conflicts in the role of the public health nutritionist as regulator as opposed to consultant to group facilities be addressed?
- What skills are needed to work with culturally diverse food service employees?
- What are the practice liability issues for public health nutritionists who provide services to group care facilities?

HELPFUL WEB SITES

American Camp Association: www.acacamp.org
American Correctional Association (ACA): www.aca.org
Agency for Healthcare Research and Quality: www.ahrq.gov
CARF – The Rehabilitation Accreditation Commission: www.carf.org
Centers for Medicare & Medicaid Services: www.cms.hhs.gov
Computrition: www.computrition.com
Consultant Dietitians in Health Care Facilities (CD-HCF):
　www.cdhcf.org
DO-Online!: www.do-online.osteotech.org
ESHA Research: www.esha.com
GeriMenu – Long-Term Care Foodservice Software: www.gerimenu.com
Joint Commission on Accreditation of Healthcare Organizations:
　www.jcaho.org

National Association for the Education of Young Children:
www.naeyc.org
National Association for Family Child Care (NAFCC):
www.nafcc.org/include/default.asp
Nutritionist Pro: www.nutritionistpro.com
Professional Nutrition and Fitness Software Site: www.nutribase.com

NOTES

1. Kaufman M. *Nutrition in Public Health: A Handbook for Developing Programs and Services*. Gaithersburg, Md: Aspen Publishers; 1990:243–244.

2. Kaufman M. *Nutrition in Public Health: A Handbook for Developing Programs and Services*. Gaithersburg, Md: Aspen Publishers; 1990:246.

3. Kaufman M. *Nutrition in Public Health: A Handbook for Developing Programs and Services*. Gaithersburg, Md: Aspen Publishers; 1990:246.

4. Kaufman M. *Nutrition in Public Health: A Handbook for Developing Programs and Services*. Gaithersburg, Md: Aspen Publishers; 1990:246.

5. Consultant Dietitians in Health Care Facilities (CD-HCF). *Pocket Resource for Management 2000*. Chicago, Ill: CD-HCF; 2000:124.

6. Consultant Dietitians in Health Care Facilities (CD-HCF). *Pocket Resource for Management 2000*. Chicago, Ill: CD-HCF; 2000:122.

7. McCargar L, Soneff R, McGeachy F, Davison K, Therein G. Effectiveness of two training methods to improve the quality of food service in small facilities for adult care. *J Am Diet Assoc*. 1994;94:869–873.

8. Kaufman M. *Nutrition in Public Health: A Handbook for Developing Programs and Services*. Gaithersburg, Md: Aspen Publishers; 1990:246–247.

9. Kaufman M. *Nutrition in Public Health: A Handbook for Developing Programs and Services*. Gaithersburg, Md: Aspen Publishers; 1990:247.

10. Kaufman M. *Nutrition in Public Health: A Handbook for Developing Programs and Services*. Gaithersburg, Md: Aspen Publishers; 1990:247.

11. Institute of Medicine. *Dietary Reference Intakes: Applications for Dietary Planning*. Washington, DC: National Academies Press; 2003.

12. Kaufman M. *Nutrition in Public Health: A Handbook for Developing Programs and Services*. Gaithersburg, Md: Aspen Publishers; 1990:247.

13. US Dept of Agriculture. *Dietary Guidelines for Americans 2005*.

14. Consultant Dietitians in Health Care Facilities (CD-HCF). *Pocket Resource for Management 2000*. Chicago, Ill: CD-HCF; 2000:155.

15. American Dietetic Association. Liberalized diets for older adults in long-term care. *J Am Diet Assoc*. 2002;102:1316–1323.

16. Kaufman M. *Nutrition in Public Health: A Handbook for Developing Programs and Services*. Gaithersburg, Md: Aspen Publishers; 1990:248.

17. Kaufman M. *Nutrition in Public Health: A Handbook for Developing Programs and Services.* Gaithersburg, Md: Aspen Publishers; 1990:248.

18. Kaufman M. *Nutrition in Public Health: A Handbook for Developing Programs and Services.* Gaithersburg, Md: Aspen Publishers; 1990:249.

19. Kaufman M. *Nutrition in Public Health: A Handbook for Developing Programs and Services.* Gaithersburg, Md: Aspen Publishers; 1990:249.

20. Kaufman M. *Nutrition in Public Health: A Handbook for Developing Programs and Services.* Gaithersburg, Md: Aspen Publishers; 1990:249.

21. Consultant Dietitians in Health Care Facilities (CD-HCF). *Dining Skills: Practical Interventions for the Caregivers of Eating Disabled Older Adults.* Chicago, Ill: CD-HCF; 1992.

22. Dept of Health and Human Services, Center for Medicare & Medicaid Services. 42 CFR Parts 483 and 488, Medicare and Medicaid Programs; requirements for paid feeding assistants in long-term care facilities. Federal Register: September 26, 2003 (Volume 68, Number 187) [Rules & Regulations]

23. Baer MT, and Harris AB. Pediatric nutrition assessment: identifying children at risk. *J Am Diet Assoc.* 1997;97: S107–S115.

24. Consultant Dietitians in Health Care Facilities (CD-HCF). *Steps to Success for Consultant Dietitians.* Chicago, Ill: CD-HCF; 1998:8–14.

25. Consultant Dietitians in Health Care Facilities (CD-HCF). *Steps to Success for Consultant Dietitians.* Chicago, Ill: CD-HCF; 1998.

26. Kaufman M. *Nutrition in Public Health: A Handbook for Developing Programs and Services.* Gaithersburg, Md: Aspen Publishers; 1990:250.

27. Kaufman M. *Nutrition in Public Health: A Handbook for Developing Programs and Services.* Gaithersburg, Md: Aspen Publishers; 1990:250.

28. Kaufman M. *Nutrition in Public Health: A Handbook for Developing Programs and Services.* Gaithersburg, Md: Aspen Publishers; 1990:250.

29. Kaufman M. *Nutrition in Public Health: A Handbook for Developing Programs and Services.* Gaithersburg, Md: Aspen Publishers; 1990:250.

30. Kaufman M. *Nutrition in Public Health: A Handbook for Developing Programs and Services.* Gaithersburg, Md: Aspen Publishers; 1990:250.

31. Kaufman M. *Nutrition in Public Health: A Handbook for Developing Programs and Services.* Gaithersburg, Md: Aspen Publishers; 1990:250.

32. Consultant Dietitians in Health Care Facilities (CD-HCF). *Steps to Success—The Business of Consulting.* Chicago, Ill: CD-HCF; 2002:7–8.

33. Kaufman M. *Nutrition in Public Health: A Handbook for Developing Programs and Services.* Gaithersburg, Md: Aspen Publishers; 1990:251.

34. Elbe D. Six ways to use the Internet to improve your dietetic practice. *Consultant Dietitian.* 2002;27:1,7–10.

35. Kaufman M. *Nutrition in Public Health: A Handbook for Developing Programs and Services.* Gaithersburg, Md: Aspen Publishers; 1990:251.

36. Kaufman M. *Nutrition in Public Health: A Handbook for Developing Programs and Services.* Gaithersburg, Md: Aspen Publishers; 1990:252.

37. Kaufman M. *Nutrition in Public Health: A Handbook for Developing Programs and Services.* Gaithersburg, Md: Aspen Publishers; 1990:252.

38. Kaufman M. *Nutrition in Public Health: A Handbook for Developing Programs and Services.* Gaithersburg, Md: Aspen Publishers; 1990:252.

39. Kaufman M. *Nutrition in Public Health: A Handbook for Developing Programs and Services.* Gaithersburg, Md: Aspen Publishers; 1990:252.

40. McKee J. The role of the dietitian in avoiding litigation. *Consultant Dietitian in Health Care Facililties.* 2002;2.

BIBLIOGRAPHY

Consultant Dietitians in Health Care Facilities (CD-HCF). *Pocket Resource for Management 2000.* Chicago, Ill: CD-HCF; 2000.

Institute of Medicine. *Dietary Reference Intakes: Applications for Dietary Planning,* Washington, DC: National Academies Press; 2003.

US Dept of Agriculture. *Dietary Guidelines for Americans 2005.* Home and Garden Bulletin.

American Dietetic Association. Liberalized diets for older adults in long-term care. *J Am Diet Assoc.* 2002;102:1316–1323.

CHAPTER 13

Protect the Food Supply

Mildred M. Cody

Reader Objectives

- Identify current food safety issues.
- Differentiate food safety risks for vulnerable populations.
- Integrate food safety into nutrition guidance.
- Review federal, state, and local food safety systems.
- Identify and describe consumer-focused food safety programs.
- Explore future food-safety issues.
- Suggest resources for public health professionals, food service workers, and consumers.

FOOD SAFETY AS A PUBLIC HEALTH NUTRITION ISSUE

A safe, nutritious, accessible food supply is the foundation for individual and community health. The primary food safety issues—presence of toxic agents in the food supply and efforts to reduce or eliminate those agents—remain constant, while the specific problems change over time. The food-borne illnesses of the early 1900s included typhoid fever, tuberculosis, botulism, scarlet fever, and trichinosis none of which are major food-borne illnesses in this century.[1] These diseases are less commonly food-borne today, because research identified their sources and characteristics, and public health programs were developed to control them. Two primary barriers to food-borne illnesses—pasteurization and refrigeration of milk—virtually eliminated food-borne typhoid fever, tuberculosis, and scarlet fever. Although the innovations of the 1900s are taken for granted today, they were hotly debated early in the century, and it took decades to pass and enact the legislation for pasteurization and to manufacture and distribute the refrigeration equipment now taken for granted.

Today's public health efforts are presented in *Healthy People 2010: Objectives for Improving Health*, the blueprint for current public health efforts in the United

States. *Objective 10: Food Safety* lists the present issues.[2] The food safety goal is to "Reduce food-borne illnesses." Under this goal are targets for the objectives supported by baseline data (see Table 13–1). Developmental objectives establish baselines for *Healthy People 2020.*

All people are susceptible to food-borne illnesses.[3] Some groups are more susceptible to pathogens than others, because of reduced immune function at certain stages of life health conditions, or their treatment.[3–5] People at risk due to their stage of life are fetuses and infants, young children, pregnant women, and the elderly. People at greater risk through disease or its treatment include those with HIV/AIDS or damaged organ systems (especially liver, kidney, or gastrointestinal tract) and those whose treatment includes chemotherapy or radiotherapy (see Table 13–2). At-risk people are more likely to develop food-borne illnesses and suffer more severe outcomes. The Centers for Disease Control and Prevention (CDC) estimates the annual health and economic costs of food-borne illness in the United States are 76 million illnesses, 325,000 hospitalizations, 5000 deaths, and $23 billion in costs (includes health care costs and opportunity costs).[6]

Food safety programs, similar to other public health programs, need to collaborate with many different stakeholders. The responsibility for safe and nutritious food involves all players in the food system. The challenge is to build comprehensive food protection systems that ensure continuing responsibility and commitment from the farm or ship, through food marketing, commercial preparation, and service. Federal and state public health regulations guide and oversee production of safe food for consumers. Locally, public health agencies share responsibility to educate and guide food producers, marketers, food service personnel, and consumers to prepare and serve safe and nutritious food.

CURRENT FOOD SAFETY ISSUES

Although food is essential for life, it can also serve as a vehicle for toxic agents to enter the body. Potential toxic agents include pathogens and toxic chemicals. Both may unintentionally become a part of food during production, marketing, or preparation, or can be added to food by intentional poisoning or bioterrorism. Pathogens are organisms that cause disease through infection or the production of toxic chemicals. Toxic chemicals, either produced by pathogens growing in food or introduced into the food through other means, cause illnesses called intoxications. Most food-borne illnesses are acute, causing short-term symptoms, such as vomiting or diarrhea, that appear shortly after the contaminated food is eaten. Some illnesses are chronic, such as food-borne hepatitis. A few food-borne illnesses have sequelae, [subsequent disease(s)], that follow the acute symptoms of infection, such as reactive arthritis that may occur after the acute infection stage.

Table 13–1   Healthy People 2010 Food Safety Objectives

Objective Number	Objective	1997 Baseline[1]	2010 Target[1]
10-1	Reduction in infections caused by microorganisms.		
		Per 100,000	
10-1a	*Campylobacter* species	24.6	12.3
10-1b	*Escherichia coli* O157:H7	2.1	1.0
10-1c	*Listeria monocytogenes*	0.5	0.25
10-1d	*Salmonella* species	13.7	6.8
10-1e	*Cyclospora cayetanensis*	Developmental	
10-1f	Postdiarrheal hemolytic uremic syndrome (HUS)	Developmental	
10-1g	Congenital *Toxoplasma gondii*	Developmental	
10-2	Reduce outbreaks of infections caused by key food-borne bacteria.		
		Outbreaks per year	
10-2a	*Escherichia coli* O157:H7	22	11
10-2b	*Salmonella* serotype Enteritidis	44	22
10-3	Prevent an increase in the proportion of isolates of *Salmonella* species from humans and from animals at slaughter that are resistant to antimicrobial drugs.		
		Percent of isolates	
	Salmonella from humans that are resistant to:		
10-3a	Fluoroquinolones	0	0
10-3b	Third-generation cephalosporins	0	0
10-3c	Gentamicin	3	3
10-3d	Ampicillin	18	18
10-4	Reduce deaths from anaphylaxis caused by food allergies.	Developmental	
10-5	Increase the proportion of consumers who follow key food safety practices.	72%	79%
10-6	Improve food employee behaviors and food preparation practices that directly relate to food-borne illnesses in retail food establishments.	Developmental	
10-7	Reduce human exposure to organophosphate pesticides from food.	Developmental	

Source: Mildred Cody, PhD, MS, RD, LD, Associate Professor, Dept. of Nutrition/Dietetics, Georgia State University, Atlanta, GA; and *US Dept. of Health and Human Services Healthy People 2020*, 2nd ed. Oct. 2002. "Objectives for Improving Health, Part A: Food Safety Objectives," p. 10:3–10:6.

Pathogens

Food-borne pathogens include bacteria, parasites, viruses, and prions. Extensive descriptions of bacteria, parasites, and viruses that cause food-borne illness are available from the FDA's *Bad Bug Book*.[3]

Table 13–2 Examples of Food Safety Problems That Target Individuals in At-Risk Categories

Population	Toxic Agents	Comments
Pregnant women and their fetuses	Listeria monocytogenes Toxoplasma gondii Methyl mercury	Advice to pregnant women is usually given to protect fetuses, which are at greater risk because of their developmental stage and small size. L. monocytogenes, most typically found in soft, unpasteurized cheeses and precooked meats (deli meats, hotdogs, etc.), can cause stillbirth, miscarriage, and fetal meningitis without causing severe symptoms in the woman. T. gondii, a parasite carried by raw or undercooked meat and cat litter, can cause serious physical and mental conditions in fetuses. Methyl mercury can cause neurological problems.
Infants	Clostridium botulinum	Infant botulism occurs when Cl. botulinum spores, largely from honey, outgrow in the gut to produce botulin toxin. This happens because infant gastrointestinal tracts are not below pH 4.6. Symptoms include loss of head control and possible death.
Children	Campylobacter jejuni Escherichia coli O157:H7 Shigella Cryptosporidium parvum Giardia lamblia Rotavirus Methyl mercury	All of these organisms cause severe diarrhea. Children and young adults are more often affected by campylobacteriosis than other healthy individuals; the food vehicle is most often undercooked poultry. E. coli infections in children cause a bloody diarrhea and are the most common cause of kidney failure in that age group; common food vehicles include undercooked ground beef and unclean raw produce. Shigellosis is more likely to occur in toddlers than in other healthy persons because the typical mode of transmission is the fecal-oral route. C. parvum, G. lamblia, and rotavirus are usually transmitted person-to-person and through contamination of ready-to-eat foods. At hazardous levels methyl mercury can cause neurological problems.

Table 13–2 continued

Population	Toxic Agents	Comments
Elderly	Many organisms that cause infections	The elderly can be more susceptible or exhibit more severe symptoms, because of reduced immune function, and because of damage to organs. Healthy elderly, i.e., those not undergoing chemotherapy, are typically less susceptible. Elderly in care settings may be exposed to more organisms that are transmitted by the fecal-oral route, or person-to-person, and they may be exposed to *Cl. perfringens* more often, since it grows in foods prepared in large batches several hours before serving.
Immune-suppressed people (from either disease or treatment)	All organisms that cause infections	Without healthy immune systems, these people cannot fight infections without antibiotics. *Cryptosporidium*, although more often waterborne than food-borne, is a greater problem than many other food-borne infections because it is harder to treat.
People with liver damage	*Vibrio vulnificus*	In people with liver damage, *V. vulnificus* can enter the blood stream and cause septic shock, characteristic blistering skin lesions, and death (about 50% of cases). Contaminated raw or undercooked shellfish are the common food vehicles.
People with reduced gastric acidity	*Clostridium botulinum* *Listeria monocytogenes* *Vibrio*	Strong stomach acid is the body's first defense against pathogens.

Source: Mildred Cody, PhD, MS, RD, LD, Associate Professor, Dept. of Nutrition/Dietetics, Georgia State University, Atlanta, GA. Compiled from references 3, 11–13.

Some bacteria, such as *Salmonella, Campylobacter jejuni, Listeria monocytogenes, Shigella*, and *Escherichia coli* O157:H7 cause food-borne infections. Other bacteria, such as *Staphylococcus aureus* and *Clostridium botulinum*, produce toxic chemicals when they grow in food. These chemicals can cause intoxications. All of the food-borne diseases caused by parasites and viruses are infections. Although bacteria cause most diagnosed food-borne illnesses in the United States, viruses may actually cause more food-borne illness. However, viral illnesses are usually less severe and are less likely to be diagnosed or reported through surveillance channels than other infections.

Plant foods, which include fruits, vegetables, nuts, and grains, can be contaminated with bacteria, parasites, and viruses during growth. Organisms may be in the soil, contaminated water, or untreated animal fecal material. Animal foods, including meat, fish, poultry, milk, and eggs can become contaminated when the live animal is exposed to pathogens through consumption of contaminated foods or through environmental contamination. Contamination can also be introduced to meat and poultry during processes associated with slaughter. All foods can be contaminated through unsanitary handling after harvest, during shipping, at the processing plant, or in the food market.

Prions

Prions are proteinaceous infective agents, less well understood than other pathogens, but apparently produced in brain tissue by a process called *recruitment* in which brain proteins assume inactive conformations following the pattern of a prion template. Prions cause infectious brain disorders that result in behavior changes, ataxia, progressive dementia, and death over a long presentation time (almost a decade). These diseases include bovine spongiform encephalopathy (BSE or "mad cow disease"), scrapie in sheep and goats, and chronic wasting disease in deer and elk. Mad cow disease, in humans more technically called *variant-Creutzfeldt-Jacob disease*, has not been seen in the United States. It has been diagnosed in Europe, and infected cows have been found in the United States. Public health precautions to reduce population exposure include prohibitions against animal feed containing spinal cord tissue, restrictions on importing agricultural stock, and screening of cattle before they go to market.[7] Prions are not associated with plant foods.

Bacteria

Although all types of pathogens can contaminate food and cause disease, only bacteria grow in food. Foods that support rapid growth of bacteria or toxin production by *Clostridium botulinum* are called potentially hazardous foods.[8] Potentially hazardous foods characteristically have water and nutrients available for bacterial growth and environmental conditions that favor growth such as low acid (pH above 4.5). Examples of potentially hazardous foods include raw and cooked meats, milk, and cooked vegetables. The food preservation techniques employed to keep food safe over long storage periods alter the factors that make foods potentially hazardous. Foods are dried to remove water, such as powdered milk, dried fruits, or dried beans. Water may be bound to the food ingredients so that it is not available to bacteria, as in jellies made with sugar. Foods can be acidulated to prevent toxin production by *Cl. botulinum,* as in pickles or acidulated mixtures containing garlic or herbs in oil. Canning destroys pathogens and their spores, including *Cl. botulinum* and holds food in a container that cannot be penetrated by contaminants. Once the can is opened or damaged enough to cause an opening, the food is potentially hazardous. Potentially hazardous foods must be held at a controlled temperature to keep them out of the "danger zone" (40°F to 140°F or 4°C to 60°C). During serving periods, this means keeping hot foods hot, above 140°F (60°C). Safe storage requires that foods be stored in the refrigerator at temperatures below 40°F (4°C) or in a freezer at a temperature below 32°F (0°C).

Toxic Chemicals

Although any chemical can be toxic or cause harm, few chemicals in foods are hazardous when consumed at the expected levels in food. Toxic chemicals present in food at very low levels are not typically consumed in sufficient quantity to cause harm. Naturally occurring toxicants in vegetables and fruits include solanine in potatoes; cyanogenic glycosides in fruit seeds, lima beans, and black-eyed peas; and goitrogens in cruciferous vegetables.[9] Residues from registered pesticides and cleaning agents are examples of toxicants that become part of foods during production, marketing, and handling. When a toxic chemical is consumed, the digestive system and auxiliary organs help to protect the body. For example, the gastrointestinal tract does not allow absorption of all chemicals, the liver detoxifies many chemicals, and the kidney helps to excrete metabolic products from the liver. Scientists study toxicants to describe their sources, their effects on the body, and to develop methods of controlling human exposures to reduce hazards in the food supply.

To accurately report toxicity, it is important to identify the dose of the chemical and the circumstances of exposure. A complete toxicity statement includes the name of the agent as a purified chemical, its dosage, route of administration, symptom(s), and species affected. The gastrointestinal tract offers several barriers to chemical absorption not presented by other routes of administration, such as injection or inhalation. This means that oral routes of administration may be less hazardous than other exposure routes. Although data from other species can provide important information on the potential effects of a toxic chemical, data from mammals, especially other primates, more closely relate to human effects.

Scientists describe toxic chemicals considering several different factors including chemical nature, source, and action. Toxic chemicals in foods may be naturally occurring—such as seafood toxins and mushroom toxins—or added to food— such as residues from pesticides or cleaning agents. Toxins may be produced by molds growing on foods, such as aflatoxins and other mycotoxins. Toxins may become part of food through environmental contamination by chemicals such as mercury and lead. Toxins may cause different types of harm. Physical symptoms include vomiting and diarrhea. Biochemical effects include inhibition of enzymes. Mutagenic examples include carcinogens and teratogens. Their chemical nature describes the chemical structure, such as an organic acid. For example, methyl mercury is an organic heavy metal complex (chemical nature) found in some large fish (source) that can cause damage to the nervous system (action).

Two units of measurement are important for expressing amounts of chemicals in food safety contexts. The first is dosage, which is the amount of a toxic agent consumed by an individual. Dosage is expressed as the amount of the chemical per unit of body mass, for example, milligrams (mg) of chemical/kilogram (kg) of body mass. The second measurement is concentration, the amount of the toxic substance in relation to the total weight of the food, for example, percent, or parts per million (ppm), or parts per billion (ppb). Examples of these measurements can be seen in Figure 13–1. Understanding these measurements make it easier to interpret reports in professional and popular papers, especially when needed to compare a concentration of a chemical in a food product to a dose for an individual.

Naturally Occurring Chemicals and Environmental Food Contaminants

Seafood toxins, mushroom toxins, and heavy metals are all included in United States food-borne illness outbreak reports.[10] Mycotoxins are chemicals produced by molds growing on foods or feed and have caused international food-borne illnesses throughout history.[3] Mycotoxins are not specifically listed in United States outbreak reports, because they are not typically responsible for intoxications in the United States. These toxins are sometimes considered naturally occurring, because mold growth is common, but the toxin is produced by the mold and not by the infected plant.

Animals that consume contaminated feed can concentrate mycotoxin contaminants, and their metabolites can occur in the animal's milk, which is one of the reasons that animal feed is regulated. There are over 50 different mycotoxins. These compounds have a wide range of structures and activities. The most studied mycotoxin group is aflatoxins. These chemicals produce acute liver necrosis and cirrhosis in mammals.[3] Chronic consumption, especially by people who consume heavily contaminated grains during food shortages, is associated with liver cancer, especially in populations predisposed by alcoholism and hepatitis B. Because of the abundant food supply in the United States, it is unlikely that most people would consume enough mycotoxin to cause acute intoxication. Instead, the US concern is for low-level, chronic consumption from common foods such as soybeans, rice, corn, peanuts and peanut butter, and milk of cattle consuming contaminated feed. These products are closely monitored for aflatoxin contamination.

Dosage is the amount of chemical per unit of body mass.

For example, if an individual who weighs 150 pounds consumes 1 ounce of a chemical, his or her dosage would be 1-ounce chemical/150 pounds body weight. This would usually be converted to the metric system (28.4 g chemical/68.1 kg body weight) and simplified to 0.4 g chemical/kg body weight or 400 mg chemical/kg body weight.

Concentration is the amount of chemical as a portion of the total product.

For example, if 100 pounds of apples contains 1 gram of a contaminant, the concentration of the contaminant would be 1 g/100 lb. This would be converted to the metric system (1 g/45.4 kg) and simplified to (0.022 or 2.2% or 22,000 ppm).

Example 1: CR, who weighs 165 lb, consumed 100 g reconstituted orange juice that contained 10 mg lead.

What is the concentration of lead in the juice?

Concentration	=	10 mg lead/100 g juice
	=	10 mg lead/(100 g juice)(1000 mg/g)
	=	10 mg lead/100,000 mg juice
	=	[10 mg lead/100,000 mg juice][10/10]
	=	100 mg lead/1,000,000 mg juice
	=	100 ppm lead in the juice

What was the dosage that CR consumed?

Dose	=	10 mg lead/165 lb
	=	10 mg lead/74.9 kg
	=	0.013 mg lead/kg
	=	13 μg lead/kg

Example 2: JK, who weighs 125 lb, consumed 100 g reconstituted orange juice that contained 10 ppm lead.

How much lead did JK consume?

Amount = (100 g juice)(10 ppm lead)	=	(100 g)(0.000010) lead
	=	0.0010 g lead
	=	1 mg lead

What was JK's dose of lead?

Dose	=	1 mg lead/125 lb
	=	1 mg lead/56.75 kg
	=	0.02 mg lead/kg or 20 μg lead/kg

Figure 13–1   Units of Measurement in Food Safety

Mushroom toxins include over 50 different chemicals that are tasteless and odorless, and their physiological effects generally categorize them.[3] For example, protoplasmic poisons destroy cells and cause organ failure, and neurotoxins cause profuse sweating, convulsions, hallucinations, depression, and blurred vision.

Although many mushrooms are edible, gathering wild mushrooms is risky, because edible and poisonous species often look alike and are undistinguishable, even with a plant key. Also, toxin accumulation in a species can be variable, making a safe species toxic in some instances.

Seafood toxins and mushroom toxins are naturally occurring toxins. Seafood toxins, mycotoxins, and environmental toxins can be bioamplified through progression in the food chain. In the case of seafood toxins the bioamplification occurs as filter-feeding shellfish concentrate the toxins from toxic algae or when large finfish consume smaller fish that have consumed toxic algae. Seafood toxins are produced by dinoflagellates (marine algae), by bacteria growing on fish during storage, and by fish themselves.[3] Dinoflagellate-caused seafood poisoning syndromes present a variety of physical symptoms including vomiting, nausea, diarrhea, cardiac arrhythmia, and biochemical symptoms (largely neurological). Extreme cases result in coma and death. Scombroid poisoning is caused by bacterial decomposition of fish flesh during storage. This process produces histamine and other biogenic amines, which contribute to the toxicity of the histamine by competing for histamine-metabolizing enzymes during digestion. Symptoms are generally mild and include headache, gastrointestinal discomfort, hypotension, and hives. Severe cases may lead to respiratory distress and shock. Tetrodotoxin (puffer fish) and Haff disease (buffalo fish) are less well understood, but they appear to be caused by chemicals produced, at least in part, by the fish themselves.

Heavy metals are usually considered contaminants that become a part of food through environmental exposure. Mercury and lead are both heavy metal contaminants of food. Over-consumption of these heavy metals causes neurological problems.[11–14] Mercury levels in fish reflect mercury levels in their environment. Mercury is bioconverted as it moves through the food chain into an organic-heavy metal complex called methyl mercury that is absorbed more quickly and is more toxic than the metal itself.[11] Larger, long-lived fish accumulate more methyl mercury in their tissues. Fetuses exposed to hazardous levels of methyl mercury may exhibit developmental delays or symptoms that resemble cerebral palsy. Lead enters food through several routes, including water from corroded pipes and solder and leaching from lead-containing ceramic food containers. In addition to neurological symptoms, lead toxicity presents with anemia, changes in kidney function, and high blood pressure. Lead levels in foods have decreased as solder was banned from cans used to preserve foods and from gasoline.

Approved Chemicals Added to Food

Approved food additives, GRAS (generally recognized as safe) substances, and prior-approved ingredients are categories of intentional food additives.[15] Pesticide residues and cleaning agent residues are examples of approved chemicals that become a part of food during its production or marketing.[16] Regardless of their technical names, approved chemicals added to foods must be safe and effective. Added chemicals cannot be used to mask food spoilage. These chemicals must be used at the lowest level required to achieve their intended effects.

Regulations apply to chemicals purposely added to foods, called *regulated food additives*. Regulations also apply to chemicals that can be reasonably expected to become a part of food, such as residues from detergents, sanitizers, and pesticides. Federal regulation includes approval of food additives by the Food and Drug Administration (FDA) and registration of pesticides regulated by the Environmental Protection Agency (EPA). In approval or registration, the safety of the chemical is assessed by the regulatory agency based on results from a variety of studies:

- Subacute toxicity—Consumption levels at which no harm is observed
- Acute toxicity—High consumption levels at which harm is observed over a short time
- Chronic toxicity—Lower consumption levels of the chemical over the lifespan
- Pharmacokinetic properties—Absorption, distribution in the body, metabolism, and elimination of the chemical and its metabolites
- Reproductive effects

The regulatory agency assesses exposure data to determine how much of the chemical would likely be consumed by an individual from all sources. The outcome of approval or registration describes the specific chemical and its permitted-use level on specific foods. Illegal use of a chemical occurs when the chemical is not approved or when it is used for a purpose for which it has not been approved. For example, a pesticide may be approved for use on apples, but not on pears.

Although testing is rigorous and answers many questions about chemical use, it is open to interpretation. The primary concern expressed is that the tests are not performed on free-living human beings over several generations. Although this is not practical, it does raise questions about the effectiveness of the testing and its interpretation. Examples of data interpretation issues include the following:

- Application of animal data to human exposure
- Use of purified chemicals fed to animals under controlled laboratory conditions as opposed to consumption of a mixed diet by free-living humans
- Use of predictive tests to determine carcinogenicity
- Effects of chronic exposures or bioaccumulation
- Synergistic effects of chemicals or combined effects of chemicals with similar structures

These issues are considered by the regulators who review the data. Approval or registration can be withdrawn if safety problems are later confirmed or when less toxic alternatives become available.

Food Allergies

Idiosyncratic reactions are individual reactions to certain food ingredients. These include food allergies, intolerances, and sensitivities. Adverse reactions happen only to predisposed people due to of immune sensitivities or enzyme deficiencies. The most common reaction is lactose intolerance, the inability to digest lactose, the naturally occurring sugar in milk and milk-containing foods. The most severe idiosyncratic reaction is a food allergy, an immunologically mediated reaction to a food protein.[17] These reactions typically are evidenced in the following:

- Gastrointestinal tract—Swelling and itching in the mouth area, nausea, and diarrhea
- Skin—Hives, rashes, and eczema
- Respiratory tract—Sneezing, shortness of breath, laryngeal edema, or asthma
- Circulatory system—Hypotension, angioedema, or anaphylaxis

Peanuts, tree nuts, seafood, eggs, and milk are foods most frequently associated with allergies. Eating even small quantities of these foods can result in death for allergic people. It is important that nutrition professionals educate clients on the products likely to contain the allergen, ingredient names for the allergen as it might appear on food labels, and ways that the allergen might enter foods through cross-contamination. New federal legislation will require clear, easily understood ingredient labels to identify common allergens in food. Because several foods frequently associated with allergies are WIC-approved foods, it is urgent to bring this to the attention of clients who have allergic family members so that they can take necessary precautions.

Newer Processes and Programs

Today's headline issues are the risks and benefits of natural and organic foods, genetically engineered foods, and irradiation of foods to reduce pathogen exposure. Each of these processes has proponents and detractors. Because many consumers and collaborating health agencies look to public health nutritionists for guidance on food safety issues and on issues affecting the nutrient content of the food supply, it is important for public health nutritionists to understand the issues behind these newer processes and programs. Separating fact from belief can be difficult for these issues. It is important to understand the evidence on all sides, as these policy issues affect everyone, and public health nutritionists influence many consumers and other professionals.

Although there is no regulatory definition for the term *natural*, there is a regulatory definition for the term *organic*.[18] Organic foods are produced under a certification process to ensure that farmers and food processors who produce foods labeled organic follow specific rules, including the following:

- Organic meat and meat products are produced from animals who are given no antibiotics or growth hormones.
- Organic plant foods are produced without using most conventional pesticides, without fertilizers made with synthetic ingredients or sewage sludge, and without bioengineering or use of ionizing radiation.

The USDA does not claim that organically produced foods are safer or more nutritious than conventionally produced foods. Their National Organic Program is a marketing certification program. Certified producers can voluntarily label foods that are at least 95% organic with the USDA organic seal: a circle with *USDA ORGANIC* written inside. Natural does not mean organic. Organic does not mean safer.

Genetically engineered foods are produced using techniques that alter the genetic material of the parent organism so that the desired traits are expressed.[19] The techniques that have been used successfully require removing a single section of DNA (a gene) from one organism and splicing it into the DNA of another organism, masking a gene so that it cannot be expressed as a trait, or making multiple copies of a desirable organism (cloning). These techniques differ from traditional breeding programs in two major ways: traits can be transferred among unrelated organisms, and the outcomes are not random. These foods are regulated in the same way that traditional counterparts are regulated.

To date, the market products of genetic engineering resemble the products produced by traditional breeding methods. For example, a newly developed, genetically engineered rice has higher levels of vitamin A and more bioavailable iron. Future products may display greater differences, especially if cross-species traits are transferred; such as transferring cold tolerance from a fish species to a fruit species. For philosophical reasons, some stakeholders are concerned about the concept of genetic modification. Some stakeholders are concerned about environmental issues such as development of "super weeds." Others are enthusiastic about the potential for foods that can be produced under adverse conditions or that can be altered to produce improved nutrient profiles. These issues and others are being explored by scientists and elected and appointed public policy makers.

Irradiation of foods is a method of food processing included in the 1958 Food Additives Amendment. Instead of energy being transmitted as heat, as it is in cooking, canning, and heat pasteurization, high-energy radiation is transmitted through air in the form of gamma rays, X-rays, or an electron beam. The levels used are much lower than those used for radiotherapy. In the United States, ionizing radiation is approved to control bacterial pathogens and parasites, to extend shelf life of foods by eliminating insects in produce and spices, and to inhibit sprouting of vegetables. In the United States, foods currently approved for irradiation include red meats, poultry, and pork; fruits and vegetables; spices and seasonings; enzyme preparations; eggs; and wheat. Irradiation of shellfish and processed meats is under review. Since the middle of the 1900s, the benefits and risks of irradiation have been discussed actively by regulatory, scientific, and consumer groups.

The primary potential benefit of food irradiation is to reduce food-borne illness through use of pasteurized products and to reduce cross-contamination of foods that might have been exposed to unpasteurized products. The estimated net benefit from irradiation pasteurization of 50% of poultry, ground beef, pork, and processed meats in the United States is prevention of "nearly 900,000 cases of infection, 8500 hospitalizations, over 6000 catastrophic illnesses, and 350 deaths each year."[20] Limitations of irradiation as opposed to heat treatment include potential recontamination of irradiated product after packaging is removed and relative resistance of bacterial spores and viruses to pasteurization by irradiation. At the doses used in foods, radiation does not destroy prions and toxic chemicals. Arguments against irradiation focus on potential chemical changes in irradiated foods. These changes include creating undesirable chemicals during processing, such as 2-alkylcyclobutanones, and destroying sensitive nutrients, such as thiamin. While considering these concerns, federal agencies, including the USDA, the FDA, and the CDC, as well as The American Dietetic Association among many other organizations, support use of irradiation to improve the safety of the US food supply.[20,21]

INTEGRATE FOOD SAFETY INTO NUTRITION GUIDANCE

Nutrition education guidelines classify foods into groups based on similar nutrient contributions to the diet. These groupings may also be useful for making food safety recommendations. Nutrient content is one of the factors governing bacterial growth in foods. Foods grouped together may share other characteristics, such as level of acidity and availability of water. Foods that are not potentially hazardous can be held safely at normal room temperatures without supporting the rapid growth of bacterial pathogens, although all foods may remain in good condition longer when refrigerated or frozen. Potentially hazardous foods should not be held in the danger zone, 40°F to 140°F or 4°C to 60°C, for longer than two hours. The USDA also recommends storage times and temperatures for foods.[22] Inappropriate handling can contaminate any food, whether it is potentially hazardous or not.

Breads, Cereals, Rice, and Pasta

This group includes both dry grains and grain products, such as ready-to-eat cereals, ready-to-cook cereals, rice, and dry pastas. These foods do not contain enough water to support bacterial growth and are not potentially hazardous foods. When cooked, these foods are potentially hazardous foods, because they contain enough water to support rapid bacterial growth. Unbaked batters, dough, and fresh pastas are potentially hazardous foods, because they are high in water content. After baking, batters and doughs are not potentially hazardous unless they contain potentially hazardous foods, such as custards or similar fillings.

Fruits and Vegetables

This category includes a variety of different plant parts. Three primary food safety considerations determining whether fruits and vegetables are potentially hazardous are whether the item is cut or whole, cooked, or acidic. Additionally, these items may be contaminated on their surfaces with pathogens or chemicals. Whole fruits and vegetables should always be washed thoroughly in cool, running water before peeling, cutting, or cooking. Most whole, uncooked produce items are not potentially hazardous foods as peels and skins protect their nutrients from bacteria. Fresh cut produce in a sealed bag labeled "ready-to-eat," "washed," or "triple washed" need not be rewashed. Cooking breaks cells and makes nutrients more available to bacteria, promoting rapid growth. This makes cooked fruits and vegetables (and opened cans of fruits and vegetables) potentially hazardous foods, unless they are high-acid foods (pH below 4.6) or have very little water available for bacterial growth. *Cl. botulinum* cannot grow and produce botulin toxin at pH levels below 4.6. Fruits are typically in this pH range, although a few, such as overripe fruits and figs, may not be. Although high-acid foods do not promote rapid bacterial growth, they can be contaminated at high enough levels to cause food-borne illness. For example, pathogens survive in fruit juices without reproducing rapidly. Because raw fruit juices are frequently contaminated with pathogens, commercial juices are usually pasteurized. Most cooked or processed vegetables contain enough water to support rapid bacterial growth, but dried vegetables and vegetable chips do not. Pathogens from unwashed melon surfaces have contaminated cut melons, which is why cut melons are specifically listed as potentially hazardous foods. Raw sprouts are listed as potentially hazardous foods in the Food Code, because they have frequently been found to be contaminated with high levels of pathogenic bacteria. If the seeds are contaminated before sprouting, the sprouting process in warm, moist conditions speeds bacterial growth. Pasteurizing the seeds would prevent sprouting.

Milk, Milk Products, Yogurt, and Cheese

These items are potentially hazardous foods, because they are high in both nutrients and water. However, some of these products have barriers to retard bacterial growth: cultured dairy products, such as yogurt and sour cream, have lower pH values than fresh fluid milk, and some hard cheeses and dried milk do not have enough water to support bacterial growth. Most milk in the United States, including the milk used to make cheese, ice cream, and other products, is pasteurized to destroy pathogens.

Meat, Poultry, Fish, Beans, Eggs, and Nuts

This category contains a variety of different foods, all high in protein and minerals. Raw and cooked meat, poultry, fish, and eggs are considered potentially hazardous foods, because all contain the nutrients and water required for rapid bacterial growth, with pH levels not low enough to retard bacterial growth. Canned meat and fish are potentially hazardous once cans are opened. Dried meats may not be potentially hazardous, depending upon the specific product. Processed meats, including most hams and cold cuts, are potentially hazardous foods. Irradiation can reduce or eliminate pathogens on raw meats and poultry, but these products can be recontaminated once their packaging is opened. Although not currently approved for this purpose, irradiation of cooked or processed meat products, such as hotdogs and deli meats, could destroy contaminating pathogens.

Dried beans are not potentially hazardous foods until cooked, because they do not have enough available water to support bacterial growth. Nuts are not potentially hazardous, because they do not have much available water. Tofu and other moist protein curds made from beans are potentially hazardous foods. Shelf-stable tofu products are potentially hazardous foods once the packages are opened.

Take-Home and Take-Out Foods

Prepared and/or cooked take-home and take-out foods should always be treated as leftovers. These foods should not be kept at room temperature for more than two hours, including time for preparation of mixed salads and other ready-to-eat foods and time after cooking hot foods. Cooked foods should be reheated to 165°F, even if the original recommended internal temperature for cooking is lower. Handling may add pathogens to the food, and bacteria grow rapidly in foods with broken cells that have released nutrients. Plated leftovers are likely contaminated, because eating utensils have cross-contaminated, foods and have contaminated foods with pathogens from the mouth. When a restaurant meal is too large to eat, it is safer to package the leftovers before beginning to eat or to separate the food into servings so that the leftovers are not contaminated.

SYSTEMS TO PROTECT THE FOOD SUPPLY

Federal, state, and local government agencies each have responsibilities for protecting the food supply. Additionally, the Joint Commission of Accreditation of Healthcare Organizations (JCAHO) works with its constituent organizations to improve food safety in health care institutions, and the United Nations' *Codex Alimentarius* establishes food safety regulations for international trade.

Food Safety Laws

There are many food safety laws in the United States.[23] The Constitution, through the commerce clause, empowers the federal government to regulate interstate commerce, including the production and marketing of foods. The USDA has authority for most animal products under a variety of laws governing meat, poultry, and their products. The FDA has authority for most other foods under the Federal Food, Drug, and Cosmetic Act of 1938, the Public Health Service Act of 1944, and their extensions and amendments. The EPA has responsibility for pesticides, cleaning agents, and other chemicals used in food production and preparation under the Federal Insecticide, Fungicide, and Rodenticide Act of 1947 and the Food Quality Protection Act of 1996. States have laws that govern foods produced and sold exclusively within their borders and food sales establishments within their borders. State and local laws govern food service establishments within their jurisdictions.

The FDA Food Code is a model for food safety regulations. However, it is not law unless it is adopted by the state or local jurisdiction. This code has been adopted, at least in part, by many state, local, and military jurisdictions. Food processors, food markets, and food service establishments are responsible for meeting their state and local laws. Laws are interpreted through regulations that are established after public hearings to discuss how laws are implemented. Regulations implement laws. Monitoring systems by local health agencies are a part of the implementation of food safety laws.

Surveillance Programs

Food safety surveillance systems are continuous monitoring systems. These systems provide baseline data that help public health professionals to determine problem areas and to track successes and breakdowns of food safety programs. Surveillance data include information on pathogens and chemicals in the food supply. Combined with data on food consumption patterns, industry practices, and consumer food handling, surveillance data are used to make public health decisions to improve food and water safety in the United States. Surveillance systems monitor both domestic and imported foods. Each surveillance system provides slightly different data, based on the collection protocol. Some of these surveillance systems, such as Surveillance for Food-borne-disease Outbreaks (CDC), the Total Diet Study (FDA), and several pesticide residue programs (EPA, FDA, and USDA) have been in place for decades, giving public health professionals longitudinal data on food safety problems. Others, such as FoodNet (Food-borne Diseases Active Surveillance Network) and PulseNet (National Molecular Subtyping Network for Food-borne-Disease Surveillance, CDC, USDA, FDA, states), are programs based on newer technologies that allow rapid responses to specific problems, as well as longitudinal data collection.

Pathogen Surveillance

Three primary surveillance systems are in place to monitor pathogen-caused food-borne illness. These include the CDC Surveillance for Food-borne-disease Outbreaks, FoodNet, and PulseNet. These surveillance programs can only count reported cases that are severe enough for an individual to seek medical treatment and for the physician to diagnose the condition using laboratory analysis. Outbreak and FoodNet data may include cases that are not food-borne, as many diseases that can be food-borne are also transmitted person-to-person or through environmental contaminants. Even with their limitations, these surveillance systems allow public health professionals to target important national food safety problems and to track improvements when controls are implemented. FoodNet and PulseNet programs have improved quality assurance and reduced response time for investigation of food-borne illness outbreaks and implementation of controls, such as food recalls. Rapid response usually leads to fewer cases of food-borne illness, demonstrated in the program results described below.

The CDC Surveillance for Food-Borne-Disease Outbreaks   This is a passive system that collects, compiles, and reports information from state and local health departments, federal agencies, and private physicians on occurrences and causes of food-borne-disease outbreaks.[10] Data include food vehicles, etiologic agents, morbidity/mortality cases, and practices that contributed to outbreaks. Although data reports are only issued every five years, intervening data are available, and data can be searched by etiology (bacterial, chemical, parasitic, viral, unknown), specific etiology, (year/month, region/state, and location, i.e. daycare, hospital, grocery store, private home, restaurant, etc.). Data from 1997 to 2001 show larger numbers of confirmed outbreaks from viruses, which may represent better confirmation methods for this etiological group. Based on current data, *Healthy People 2010* objectives to reduce outbreaks of food-borne infections caused by *E. coli* O157:H7 and *Salmonella* serotype Enteritidis may not be met.

FoodNet   A component of CDC's Emerging Infections Program (EIP), FoodNet provides a collaborative network for regional and national monitoring and quantification of nationally important food-borne diseases caused by enteric pathogens.[24] Data are actively sought for this program by calling diagnostic labs in the Catchment Information System to collect information on confirmed cases of infections caused by bacteria (*C. jejuni, E. coli* O157, *L. monocytogenes, Salmonella, Shigella, Vibrio, Yersinia enterocolitica*) and parasites (*Cyclospora cayetanensis* and *Cryptosporidium parvum*).

Collaborators for this program include the USDA, the FDA, and EIP sites in 10 states. The original catchment areas included parts of 5 states totaling a population of 13.2 million. The 2003 catchment area includes 41.5 million persons. Data collected in FoodNet consistently show *C. jejuni, Salmonella* and *Shigella* as the bacteria that cause the most food-borne bacterial infections in the United States. Current trends show declines over the past decade in incidence of infections caused by *C. jejuni, C. parvum, E. coli O157, Salmonella,* and *Y. enterocolitica.* These trends suggest that the *Healthy People 2010* targets for reduction in infections caused by *C. jejuni* and *E. coli O157:H7* will be met, and that the reduction targets for *L. monocytogenes* and *Salmonella* may not be met.

PulseNet   PulseNet is a network of public health laboratories (all 50 state and several local public health department laboratories, FDA laboratories, and the USDA FSIS laboratory).[25] These laboratories subtype or "fingerprint" organisms isolated from suspect foods and from human specimens to confirm food vehicles in cases or outbreaks of food-borne illness. The network permits rapid comparisons of these fingerprints through a CDC electronic database to allow for early recognition and detection of cases related to a common food vehicle. For example, in 2001, two simultaneous outbreaks of *E. coli* O157:H7 infections were reported in Michigan. Analysis revealed two distinct clusters of cases plus two cases that were unrelated to either cluster. The first cluster was linked to home-prepared ground beef purchased at different food markets. Traceback revealed a likely common meat-processing plant. The same fingerprint was identified in *E. coli O157:H7* samples from Wisconsin and Illinois. USDA tests of warehoused samples of the implicated ground beef confirmed contamination with *E. coli O157:H7* having the same fingerprint identified in the Michigan, Wisconsin, and Illinois laboratories, lead to a recall of ground beef products from the plant. While the other cluster also implicated home-prepared ground beef, the product was from a different plant. PulseNet was able to separate the two outbreaks and identify two cases that were unrelated to the outbreaks. This differentiation allowed faster action, possibly reducing the numbers of cases associated with the outbreaks. In other examples, PulseNet has helped in multistate tracebacks of *E. coli O157:H7* in lettuce and apple juice, *Salmonella* in ready-to-eat toasted oat cereal, and *L. monocytogenes* in contaminated hotdogs and deli meats.

Chemical Surveillance

Federal regulatory agencies monitor different types of chemicals in the food supply, including pesticide residues, industrial chemicals, radionucleotides, heavy metals (elements), and nutrients. Because chemicals may change during food production, marketing, and handling, these programs measure levels of residues, not simply levels of the original chemical. For registered (approved) chemicals that are added to food or that may become a part of food during its production, marketing, or handling, regulatory agencies set tolerances for the maximum amounts of residues permitted in or on a specified food. Tolerances are set for specific residues on specific foods. If a residue exceeds its tolerance on a specific food, or if there is a residue on a food for which there is no tolerance established, the residue is described as violative or contaminated. In some cases, commodities can be contaminated with residues for which they are not registered through spray drift, crop rotation, or production errors. In many cases, these are not of regulatory concern, because the levels are sporadic and not hazardous. If samples are violative and there are regulatory concerns, sanctions can be imposed. Sanctions may include seizure for domestic products. Imported food products can be refused entry without examination if previous examinations have detected a violative sample and there is reason to believe that other food lots during the same shipping season will be the same.

FDA's Total Diet Study (Market-Basket Study: TDS), the FDA Pesticide Program, and the USDA Pesticide Data Program monitor pesticide residues in the food supply. These programs measure pesticide residues in domestic raw commodities at locations close to the point of production or distribution. Pesticide residues in imported commodities are measured at port of entry. In contrast, the TDS determines residue levels in foods, as they would be prepared for consumption. The analytical methods used by TDS are usually more sensitive, because this analysis is used to determine incidence, not to check compliance with regulatory requirements. Residue levels are usually measured in parts per billion (ppb).

The Total Diet Study (TDS)[26]   TDS is a chemical analysis of foods collected from neighborhood food markets and prepared using household practices. Each quarterly market basket contains about 280 foods selected based on national food consumption data and represent major components of the US diet. Each region of the country (West, North Central, South, and Northeast) is sampled once a year. The foods are examined for pesticide residues, industrial chemicals, elements, radionucleotides, and folate.

Over 300 different chemicals can be determined by the analytical methods used. The five most frequently observed chemicals for the past several years are the pesticides DDT, chlorpyrifos-methyl, malathion, endosulfan, and dieldrin. These and other pesticides were found to be well below regulatory limits. DDT and dieldrin (residue of aldrin) are no longer registered, but they persist in the environment. Chlorpyrifos-methyl is being phased out of use through voluntary cancellation. Since chlorpyrifos-methyl is an organophosphate pesticide, this cancellation may contribute to the *Healthy People 2010* Objective 10.7: Reduce human exposure to organophosphate pesticides from food (developmental).

FDA Pesticide Program (Regulatory Component)[27]   This program measures pesticide residues in both domestic and imported commodities and processed products near the point of production or entry into the United States. In the three most recent reporting years, approximately 1% of domestic samples and 4% of imported samples contained violative residues, and most of these violative samples were for fruits and vegetables. The values do not directly reflect consumer exposures, because the products are not sent through the marketing system to allow for degradation during transit and storage or preparation (washed, peeled, or cooked). However, these data are useful for EPA estimates of dietary exposures for reregistration of agricultural chemicals and for assessing potential cumulative exposures.

Pesticide Data Program (PDP)[28] The PDP is a national pesticide program that focuses on foods most commonly consumed by infants and children, including fresh and processed fruits and vegetables, fruit juices, whole milk, grains, corn syrup, poultry, beef, and drinking water. Samples are collected in consumer food markets at the point of purchase to take into account pesticide degradation during transit and storage. The values do not directly reflect consumer exposures, because they are not prepared (washed, peeled, or cooked). These data, like the FDA surveillance data, are useful for EPA estimates of dietary exposures for reregistration of agricultural chemicals and for assessing potential cumulative exposures. Similar to the FDA Pesticide Program data, few residues exceed tolerances (much less than 1%), and less than 3% of the commodities are contaminated with residues with no established tolerances. These data also show that fruits and vegetables are much more likely to be contaminated with pesticide residues than are other agricultural commodities, such as grains and meats.

EDUCATE CONSUMERS AND FOOD HANDLERS TO ASSURE SAFE FOOD

Food safety education for the public and food service workers includes media messages on selecting, preparing, and serving food; specific messages on food labels directed to people; and food-safety certification programs. Currently food safety messages emphasize four common food-handling practices: clean, chill, separate, and cook. Specific messages directed to high-risk people include warnings for those with phenylketonuria when products contain the artificial sweetener aspartame and food labels on processed foods that may contain common allergens such as milk, eggs, peanuts, and their products. Food safety certification programs include local food handler training and national training programs, such as ServSafe from the National Restaurant Association Education Foundation. Food safety education helps consumers and food service personnel meet their responsibilities to keep safe the foods they prepare, serve to others, and eat themselves.

The general food safety messages—clean, chill, separate, and cook—originated from the Partnership for Food Safety Education (FightBAC!), a nonprofit organization that includes governmental agencies (CDC, FDA, USDA), trade associations and commodity groups, and consumer and professional associations.[29] These messages form the basis of *Healthy People 2010* Objectives 10-5 and 10-6 on improving key food preparation practices for food service personnel and consumers. The messages are based on data from food safety surveillance programs, which track practices that contribute to food-borne illness. The messages describe the practices needed to reduce contamination of foods purchased in food markets, restaurants, and fast-food outlets, as well as those prepared and served at homes. The general messages are to reduce contamination of ready-to-eat foods in retail establishments and homes (separate), reduce growth of bacteria on potentially hazardous foods (chill), remove surface pathogens from food contact surfaces, hands, and raw fruit and vegetable surfaces (clean), and inactivate pathogens in foods (cook). The messages are general, but can be made more specific to give advice to specific audiences in specific settings. For example, the *Home Food Safety—It's in Your Hands* food safety campaign targets food preparers with these messages:

- Wash hands often—clean
- Refrigerate promptly below 40°F—chill
- Keep raw meats and ready-to-eat foods separate—separate
- Cook to proper temperatures—cook[30]

These general messages are also being publicized through coalitions of stakeholders, such as the National Coalition for Food Safe Schools and the Clean Hands Campaign. Public health nutritionists should collaborate with environmental health specialists in their communities to educate both consumers and commercial food handlers using the "clean-chill-separate-cook" messages.

With the public eating more commercially prepared meals and snacks, public health nutritionists in partnership with environmental health specialists should offer periodic food safety training for food handlers as part of their agency's health improvement plan. These collaborative, unified, local efforts can improve the safety of foods from food sales establishments, food service establishments, and consumer kitchens. Coalitions and collaborations work to integrate and publicize best practices into their communities. Food safety messages—specific and general—must reach consumers and food service workers in every community in the United States every day.

Recent surveys of food safety knowledge, attitudes, and practices show that consumers recognize many food safety problems and their own responsibilities. For example, in free response to the question, "When food is prepared at home, what do you think are the most common things people do that might cause food poisoning?" respondents named behaviors that are considered in the FightBAC program, such as inadequate cleaning and sanitation (61%), improper refrigeration (49%), undercooking (26%), and cross-contamination (18%).[31]

Most people know many of the factors that contribute to food-borne illness, such as improper refrigeration, but there are large gaps in their knowledge of specific recommendations, such as the temperature recommended for refrigeration of food and the need for a thermometer to monitor home refrigerator temperatures.[31] People do not always follow recommended practices as demonstrated by both observation and self-reports.[31,32] Based on self-reported behaviors, the public has exceeded *Healthy People 2010* expectations for chill (86%), clean (90%), and separate (82%).[31] Most consumers do not report meeting the recommendations for cook (25%). Additionally, few people report that they follow all of the recommended behaviors almost all of the time, and the actual practices are not always met, even when people report knowing appropriate practices.[31,32] Two specific practices that require improvement are hand washing and cooking foods to recommended internal temperatures. For hand washing, although people report the appropriate practice, they frequently do not complete the process properly (scrubbing with soap and water for 20 seconds, followed by thorough rinsing and drying on a clean surface) or they do not wash their hands at all of the recommended times, such as between preparations of different foods. In a recent national survey, less than one third of respondents thought it common for people to become sick as a result of home food-handling practices, and most gave themselves high marks for their own food safety behaviors.[31] These attitudes of low risk and high control may make it difficult for food safety messages to reach consumers effectively to improve practices to meet recommendations. Although continued improvement in food safety practices is important for everyone, it is especially important to the growing number of people in the at-risk groups. Using the same messages in various formats to reach a wide variety of audiences must continue to penetrate both at-risk and general populations, particularly those whose job responsibilities are to prepare and serve food to the public.

FUTURE FOOD SAFETY ISSUES

Continuous improvement of the food supply to make it safer, more nutritious, and more accessible shows a history of continuing success, with challenges continuing to confront public health systems. Will newer technologies, such as irradiation and genetic engineering, be used to improve the safety and accessibility of our food supply? Will current food safety messages expand to include a specific focus on checking foods for expiration dates, package integrity, and visible signs of tampering? Will labeling messages expand to include "soft" messages to inform consumers of the presence of organic or genetically modified ingredients? The challenge is to use cutting-edge scientific evidence, information dissemination through the media and Internet, and evaluation to continue to improve the safety of the food supply for all people throughout the United States.

POINTS TO PONDER

- What is the role of labeling in alerting consumers to potential risks and concerns?

- How are scientific measures of risk different from consumer risk perceptions?
- How can consumers balance food safety risk issues with nutrient and cost issues?
- What are the most authoritative sources for consumer food safety information?
- How can public health professionals use authoritative sources of food safety information when consumers cite misinformation?
- What is the role of the nutrition professional in including food safety information as a part of food guidance?
- What are the best ways to target vulnerable populations with the food safety information they need?

HELPFUL WEB SITES

General Information

General food safety information is available through government and university gateway sites. Most of these sites are searchable and contain training aids and consumer education materials.

CDC Food Safety Office: www.cdc.gov/foodsafety
Database: www.nal.usda.gov/fnic/food-borne/wais.shtml
FDA Recalls and Safety Alerts: www.fda.gov/opacom/7alerts.html
Food Safety Modules (Online) Project: www.gsu.edu/~wwwfsm
Government gateway to food safety information: www.foodsafety.gov
Meat and Poultry Hotline (1-800-535-4555:
    www.fsis.usda.gov/mph/index.htm
University and Cooperative Extension food safety sites listing:
    www.foodsafety.iastate.edu/links/index.cfm?categoryid=42
USDA/FDA Food-Borne Illness Information Center Training Material
    USDA Food Safety Education and Consumer Information:
    www.fsis.usda.gov/OA/consedu.htm
USDA Recall Information Center: www.fsis.usda.gov/Fsis_Recalls/

Information on Food Safety Goals and Supporting Data

Healthy People 2010 (HP2010) outlines the national food safety goals. Data from surveillance programs are also available online.

CDC Food-Borne Outbreak Response and Surveillance Unit:
    www.cdc.gov/food-borneoutbreaks
FDA Pesticide Program: www.cfsan.fda.gov/~dms/pesrpts.html
FDA Total Diet Study: www.cfsan.fda.gov/~comm/tds-toc.html

FoodNet: www.cdc.gov/foodnet
Healthy People 2010:
    www.health.gov/healthypeople/Document/pdf/Volume1/10Food.pdf
PulseNet: www.cdc.gov/pulsenet
USDA Pesticide Data Program: www.ams.usda.gov/science/pdp

Online Books and Journals That Focus on Food Safety:

Bad Bug Book: www.cfsan.fda.gov/~mow/intro.html
Emerging Infectious Diseases (journal):
    www.cdc.gov/ncidod/EID/index.htm
FDA Food Code: www.cfsan.fda.gov/~dms/foodcode.html
FDA Consumer Magazine: www.fda.gov/fdac
Morbidity and Mortality Weekly Reports (journal): www.cdc.gov/mmwr

Programs and Organizations:

Clean Hands Campaign: www.washup.org
Home Food Safety—It's in Your Hands: www.homefoodsafety.org
National Coalition for Food Safe Schools: www.foodsafeschools.org
National Food Safety Education Month: www.nraef.org/nfsem
Partnership for Food Safety Education (PFSE): www.fightbac.org

---

NOTES

1. Achievements in public health, 1900–1999: safer and healthier foods. *MMWR.* 1999;48:905–913. Available at: http://www.cdc.gov/mmwr/PDF/wk/mm4840.pdf. Accessed June 12, 2004.

2. US Department of Health and Human Services. Food safety. In: *Healthy People 2010.* 2nd ed. With Understanding and Improving Health and Objectives for Improving Health. 2 vols. Washington, DC: US Government Printing Office, November 2000:10.3–10.9. Available at: http://www.health.ogv/healthypeople/Document/pdf/Volume1/10Food.pdf. Accessed June 30, 2004.

3. US Food and Drug Administration Center for Food Safety & Applied Nutrition. Bad Food Book Food-borne pathogenic microorganisms and natural toxins handbook. Available at: http://www.cfsan.fda.gov/~mow/intro.html. Accessed June 30, 2004.

4. Helms M, Vastrup P, Gerner-Schmidt P, Molbak K. Short- and long-term mortality associated with food-borne gastrointestinal infections: registry-based study. *Brit Med J.* 2003;326:357–361.

5. Kaplan JE, Masur H, Holmes KK. Guidelines for preventing opportunistic infections among HIV-infected persons—2002: recommendations of the US Public Health

Service and the Infectious Diseases Society of America. *MMWR*. 2002;51 (RR-08):1–82. Available at: http://www.cdc.gov/mmwr/PDF/RR/RR4910.pdf. Accessed June 30, 2004.

6. Mead PS, Slutsker L, Dietz V, et al. Food-related illness and death in the United States. *Emerging Infectious Diseases*. 1999;5:607–625.

7. US Department of Agriculture. BSE information and resources [USDA Web site]. Available at: http://www.usda.gov/BSE/. Accessed June 30, 2004.

8. US Food and Drug Administration. 2001 Food Code with errata sheet and supplements. [FDA Web site]. Available at: http://vm.cfsan.fda.gov/~dms/foodcode.htm. Accessed June 30, 2004.

9. Beier RC, Nigg HN. Toxicology of naturally occurring chemicals in food. In: Hui YH, Gorham JR, Murrell KD, Cliver DO, eds. *Food-borne Disease Handbook*, vol. 3. New York, NY: Marcel Dekker, Inc; 1994:1–186.

10. US Centers for Disease Control and Prevention. US food-borne disease outbreaks [CDC Web site]. Available at: http://www2.cdc.gov/ncidod/food-borne/fbsearch.asp. Accessed June 30, 2004.

11. US Food and Drug Administration. Backgrounder for the 2004 FDA/EPA consumer advisory: what you need to know about mercury in fish and shellfish [FDA Web site]. Available at: http://www.fda.gov/oc/opacom/hottopics/mercury/backgrounder.html. Accessed June 30, 2004.

12. US Centers for Disease Control and Prevention, Agency for Toxic Substances and Disease Registry. ToxFAQs for mercury [CDC Web site]. 1999. Available at: http://www.atsdr.cdc.gov/tfacts46.html. Accessed June 30, 2004.

13. US Centers for Disease Control and Prevention. CDC Health Topic: lead [CDC Web site]. Available at: http://www.cdc.gov/health/lead.htm. Accessed June 30, 2004.

14. US Environmental Protection Agency. Lead in paint, dust, and soil [EPA Web site]. Available at: http://www.epa.gov/lead/. Accessed June 30, 2004.

15. US Food and Drug Administration. EAFUS: a food additive database [FDA Web site]. Available at: http://www.cfsan.fda.gov/~dms/eafus.html. Accessed June 30, 2004.

16. US Environmental Protection Agency. Pesticide fact sheets [EPA Web site]. Available at: http://www.epa.gov/pesticides/factsheets/index.htm. Accessed June 30, 2004.

17. US Department of Health and Human Services, National Institute of Allergy and Infectious Diseases. Food allergy and intolerances [NIH Web site]. 1999. Available at: http://www.niaid.nih.gov/factsheets/food.htm. Accessed June 30, 2004.

18. US Department of Agriculture. National organic program [USDA Web site]. Available at: http://www.ams.usda.gov/nop/indexIE.htm. Accessed June 30, 2004.

19. Cornell University, College of Agricultural and Life Sciences. Agricultural biotechnology: informing the dialogue. Available at: http://www.nysaes.cornell.edu/comm/gmo/PDF/GMO2002.pdf. Accessed June 30, 2004.

20. Tauxe RV. Food safety and irradiation: protecting the public from food-borne infections. *Emerg Infect Dis*. 2001;7(Suppl):516–521. Available at: http://www.cdc.gov/ncidod/eid/vol7no3_supp/tauxe.htm#Figure. Accessed June 30, 2004.

21. Osterholm MT, Norgan AP. The role of irradiation in food safety. N *Engl J Med*. 2004;350:1898–1901.

22. US Department of Agriculture. Basics for handling food safely [USDA Web site]. 2003. Available at: http://www.fsis.usda.gov/oa/pubs/facts_basics.pdf. Accessed June 30, 2004.

23. Pina KR, Pines WL. *A Practical Guide to Food and Drug Law and Regulation*. Washington, DC: FDLI; 1998:1–351.

24. US Centers for Disease Control and Prevention. FoodNet [CDC Web site]. Available at: http://www.cdc.gov/foodnet/default.htm. Accessed June 30, 2004.

25. US Centers for Disease Control and Prevention. The national molecular subtyping network for food-borne disease surveillance [CDC Web site]. Available at: http://www.cdc.gov/pulsenet/. Accessed June 30, 2004.

26. Food and Drug Administration. Total diet study [FDA Web site]. Available at: http://vm.cfsan.fda.gov/~comm/tds-toc.html. Accessed June 30, 2004.

27. Food and Drug Administration. FDA pesticide program residue monitoring 1993–2002 [FDA Web site]. Available at: http://vm.cfsan.fda.gov/~dms/pesrpts.html. Accessed June 30, 2004.

28. US Department of Agriculture. Pesticide Data Program (PDP) [USDA Web site]. Available at: http://www.ams.usda.gov/science/pdp/. Accessed June 30, 2004.

29. The Partnership for Food Safety Education Web site. Available at: http://www.fightbac.org/main.cfm. Accessed June 30, 2004.

30. Home Food Safety—It's in Your Hands Web site. Available at: http://www.homefoodsafety.org/index.jsp. Accessed June 30, 2004.

31. Cody MM, Hogue MA. Results of the Home Food Safety—It's in Your Hands 2002 Survey: comparisons to the 1999 benchmark survey and *Healthy People 2010* food safety behaviors objective. *J Am Diet Assoc*. 2003;103:1115–1125.

32. Anderson JB, Shuster TA, Hansen KE, Levy AS, Volk A. A camera's view of consumer food-handling behaviors. *J Am Diet Assoc*. 2004;104:186–191.\

Plan, Implement, and Evaluate Public Health Nutrition Services

Mildred Kaufman

Reader Objectives

- List the values of writing a plan for nutrition services.
- Compare and contrast structure, process, and outcome objectives.
- Write nutrition outcome objectives for the agency's health improvement plan.
- Compare and contrast measures used in nutrition and health program evaluation.

UNDERSTAND PLANNING

Healthy People 2010 states:

Planning is central to improving public health in any state or community. A health improvement plan (HIP) is a long-term systematic effort to address health problems identified in the community needs assessment. This plan is used by health agencies with other education and human service agencies to collaborate as community partners. It sets priorities and coordinates and targets resources. Available baseline data showed that in 1997, 78% of state health agencies and in 1992–1993 only 32% of local jurisdictions had a health improvement plan linked to their state plan. Objective 23-12 in *Healthy People 2010* is to increase the proportion of tribes, states, and the District of Columbia that have a health improvement plan to 100% and the proportion of local jurisdictions that have a health improvement plan linked to their state plan to 80% by 2010.[1]

To learn more see www.health.gov/healthypeople.

MAP-IT (Mobilizing for Action through Planning and Partnerships)

MAP-IT maps out a path toward creating a healthy community:

- *Mobilize* individuals and organizations that care about the health of your community into a coalition.
- *Assess* the areas of greatest need in the community, as well as the resources and other strengths you can tap into, to address those areas.
- *Plan your approach.* Start with a vision of where you want to be as a community, then add strategies and action steps to help achieve that vision.
- *Implement your plan* using concrete action steps that can be monitored and that will make a difference.
- *Track your progress* over time.[2]

A Strategic Approach to Community Health Improvement: The MAPP Field Guide

The MAPP field guide summarizes the action cycle as:

- *Planning*—Determining what will be done, who will do it, and how it will be done
- *Implementation*—Carrying out the activities identified in the planning stage
- *Evaluation*—Determining what has been accomplished[3]

To learn more see: www.naccho.org

Nutritionists must sit at the table with the agency planners who write and periodically update the agency's health improvement plan. In Chapter 19 of *Healthy People 2010,* "Nutrition and Overweight," nutrition-related objectives are listed in 13 of the 27 focus areas.[4] Adapting these objectives to local community needs should be integrated and be clearly visible in both the state and local health improvement plans.

Whether or not the health agency uses a formal process for planning its public health program, some tips are suggested here to establish the health priorities upon which to build nutrition interventions:

- Where a health improvement plan exists, select the nutrition-related health priorities as identified in the community assessment (see Chapter 3).
- Work with the health planning team and advocate nutrition priorities in the context of community health problems.

- Address the health problems that are articulated by community members and leaders to ensure the success of current and future interventions.
- Determine how large the problem is in numbers of people affected or numbers of deaths attributed to the health problem and consider how the problem will grow without intervention.
- Assess the seriousness of the nutrition-related health problem to individuals and society, considering the extent of social disruption and economic loss.
- Recommend interventions that are cost-effective.
- Consider the political support available to address the priority.
- Compare the magnitude of the health problem with available resources.[5]

As a midlevel manager, the public health nutritionist contributes to the agency's health improvement plan by taking responsibility to develop and implement the plan for nutrition services. An effective nutrition program planner speaks the language and uses recognized methods of program planning and evaluation. Planners know that while the plan is the blueprint for action, it must be continuously critiqued and the services evaluated as the plan is put into action. Monitoring and evaluating are integral to planning: observing needs for new directions, reviewing the literature for cutting-edge research evidence that may alter practices; testing innovative interventions including state-of-the-art technologies; reaching out to more diverse populations; focusing on emerging problems; reallocating resources; and activating alternative networks are all parts of the planning process. Continuous monitoring and feedback makes it possible to fine-tune, or even overhaul the plan as new problems are observed in the community, or as conditions in the agency or available resources change. In the current economy, successful planners understand that resources are finite and that program survival requires active competition with colleagues who may offer equally important and appealing plans. Funds must be used wisely to demonstrate measurable results. Effective marketing maintains popular support (see Chapter 15).

The health improvement plan and its nutrition component have several distinct, but interrelated, parts. The nature and scope of community health and nutrition-related problems are presented in a summary introduction from the community assessment (see Chapter 3). The plan includes a mission statement and goals; measurable structure, process, and outcome objectives to address the problems; an action plan of services to be delivered to reach the objectives; and an evaluation strategy to assess achievement of each objective. The plan includes a line item budget with a written justification for the personnel, facilities, equipment, supplies, and travel required to carry out the action plan. It is necessary to comply with any federal or state legislation or local statutes that require or permit nutrition services in the community's health, human service, or education systems. The budget should identify and utilize available federal, national, state, local, and public foundation or private-sector funds that can be obtained to finance or reimburse for nutrition services. Developing partnerships is cost-effective. Opportunities should be sought to contract with other community agencies to provide them with nutrition services on one hand or purchase nutrition services from private practitioners on the other. In-kind services provided by volunteers, other community agencies, or donated by local businesses (such as clinic or office space, food, or incentives) should be included and assigned a realistic dollar value. The plan should improve, strengthen, and expand successful existing services and initiate new services that are justified, make the most of all available resources, and drive the program to higher levels of community service and services. Since the plan is a political as well as a professional document, it will be read with more enthusiasm and enlist more support if it is written in clear, simple language.

Planners use today's best knowledge and vision to set the direction toward an unpredictable future. Because the future is unknown the plan and its planners must be flexible. As they move from step to step in the planning process, planners weigh and balance many what-ifs and deliberate on alternative scenarios. At each step in planning, priorities must be selected from among many equally appealing alternatives.

Seek Input from Stakeholders

The public health nutrition planner can engage community insights and involvement by requesting the agency administrator appoint an advisory committee to participate in developing the nutrition services plan. This may be a subcommittee of the agency's advisory committee or a small group specifically concerned with the nutrition services.

The advisory committee contributes the diverse viewpoints of no more than 8 to 10 stakeholders. Although members of the committee should be interested and concerned about the contributions of nutrition to the public's health, they need not have a degree in nutrition. Involving a thoughtful, articulate client or consumer, an educator, an elected official, a business leader, as well as health and human service professionals, builds support and a sense of ownership for the nutrition part of the health improvement plan. A nutritionist who will participate in implementing the nutrition services should be a member of this committee.

The chairperson should be enthusiastic, articulate, objective, and organized, but not necessarily a member of the agency's public health nutrition staff. New committee members should be oriented to the planning process of the agency and its current nutrition services. Orientation includes a review of previous plans, policy and procedure manuals, budgets, annual reports, and nutrition education materials. Committee members might observe staff nutritionists at work in clinics, the agency offices, and the community.

The major role of this committee is to review and discuss the community assessment and nutrition problem list, to recommend priorities for programs and later to help "sell" the annual plan to administrators, policy makers, and community leaders. The committee members should be encouraged to seek suggestions and ideas from a wide variety of other concerned citizens and agency staff. Brainstorming and nominal group process are useful techniques for facilitating committee discussion. The committee might conduct some focus groups (see Chapter 15) among the target populations to elicit their suggestions for programs that would best meet client, consumer, and community health needs.

The Planning Process

The program development cycle in Figure 14–1 shows the interfaces in planning that involves agency administration responsible for overall policy formulation and strategy, the midlevel managers who participate in planning and who are responsible for supervising services, and the staff who deliver the services.

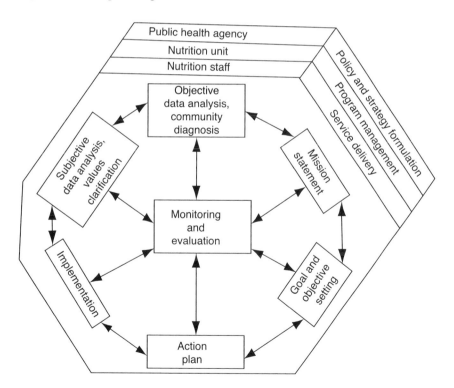

Figure 14–1 Program Development Cycle. *Source:* Prepared by Chapter Author and Editor, Mildred Kaufman.

This model visualizes the concept of management by objective in which each level in the agency has interrelated planning and service delivery functions. It sequences the series of steps that progress as the plan is developed, implemented, and evaluated and how it evolves over succeeding years.

STUDY THE COMMUNITY ASSESSMENT

The community assessment (see Chapter 3) is used to select priorities for the agency's health improvement plan and its nutrition component. This assessment includes an analysis of equally important subjective and objective data.

Subjective data provides insight into the perceived needs of the various stakeholders. It reflects community values, health and nutrition needs, and priorities as viewed by consumers, community leaders, and service providers. It compares and contrasts the views and values of people in the larger external community with those within the agency. Collection and analysis of objective data compiles published demographic (population-based) statistics, such as census data, vital statistics, and other available health statistics. Local health and clinical data can be summarized from client records in public health clinics, community hospitals, and other sources, or from results of special studies or surveys (see Chapters 3 and 16).

The advisory committee works with the health and nutrition planners to study both subjective and objective data and helps prepare the prioritized problem list. Together, they discuss the perceived needs, which may not be consistent with those suggested by the statistics. In selecting and ranking the priorities for nutrition services it is also important to look at priorities of other agency programs, other community health agencies, and health care providers, especially those who request or require nutritionists to work with them in their programs or projects. Selecting priorities must consider the competencies of the workforce (see Chapter 19) and other available resources. Trying to spread time and energy too thinly on too many health and nutrition problems will make it less possible to demonstrate quantifiable results. A few carefully selected, well-supported, well-targeted, population-based, intensive interventions will benefit the high-risk members of the community far more than scattered, fragmented, one-shot services. This means that some of the identified needs may remain unmet and some high-risk populations may not be served at this time.

WRITE THE PROGRAM PLAN

Write a Mission Statement

A mission statement concisely describes the general program thrust. The mission statement for nutrition services ties into the agency's mission statement. It describes how nutrition promotes the public's health and lists priorities for nutrition interventions. It tells who will be served and how these selected populations will benefit. A mission statement is clear, realistic, and inspiring. For example, working from a statement in *Healthy People 2010,*[6] "Increase the proportion of adults who are at a healthy weight," a mission statement adapted for the county health department might be to reduce obesity and overweight among the children and adults who live in the county. Consistent with that agency statement, the nutrition program's mission statement might read: To educate and motivate more people in the county to reduce their health risks and manage their weight by improving their food choices and increasing their physical activity.

Write Goals and Objectives

Most public health workers define goals as the guiding aspirations, ideals, or visions, which the program strives to achieve. Goals set a direction for the future. Goals are easy to write as these general statements are not required to be measurable. Goals state who will be affected and what is expected to change as a result of the program.[7] A nutrition program goal consistent with the above mission statements might read: To encourage adults and children to consume more fruits, vegetables, low-fat dairy products, whole grain cereals, and eat fewer high-fat, high-sugar, and high-calorie foods.

Objectives are measurable steps that drive the action required to reach the goal by a specified date. A well-written objective is realistic, understandable, measurable, behavioral, and achievable. Objectives target the most important population problems on which the health agency will invest staff time and resources. To prepare state or local objectives, planners should study the published *Healthy People 2010*[8] national objectives and standards for community preventive health services and determine which of these national objectives they might adapt. Also, the planners should determine any unique local health and nutrition problems that demand attention.

Cost-benefit analysis (CBA) is used to select objectives by weighing the economic worth when choosing from alternative strategies. CBA compares objectives that may target different audiences. What is the cost as opposed to the benefit of targeting interventions to schoolchildren, as opposed to women of childbearing age as opposed to older adults since the costs and benefits are defined in dollars? A program is cost-beneficial when the net dollars spent in providing the services are less than the costs to the taxpayers if the primary preventive services were not provided. Will the dollars anticipated to be saved by implementing the proposed objective prevent or reduce later client use of costly physician, hospital, or nursing home care? Estimating costs for nutrition services is discussed in Chapter 17. The challenge of CBA is estimating the economic benefits. Linkages in weight management might reflect intermediate changes that could result in health care savings by preventing such killing and crippling diseases as heart disease, hypertension, type 2 diabetes, and some types of cancer as shown in Figure 14–2.

If benefits will be achieved a time long after the program dollars have been spent, the benefits must be discounted to the present dollar value. The number of objectives selected must be manageable within the available or requested budget and staff.

Each objective must be written to specify the following:

- *What will be done?*—Action or intervention
- *Who will it benefit?*—Target population
- *How much will be achieved?*—Measure
- *When will it be done?*—Deadline date
- *What will be required?*—Resources

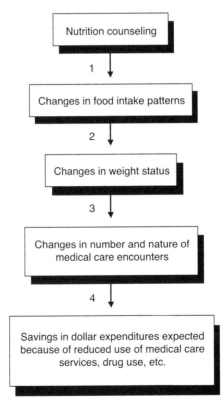

Figure 14–2   Potential Economic Benefits Associated with Nutrition Counseling in Weight Loss. *Source:* Prepared by Chapter Author and Editor, Mildred Kaufman.

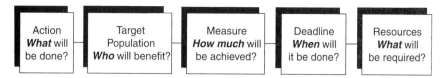

Figure 14–3 Structure of an Objective. *Source:* Kaufman MK. Plan, implement, and evaluate public health nutrition services. In: Kaufman MK, ed. *Nutrition in Public Health—A Handbook for Developing Programs and Services.* Rockville, Md: Aspen; 1990:286.

Figure 14–3 offers a framework to use to write each objective.

Inserting the appropriate words into this framework makes it easier to write objectives. Objectives should relate to the agency and the nutrition program mission and goals. They should use words easily understood by both lay and professional readers. Objectives are stated at three levels that are hierarchical. Structure objectives facilitate process objectives, which set the stage for outcome objectives that, when achieved, reach the program goals.[9]

Structure objectives set targets for budget; number, qualifications and scheduling of staff; facilities, equipment, travel, space, and so on. An example would be: By 8/1/05, the county health department in partnership with the county school district will employ one full-time equivalent (FTE) public health nutritionist to write and implement a weight management, nutrition education, and physical fitness curriculum for the county schools (Grades K through 12).

Process objectives stipulate the work to be carried out by public health and nutrition staff. These objectives are derived from research evidence and state-of-the-art practices considered essential to achieve anticipated outcomes under most conditions. An example would be: By 1/01/06 the county health department with the school board will implement a policy to replace sweetened soft drinks, candy, and chips in 100% of county high school and middle school vending machines with bottled water, full-strength fruit juice, fresh fruit, and low-fat milk or yogurt.

Examples of some action verbs to use in writing process objectives are:

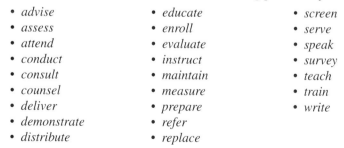

- *advise*
- *assess*
- *attend*
- *conduct*
- *consult*
- *counsel*
- *deliver*
- *demonstrate*
- *distribute*
- *educate*
- *enroll*
- *evaluate*
- *instruct*
- *maintain*
- *measure*
- *prepare*
- *refer*
- *replace*
- *screen*
- *serve*
- *speak*
- *survey*
- *teach*
- *train*
- *write*

Outcome objectives are measurable changes in attitudes, knowledge, skills, or nutritional or health status of the selected population of clients, consumers, or the public. An example would be: By 6/15/06, 3-day food intake records of 25% of the students in the three county high schools will list five or more servings of fruits and vegetables consumed on each of the preselected school days.

Examples of some action verbs to use in writing outcome objectives are

- *achieve*
- *attain*
- *choose*
- *complete*
- *consume*
- *decrease*

- *eliminate*
- *identify*
- *improve*
- *increase*
- *know*
- *list*

- *maintain*
- *participate*
- *reach*
- *reduce*
- *select*

Clear, explicit objectives organize and communicate a complex plan into a few descriptive statements. The more precise the statement of each objective, the clearer the direction of the action plan and the more easily a data system can be developed to monitor and evaluate progress.

Activate Objectives

The next step is to prepare an action plan or list of activities to implement each objective, indicating the resources required and data to be collected to monitor achievement. Interventions must be intensive enough to achieve the measurable objective by the deadline date. Intervention activities relate to the type of objective.

For structure objectives, examples of activities include the following:

- Funding requested to expand existing or develop new interventions
- Number of full-time equivalent positions (FTE) type and qualification of staff required and requested
- Facilities, equipment, and supplies requested to support new or expanded initiatives
- Advocacy activities to achieve passage of policies or legislation to support nutrition interventions

For process objectives, examples of some types of activities include the following:

- One-on-one counseling to be provided for various types of medical nutrition therapy
- Group classes on nutrition and weight management to be conducted, describing the settings and expected audiences
- Media programs directed to the public on current nutrition topics on radio, television, and the Internet
- Print media articles on nutrition and weight management or other "popular" topics in food, nutrition, and fitness to be written for newspapers, newsletters, and handouts

- Environmental changes—Consultation and technical assistance to recommend nutrient labeling, school meals, restaurant menus, changes in processed food formulation to reduce total calories, saturated fats, and refined sugar and to increase use of whole grains, fruits, vegetables, reduced-fat milk or cheese, and food fortification or enrichment.

For outcome objectives, examples of activities include measurable changes in the following:

- Client, consumer, and public awareness, attitudes, knowledge, and skills
- Client, consumer or public changes in behavior—Food choices, food preparation methods, and physical activity
- Client or population changes in health and nutritional status—Body weight, body mass index (BMI), blood pressure, biochemical tests, morbidity or mortality rates for nutrition-related health conditions for the community
- Food environment—Food safety regulations or legislation passed; food security or food access increased; use of WIC, food stamps, food pantries, congregate meals; changes in nutritional quality of meals in group care facilities; nutrient quality of processed or out-of-home prepared foods

Cost-effectiveness analysis (CEA) can be used to select from several alternative interventions. CEA is used to compare alternative interventions, assuming that the basic objective is economically worthwhile. Approaches to be compared by CEA must be measured by the same outcome. For example, the relative cost-effectiveness of a weight-loss program might compare the cost of eight weeks of intensive, one-on-one, nutritionist-to-client counseling at a health agency clinic against the cost for the same number of clients to participate in an 8-week series of group sessions in the community facilitated by a nutritionist and fitness instructor. The outcome measure of effectiveness could be measured in pounds lost or changes in body mass index (BMI) recorded for participants in both programs. The approach that achieved the greater number of pounds lost per dollar spent would be considered the most cost-effective. See Figure 14–4.

In selecting interventions, it is important to consider the number and competencies of the available or anticipated staff (see Chapter 19) and the "fit" of the proposed interventions to the needs and desires expressed by members of the target population. Most nutrition interventions strive to educate and motivate people to choose, prepare, and eat foods recommended in the current *US Dietary Guidelines* or to adhere to medical nutrition therapy prescribed by a health care professional.

When the objectives are to change food choices in a culturally diverse population, the messages must be tailored to local food preferences and be affordable to clients and families as they purchase foods available in their neighborhood food markets and family restaurants. Public health nutritionists or their trained nutrition program assistants should speak and write in the languages of the local

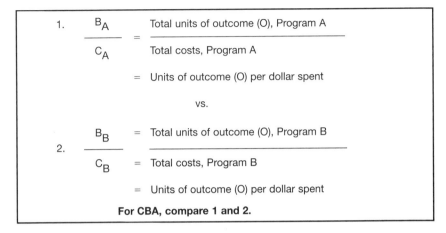

Figure 14–4   Which Alternative Provides the Greater Level of Benefits per Dollar Spent? *Source:* Prepared by Chapter Author and Editor, Mildred Kaufman.

people. To promote health literacy, printed materials must be at the reading level and in the language of most of the residents in the community. Advice that respects the cultural food habits modifies or uses the popular methods of food preparation. Effective interventions are consumer friendly.

Based on tried and tested past experiences, the choice of some interventions may be clear. For innovative interventions, a demonstration or pilot test might be designed into the plan. Before committing much money or staff time to an untested new idea, it is wise to test several different intervention approaches with different groups of people in different settings or at different times in the same setting. The test can determine the most acceptable to the audience, the most cost-effective, and the most achievable.

The interventions selected must also be realistic considering the size and competencies of the agency's workforce, facilities, budget, and potential for collaborating with other community agencies. If the needed resources do not exist or cannot be obtained through the agency budget request, it should be determined if fees can be charged for the services or if a contract or grant application written to obtain external funding.

Writing the action plan offers the opportunity for planners to brainstorm with the nutrition advisory committee and think "outside the box." The action plan should be descriptive and concise. An expanded listing of specific tasks and a Gantt chart with timelines is detailed in the operational plan written by staff when they prepare to carry out the activities. The timeline shows the planning, implementation, and data collection tasks to monitor progress over the lifetime of the program or project. A weekly or monthly calendar and schedule displays staff assignments to routine and special project duties. This schedule can be used for planning, delegating work, and assessing staff productivity. Implementation requires that adequate resources be requested through the detailed and carefully justified line item budget (see Chapter 17).

IMPLEMENT THE PLAN

Effective program implementation requires the following:

- Administrative commitment with a budget that provides a realistic number of qualified staff, plus space, equipment, teaching aids, educational materials, supplies, travel, and so on. Staff must have a work schedule that they can accomplish within available hours of work. For new programs, time must be scheduled for training, field-testing, troubleshooting, and revising.
- Dedication of the participating staff to the goals, objectives, and interventions. Staff must be completely oriented to their responsibilities and trained to ensure their competency to perform the required tasks. They must feel comfortable that they can perform the tasks required and that their work is valued. They must be assured that their constructive suggestions will be welcomed, thoughtfully considered, and used to improve the program.
- Respect and enthusiasm of the target population who are convinced that the program will benefit them, their families, and their community. They must buy in to the program by committing their time and effort to participate. Their suggestions should be continuously sought, considered and used. Social marketing strategies (see Chapter 15) and networking (see Chapter 22) are useful to involve community participation. The advisory committee community representative and local program assistants or volunteers who are respected by their neighbors are useful liaisons with the participants.

Putting the plan into action is the "reality check." A well-designed plan for new initiatives should build in time for testing, dry runs, and trying out alternative strategies. It is important to always have a Plan B. Murphy's Law can be anticipated: "If anything can go wrong it will." Unexpected situations should not come as a shock to experienced planners. On-site changes may be required during implementation and must be documented. The need to make changes does not necessarily mean that the plan as written was ill conceived. The secrets to successful implementation are open communication, flexibility, a sense of humor shared by staff and participants, and responsive program planners and managers.

TRACK PROGRESS

As the program is implemented, it must be monitored by collecting and analyzing appropriate data on a predetermined schedule. Systematic monitoring provides continuous feedback to assess progress toward achieving process and outcome objectives. By stating each objective in measurable terms, specifying the criterion and performance level or standard, and listing deadline dates, evaluation is built into the planning cycle. Programs that spend tax dollars must be accountable and responsible for periodically analyzing and reporting their progress to both administrators and the public. Results of the findings of the periodic monitoring should be used to decide whether to continue, expand, redesign, or terminate the program.

As each activity is developed, a data system must be designed into the plan to capture information to be recorded at the beginning (baseline), at scheduled intermediate midpoints, and upon completion (end points) of the implementation. Data collection instruments must be validated to be sure that they measure what they intend to measure and are reliable in yielding the same results when used repeatedly and by different workers. The data system must be quick and easy to use, preferably designed to enter information into readily accessible computers (see Chapter 16).

Some measures used in program evaluation include the following:

- Structure objectives measure inputs, such as dollars budgeted and expended; numbers and qualifications of staff; size, location, and accessibility of facilities; and equipment available. Documentation of inputs includes budgets, organization charts, job descriptions, schedules, personnel and expenditure reports, maps indicating locations of service sites, and inventories.
- Process objectives measure outputs, such as statistical reports; logs of services provided or work performed; numbers of encounters; unduplicated counts of clients served; numbers of classes held and rosters of attendees at each; lists of educational materials purchased or printed and number distributed; number of speeches given and sizes of audiences; number and type of media presentations; logs of numbers and content of telephone calls, e-mails, letters, and so on.
- Output measures the amount of work performed, but not its quality. Some call this "bean counting."
- Outcome objectives measure quality changes in consumer health and nutrition knowledge comparing pre- and post-test scores; changes in food choices measured by before-and-after dietary intake assessments using standardized, validated methods and forms; and changes in health and/or nutritional status as measured by before-and-after changes in standardized body measures or biochemical tests.

At the client service level, changes can be monitored over time by audits of agency medical or health records; periodic reports from the Centers for Disease Control and Prevention Nutrition Surveillance systems; reviews of data in automated client information systems; or by special studies. Population outcomes can be monitored by observing trends over time in aggregated data from birth and death certificates, school and child day care (Head Start) health records, or hospital discharge reports. Changes in quality of food purchasing can be monitored by using supermarket sales data. When data are collected, analyzed, and reported, outcome evaluations provide the response to the frequently asked question, "What has the public health nutrition program actually accomplished?"

When output and outcome data are collected, some correlations can be made to show the following:

- Program efficiency or productivity relates output to each unit of input to determine the dollar value of resources used to accomplish each stated process objective.
- Program coverage or penetration compares output or number of people actually served to the estimated number of people in the eligible target population who need the service as estimated in the community assessment.
- Program impact compares outcome data for a specified health or nutrition status measure with the number of people who are estimated to be at risk for the particular health problem as identified in the community assessment.

Client or consumer satisfaction is an important indicator of public and client awareness of nutrition services and their opinions of the usefulness, quality, and convenience of the services, in addition to the responsiveness and expertise of the staff. Client satisfaction is determined by conducting surveys of randomly selected clients and program participants at periodic intervals. Written questionnaires, personal or telephone interviews, or e-mail questionnaires may be conducted on a predetermined schedule. Results from the consumer satisfaction survey are used to improve the quality, scheduling, or location of services and to elicit suggestions for making services more user friendly. Although the satisfaction survey is by nature subjective, clients and the public may consider this the most valuable measure, because it invites them to express their opinions and make suggestions to improve services. Satisfied customers are goodwill ambassadors to the community.

In addition to these internal evaluations, some agencies arrange for a more rigorous, unbiased, external evaluation using an experimental or quasi-experimental design. For an external evaluation, the health agency usually contracts with a university or private research group known for their expertise in scientific evaluation methodology. Funding for an external evaluator may be included as a line item in grant applications to federal or foundation funders and strengthens the proposal.

Obtain Review and Comment

An early draft of the written plan in the short format shown in Figure 14–5 or the more detailed forms in the workbook and training manual of *Moving to the Future: Developing Community-Based Nutrition Services*[10] should be circulated to the administrator, peers, coworkers, and members of the advisory committee for review and comment. Suggestions should be carefully considered and incor-

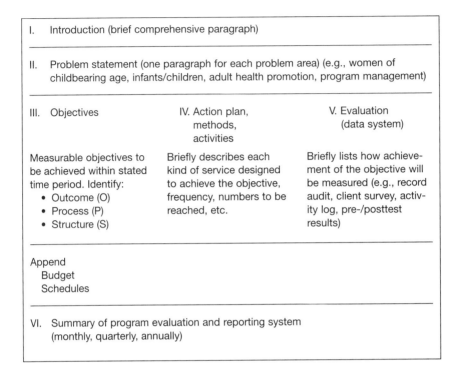

I.   Introduction (brief comprehensive paragraph)

II. Problem statement (one paragraph for each problem area) (e.g., women of childbearing age, infants/children, adult health promotion, program management)

III. Objectives	IV. Action plan, methods, activities	V. Evaluation (data system)
Measurable objectives to be achieved within stated time period. Identify: • Outcome (O) • Process (P) • Structure (S)	Briefly describes each kind of service designed to achieve the objective, frequency, numbers to be reached, etc.	Briefly lists how achievement of the objective will be measured (e.g., record audit, client survey, activity log, pre-/posttest results)

Append
  Budget
  Schedules

VI. Summary of program evaluation and reporting system (monthly, quarterly, annually)

Figure 14–5 Format for a Nutrition Program Plan. *Source:* Prepared by Chapter Author and Editor, Mildred Kaufman.

porated as appropriate. The completed plan should be widely distributed in the agency and in the community.

The written program plan shares the vision for nutrition services that are part of the health improvement plan with the agency administrator, the community, professional colleagues, and nutrition peers. It records the planning process and guides the staff as they implement and monitor their activities. The format of the plan may be dictated by guidelines from the agency administrator, health agency planners, or from funding agencies. The format is less important than the fact that there is a written plan containing all of the essential elements. The plan should be sequenced in logical order. It should be brief, clearly written in words easily understood by the public, the media, and by public health nutrition, health, and planning professionals. Professional jargon, government bureaucrat-ese, and undefined acronyms must be avoided. The plan focuses the thinking of influential stakeholders on the contributions of nutrition and diet to promote the public's health. It must make nutrition interventions tangible, visible, thought provoking, and enticing. It justifies the funds allocated to nutrition services. The written nutrition services plan as part of the agency's health improvement plan provides a frame of reference for actions that can be observed and for feedback. As a continuous, evolving process, the plan sets a direction and criteria to measure progress.

Publicize Success

Results and recommendations from the several evaluations should be summarized, analyzed, interpreted, and written at scheduled intervals. Statistical, graphic, and narrative reports are prepared according to agency guidelines. Reporting includes weekly or monthly informal feedback to the staff, administrator, and advisory committee with annual written reports to the agency board, funding agencies, partners, and the public. Many public health agencies publish annual reports to summarize their work during the year and disseminate these to health and human service agencies and interested citizens. Nutrition services should be highly visible in these reports. Successful evaluations merit wide media coverage to showcase public health nutrition accomplishments to the community.

POINTS TO PONDER

- Discuss the criteria for selecting stakeholders to involve in developing the nutrition service plan as a component of the agency's health improvement plan.
- What are the pros and cons of basing the nutrition plan on a priority list derived from the community needs assessment rather than offering nutrition services based on availability of federal or other external grants?
- What approaches can be made to community agencies that had been getting health department nutrition services at no cost to request that they contract and pay a fee for services?
- How can evaluation strategies be designed to collect meaningful data without generating excessive paperwork?
- How can time be justified for planning when there are many pressures to provide services?

HELPFUL WEB SITES

Healthy People 2010: www.health.gov/healthypeople

NOTES

1. US Department of Health and Human Services. *Healthy People 2010,* 2nd ed. McLean, Va: International Medical Publishing; 2002:23-16

2. US Department of Health and Human Services. *Healthy People 2010 Planning Guide.* Washington, DC: US Government Printing Office; 2001:2.

3. *A Strategic Approach to Community Health Improvement: The MAPP Field Guide,* p 22, 23

4. US Department of Health and Human Services. *Healthy People 2010,* 2nd ed. McLean, Va: International Medical Publishing; 2002:19–46,19–47.

5. Association of State and Territorial Public Health Nutrition Directors (ASTPHND). *Moving the Future: Developing Community-Based Nutrition Services.* 1996;21-22.

6. US Department of Health and Human Services. *Healthy People 2010,* 2nd ed. McLean, Va: International Medical Publishing; 2002. http://www.healthypeople.gov/default.htm. Accessed May 5, 2006.

7. McKenzie JE, Smeltzer JL. *Planning, Implementing and Evaluating Health Promotion Programs: a Primer.* 3rd ed. Boston, Mass: Allyn and Bacon; 2000;124.

8. US Department of Health and Human Services. *Healthy People 2010,* 2nd ed. McLean, Va: International Medical Publishing; 2002:19–1. http://www.healthypeople.gov/default.htm. Accessed May 5, 2006.

9. ASTPHND. *Moving the Future: Developing Community-Based Nutrition Services.* 1996;23. aspe.os.dhhs.gov/PIC/pdf/6179.PDF. Accessed May 5, 2006.

10. ASTPHND. *Workbook and Training Manual of Moving to the Future: Developing Community-Based Nutrition Services.* 1997. http://aspe.os.dhhs.gov/PIC/pdf/6179.PDF. Accessed May 5, 2006.

BIBLIOGRAPHY

Kaufman M. *Nutrition in Public Health: A Handbook for Developing Programs and Services,* Rockville, Md: Aspen Publishers, Inc; 1990.

McKenzie JF, Smeltzer JL. *Planning Implementing and Evaluating Health Promotion Programs: A Primer.* 3rd ed. Boston, Mass: Allyn and Bacon; 2001.

National Association of County and City Health Officials, Centers for Disease Control and Prevention. *A Strategic Approach to Community Health Improvement: MAPP.* Washington, DC: undated.

Office of Disease Prevention and Health Promotion. *Healthy People in Healthy Communities: A Community Planning Guide Using Healthy People 2010.* Department of Health and Human Services, Rockville, Md: 2001.

Probert KL, ed. *Moving to Future: Developing Community-Based Nutrition Services.* Association of State and Territorial Public Health Nutrition Directors, Health Resources and Services Administration, US Department of Health and Human Services; 1996.

Public Health Foundation. *Healthy People 2010 Toolkit.* Washington DC: Public Health Foundation; 2002.

Rohrer JE. *Planning for Community-Oriented Health Systems.* 2nd ed. Washington, DC: American Public Health Association; 1999.

Scutchfield FD, Keck CW. *Principles of Public Health Practice.* 2nd ed. Clifton, NY: Delmar Learning; 2003.

Timmreck TC. *Planning, Program Development and Evaluation: A Handbook for Health Promotion, Aging and Health Services.* 2nd ed. Sudbury, Mass: Jones and Bartlett Publishers; 2003.

Turnock BJ. *Public Health: What It is and How It Works.* Sudbury, Mass: Jones and Bartlett Publishers; 2004.

CHAPTER 15

Market Nutrition Programs to the Public

Diane R. Wilson

Reader Objectives

- Compare and contrast social marketing with business marketing.
- Discuss types of market research and how these can be used in preparing a plan for a public health nutrition program.
- List and define the *P*s of social marketing.
- Discuss the ethics of marketing

DEFINE MARKETING

Slick television advertisements promote carbonated beverages; pop-up ads on Web sites offer nutritional supplements; and glossy free-standing inserts (FSIs) in Sunday newspapers offer free merchandise in return for food product labels. Highway billboards advertise weight-control products, and public speaking engagements by celebrities sponsored by food manufacturers are examples of marketing tactics. Marketing has come into vogue to describe many activities related to the field of communication. However, marketing consists of much more than these tactics. Health professionals and organizations now realize the value of marketing to reach their desired objectives. The public health nutritionist must understand marketing and use its concepts to develop and implement an effective nutrition program plan.

Marketing is defined as satisfying the needs of the consumer through a product or service. It is the packaging, positioning, pricing, promotion, distribution, and selling of a product or service.[1] Marketing starts with the consumer's actual or perceived wants and needs, not with the product or service.

353

Business Marketing vs. Social Marketing

When people buy products or services, they are really purchasing satisfaction. Their definition of marketing applies to business marketing in which an exchange of goods or services occurs between a buyer and a seller. Business marketing is also known as commercial, conventional, or traditional marketing. Is there a role for business-type marketing in situations in which consumers are not satisfying their own needs, but in which society or a health and human service agency believes that behavioral changes are in the consumers' best interests? Many health professionals believe that there is an important role for so-called social marketing.[2]

In the early days of television, this question was asked: "Why can't you sell brotherhood and rational thinking like you sell soap?"[3] The nutritionist could ask: "Why can't we sell good nutrition like food manufacturers sell cereal?" These questions were answered in 1971 when the term *social marketing* was introduced.[4] Since then, variations of the term *social marketing* and the *social marketing approach* to changing behavior have developed. They are sometimes referred to as *community-based marketing, cause marketing, cause-related marketing*, or *social norms intervention*.

Social marketing is defined as "the design, implementation, and control of programs calculated to influence the acceptability of social ideas and involving considerations of product planning, pricing, communication, distribution, and marketing research."[5] This definition describes the activities of the public health nutritionist who designs, implements, and controls programs to change eating behavior. Business marketing focuses on fulfilling customers' needs and desires. Social marketing focuses on changing personal or social behaviors, including the use of needed health products or services, for the benefit of the public, even when the public neither recognizes their need nor desires the change.
Social marketing most often is used to accomplish three objectives:

1. Disseminate new data and information on practices to individuals.
2. Offset the negative effects of a practice or promotional effort by another organization or group.
3. Motivate people to move from intention to action.[6]

Examples of ways nutritionists might use social marketing in a program plan include the following:

- Motivate clients to control their weight.
- Inform the public about the role of dietary saturated fats and cholesterol in the prevention of heart disease.
- Offset the promotion of megavitamin supplements.

Use of social marketing in the development of a nutrition program plan requires the following:

- Adequate resources
- Strong support from the sponsoring agency's administrators and community leaders
- Marketing skills
- Clear authority to make the necessary marketing decisions and implement them in a timely fashion.[7]

All of these conditions must be present for the program to succeed.

The first step in developing a nutrition program plan is to identify the problem or opportunity. Chapter 3 reviews the steps in assessing community nutrition needs and setting priorities for satisfying these needs. This community assessment includes efforts to identify the target consumer group's values, attitudes, habits, or customs as they relate to the assessed need. This can be done through market research. Goals and objectives for the nutrition program are then determined (see Chapter 14).

MARKET RESEARCH

Market research is information gathering and uses observation, primary data, and secondary data, all of which are also used in community assessment for the nutrition program plan (see Chapters 3 and 14). The decision on the type of market research to perform is based on the type of program being planned and the available time, staff, and money. The cost of market research increases as it progresses from observation to the collection of secondary data, to the use of primary data collection techniques.

Observation

Watching and listening to customers as they find and use food products provides useful information in planning a nutrition program. Observation does not provide strong or systematic evidence, but it suggests a helpful starting point in thinking about strategies and tactics.[8] Visits to a food market where the target population shop provide insights into what foods and beverages they purchase and how a program on weight management can build on local preferences.

Primary Data

Information gathered, recorded, and used for the first time is primary data. Common techniques for gathering primary data include the following:

- Internet surveys
- Personal or telephone interviews

- Focus groups
- Client panels
- Mail surveys
- Questionnaires

Primary data are used more frequently than secondary data to develop strategies and tactics specific to the targeted population. For this reason, primary data are frequently used in social marketing. Techniques to collect primary data focus on local needs, trends, and behaviors. A client questionnaire can provide a tremendous amount of information useful in identifying clients' awareness and knowledge of a specific nutrition issue.

Secondary Data

Secondary data are secondhand bits of information gathered by other agencies, organizations, and individuals. Such data can be internal (found within the health agency) or external (obtained from outside sources). Examples of internal data include medical records, clinic attendance records, correspondence, and the log of telephone requests for services. External sources of available data are federal, state, and local governmental or university publications and reports, professional journals, trade association publications, and the wealth of information found in agency, public, and university libraries.

Secondary data, other than observational information, are the easiest and least expensive sources of useful information. Secondary data provide the program planner with ideas of directions and trends. However, this data may not be relevant to assessing the local situation or determining the targeted population's specific needs and behaviors. Secondary data are used as the basis for the community nutrition needs assessment discussed in Chapters 3 and 16.

Market Segmentation

The objectives in the community nutrition plan specify the audience or market for specified nutrition services—women of childbearing age, schoolchildren, adults with diabetes, athletes, or other population groups. Within each broad market, there are subgroups or segments with particular characteristics or consumer profiles that are similar and with needs that can be met through social marketing. Figure 15–1 reviews major market segmentation categories. Market research techniques collect primary data within each category.

The specific data to collect depend on the objectives of the nutrition program and how narrowly or specifically targeted the audience needs to be. For example, a process objective of a program for teen weight control could be to increase

Demographic	Geographic	Psycographic	Consumer-Behavioral
Age	Country	Feelings	Rate of usage
Sex	Region	Opinions	Benefits sought
Income	State	Beliefs	Reliability
Occupation	County	Prejudices	Health
Religion	City	Needs	Method of usage
Ethnicity	Zip code	Desires	Frequency of usage
Education	Climate	Aspirations	Comfort
Family status	Size of population	Hopes	Safety

Figure 15–1 Market Segmentation Categories. *Source:* Diane R. Wilson, Chapter Author.

awareness about this service among teenage girls. Data on age, ethnicity, education, residence, media use, and sources of physical education activities in the community are useful. Other data, such as sources of nutrition information or willingness to use the service, could also be collected. If the marketing objective is to increase awareness of this weight control program among teenage family planning clients attending a specific public health center, then age, ethnicity, education, residence, and employment data may not be needed, because the young women are already enrolled in the health center and the data are available.

The advantage of market segmentation is that social marketing strategy and tactics can be planned to fit the specific consumer profile. Targeting the group enhances program cost effectiveness and success.

Social Marketing Mix

The components of a business marketing plan are known as the marketing mix, or the four *P*s of marketing: product, place, price, and promotion.[9] In thinking through the *P*s of marketing, the four *C*s of marketing have been suggested as the platform upon which to base the four *P*s. The four *C*s are customer value, cost to the consumer, convenience, and communication.[10] All of these components are also used in the social marketing plan. The marketing mix can fit into the overall nutrition program plan.

The framework for developing a marketing plan is quite similar to that used in preparing a health improvement plan or a nutrition program plan. The steps to an effective marketing program include the following:

- R—Research (market research)
- STP—Segmentation, targeting, and positioning
- MM—Marketing mix (the Ps and Cs of marketing)
- I—Implementation
- C—Control, getting feedback, evaluating results, revising and improving STP and MM[11]

Product

Unlike the product of most businesses, the product in public health nutrition programs is not always tangible. It can be a service like nutrition information dissemination, diet counseling, or food service consultation. It can also be a practice like encouraging eating more fruits and vegetables. The product deals with awareness, knowledge, or motivation.

In social marketing, the product is often an available service the client needs to be successful, but is not viewed by the client as a need, because it is not a socially accepted or 'usual' practice. For example, all mothers attending a child health clinic may be referred to the nutritionist as a matter of clinic policy, not because they want the service. Others may be aware of the nutritional needs of their children, but may not see the benefit of seeking help. The product, child nutrition counseling, must be defined in a way to bring about a behavior change or action that is acceptable to the consumer. An example of a product that has gained consumer acceptance is a healthy weight program for black women ages 18 and over to encourage physical activity and eating healthier foods.[12]

Designing the Product Factors to consider in designing the nutrition program's product include:

- Branding
- Packaging
- Differentiating the product from others in the market
- Considering the life or length of usefulness
- Planning ahead for revision
- Developing new products or line extensions

A series of classes for clients on how to restrict sodium in their diets may be much more appealing to them if it is titled or branded "How to Prepare Tasty Foods" or "The Low Salt Gourmet," rather than "How to Cut Back on Salt." In packaging the product, planners should remember that a cooking demonstration with a tasting party attracts consumers much more than a lecture. Differentiating the product from those of competitors in the marketplace means positioning the product in the consumers' eyes in a specific and appealing way. Knowing the competitors, the details of their products, and all of their products' related components (price, place, and promotion) are necessary in the positioning process. Information about competitors can be obtained from the Internet, Yellow Pages in the telephone directory, media advertisements, promotional literature, and clients' verbal reports. Product development requires thinking ahead. Will new technologies and research make the product obsolete in a few years? Will the current product need to be revised to maintain its appeal to consumers? Will new products or adding components to the current product be required? Strategic or forward planning is required. What works today may not work tomorrow. These elements are as important for products and services within the social marketing realm as they are for those marketing in the commercial realm.

Testing the Product   Pretesting the product or service with a sample of targeted consumers provides insight on the appropriateness of the product's name and customer appeal. Market research techniques that can be used to pretest the product have been mentioned. Changes in the product are made more easily before it is introduced to the intended audience. This can save time, energy, and cost, while increasing the likelihood of program success.

Planned evaluation throughout the nutrition program is essential to assure the social marketer that the product is meeting its intended objectives. Strategies and tactics may need to be refined as one moves through the social marketing process.

Place

The second major component of the marketing mix is distribution. Distribution means the channels through which the product becomes available to the consumer. Health departments, clinics, hospital outpatient departments, child day care centers, congregate meal sites, and other similar facilities have traditionally served as distribution channels for nutrition programs and services. The Internet is a powerful place and is reshaping how information is accessed and shared. Consumer health, including nutritional care, is one area being rapidly transformed by interactive health communication.[13]

Since distribution and promotion are so closely related in the marketing plan, alternative channels might be investigated once promotional tactics are set. For example, if awareness of nutrition services for weight control is the objective of the nutrition plan, channels of distribution could include local broadcast media, Web sites, Internet discussion groups, or public forums at community centers. Schools, libraries, recreation centers, places of worship, work sites, and meeting rooms at shopping malls might be explored as possible sites. Selecting the place should consider the convenience of the product or service to the consumer and where the consumer can obtain it most readily. Access to parking, handicapped parking, and ancillary or related services should be considered. Selection of the most appropriate site is a part of the second *P* of marketing: place.

Price

Price is the third component in both business and social marketing, but its purposes differ in the two contexts. A business marketer will set a profitable price for a product that is acceptable to both consumers and the business. The business marketer must meet the needs of consumers, but must also satisfy the financial commitments to employees, management, and shareholders. The social marketer is not interested in financial gain. The emphasis is on the value to society in terms of safety, health, or other social issues, rather than monetary cost. However, there is a cost to be considered in social marketing: Psychological or physical cost. Consider what a consumer must give up to accept a health offer. This could be time, effort, or the risk of embarrassment and disapproval.

Three different pricing strategies are used in social marketing: cost recovery, market incentives, and market disincentives.[14]

Cost Recovery   Because many public health nutrition programs receive grants, foundation funds, or federal, state, or local government financial support, a price may not need to be set for the product. However, a sliding scale fee for the service based on ability to pay may be desirable to recover a portion of the costs, to obtain funds to expand services, as well as to appear to have value to the clients. The solicitation of donations could also be considered a cost recovery strategy.

Market Incentives   Market incentives are used to stimulate the adoption of a product. Offering a product at a price below current costs, at a price lower than that of a competitor, or at no cost reflects this pricing strategy. If the objective of a sliding scale, fee-for-service, weight-control program is to increase the number of enrollees, the incentive could be $10 off the set price. The "buy one, get one free" approach appeals to many consumers. The cost of a health service or product should consider the consumer's views on benefit and perceived value. A service priced too low or offered at no cost could have a perceived low value or be viewed as being inferior.

Market Disincentives   Pricing can also be used to discourage consumers from using a product. High taxes on cigarettes and liquor are examples of attempts by the government to discourage their use. An example of a market disincentive for a nutrition program might be to price soft drinks higher than fruit juices in vending machines at schools, meal program sites, or work site cafeterias.

Promotion

The fourth *P* in the marketing mix, promotion, is usually the first that comes to mind when thinking of marketing. Promotion is the communications component of marketing. It identifies the specific tactics or activities needed to create awareness, provide knowledge, and motivate the consumer to action. A goal of promotion can be to communicate consumer benefits or to destroy or lessen the demand or perceived value of a product or behavior deemed unhealthy or unsafe. Promotion includes advertising, personal selling, public relations, and consumer incentives. The combination of these various tactics promotes *social* as well as business marketing plans. The purpose of promotion is to move the consumer through the stages from unawareness to action.

Advertising   Advertising is just one piece of a promotion. Advertising has traditionally been defined as any paid form of mass presentation and promotion of ideas, goods, or services by an identified sponsor.[15] Advertising is publicity. In social marketing, advertising differs from commercial or business advertising in the following ways: (1) the product is usually a social cause, product, or service; (2) the advertiser is not a commercial enterprise; and (3) the advertiser's motivation is to benefit the consumer or client, rather than a commercial profit to the advertiser.[16] These characteristics usually exist in a public health nutrition program.

Advertising is not a one-time activity. It must be ongoing in a planned series of activities known as an advertising campaign. To enhance the effectiveness of the promotion, the purpose of the campaign must be clear. The media and entertainment vehicles used for advertising include e-mail, Web sites, television, radio, newspapers, magazines, brochures, billboards, posters, bumper stickers, buttons, and t-shirts.

The selection of advertising media depends on local time, money, and material resources. It should be designed to achieve the greatest effect on the target audience in terms of the number of people exposed to the advertisement and the frequency or number of times the message is seen or heard.

Advertising must always be informative, accurate, tasteful, clear, and valid. It can be entertaining, amusing, or serious, but it must always be credible, competitive, and leave a pleasing and lasting impression on the consumer.

Personal Selling   Salesmanship is the art and science of persuading another person to do something when direct power to cause the action does not exist.[17] Any direct contact to promote a program or service to a consumer or group of consumers is selling. Contacts can be through letters, telephone calls, e-mails, one-on-one client encounters, or group classes. A number of personal selling situations have been described as population-based interventions in Chapter 18. In any buyer-seller or user-provider situation, establishing and maintaining warm relationships are essential. Seller/provider actions that promote good relationships include the following:

- Initiate positive contacts, not negative situations.
- Be reliable, not unavailable.
- Make recommendations, not demands.
- Use candid, not accommodative, language.

- Use "we" problem-solving, not "I want" language.
- Use easily understood words or local jargon, not long, scientific explanations.
- Show respect and concern, not disdain, hostility, or indifference.
- Be courteous, not abrupt.
- Be attentive; do not interrupt.

Public Relations   Public relations is considered free publicity and an image builder for a service, idea, or individual. It can stimulate the demand for a product. Public relations is a valuable promotional tool in social marketing since it is free. Airtime and print space are provided as a public or community service. Although public relations activities involve time and materials, local companies, the media, or individuals can donate these.

The paying advertiser controls the message and the time in which the customer receives the message. Public service channels usually do not allow such controls. Press releases, media interviews, and articles can and usually are edited by the publisher or producer. Nevertheless, public relations can be effective in promotion. Planned activities could include sponsorship of a special community event such as a fun-run, cosponsorship of a health fair with another group such as the local diabetes association, press briefings or conferences to present new nutrition research findings, public speaking engagements with community groups, and a visit to the office of a local legislator. Many population-based interventions addressed in Chapter 18 are public relations.

Media advocacy programs are important tools to consider in social marketing. One form of media advocacy is through public service announcements (PSAs). Because PSAs are often aired late at night or during the early morning hours, they have been referred to jokingly as "People Sound Asleep."[18] Effective networking with staff of local television and radio stations may help to obtain more prime viewing or listening times for PSAs and other public relations messages. Radio stations may be more willing than television stations to provide prime time.

The image-building aspect of public relations also deals with the environment in which services or products are delivered. Attractive and comfortable client waiting rooms, colorful and current educational materials, friendly and caring professional staff, and convenient locations project a powerful positive message to consumers about the importance of the program or service.

Promotional Tools   In addition to advertising, personal selling, and public relations, sales promotional tools that can be included in a nutrition program plan include the following:

- Food demonstrations and tasting parties at schools, places of worship, work sites, service club meeting sites, congregate meal sites, supermarkets, and malls
- Booths and exhibits at malls, libraries, recreation centers, and fairs

- Internet or media-based recipe contests with prizes for recipes that demonstrate ways to prepare health-promoting foods
- Public recognition programs and testimonials in cooperation with the media for those who achieve weight-control successes
- Nutrition poster contests for children through their schools
- Health promotion and food fairs in parks, malls, or recreation centers
- Promotion of National Nutrition Month with a multimedia campaign of community activities

The purpose of sales promotion is to support, supplement, reinforce, or complement the other promotional tactics. Promotion cannot exist in a vacuum, but must be integrated into the overall plan.

Ps Unique to Social Marketing

In addition to the four *P*s of business marketing that can be adapted for social marketing purposes, social marketing also includes additional *P*s: publics, partnerships, policy, and purse strings.[19]

Publics   Publics are the internal and external people involved in social marketing programs. Internal publics are people involved with the approval and implementation of a program. External publics include the targeted customers and their influencers such as a parent, spouse, child, or staff. Secondary customers include elected officials, policy makers, and gatekeepers who have an interest in the program's goals, outcomes, and finances. The early support and involvement of publics is necessary and often crucial to planning and implementing a social marketing program, especially if the issue is controversial.

Partnerships   Nutrition services are one part of an overall and complex health improvement plan requiring interaction with many other colleagues, organizations, and agencies. Teaming up with those who have similar goals and objectives can help to reach targeted publics more effectively. Advantages of collaborating are numerous and include cost sharing, more effective use of staff, and wider dissemination of promotions, community support, or even enhanced credibility by publics.

Policy   Unless the social marketing program has supportive policies to sustain individual and population behavioral change, the program will not achieve long-term success and the individual and target population will revert to their old unhealthy food habits. If policy changes are needed, media advocacy programs as part of the promotional mix are useful. Examples of nutrition policy changes are the removal of soft drink vending machines from schools and insurance coverage for weight-control programs.

Purse Strings   Unlike business marketers who have financial resources from company assets, entrepreneurs, or financial institutions, the social marketer usually relies on government grants, foundations, or donations for program expenses. Pricing has been discussed previously in this chapter. However, even social marketing products that have a price to the target population will require other sources of funding. A question that must be addressed early in planning the nutrition program is: Who has the purse strings to support the program?

INTEGRATE THE MARKETING MIX INTO THE HEALTH IMPROVEMENT PLAN AND NUTRITION PROGRAM PLAN

"People change their food habits when two prerequisites are satisfied. First, the individual believes that such a change will help achieve some personally desired goal: weight loss, better health, more physical attractiveness, etc. Second, the mechanism of the change process must be uncomplicated and easily activated."[20]

Considering each of the *P*s of marketing, both business *P*s and social marketing *P*s helps develop an action-oriented and effective health improvement plan and nutrition services plan. A quality product offered in a convenient place at an acceptable price and promoted with an appealing message and planned with publics, partners, and appropriate policies in place and with adequate funding (purse strings) will be successful.

MARKETING ETHICS

It has been said "When judging social marketing from an ethical standpoint, it appears to be difficult to separate the ethics of applying marketing techniques to social ideas and programs from the ethics of the ideas themselves."[21] *The Code of Ethics for the Profession of Dietetics*[22] and the *Position of the American Dietetic Association: The Role of Dietetics Professionals in Health Promotion and Disease Prevention*[23] should guide the conduct of the nutritionist.

Just as the business marketer can be accused of selling or promoting a product in an unethical way, so can the social marketer who misuses marketing tools to compound a social abuse or manipulate public opinion. Social marketing should inform, educate, or bring about a change in behavior to improve health or quality of consumer and community life. It differs from business marketing, which responds to needs and wants of consumers who are pursuing their own self-interests. Regardless, any marketer must understand ethics and the social consequences of any marketing action.

Public health nutritionists can learn to think and plan like marketers. They must listen and seek out the nutrition wants and needs of the public and then create, develop, or redesign services and programs to meet these wants and needs.

Targeting services to a specific population group is critical. The business marketer's approach to planning and using market research techniques, product concepts, distribution channels, pricing strategies, and promotional tactics can be successfully applied to the nutrition program planning process.

POINTS TO PONDER

- How can a public health nutritionist promote healthful eating practices in a community where these recommendations are contrary to well-entrenched regional or ethnic food habits?
- How can and should a tax-supported public health agency market a weight-management program that competes with for-profit weight loss programs?
- What pricing strategies are appropriate for a public health agency offering a new nutrition service directed to middle- and upper-income taxpayers?
- How can a public health agency respond to the results of a satisfaction survey that indicate consumers' frustration with the excessive waiting time and hours lost from work required to obtain health and nutrition services?

HELPFUL WEB SITES

Center for Advanced Studies in Nutrition and Social Marketing, Department of Public Health Sciences:
www.socialmarketing-nutrition.ucdavis.edu
Social Marketing Institute: www.social-marketing.org
Social Marketing Institute, Weinreich Communications:
www.social-marketing.com
Society of Nutritional Education: www.sne.org
Turning Point National Program Office, University of Washington:
www. turningpointprogram.org

NOTES

1. Marconi J. *Future Marketing: Targeting Seniors, Boomers and Generation X and Y.* Chicago, Ill: NTC Business Books; 2001:5.

2. Wiebe GD. Merchandising commodities of citizenship on television. *Public Opinion Quarterly.* Winter 1951:679.

3. Wiebe GD. Merchandising commodities of citizenship on television. *Public Opinion Quarterly.* Winter 1951:679.

4. Kotler P, Saltman G. Social marketing: an approach to planned social change. *J Marketing.* 1971;35:5.

5. Kotler P, Saltman G. Social marketing: an approach to planned social change. *J Marketing.* 1971;35:5.

6. Fox KFA, Kotler P. The marketing of social causes: the first 10 years. *J Marketing.* 1980;44:26–27.

7. Population Information Program. Social marketing: does it work? *Population Reports.* January 1980;Series J(21):J394.

8. Kotler P. *Kotler on Marketing: How to Create, Win and Dominate Markets.* New York, NY: The Free Press; 1999:88.

9. McCarthy EJ. *Basic Marketing: A Managerial Approach.* Homewood, Ill: Richard D. Irwin; 1968:32.

10. Lauterborn R. New marketing litany: 4 P's passe, C-words take over. *Advertising Age.* October 1, 1990:26.

11. Kotler P. *Kotler on Marketing: How to Create, Win and Dominate Markets.* New York, NY: The Free Press; 1999:30.

12. National Institute of Diabetes & Digestive & Kidney Disease. *Sisters Together: Move More, Eat Better.* Available at: http://www.niddk.nih.gov/health/nutrit/sisters/sisters.htm. Accessed March 28, 2004.

13. National Research Council. *Networking Health: Prescription for the Internet. Committee Enhancing the Internet for Health Applications: Technical Requirements and Implementation Strategies.* Washington, DC: National Academies Press; 2000.

14. Muskkate M Jr. Implementing public plans: the case for social marketing. *Long Range Planning.* August 1980;13:27.

15. Alexander RS, Committee on Definitions of the American Marketing Association. *Marketing Definitions: A Glossary of Marketing Terms.* Chicago, Ill: American Marketing Association; 1963:9.

16. Crosier K. The Advertising Dimension of Social Marketing. *Advertising.* Autumn 1978:33.

17. Russell FA, Beach FH, Buskirk RH. *Textbook of Salesmanship.* New York, NY: McGraw-Hill Book Co; 1974:3.

18. Manoff RK. Marketing not society's enemy. *Advertising Age.* July 15, 1985:18.

19. Weinrich NK. *What is Social Marketing?* Weinrich Communications. Available at: http://www.social-marketing.com.htm. Accessed March 23, 2004.

20. Sorenson AW, Hanson RG. Index of food quality. *J Nutr Ed.* 1972;7:53.

21. Laczniak GR, Lusch RF, Murphy PE. Social marketing: its ethical dimensions. *J Marketing.* Spring 1979;43:30.

22. American Dietetic Association. Code of ethics for the profession of dietetics. *J Am Diet Assoc.* January 1999;99:109.

23. Hampl JS, Anderson JV, Mullis R. Position of the American Dietetic Association: the role of dietetics professionals in health promotion and disease prevention. *J Am Diet Assoc.* November 2002;102:1680.

CHAPTER 16

Understand, Interpret, and Use Data

Carole B. Garner

Reader Objectives:

- Discuss the role data contributes in the core public health functions.
- Specify the types of data to use for community assessment.
- Link the many sources of data available from federal and state agencies useful to plan public health nutrition programs.
- Discuss the steps to collect new data.
- Describe the advantages and disadvantages of the existing survey tools.

DATA WITHIN CORE PUBLIC HEALTH FUNCTIONS

Sir Arthur Conan Doyle said, "It is a capital mistake to theorize before one has data. Insensibly one begins to twist facts to suit theories, instead of theories to suit facts."[1] Accountability, effectiveness, and efficiency require quality data. Data plays a key part throughout the range of core public health functions. Background data guide development of policies such as recommending the ratio of healthier foods and beverages to less healthy items offered in school vending machines. Having data can aid a school board's decision on product mix. Assessing the population's weight status documents the growing trend indicating a public health problem with overweight and obesity. Measures showing the staff nutritionists limited knowledge of appropriate physical activities for the elderly help develop an education program to assure a competent workforce.

Community Assessment

Clinical dietitians gather objective and subjective data and assess individual clients as the basis to work with each individual to develop a care plan. In public health programs where the community is the patient, the same process is used for the community assessment. Objective data includes information to describe the population by age, gender, education, economic status, and race and ethnic distribution. Public health nutritionists also relate health, nutrition, and physical activity status indicators to environmental factors such as urban sprawl. Subjective data look at the perceived needs or how the community views its collective health concerns.

Source accessibility varies depending on the available technology. Increasing access to the Internet with its expanding number of postings of data sets by various governmental and nongovernmental agencies and organizations now make it easier to access the information needed to plan and evaluate programs.

For more information go to FEDSTATS at www.fedstats.gov. This site links over 70 agencies that collect statistics. If alternative or additional sources are needed to locate desired information, state, county, or local government agencies, libraries, and universities usually have census data. Federal publications and other information products are available free for public use in federal depository libraries located throughout the United States. Vital statistics, such as the number of births and deaths and hospital discharge information, can be found at state and local public health departments. Data sources discussed in the subheadings of this chapter include surveillance systems, surveys, and other readily available sources of information. Those that include nutrition, physical activity, and related data tabulated for state and/or local populations are listed in the section on program management. As with all research, the user must be certain that the data is from a reputable source.

Demographic and Socioeconomic Characteristics

Knowing the frequent associations between health risks and demographic characteristics suggests the indicators that provide clues to potential problems. For example, the incidence of obesity has been found to be higher in low-income populations and in some minority groups. A community with a profile that indicates a high number of families in poverty might be expected to have a greater probability of overweight and obesity among its population.

The US Census Bureau provides online links to data summarized from a variety of surveys and censuses.[2] The decennial census is conducted every 10 years. Population information used in the community assessment (see Chapter 3) includes age, gender, race, ethnicity, income, education, household composition, language spoken at home, and occupation. Tables and demographic profiles from the decennial census vary depending on the entity for which information is requested, such as state, county,[3] township, city, census tract, congressional district, or metropolitan statistical area.[4] The American Community Survey initiated in 1996 as an annual national survey, collects similar population and housing information as the census long form.[5] The Population Estimates Program publishes population estimates for each year between the 10-year censuses.[6]

Health Status

Traditionally, the health status indicators used for community assessment have been mortality figures. Tabulated data also monitor health risk behaviors, incidence of specific diseases, as well as reasons for hospitalization. For example, the use of hospital discharge data by diagnostic codes and costs suggests hospitalization expenses for obesity-related diseases by payment source.

The National Center for Health Statistics (NCHS) publishes a variety of data tabulated by state. Items in the National Vital Statistics Reports include recorded births, deaths, (including infant deaths), marriages, and divorces. These reports can be obtained from the NCHS Web site or by contacting the state health department's interactive Web site *Healthy Women: State Trends in Health and Mortality* accessed at www://209.217.72.34/healthywomen/eng/ReportFolders/Rfview/explorerp.asp. This site displays tables that document the health of people in each state by gender, race, and age. Although the title is "Healthy Women," data is also provided for men. Current mortality tables and health behavior and risk factor tables can be accessed. These are grouped in several categories including those used in the *Healthy People 2010* objectives. Users can choose to view whichever parameters they may need for their assessment. The data useful to create the tables for the community assessment comes from the Behavioral Risk Factor Surveillance System and mortality data sets.

State health department statisticians collect data on defined populations. Hospital discharge information provides patient demographics, diagnosis codes for the individuals who have been hospitalized, services provided to them, as and total cost for the services and payment source. Disease registries (such as cancer registries) monitor the number of people with a specific disease and their survival rates. Depending on the size of the population and number of cases, the information may further differentiate site-specific cancer incidence rates. Some states maintain a birth defect register to list birth defects diagnosed in all infants. The state health department may provide online or hard copy reports. Some of the online reports are interactive, similar to the NCHS Healthy Women site noted above.

National Health Interview Survey (NHIS)

The annual *National Health Interview Survey* (NHIS), a part of the National Health Survey, is a cross-sectional household interview survey. Questionnaires are administered at a personal visit. Although the survey sample is drawn from each state, the numbers interviewed in each state are too small to provide precise individual state data. The basic module for the NHIS was redesigned in 1997. The NHIS includes three core questionnaires: family, adult, and child.

Table 16–1 National Health Interview Survey Supplements, 1997–2005

1997	Adult and child immunization
1998	Prevention: health behaviors
	Adult and child immunization
1999	Chronic conditions
	Cancer screening
	Health care access and utilization
	Adult and child immunization
2000	Cancer control
	Adult and child immunization
2001	Children's mental health
	Emergency access to care
	Access to care
	Disability and secondary conditions: social support
	Heart disease, CPR, and stretching exercises
	Stroke warning signs
	Adult and child immunization
2002	Complementary and alternative medicine
	Hearing
	Vision
	Arthritis
	Asthma
	Disability and secondary conditions: Assistive technologies and environmental barriers
	Environmental health—lead paint
	Children's mental health
	Adult and child immunization
2003	Children's mental health
	Diabetes
	Asthma, heart, and respiratory disease
	Cancer screening and sun protection
	Smoke and fire alarm
	Adult and child immunization
2004	Children's mental health
2005	Cancer control

Source: Centers for Disease Control and Prevention, National Center for Health Statistics.

Each year, special topic supplements are added to the core questions. Table 16–1 lists the areas of focus from 1997 to 2005. National statistics summarizing these findings are available online.

Nutritional Status

Population-based systems investigate food availability, food expenditures, and food security. Surveys to assess individual intakes use tools such as the individual 24-hour diet recall, food frequency, and 3- to 7-day food record or diet history.

"National surveys estimate dietary intakes representative of the national population, but are not designed to provide measures representative of any particular locality."[7] Synthetic estimates are one way to use national data to develop a profile for a state or community. The most basic approach is to apply national estimates for the demographic characteristics, usually age distribution, gender, race/ethnicity, and socioeconomic status, that best match the state and local community. For example, the national prevalence rate for a particular health condition for African-American males between ages 18 and 24 may be 10%. If the community being studied has 10,000 African-American men, then it could be estimated that 1000 of these men might have the given condition. Unfortunately, this approach does not account for individual variability and the community's potential risk factors. Synthetic estimates may extrapolate survey results to the local community, but are not as accurate as data derived from the community's population. For assistance with this type of analysis, statisticians or epidemiologists at the state or local health department, college, or university might provide helpful advice.

National Health and Nutrition Examination Survey (NHANES)

The *National Health and Nutrition Examination Survey* (NHANES) is a population-based survey that collects information on the health and nutritional status of US households. From 1971 to 1994 NHANES was conducted periodically. Beginning in 1999, NHANES became a continuous, annual survey. Survey data are published every two years titled "NHANES 1999–2000," "NHANES 2001–2002," "NHANES 2003–2004," and so on. The NHANES 1999–2000 oversampled low-income adolescents, ages 12–19; individuals sixty years of age or older; and Mexican-Americans and African-Americans. NHANES 2001–2002 included these groups and also included oversampling of pregnant women. The National Center for Health Statistics NHANES Web site www.cdc.gov/nchs/nhanes.htm provides the analytic guidelines used, data sets, and related documentation for each series release. It also reports and includes a bibliography of articles that present an analysis of various portions of the NHANES data.

There are two parts to the NHANES survey: the findings of the home interviews and the findings of the individual health examinations. The in-home interview asks questions about each individual's health status, disease history, diet, and nutrient supplement use; physical activity and fitness; and weight history of household members. The individual health examination includes physical assessments such as muscle strength, body composition, cardiovascular fitness, as well as a physical examination and a 24-hour diet recall. It also asks interviewees about their immunization status, any diagnosis of diabetes, tobacco use, and results of laboratory tests for blood lipid profiles, hematologies, and so on.

The dietary components of NHANES and the USDA Continuing Survey of Food Intakes by Individuals (CSFII) are now integrated and named *What We Eat in America, NHANES*. The benefit of merging these surveys is to link the diet and health data of NHANES with the two days of 24-hour dietary recall data collection procedures of CSFII. Questionnaires specific to the amount of drinking water and another on fish and shellfish consumption are included. A 23-page food propensity questionnaire (FPQ) was added to the survey in 2003. This is a modification of the National Cancer Institute (NCI) Diet History Questionnaire. The FPQ collects much of the same information as a food frequency, except without portion sizes. FPQ forms are mailed to the participants. A statistical model that uses the FPQ and dietary recall data to estimate usual food consumption patterns has been developed by the NCI. The *Diet and Health Knowledge Survey* previously conducted by USDA is no longer used.

Food Consumption (Per Capita) Data System

The USDA Economic Research Service annually calculates the data on amount of food and nutrients available for human consumption in the United States. This data obtains information from food producers and distributors rather than consumers. It can be obtained at no cost at the ERS-USDA Web site www.ers.usda.gov/data/FoodConsumption/ or via reports at the online version of *Amber Waves* www.ers.usda.gov/Amberwaves/. It also can be purchased from ERS-NASS, 5285 Port Royal Road, Springfield, VA 22161.

Consumer Expenditure Survey (CEX)

The annual *Consumer Expenditure Survey* conducted by the US Census Bureau for the Bureau of Labor Statistics collects information on consumer buying habits. This survey is in two parts. Survey participants are asked to keep a diary for two consecutive 1-week periods to record their expenditures of their small routine purchases such as food, beverages, tobacco, nonprescription drugs, entertainment, and personal and household care products. The second component is a series of interviews asking these participants to list large recurring expenditures such as rent or mortgage payments, household utilities, insurance premiums, and car expenses. The data is tabulated in a variety of participant categories including income, age, race and ethnicity; the size and composition of their household; whether they own or rent their home and if it is in an urban or rural area; and by section of the United States. Areas of most interest to nutritionists include expenditures on food eaten at home subdivided into cereals and bakery products; dairy products; fruits, and vegetables; meat, fish, poultry, and eggs; and other foods. Respondents are also are asked about their expenditures for food they eat away from home.

Physical Activity Status

Data on physical activity is a component of several ongoing surveys and surveillance systems. The *National Health Interview Survey* (NHIS) basic module questions adults concerning their physical activities. These questions ask about leisure activities such as exercise and sports. They are asked to estimate duration and the intensity of each activity as vigorous, moderate, or light. These are differentiated by the amount of sweating and increases in breathing or heart rate. In addition to the cardiovascular-enhancing activities participants are queried about lifting weights and other actions that strengthen their muscles.

The home interview component of NHANES includes a set of questions similar to the leisure activities in the NHIS using prompts, such as the number of push-ups and sit-ups with the muscle strengthening series, contrasted to the hours spent watching television and nonwork computer use. Further questions explore transportation-related activities of walking and bicycling to work, school, or for errands. The activity profile also asks about household and yard tasks such as heavy cleaning, mowing the lawn, and raking leaves. The NHANES health examination provides a physical activity monitor for persons six years of age and older. Participants are asked to wear the monitor (accelerometer) during their waking hours for seven days. The monitor records activity intensity and duration and the number of steps traveled.

The scope of physical activity is more than how much and in what ways people move, but also their limitations. The three core questionnaires, the family, child, and adult, of the National Health Interview Survey ask about any mobility problems. These include each interviewee's needs for assistance with personal care, handling household chores, shopping, and conducting necessary business. They report any degree of difficulty they may have in walking, standing, and lifting or carrying. Year-specific supplements ask about other potential physical activity barriers due to arthritis or injuries. NHIS and NHANES include similar questions about physical function.

Environmental Indicators

The environment can affect health through physical activity and nutrition. Within the scope of public health concerns related to the environment, the topics that typically emerge first are areas such as air and noise pollution, water quality, and toxic chemicals.

A review of the community environment includes availability, use, and condition of sidewalks and other locations for safe walking; convenience of recreational facilities such as gymnasiums, swimming pools, and playgrounds; and bike paths or bike lanes. *Measuring the Health Effects of Sprawl: A National Analysis of Physical Activity, Obesity, and Chronic Disease* reports on residential density, street connectivity, distance from residential areas to shopping and service areas, and data from the CDC Behavioral Risk Factor Surveillance System.[8] Data tables for several counties in each state relate their sprawl score to the expected BMI and probability of obesity and hypertension for their population.

Collecting data on the nutrition environment records factors that influence the eating habits and health outcomes that are assessed with surveys such as NHANES. Foods available in different locations can provide a picture of a community's assets or problems. Questions include the food and beverage choices available to the public in vending machines, snack bars, and cafeterias in schools, work sites, and recreational areas; the variety, quality, and cost of food items at grocery stores, farmers markets, food marts, and discount outlets; and the number and location of the various types of cafeterias, restaurants, and fast-food outlets and the items each offers.

Perceived Needs

In addition to the objective data, public opinion and what influences that opinion are useful to understand the nutrition and physical activity concerns of the community's population. Opinion surveys, intercept studies, key informant interviews, and focus groups are some methods to use to determine the issues. Questions ask respondents to rank in order of priority their opinions of the main health, nutrition, and/or physical activity problems of the community. Do the respondents believe nutrition and physical activity contribute to obesity and overweight as a public health issue? Questions on possible ways to address the problems along with opportunities and barriers complete the survey. Media can influence the people's nutrition and physical activity. A survey of media outlets includes several areas. Suggestions from *Moving to the Future: Developing Community-Based Nutrition Services* include magazines; local and national newspapers, radio stations, and television stations/networks and their Web sites; and publications produced by nonprofit advocacy organizations[9] (see Table 16–2). Community coalitions, initiatives, or other organizations can be sources of existing data for opinion surveys, focus groups, and media.

PROGRAM MANAGEMENT

Data is also used to develop program plan objectives and then monitor and evaluate achievement of activities addressing the objectives. Objectives should be SMART: specific, measurable, appropriate, realistic, and time specific. Whether objectives address outcomes, processes to reach the outcomes, or the structure needed to implement the processes, objectives indicate what action might be used for each population, what time period, and the measured indicator of change (see Chapter 14).

For example, a school district wellness advisory committee decides to make incremental changes to the nutrition quality of foods offered in their schools as one way to improve the health of students. At the start of the school year, an outcome

Table 16–2 Example of Media Activity Summary Chart

Media Chart

Use this table to track the results of your media survey

Media Outlet	Type of Coverage/Topic	Frequency	Audience/No. Reached	Contact
Example: Channel 12 News	Features on diabetes	2-min. segment (aired 3 X)	Local viewers (24,000)	

Summary of findings

1) What health issues are receiving the most media coverage in your community (both in terms of frequency and audience reached)?

2) Which media outlets might help you reach your community?

Source: Probert, K.L. (Ed.). 1996. Moving to the Future: Developing Community-Based Nutrition Services. Washington DC Association of State and territorial Public Health Nutrition Directors.

Table 16–3   Table Shell—Vending Machines in Middle Schools Containing 100% Healthy Options and in High Schools Containing 75% Healthy Options at Start of School Year, Midterm and End of School Year.

Schools in District	Total Number of Vending Machines	Vending Machines Meeting Goal					
		Start of School Year		Midterm		End of School Year	
		N	%	N	%	N	%
Middle School A							
Middle School B							
Middle School C							
Middle School D							
High School A							
High School B							

Source: Arkansas Department of Health.

objective is stated relative to the vending machines in the school district: "By June 1, 2008, all middle schools' vending machines will contain 100% healthy choices, and all high schools' vending machines will contain at least 75% healthy choices." With the objective developed a table shell is prepared (Table 16–3).

This table has a title and is labeled, but does not contain data. A series of table shells should be developed as a guide for the analysis.[10] The blank spaces indicate additional information to collect. As in this example, to determine the percent of healthy choices available to students, another table shell is needed (Table 16–4).

Subsequently, more detailed tables would be developed for use at each school. The *School Foods Tool Kit* provides a sample form for school vending machine survey. The kit can be found on the Web at www.cspinet.org/schoolfoods or by contacting the Center for Science in the Public Interest in Washington, DC.

STATE HEALTH INFORMATION

Federal, state and local governments, as well as other funding sources, require program accountability. Performance measures may need process data, outcome data, or both. An agency-integrated health information system focuses on all of their programs and clients. This collected data may be combined into a single report or subdivided into individual categories or programs. Maternal and child health would include family planning, prenatal care, WIC, infant, and child health. Health promotion and disease prevention includes adult health promotion, work-site wellness, 5-a-day, obesity prevention, communicable disease prevention and immunization, and food safety.

Table 16–4 Table Shell—Healthy and Other Options Available in Vending Machines in Middle Schools and High Schools

Schools in District	Beverages			Food Items			All Choices		
	Healthy N	Other N	Healthy %	Healthy N	Other N	Healthy %	Healthy N	Other N	Healthy %
Middle School A									
Middle School B									
Middle School C									
Middle School D									
High School A									
High School B									

Source: Arkansas Department of Health.

Encounter systems track clinic services provided to individual clients with their demographic profile. Data items usually include age, gender, race, ethnicity, and education, as well as diagnosis, type of clinic attended, service provided, type of health care provider, anthropometrics measures, and lab tests completed.

Program-specific data items expand upon the general encounter. Items included in the collection system are required by the funding source. Table 16–5 and Table 16–6 illustrate the computer data entry screens used by the Arkansas WIC Program.

The base data screen is similar to a general encounter form, asking for demographics adding contact and identifier information. WIC management data collects information on the participant and family income, employment, participation in other assistance programs, household size, and migrant status. This information is required for the *WIC Participant and Program Characteristics Survey.* Certification data is needed to establish nutrition risk factors. It includes height,

Table 16–5   Arkansas Department of Health WIC Data Entry Screen—Base and Management

WIC Patient Management (Base Data)	Arkansas Department of Health
Add Patient (Auto)	Arkansas WIC Program ADHVS001

Pick Up Clinic	___		
Patient Name	___	Date of Birth	___
Patient Sex	___	Patient Race	___
Marital Status	___	Education	___
Patient Number	___	Social Security	___
Medicaid Number	___	Case Management	___
Patient Address	___		
	___		
City, State, Zip	___ AR ___		
Phone No (Work)	___-___-___ (Home) ___-___-___ (Message) ___-___-___		
Residence County	___		
Responsible Adult	___		
Mother Maiden Name	___		
Comment	___		

Press Enter to Update Patient Record or Select:

1) Assign Manual Patient No		10) Pick County	
2) Income Calc	8) Pick Mar Status	11) Pick Race	15) Print
3) Imm Eval	9) Pick Sex		16) Exit

WIC Patient Management (Management Data)	Arkansas Department of Health
Add Patient (Auto)	Arkansas WIC Program ADHVS001

       Patient No **********   Patient Name X

Is Head of Household a Farmworker	___	Is Head of Household a Female	___
Is Head of Household Employed	___	Does Applicant Have Private Insurance	___
Is Applicant Under Foster Care ...	___	Is Applicant a Migrant	___
Is Applicant Homeless	___	Is Applicant Disabled	___
Is Applicant a Medicaid Recipient	___	Is Family Member a Medicaid Recipient	___
Is Applicant on ARKids First	___	Is Applicant Receiving TEA	___
Is Family Member Receiving TEA ...	___	Is Anyone in Family on Food Stamps ..	___

     Current Household Size/Income ___ ___ and at WIC Cert ___ ___

WIC/Medicaid ___	WIC/TEA ___	WIC/Food Stamps ___
Category	Priority	High Risk Flag

Press Enter to Continue or Press the Appropriate PFKey to Select:

2) Income Calc	15) Print
3) Imm Eval	16) Exit

Source: Carole Garner, Arkansas Department of Health, Arkansas WIC Program.

Table 16–6   Arkansas Department of Health WIC Data Entry Screen—Base and Management, / Certification and Food Package

WIC Patient Management (Certification Data)	Arkansas Department of Health
Add Patient (Auto)	Arkansas WIC Program ADHVS001

Patient No _____   Patient Name X   Date First Entered System _/_/___

Eval. Clinic	____			Cert Ends	_/_/___
Measure Date	_/_/___	Cert Date	_/_/___	Act Date	_/_/___
Status	_	Activity	_	Initial Cert Type	_
Height	_ ft _ in _ /8	Weight	_ lb _ oz	Hemoglobin	___
Hematocrit	_ %	Head Circ	__ cm	Breastfed	__ Weeks
EDC Date	_/_/___	Del. Date	_/_/___	Birth Wt.	_ lb _ oz

RiskCode 1 ___   RiskCode 2 ___   RiskCode 3 ___   RiskCode 4 ___   RiskCode 5 ___

Clerk	CPA	IR Rcvd	Food Pkg	Issue Week	Issue Day	Issue Cycle
__	__	_	__	_	_	_/_/___

Auth Rep _____ Comment _____

Press Enter to Continue or Press the Appropriate PFKey to Select:

2) Income Calc	15) Print
3) Imm Eval	16) Exit

WIC Patient Management (Food Package Data)	Arkansas Department of Health
Add Patient (Auto)	Arkansas WIC Program ADHVS001

Patient No **********   Patient Name X

Category	Item, Qty, Unit/Measure, Desc	Item, Qty, Unit/Measure, Desc
Formula	___	___
Cereal	___	___
Juice	___	___
Milk	___	___
Milk	___	___
Milk	___	___
Cheese	___	___
Eggs	___	___
Beans/Peas	___	___
Carrots	___	___
Tuna	___	___

Press Enter to Continue or Press the Appropriate PFKey to Select:

2) Income Calc	15) Print
3) Imm Eval	16) Exit

Source: Carole Garner, Arkansas Department of Health, Arkansas WIC Program.

weight, hemoglobin, and other measures, along with breast-feeding information and risk factor codes. The final screen records food package data noting what and how much each of the WIC foods the woman, infant, or child is to receive. In addition to contributing to the federal survey, this recorded data offers many possibilities for program management. For example, review of food package item choices might suggest concomitant education on lower-fat selections. Data may suggest development of breast-feeding programs to increase initiation and duration. In-service training for staff might be needed to address specific risk criteria and expanding of outreach efforts.

SURVEYS, SURVEILLANCE SYSTEMS, AND OTHER SOURCES OF EXISTING DATA

When reviewing the existing data pertinent to public health issues such as nutrition and physical activity, the basic difference of the sources must be understood. A survey is a one time questioning of a sample of the population. A surveillance system is a series of surveys, repeated at periodic intervals, to examine an issue over time to monitor trends.

The Centers for Disease Control and Prevention, the US Department of Agriculture, the Administration on Aging, and the Public Health Foundation work with state programs to collect and analyze data specific to their missions. The surveillance systems and other compilations of data aids to develop and evaluate the studies of public health nutrition programs.

Whether completing a community assessment or using data to manage and monitor programs, the most recent data available should be used. Federal program and national organization sources may provide older information than can be obtained directly from local or state programs.

CDC Surveillance Systems

The CDC surveillance systems include the Behavioral Risk Factor Surveillance System (BRFSS), Youth Risk Behavior Surveillance System (YRBSS), Pediatric Nutrition Surveillance System (PedNSS), Prenatal Nutrition Surveillance System (PNSS), and Pregnancy Risk Assessment Monitoring System (PRAMS). There are also special data subsets of BRFSS; US Physical Activity Statistics, 5-a-Day Data and Statistics, and Selected Metropolitan/Micropolitan Area Risk Trends (SMART). The states participating in one or more of these systems in 2003 are illustrated in Figure 16–1.

Annual summaries are on the CDC Web site and on many state health department Web sites. These summaries are also published in the CDC's *Morbidity and Mortality Weekly Report* and can be obtained by contacting state health departments.

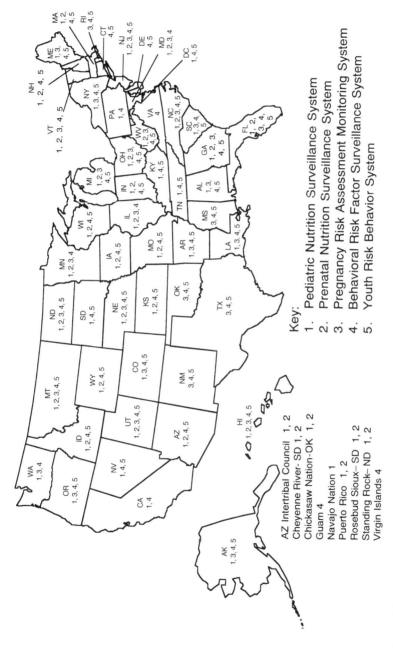

Figure 16–1 Participating State, Territorial and Tribal Health Agencies, 2003 CDC Surveillance Systems. Source: Centers for Disease Control and Prevention (CD). *CDC Surveillance Systems.* Atlanta, Georgia: U.S. Department of Health and Human Services, Centers for Disease Control and Prevention, 2003.

An example of one method of presenting surveillance data is the series of maps of the United States used by CDC to graphically present the trends in the prevalence of obesity (www.cdc.gov/nccdphp/dnpa/obesity/trend/index.htm) and diabetes (www.cdc.gov/diabetes/statistics/maps/index.htm).

Behavioral Risk Factor Surveillance System (BRFSS)

The BRFSS is a population-based survey conducted by the official health departments of each state, the District of Columbia, Puerto Rico, the Virgin Islands, and Guam. The BRFSS's focus examines health-related behaviors linked with the leading causes of death including heart disease, cancer, stroke, diabetes, and injury. States use standard core questions and procedures to collect data through telephone interviews with adults ages 18 years and older. States may also include questions they develop to study their specific concerns. In addition to a series of demographic questions, core behavior questions include use of periodic screenings such as colonoscopy, Pap tests and mammograms; health care access and insurance; diagnosis of asthma, diabetes, and arthritis; alcohol consumption; smoking; weight and height; intake of fruits and vegetables; physical activity; seat belt use; dental care; and up-to-date flu shots. The data generally uses state-level statistics. Some states modify their sampling procedures or combine several years of data to provide county profiles. States use BRFSS data in a variety of ways to identify their health problems so they can develop policies and programs and evaluate efforts. For some examples see the CDC Web site; www.cdc.gov/brfss/dataused.htm.

An interactive mapping application graphically displays the prevalence of behavioral risk factors at the state and metropolitan/micropolitan statistical area (MMSA) level. It is available at the BRFSS Web site www./apps.nccd.cdc.gov/gisbrfss/. Combining GIS mapping technology and BRFSS data, the Web site visually compares prevalence data for states, territories, and local areas. State and MMSA data layers can be displayed independently or combined to form regional patterns.

US Physical Activity Statistics

Physical activity data are derived from the BRFSS. The summaries are at the national and state level as well as for metropolitan areas with at least 500 respondents. The categories rank percentages of adults into those who meet recommended levels of physical activity, those who have insufficient physical activity, those who are inactive, and those who have no leisure physical activity.

5-a-Day Data and Statistics

The 5-a-Day surveillance questions average daily fruit and vegetable consumption. An interactive tool on the Web site www.apps.nccd.cdc.gov/5ADaySurveillance view trends over time and compares each state with others or the nation as a whole.

Fruit and vegetable intake can also be compared to BMI, physical activity, age, race, gender, education, and income.

Selected Metropolitan/Micropolitan Area Risk Trends (SMART)

Due to the increase in BRFSS respondents, CDC is able to perform analysis on smaller geographical areas that meet specific population density criteria. The 2002 BRFSS state data is the first to include SMART BRFSS. This project produced data for 98 MMSAs. It provides health officials and workers with access to local-level data that are comparable across the nation.

Youth Risk Behavior Surveillance System (YRBSS)

The Youth Risk Behavior Surveillance System established in 1990 is a composite of national, state, and local biennial school-based surveys of representative samples of high school students (grades 9-12). CDC conducts the national survey. State and local surveys are conducted by state and local health and education departments. It monitors six categories of health-risk behaviors that significantly contribute to death, disability, and the social problems of youth. These health-risk behaviors include or contribute to tobacco use, food habits, alcohol, and drug use; physical activity; violence and unintentional injuries, and unintended pregnancy and sexually transmitted diseases (STDs). Current YRBS physical activity questions measure factors related to physical activity participation (including moderate-intensity, vigorous-intensity, and muscle strengthening and flexibility), physical education class attendance and availability, and television viewing habits. Nutrition-related questions include consumption of milk, fruits, and vegetables. Self-descriptions of weight status and weight control efforts such as exercise, restricting intake of fat, skipping meals, taking diet pills, using laxatives, or vomiting are also asked. Survey results are published in the CDC's *Morbidity & Mortality Weekly Report* and are online at the CDC.

YRBSS: Youth Online

This Web site (www.apps.nccd.cdc.gov/yrbss/) presents the results of the Youth Risk Behavior Survey for each year since 1991. The data can be viewed in several ways: individual questions within each health topic; by national, state, or local level; or as comparisons, as in one location and two survey years, two locations for all health topics and selected years, or all locations for each risk behavior and selected years.

Global School-Based Student Health Survey (GSHS)

The Global School-Based Student Health Survey, www.cdc.gov/gshs, is a school-based survey developed by the World Health Organization (WHO) in collaboration with United Nations' UNICEF, UNESCO, and UNAIDS, with technical assistance from CDC. The survey is conducted primarily among students aged 13–15 years. GSHS uses core, core-expanded, and country-specific questions in a self-administered questionnaire similar to the YRBSS. Topic areas include dietary behaviors, physical activity, tobacco use, sexual behaviors, violence and unintentional injury, as well as others comparable to the YRBSS.

Pediatric Nutrition Surveillance System (PedNSS)

PedNSS is a program-based surveillance system. States submit data to the CDC collected from health, nutrition, and food assistance programs for infants and children. The 2003 data, represented nearly 5,100,000 children, mainly participants in Special Supplemental Nutrition Program for Women, Infants, and Children (WIC 81%); Early Periodic Screening, Diagnosis and Treatment (EPSDT 11%); clinics funded by Maternal and Child Health Program (MCH block grants 3%) and other sources 5%. Data items include age, gender, race/ethnicity, geographic location, birth weight, height/length and weight, hemoglobin and/or hematocrit, and initiation and duration of breast-feeding. In 2004 race/ethnicity items were revised to comply with the 1997 Office of Management and Budget revised government-wide standards for collection of data on race and ethnicity. WIC Program descriptor for race/ethnicity allows reporting one ethnic and two racial categories for each participant. An optional contributor-specific race/ethnicity description such as Korean or Vietnamese permits PedNSS contributors to target particular groups in their PedNSS analysis. Household size and income, migrant status, food assistance program participation, and infant age at which food other than breast milk was introduced were included. Also asked was TV viewing time of children two years of age or older and smoking products used in the household. Calculation of weight status for children two years of age and older are based on the year 2000 CDC growth chart percentiles for BMI-for-age. The 85th to less than 95th percentile (85th to < 95th) category identifies children at risk for overweight; above the 95th percentile ($\geq$ 95th) category identifies children who are overweight. The system has expanded from 5 states in 1972 to 44 states and territories, 7 tribal governments, and the District of Columbia in 2003. Annual results are analyzed at the national, state, county, and local health unit or WIC agency level. The state health department or CDC can provide these reports.

Pregnancy Nutrition Surveillance System (PNSS)

The Pregnancy Nutrition Surveillance System is also a program-based surveillance system. State and territorial health departments and Indian health agencies, submit information to CDC. Of the nearly 730,000 records submitted in 2002, almost 99% were from the WIC Program. The remaining 1% was from other programs. Population items include age, race/ethnicity, education, household size and income, geographic location, migrant status, and food assistance program participation. Client descriptions include WIC enrollment; height; pregravid weight and weight gain during pregnancy; hemoglobin and/or hematocrit; parity and intervals between pregnancies; medical care; smoking households; and alcohol consumption. It also includes the infant's birth weight, if preterm or multiple births, and breast-feeding initiation. Items added in 2004 include the same race/ethnicity descriptors as PedNSS, diabetes or hypertension during pregnancy, and multivitamin use prior to and during pregnancy. PNSS data monitors trends in prenatal risk factors that may predict low birth weight and/or infant mortality. In 2003, this system gathered data in 25 states, one territory, and five tribal governments. Annual results are analyzed at the national, state, county, and local health unit or WIC agency level. State health departments or CDC can provide these reports.

Pregnancy Risk Assessment Monitoring System (PRAMS)

PRAMS started in 1987 to document low birth weight and infant mortality. As with the BRFSS, PRAMS consists of a core set of questions to compare the 31 participating states and ordered state-specific questions to address individual needs. The goal of the PRAMS project is to improve the health status of mothers and their infants and reduce adverse outcomes such as low birth weight, infant mortality and morbidity, and maternal morbidity. PRAMS provide state-specific data to plan and assess health programs and describe maternal experiences that may contribute to improved maternal and infant health. This monitoring system collects state-specific, population-based data on maternal attitudes, risk factors, and experiences prior to, during, and immediately following pregnancy. Questions explore breast-feeding, smoking, alcoholic beverage use, physical abuse, unintended pregnancy, prenatal care, infant health, and knowledge of the benefits of folic acid. PRAMS participants are a sample of women who have had a recent live birth and are drawn from the state's birth certificate file. Examples of PRAMS data use by states is provided on CDC's Reproductive Health Web site www.cdc/gov/reproductivehealth/srv_prams_examples.htm.

National Immunization Survey (NIS)

Since 1994, CDC has conducted the National Immunization Survey (NIS) in all states, the District of Columbia, and selected geographic areas within the states. The NIS has two parts—the household telephone survey and the vaccination provider survey. It collects information on vaccination coverage rates for children aged 19 to 35 months. The addition of breast-feeding questions were piloted in 2001 and became part of the 2003 household telephone survey for all participants. NIS results provide national estimates for the initiation, duration, and exclusivity of breast-feeding by sociodemographic characteristics and by geographically specific areas. Tables and maps can be accessed on the CDC NIS Web site www.cdc.gov/breastfeeding/NIS_data.

School Health Profiles

The School Health Profiles assists state and local education and public health agencies to monitor and assess the status of school health programs and policies of middle/junior and senior high schools. With technical assistance from the CDC, state and local education and health agencies conduct the survey biennially. The confidential, voluntary questionnaires are mailed to the principals and the school's lead health education teacher. Data is collected on school health education curricula; the physical education curriculum; asthma management activities; school health policies related to tobacco-use prevention, violence prevention, HIV/AIDS prevention, physical activity, and nutrition and food service; and family and community involvement in schools. Nutrition and food service questions include policies related to and items sold at school stores, snack bars, canteens, and vending machines. Physical education questions include requirements and exemptions, intramural sports, and use of school facilities for community-sponsored sports teams or physical activity programs. Reports are available from CDC online at www.cdc.gov/HealthyYouth/profiles. State specific data is in the tables at the end of the reports.

State and Local Area Integrated Telephone Survey (SLAITS)

The State and Local Area Integrated Telephone Survey (SLAITS), www.cdc.gov/nchs/slaits.htm, was developed by the National Center for Health Statistics (NCHS). It collects health care data at state and local levels. It supplements current national data collection providing in-depth state and local area data. Funding is provided through sponsorship from government agencies and non-profit organizations for specific questionnaire modules. Among the questions in the 2003 National Survey of Children's Health SLAITS module are items on breast-feeding practices, meals eaten together as a family group, and physical activities of the children and their parents.

US DEPARTMENT OF AGRICULTURE (USDA)

The US Department of Agriculture administers and funds many of the food and nutrition programs and provides reports and statistics on program participation, food consumption, food expenditures, and areas of agriculture production.

USDA Food Assistance Programs Map Machines

Food Stamp Program (FSP) Map Machine

The Food Stamp Program Map Machine is an interactive mapping program that shows Food Stamp Program participation and benefits by county, state, and national levels. The maps provide both pictorial and tabulated data on per capita participation, per capita benefits, per capita poverty, monitor changes over time, and average benefits.

Summer Food Service Program (SFSP) Map Machine

The Summer Food Service Map Machine is an interactive mapping program that profiles the SFSP sites by neighborhood, county, state, and national levels. Pictorial illustrations show site locations in relation to areas of child poverty and school locations. Additional parameters can be selected. Tabulated data is available.

Current Population Survey—Food Security Supplement (CPS-FSS)

The CPS-FSS, initiated in 1995, is the source of national and state data on food insecurity and hunger. It is used in USDA's annual reports on household food insecurity. The US Census Bureau conducts the initial Current Population Survey (CPS) for the US Bureau of Labor Statistics. The CPS data include employment, annual income, and other characteristics of the labor force. The annual CPS-FSS questions food security, food expenditures, and use of nutrition and food assistance programs. Data files along with technical documents and questionnaires are available from the US Census Bureau or the Economic Research Service (ERS) of the USDA. To use the raw data, knowledge of the subject matter, survey methods, data format, and data analysis are essential. The compiled data are available online at the ERS-USDA Web site.[11]

WIC Participant and Program Characteristics

The WIC Participant and Program Characteristics reports have been compiled biennially since 1992. Data elements are collected by WIC state management information systems on all individuals enrolled in WIC, not just participants defined by WIC administrative funding regulations or those who actually redeem their vouchers. All states are expected to submit a minimum data set. The state health department, WIC agency, or USDA Food and Nutrition Service Web site shows this information, most of which is included in the CDC pregnancy and pediatric surveillance systems described earlier in this chapter.

The National School Lunch Program (NSLP) and School Breakfast Program

The National School Lunch Program established in 1946 is the federally assisted meal program serving nutritious lunches in public and nonprofit private schools and residential child care institutions. It provides funds and guidelines for nutritionally balanced, low-cost or free lunches to children each school day. The School Breakfast Program assists states to offer nonprofit breakfast programs in schools and residential child care institutions. State-level information on the number of participating students can be found at the USDA's Food and Nutrition Service Web site or by the state's education or agriculture agency. Local school districts must keep records of student participation for their specific programs.

Older American Nutrition Program

This nutrition program is authorized under Title III and Title VI of the Older Americans Act and administered by the Administration on Aging of the federal Department of Health and Human Services (see Chapter 10). It provides grants to support congregate meals and home-delivered meals to eligible older people throughout the country. Its purpose is to improve the nutrient intakes of participants with meals and nutrition education. Nutrition assessment and counseling services are also available. For information on the number of older adults participating in each state, contact the state's Agency on Aging.

PUBLIC HEALTH FOUNDATION (PHF)

The Public Health Foundation (PHF) is the national nonprofit organization that enhances and builds the infrastructure of the public health system through research, training, and technical assistance. Assessment tool kits to enhance performance management and *Healthy People 2010* objectives are available at their Web site www.phf.org/index.htm.

OTHER SURVEYS

In addition to the federal-state collaborative systems, some health state departments, university schools of public health, health policy organizations, and institutes conduct surveys specific to their mission. Survey results, questionnaires, and their data collection tools may be available. Examples include the University of California Los Angeles, UCLA's California Health Interview Survey www.chis.ucla.edu/chis_questionnaires.html, the Public Health Institute's California High School Fast-Food Survey, www.phi.org/pdf-library/fastfoodsurvey2003.pdf, and the California Department of Health Service's California Dietary Practices Survey, www.dhs.ca.gov/cpns/research/rea_surveys.htm.

Other states, such as the Arkansas Center for Health Improvement has BMI-for-age percentiles for all of the public school children and reports for school districts and the state, www.achi.net. The South Dakota Department of Health has height and weight data on their school-age children available at www.state.sd.us/doh/Stats/index.htm. North Carolina's Division of Public Health has a Nutrition and Physical Activity Surveillance System (NC-NPASS).

LOCAL PROGRAMS

Within the Department of Health and Human Services (DHHS) Health Resources and Services Administration (HRSA), the Maternal and Child Health Bureau (MCHB) funds many maternal and child health services including nutrition services. States submit data on key measures of maternal and child health as part of their annual Title V Social Security Act Block Grant application, www.performance.hrsa.gov/mchb/mchreports/Search/program/prgmenu.asp. The information on mothers, other women of reproductive age, infants, children, and children with special health care needs compares each state to national performance and outcome measures, www.performance.hrsa.gov/mchb/mchreports/Search/core/corsch01p.asp. It lists state performance and outcome measures. An example of national performance measure is the number of mothers who breast-feed their infants at hospital discharge and how long they continue. Most states report on at least one measure relating to diet and physical activity, including children who are overweight or obese. The reports may also include prenatal folic acid intake, prenatal weight gain, baby-bottle tooth decay, breast-feeding duration, fruit and vegetable consumption, and/or food security. Go to www.performance.hrsa.gov/mchb/ mchreports/Search/neg/negmenu.asp.

Health care utilization and access data items are summarized by national total, each HRSA region, and each state. Categories include numbers of women, infants, and children served; the payment source for services, such as Medicaid (Social Security Act Title XIX), State Children's Health Insurance Program (CHIP, or Title XXI), private or other coverage; or no insurance. Number of deliveries and infants served by Title V and eligible for Medicaid are further subdivided by race and ethnicity. Additionally, the number of infants' screened for metabolic errors such as phenylketonuria, congenital hypothyroidism, galactosemia, and sickle cell disease are tabulated. The number of screenings performed for each condition is related to the total number of births to determine the percentage of newborns screened, number of cases found, and treated.

States health agencies also report health systems capacity indicators that are considered key indicators of maternal and child health systems and their program capacity. Indicators list selected services, use of these services, and health outcomes compared to the total state Medicaid and SCHIP populations, with outcome data linked to capacity.

Comparing the various services, screening, and capacity categories measures program utilization and effectiveness, such as when comparing the data item number of pregnant women receiving Medicaid who entered prenatal care in the first trimester from the MCHB health capacity indicator list to the number from the WIC Participant Characteristic Survey. Do the numbers match? Could either or both programs provide information and referrals to enhance their participants' access to services and health outcomes?

Research suggests that breast-fed infants are at reduced risk of becoming overweight later in life. This suggests that an early intervention for an obesity-prevention program might promote and support breast-feeding. Compare the state breast-feeding performance measure goal and prevalence to both the state-specific breast-feeding rates from the National Immunization Survey to the percentage of infants ever breast-fed in the WIC program. Where are the rates the lowest? Where is action needed? This data can be accessed through the MCH Title V Information System (TVIS) Web site at www.performance.hrsa.gov/mchb/mchreports/Search/search.asp or by contacting the state health department.

Creating an annotated list of data resources is a useful tool for current and future activities. It can also be shared with colleagues, coalition members, and other partners.

Collect New Data

Gathering new data to plan new and available interventions, write reports, assess service cost-effectiveness, and other aspects of program management is costly and time consuming. The first step is to check availability and usefulness of existing information. If new data is needed, a statistician or epidemiologist should be appointed to the survey team. A survey is only as good as the quality of the data it collects. Herold and Peavy in *Field Epidemiology* emphasize the need for a detailed protocol or plan before any survey is started.[12] Each step of the survey requires careful thought and planning. The survey sample design and size depend on the budget and the plan for analysis. The sample size affects the analysis and type of survey. The type of survey influences the length and format of the questionnaire, which is limited by the budget. The main sections of the survey protocol includes the measurable objectives, methods, analysis plan, implementation logistics, budget, and timeline. The protocol checklist includes specific survey steps, completion deadlines, and responsible persons (see Table 16–7). This checklist can be expanded to include more detail.

Health Insurance Portability and Accountability Act (HIPAA)

The Health Insurance Portability and Accountability Act (HIPAA) was enacted in 1996. Its regulations restrict use and disclosure of health information, lists consumer rights, and imposes penalties and redress for misuse of the information. A summary of this act is available from CDC at www.cdc.gov/privacyrule/privacy-HIPAAfacts.htm. When planning to collect new data it is important to check with the agency's interpretation and use of HIPAA. The health agency also

Table 16–7 Survey Steps Checklist

Steps	Planned Completion	Responsible Person(s)
1. Develop survey objective(s).		
2. Determine information to be collected.		
3. Select survey type.		
4. Develop questionnaire; pretest and revise as needed.		
5. Design and select sample.*		
6. Train interviewers (if needed for survey type).*		
7. Collect data.*		
8. Enter data and edit.*		
9. Analyze data.*		
10. Write report.		
11. Present report.		

*Provide for quality assurance monitoring.
Source: Carole Garner, Arkansas Department of Health.

may have its own internal review board (IRB). Any interventions and/or data collection must include signed participant consent forms.

Methods to Collect Data

Data collection methods include person-to-person interviews, self-administered surveys, and chart reviews. Person-to-person techniques include face-to-face interviews and telephone surveys. Self-administered designs include mailed questionnaires; electronic mail surveys; interactive voice response to taped telephone messages[13]; in-person individual and group self-assessments; magazine, journal and newsletter polls; and online surveys. Each data collection method has advantages and disadvantages relative to cost, potential bias, and questionnaire format and response rate.

A key advantage of face-to-face interviews is a high response rate. Questionnaire format may be more complex and tailored to each respondent by incorporating filter questions and skip questions. With computer-based questionnaires, prompts can be incorporated to assist the interviewer elicit more specific answers. Disadvantages of face-to-face interviews include the costs of interviewers' salaries and training and the potential for interviewer bias.[14]

Telephone surveys are quicker and cost less than face-to-face interviews but tend to have a lower response rate. Technological advances allow for an alternative to the use of a "live" interviewer. Touch-tone data entry (TDE) and interactive voice response (IVR) incorporate prerecorded questions, answer categories, and response instructions. As with other survey methods, TDE and IVR each have disadvantages that include question clarity and speed of question sequence. The public's displeasure with telephone solicitations is shown by the growth of "Do not call" lists. Cooperation of the public to telephone and mailed surveys has also declined. Developing the list to select the sample can be a problem. Although most households have phones, increasingly those are cell phones rather than land-lines. Cell phones may or may not be linked to physical addresses. Of those households that still use landlines, not all are listed, and others are listed multiple times with lines for children or dedicated to facsimile machines. Some biases also arise related to segments of the population who cannot afford a phone or do not choose to have one.

Mail surveys are the least expensive way to collect new data. Along with less cost generally comes lower response rate. Techniques that may improve response rate are respondent-friendly questionnaires, multiple contacts, personalized corre-spondence, and offering incentives.[15] Sources for addresses to mail surveys to the general population are commonly not complete. Problems with telephone direc-tory listings are noted above. Motor vehicle departments have lists of licensed drivers, but not everyone has a driver license. Private companies develop lists for their corporate uses such as niche marketing. They may combine several informa-tion sources. These might be the two examples cited plus credit card lists, mem-bership lists, real estate lists, subscription lists, and pet license lists. These compilations may sometimes be useful for public health surveys. Targeting spe-cific groups rather than the general public may yield more complete lists and bet-ter returns.

Electronic survey methods offer many advantages ranging from decreased costs of printing and mailing questionnaires to easier and less data entry time to implement. Web surveys add the advantages of providing visual stimulation with color, animation, and sound. They also offer interactive formats. However, ques-tionnaires posted on Web sites or distributed via e-mail are limited to use by pop-ulations that have access to a computer with the required operating system(s), have computer skills to complete the survey, and trust the security of the data transmis-sion. These limitations may decrease as technology improves and becomes more accessible.

In *Mail and Internet Surveys* Dillman addresses the strengths and weaknesses of alternative questionnaire delivery.[16] Group administration has the advantages of reduced costs and minimizes no responses. By contrast, the incorporation of a questionnaire into a publication, such as a newsletter or magazine, tends to result in lower response rates and greater response bias.

Periodic systematic review of client charts and the recorded data are useful to develop and evaluate a program plan. This data relates to the individuals served by the agency clinic or program, but does not apply to the population at large.

HIPAA regulations govern what information may be extracted and by whom. Although client charts usually follow a specified format, retrospective analysis may run into problems, such as missing data.

Develop the Questionnaire

When developing a questionnaire there are several considerations, including the specific information needed, the method to be used to analyze the data, and the type of survey to use to collect the data. Questions should be objective, concise, understandable, and have a clear time reference. The sequence of questions places strategic, sensitive questions along with buffer questions.[17] Question format can be closed ended, such as multiple choices or true/false. Open-ended questions allow respondents to reply in their own words. Interviewer-assisted questionnaires can be precoded and open ended.[18] Page layout also influences responses to the questionnaire. Print should be clear, easy to follow, and well spaced. The final draft of the questionnaire should be pretested with individuals from the population to be surveyed to check their understanding of questions, question flow, and ease for them to complete. Necessary adjustments can then be made before launching the full survey.

Sample Selection

For the program management plan, the objectives of the survey guide the selection of the sampling method. A complete or census type survey may be used when the study group is relatively small. A sample may be used when the population is larger. When the objective is to document time allocation for 35 clinic staff members, it is feasible to collect data from all of the staff. When the objective is to determine the physical activity levels of employees at a large work site, a sample of the population is the practical option.

The easiest method is to use a convenience sample, selecting individuals who are easy to reach and within close proximity. However, the characteristics of this convenience sample may not reflect the characteristics of the larger group of which they are a part. A survey of women attending a WIC clinic questioned about the benefits and barriers they perceive to breast-feeding their infants would provide information that could be used for an intervention with women who attend that clinic. However, it may not reflect the attitudes of women in the area who do not choose to participate in WIC. The use of a convenience sample is inherently biased, and while it may help explore ideas or opinions, it cannot be used to draw conclusions about the population as a whole.

With random sampling, everyone on the population list has an equal chance to be selected. A newer way to select the individuals to survey is to use a computer program that numbers and randomly selects the respondents. If the entire population cannot be listed or if simple random sampling does not provide sufficient numbers of individuals in subgroups, additional sampling techniques can be used, such as cluster sampling and stratified sampling.[19] Statisticians at the health department or local university can be knowledgeable consultants.

Data Entry

The quality and completeness of the data entered for analysis affects the reliability of the survey results. Before any data is keyed or scanned into a computer, the questionnaires must be reviewed for completeness, clarity, and acceptability. Software, such as Epi Info, edits data as it is entered. The questionnaire becomes the data entry screen, avoiding the need to code responses before entry. In addition, allowable code ranges can be set for the questions such as preschoolers' height of 31–46 inches or requiring an alpha code of a yes/no answer. For other types of keyed analysis programs, responses must be coded prior to entry. Interviewer-assisted questionnaires such as the Behavioral Risk Factor Surveillance System are precoded to assist with data entry (see Table 16–8). Self-administered questionnaires are generally coded after the respondent's complete the questionnaire to avoid a cluttered, confusing appearance of the form. Periodic comparisons of sample questionnaires with entered data can catch miskeyed items.

Scanning questionnaires into an analysis program may be as cost-effective as paying for keyed data entry. Local universities and businesses may provide this service for a fee. Advantages include the ability of multiple people to view the scanned questionnaires at the same time and not needing to code the questions.

Data Analysis

The objectives developed in the survey protocol guide the choice of data analysis methods to be used to describe the population or program. For example, an intervention aimed at heart disease prevention assesses local milk consumption. The survey includes a question to determine overall milk consumption with the analysis addressing the average number of people who drink milk, the frequently occurring observation, and the standard distribution. Another question determines the type of milk with responses analyzed by grouping percentages of respondents who use whole, reduced-fat, low-fat, or fat-free milks. A third question may ask about the quantity with the hypothesis that whole milk is consumed by most people. This theory can be addressed with a contingency table. The statistician or epidemiologist on the survey team can provide consultation in analysis selection and calculation.

Table 16–8   Example of a Precoded Survey Tool

Section 18: Physical Activity

If "employed" or "self-employed" to core Q14.8 continue. Otherwise, go to Q18.2.

18.1   When you are at work, which of the following best describes what you do?
Would you say?

(173)

If respondent has multiple jobs, include all jobs.

Please read:

1   Mostly sitting or standing
2   Mostly walking

Or

3   Mostly heavy labor or physically demanding work

Do not read:

7   Don't know/Not sure
9   Refused

We are interested in two types of physical activity—vigorous and moderate. Vigorous
activities cause large increases in breathing or heart rate while moderate activities cause
small increases in breathing or heart rate.

18.2   Now, thinking about the moderate activities you do **[fill in "when you are not
working," if "employed" or "self-employed"]** in a usual week, do you do
moderate activities for at least 10 minutes at a time, such as brisk walking,
bicycling, vacuuming, gardening, or anything else that causes some increase in
breathing or heart rate?

(174)

1   Yes
2   No   **[Go to Q18.5]**
7   Don't know/Not sure   **[Go to Q18.5]**
9   Refused   **[Go to Q18.5]**

18.3   How many days per week do you do these moderate activities for at least 10
minutes?

(175–176)

— —   Days per week
7 7   Don't know/Not sure   **[Go to Q18.5]**
8 8   Do not do any moderate physical activity for at least 10 minutes
         at a time
                                        [Go to Q18.5]
9 9   Refused   **[Go to Q18.5]**

Source: Behavioral Risk Factor Survey: Centers for Disease Control and Prevention, National Center
for Health Statistics.

Reporting

The decision to gather specific information was based on the reason the information was needed. The protocol includes written objectives and procedures. To ensure the objectives are met and data is shared, a report must be presented orally, in writing or both. The method and style of the report should keep the audience in mind. The results should propose recommendations that are clear and easy to understand.

Collection, analysis, and interpretation of data must be communicated effectively. To summarize the data, the report can include numbers and rates to document the health condition in any one or combination of three dimensions: time, place, and person. Time refers to change in occurrence and is usually displayed graphically. Place shows boundaries, which can be illustrated with maps. Person data appears as tables or graphs and includes demographics and other personal characteristics.[20] Figure 16–2 shows obesity data in each of these three ways. Software programs are available to easily create charts, tables, and maps. These might allow for the insertion of photographs and creation of presentations and production of text documents.

COLLECT DIETARY DATA

To collect dietary information, several options are available. Each option offers preferred uses and related advantages and disadvantages. The traditional 24-hour diet recall documents the variety of foods and actual amounts eaten by each individual on one or more specific days. In contrast, food frequencies record individual intake over an extended period.

The 24-hour dietary recall relies on the respondent's short-term memory and the skills of the interviewer to obtain complete and accurate information. The period relates to the day of the interview from either midnight to midnight of the previous day or the immediate past 24 hours. To improve portion size estimates, illustrative tools are used, such as standard-sized measuring cups or spoons; standard-sized bowls, glasses; food models; or two-dimensional drawings, photographs, and geometric shapes. The open-ended recall allows for any food or food combination consumed and can capture culturally diverse food items. Standardized measures can be used with low-literacy populations. The USDA developed the multiple-pass 24-hour dietary recall to limit the amount of underreporting that often occurs with self-reported food intake. This method consists of five steps: a "quick list" of everything eaten the previous day; a "forgotten list" using interviewer probes; a "time and occasion" check on when and where the food was eaten; a "detailed cycle" specific to each food and portion size; and last a "final review probe."[21] This multiple-pass 24-hour dietary recall has been shown to provide similar results if administered face-to-face or by telephone.[22]

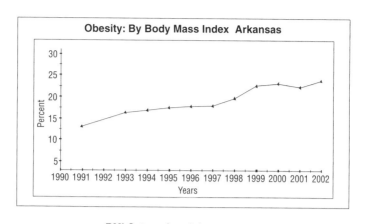

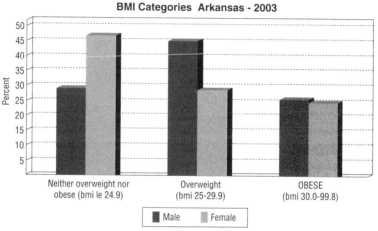

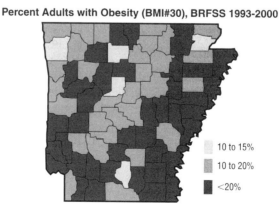

Figure 16–2 Obesity data for Arkansas, Trends 1991–2002, prevalence by Gender 2003 and County Specific (1993–2000). *Source:* Centers for Disease Control and Prevention (CDC). *Behavioral Risk Factor Surveillance System Survey Data.* Atlanta, Georgia: U.S. Department of Health and Human Services, Centers for Disease Control and Prevention, 2002.

The food record does not rely on memory. It requires a literate, motivated respondent. Typically the written record is kept for three to seven days and often requests the respondent to measure and record serving sizes. Bias may be introduced when the recording of intake leads respondents to change their usual food choices and amounts.

Food frequency questionnaires (FFQ) consist of a food list, a section to note how often the food is eaten, and another section for the amount. The list of foods must be specific to cultural food habits of the population. Several proprietary questionnaires such as the Block98 and Willett FFQs have been developed and modified for use in research studies. As with the 24-hour diet recall, the FFQ uses self-reported information, which tends to be underreported. Though some FFQs have been validated for use with adults, their use with children have been questioned.[23,24] Development of specific FFQs for youth continues,[25] and review of newer research may provide useful examples.

The National Cancer Institute's Diet History Questionnaire (DHQ) is a food frequency questionnaire developed in 1998 and validated by the Eating at America's Table Study (EATS).[26] A Spanish translation of the DHQ and an updated version was completed in 2002. A sample can be downloaded from the NCI Web site at www.riskfactor.cancer.gov/DHQ/forms. The format varies depending on the computer-assisted interviews method of analysis, scanning, and data entry. DHQ options include file formats designed for specific scanners. Diet*Calc PC software is available at no cost. The analysis package generates nutrient and food group intake estimates.

Collect Physical Activity Data

Traditionally, nutritionists have focused on food intakes of individuals and populations. The epidemic of obesity and increasing awareness of the need for overall healthy lifestyles broadens that perspective to also include physical activity. Multiple tools to assess physical activity have potential problems with validity, reliability, and sensitivity. A literature review by Shepard assessed questionnaires of type, intensity, frequency, and duration of physical activity.[27] Recommendations include developing standardized instruments to account for low intensity of activities and to use consistent definitions for light, moderate, and heavy exercise.

Commonly used questionnaires include recalls of 24-hour physical activity and 7- to 30-day records. As with food intake, weekdays and weekends differ, and memory influences reliability of recall. In addition to the surveys noted earlier that include physical activity questions, others used in various research studies include the Stanford Seven-Day Physical Activity Recall,[28] the EPIC Physical Activity Questionnaire,[29] the Yale Physical Activity Survey for Older Adults,[30] and the Self-Administered Physical Activity Checklist (SAPAC).[31] Each questionnaire has advantages and limitations to consider before deciding if it is useful and appropriate.

Does the built environment offer safe places to walk or play? Some tools developed and assessed for reliability measure social and physical environment characteristics that support physical activity.[32] These include the Neighborhood Environment Walkability Survey from San Diego, the South Carolina instrument, and the St. Louis instrument.

Software and Online Services

CDC has a variety of free software programs to use in program management. Some of these software systems help with community assessment and evaluation of intervention. Others assist with analyzing personnel use and client time in clinic settings.

Epi Info

Epi Info is a software program that records and organizes epidemiologic information on a computer. It includes word processing, a database, and a statistical system. The forms and questionnaires are also in the format through which the data is entered. As the forms and questionnaires are developed, the software automatically creates a database. The analysis component can produce lists, frequencies, tables, statistics, graphs, and charts. One of the features is NutStat, a nutrition anthropometry program that calculates percentiles and z-scores using the 2000 CDC growth chart reference. Epi Map displays numeric data in relation to geographic map boundaries.

In addition to Epi Info, other descriptive statistic software packages include Statistical Programs for the Social Sciences (SPSS) and Statistical Analysis System (SAS).

Patient Flow Analysis (PFA)

Patient Flow Analysis (PFA) is a computer application that documents personnel use and patient flow in health service clinics. It provides clinic managers with data and graphics of a clinic session. Managers can use the data to identify problems in patient flow, determine personnel and space needs, and document personnel costs per patient visit.

Food Intake Analysis System (FIAS)

Food and nutrient analysis of 24-hour dietary recalls and food records can be complicated. When selecting a nutrient analysis program, it must suit program needs and have a quality nutrient database.[33] Programs may vary in the research used to support the nutrient database, the number of food items included, and number of nutrients for each food item. Some features allow the addition of recipes and the entry of portions in various formats from ounces to food-specific units such as "slice." Two nutrient analysis programs cited in several nutrition research articles are described here. Others are also available.

The Food Intake Analysis System (FIAS), developed by the University of Texas School of Public Health, Human Nutrition Center, is a nutritient analysis software package designed to analyze individual food records or 24-hour dietary recalls. The FIAS system includes nutritional analysis programs, nutrient data files, sample food intake and recipe forms, as well as reproducible selected two-dimensional food models. The FIAS Survey Nutrient Data Base (Survey NDB) was developed by the USDA Agriculture Research Service and was used for the 1998 USDA Continuing Survey of Food Intakes by Individuals (CSFII).

Nutrition Data System (NDS)

The University of Minnesota Nutrition Coordinating Center first released the Nutrition Data System (NDS) DOS-based system in 1988. A Windows-based version was made available in 1998. The software calculates the nutrients for individual 24-hour dietary recalls, food records, or menus, and recipes. This NDS uses the USDA database and addresses market changes by updating nutrient values as published. It contains over 18,000 foods, and 8000 brand name food products.

Proprietary online survey programs allow the users to design their surveys, collect the responses, and analyze results. The design tools offer a variety of question types such as single or multiple choice, as well as rating scales. Designs include skip logic options and other customizing features. Results may be analyzed and displayed as data tables, charts, and/or graphs in addition to raw data exportability to various analytical programs. Features, accessibility, and cost vary. Check online for the many available programs such as *Survey Monkey, SurveyCrafter, Active Websurvey, Zoomerang,* and *Infopol.*

Use of appropriate data is essential to develop, evaluate, maintain, and expand effective public health nutrition programs. Technological advances improve the approaches to obtain, assess, and present information. When trying to fill in the gaps between existing data and data needed to update and expand program efforts, it can be cost-effective to consult with a statistician or expert knowledgeable in survey design, sampling, and analysis.

POINTS TO PONDER

- Are there a core set of data items applicable to all public health nutrition programs, or are programs too specialized to be able to use a generic base?

- Are expectations of data accuracy beyond the scope of currently available collection and analysis tools?
- Do public health nutritionists views of the value of data mesh with those of their public health colleagues and policy makers?

HELPFUL WEB SITES

California Health Interview Survey: www.chis.ucla.edu
California High School Fast Food Survey:
    www.phi.org/pdf-library/fastfoodsurvey2003.pdf
California Department of Health Service's Cancer Prevention and Nutrition Section (CPNS) Statewide Surveys:
    www.dhs.ca.gov/cpns/research/rea_surveys.htm
CDC Overweight and Obesity – Obesity Trends:
    www.cdc.gov/nccdphp/dnpa/obesity/trend/index.htm
CDC Diabetes Public Health Resource – Diabetes Maps:
    www.cdc.gov/diabetes/statistics/maps/index.htm
CDC Behavioral Risk Factor Surveillance System:
    www.cdc.gov/brfss/dataused.htm
CDC Behavioral Risk Factor Surveillance System Maps:
    apps.nccd.cdc.gov/gisbrfss
CDC Global School-Based Student Health Survey: www.cdc.gov/gshs
CDC Healthy Youth – School Health Policies:
    www.cdc.gov/HealthyYouth/ profiles
CDC HIPAA Basic Facts: www.cdc.gov/privacyrule/privacy-HIPAAfacts.htm
CDC National Center for Health Statistics – State and Local Area Integrated Telelphone Survey: www.cdc.gov/nchs/slaits.htm
Center For Science in the Public Interest – Improve School Foods:
    www.cspinet.org/schoolfoods
FedStats: www.fedstats.gov
Public Health Foundation: www.phf.org/index.htm
South Dakota Department of Health – Health Statistics:
    www.state.sd.us/doh/Stats/index.htm

NOTES

1. Doyle AC, *The Adventures of Sherlock Holmes, "Scandal in Bohemia,"* (1892). Cited in *The Columbia World of Quotations.* 1996. Available at: http://www.bartleby.com/66/68/17668.html. Accessed July 9, 2004.

2. US Census Bureau. Census Overview. Available at: http://factfinder.census.gov/jsp/saff/SAFFInfo.jsp?_pageId=gn6_datasets_intro. Accessed July 7, 2004.

3. US Census Bureau. State and County Quick Facts. Available at: http://quickfacts.census.gov/qfd/. Accessed July 7, 2004.

4. US Census Bureau. Access Data by Geography – Street Address search link. Available at: http://factfinder.census.gov/servlet/AGSGeoAddressServlet?_lang=en&_programYear=50&_treeId=420&_sse=on. Accessed July 7, 2004.

5. US Census Bureau. American Community Survey. Available at: http://factfinder.census.gov/jsp/saff/SAFFInfo.jsp?_pageId=sp1_acs. Accessed July 7, 2004.

6. US Census Bureau. Population Estimates Program. Available at: http://factfinder.census.gov/jsp/saff/SAFFInfo.jsp?_pageId=sp3_pop_est. Accessed July 7, 2004.

7. Willett W. *Nutritional Epidemiology*. 2nd ed. New York, NY: Oxford University Press; 1998:349.

8. McCann BA, Ewing R. Measuring the health effects of sprawl: a national analysis of physical activity, obesity, and chronic disease. *Smart Growth America*. September 2003. Available at: http://www.smartgrowthamerica.org. Accessed April 12, 2004.

9. Probert KL, ed. *Moving to the Future: Developing Community-Based Nutrition Services* [Electronic version]. Washington, DC: Association of State and Territorial Public Health Nutrition Directors; 1996.

10. Gregg MB, ed. *Field Epidemiology*. 2nd ed. New York, NY: Oxford University Press; 2002:136–137.

11. Economic Research Service Briefing Room. Food security in the United States: recommended readings. USDA Available at: http://www.ers.usda.gov/briefing/FoodSecurity/readings.htm. Accessed June 26, 2004.

12. Gregg MB, ed. *Field Epidemiology*. 2nd ed. New York, NY: Oxford University Press; 2002:197.

13. Dillman D. *Mail and Internet Surveys*. New York, NY: John Wiley & Sons; 2000:6.

14. Gregg MB, ed. *Field Epidemiology*. 2nd ed. New York, NY: Oxford University Press; 2002:198.

15. Dillman D. *Mail and Internet Surveys*. New York, NY: John Wiley & Sons; 2000:193.

16. Dillman D. *Mail and Internet Surveys*. New York, NY: John Wiley & Sons; 2000:245–262.

17. Brookmeyer R, Stroup DF, eds. *Monitoring the Health of Populations: Statistical Principles and Methods for Public Health Surveillance*. New York, NY: Oxford University Press; 2004:63–65.

18. Gregg MB, ed. *Field Epidemiology*. 2nd ed. New York, NY: Oxford University Press; 2002:199–200.

19. Dillman D. *Mail and Internet Surveys*. New York, NY: John Wiley & Sons; 2000:210–211.

20. Gregg MB, ed. *Field Epidemiology*. 2nd ed. New York, NY: Oxford University Press; 2002:107.

21. Johnson RK. Dietary intake—how do we measure what people are really eating? *Obesity Research*. 2002;10(Suppl 1):63S–68S.

22. Tran KM, Johnson RK, Soultanakis RB, Matthews, DE. In-person vs telephone-administered multiple-pass 24-hour recalls in women: validation with doubly labeled water. *J Am Diet Assoc*. 2000;100:777–783.

23. Wilson AMR, Lewis RD. Disagreement of energy and macronutrient intakes estimated from a food frequency questionnaire and 3-day diet record in girls 4 to 9 years of age. *J Am Diet Assoc.* 2004;104:373–378.

24. Kaskoun MC, Johnson RK, Goran MI. Comparison of energy intake by semiquantitative food-frequency questionnaire with total energy expenditure by the doubly labeled water method in young children. *Am J Clin Nutr.* 1994;60:43–47.

25. Hoelscher DM, Day RS, Kelder SH, Ward JL. Reproducibility and validity of the secondary level School-Based Nutrition Monitoring student questionnaire. *J Am Diet Assoc.* 2003;103:186–194.

26. Subar AF, Thompson FE, Kipnis V, et al. Comparative validation of the Block, Willett and National Cancer Institute food frequency questionnaires. *Am J Epidemiol.* 2001;154:1089–1099.

27. Shepard RJ. Limits to the measurement of habitual physical activity by questionnaires. *Br J Sports Med.* 2003;37:197–206.

28. Conway JM, Seale JL, Jacobs DR, Irwin ML, Ainsworth BE. Comparison of energy expenditure estimates from doubly labeled water, a physical activity questionnaire, and physical activity records. *Am J Clin Nutr.* 2002;75:519–525.

29. Wareham NJ, Jakes RW, Rennie KL, et al. Validity and repeatability of a simple index derived from the short physical activity questionnaire used in the European Prospective Investigation into Cancer and Nutrition (EPIC) study. *Public Health Nutr.* 2003;6:407–413.

30. Kruskall LJ, Campbell WW, Evans WJ. The Yale Physical Activity Survey for Older Adults: predictions in the energy expenditure due to physical activity. *J Am Diet Assoc.* 2004;104:1251–1257.

31. Sallis JF, Strikmiller PK, Harsha D, Feldman HA. Validation of interviewer- and self-administered physical activity checklists for fifth-grade students. *Med Sci Sports Exerc.* 1996;28:840–851.

32. Brownson RC, Chang JJ, Eyler AA, et al. Measuring the environment for friendliness toward physical activity: a comparison of the reliability of 3 questionnaires. *Am J Public Health.* 2004;94:473–483.

33. Buzzard IM, Price KS, Warren RA. Considerations for selecting nutrient-based calculation software: evaluation of the nutrient database. *Am J Clin Nutr.* 1991;54:7–9.

BIBLIOGRAPHY

Aschengrau A, Seage GR. *Essentials of Epidemiology in Public Health.* Sudbury, Mass: Jones and Bartlett Publishers; 2003.

Brookmeyer R, Stroup DF, eds. *Monitoring the Health of Populations: Statistical Principles and Methods for Public Health Surveillance.* New York, NY: Oxford University Press; 2004.

Brownson RC, Baker EA, Leet TL, Gillespie KN. *Evidenced-Based Public Health.* New York, NY: Oxford University Press; 2003.

Centers for Disease Control and Prevention,. National Center for Health Statistics. *Healthy Women: State Trends in Health and Mortality.* Available at: *http://www.cdc.gov/nchs/ healthywomen.htm.*

Chernick MR, Friis RH. Introductory Biostatistics for the Health Sciences. Hoboken, NJ: John Wiley & Sons; 2003.

Cohen B. *Community Food Security Assessment Toolkit.* Food Assistance & Nutrition Research Program, USDA, ERS E-FAN No, 02-013. July 2002. Available at: http://www.ers.usda.gov/publications/efan02013/.

Gregg MB, ed. *Field Epidemiology.* 2nd ed. New York, NY: Oxford University Press; 2002.

McCann BA, Ewing R. Measuring the health effects of sprawl: a national analysis of physical activity, obesity, and chronic disease. *Smart Growth America.* September 2003. Available at: http://www.smartgrowthamerica.org.

SIP 4-99 Research Group. Environmental supports for physical activity questionnaire. University of South Carolina, Norman J. Arnold School of Public Health, Prevention Research Center. Available at: http://prevention.sph.sc.edu/tools/docs/Env_Supports_for_PA.pdf.

Willett W. *Nutritional Epidemiology.* 2nd ed. New York, NY: Oxford University Press; 1998.

CHAPTER 17

Maximize Available Funds

Katherine A. Cairns

Reader Objectives

- Identify the major sources for funding public health nutrition services.
- Identify and describe major categories for a nutrition program budget.
- Specify four major components of a grant application.
- Understand cost-effectiveness and cost-benefit analyses.
- Identify major sources of third-party reimbursement for public health nutrition services.

FINANCE NUTRITION PROGRAMS AND SERVICES

Organizations, like personal or family budgets, require attention to how much money comes in and where it is spent. Every public health nutritionist who manages a program, service, or project must request, justify, and negotiate a budget, and control expenditures within the funds allocated. Fiscal management means the nutrition program manager must understand the financing and budgeting process and work closely with the following key people in the organization:

- *The agency administrator and board members* set the agency's fiscal policy and determine how the agency budget will be allocated to programs and overhead.
- *The finance/fiscal officer or business manager* maintains accounts, controls expenditures, and advises on the organization's written and unwritten fiscal policies and procedures.
- *Other program directors* request and manage budgets for programs that could and should utilize nutrition services. These directors may want to collaborate in funding nutrition services through their internal funding sources for larger

programmatic reimbursement or collaborating in writing grants to obtain external funding.

Tighter federal, state, and local government agency budgets require nutritionists to compete for the money needed to turn plans for comprehensive nutrition services into action. Convincing a governmental unit or foundation to invest money in nutrition services requires that the value of each proposal be clearly justified. Key questions to address when preparing a budget include the following:

- Are there federal, state or local requirements or mandates for components of the proposed nutrition service?
- Is there really a need for the service? Use data from the needs assessment.
- What are the competing options for the available and new money? The plan, budget, service, product, and their evaluation must stand out from the competition.
- Can cost-effectiveness data be provided for the proposed nutrition service?
- What stakeholder support and contributions are there for the proposal?
- What additional community support and media attention can be generated before, during, and following the funding decisions?
- What support does the competition have for the same funding?
- What potential does the proposed service have to generate income for the agency?
- Are federal or foundation grants available to establish and maintain the service into the future?

Competitive proposals for allocating new or ongoing funds must show evidence of support from individuals and organizations in the community who will benefit from the product or service. They can demonstrate their support by paying fees for services; making in-kind contributions of staff, volunteer time, or space in offices or clinics; writing letters of support; presenting testimony; lobbying proactively; or by donating equipment, materials, or cash contributions.

Networking and interdisciplinary teamwork increase the number of stakeholders committed to community nutrition programs. Financers prefer to fund a service that responds to a demonstrated need that can be met cost-effectively. A well-conceived budget for a new service or product details the cost per unit. Services that are costly to start-up should show a reasonable cost per unit after the start-up and within the first six months of operation. Fiscal managers from the public health agency may ask the following:

- Will the proposed service or product have a reasonable cost-to-benefit ratio? Funders compare the costs and outcomes of varying types of service delivery options.
- Will the service be carried out using the most cost-effective intervention? For example, will reducing anemia in 80% of a population group within six months of diagnosis be less costly if nutrition counseling is provided by a trained and

supervised paraprofessional rather than by a nutritionist? Although the outcome may be the same, the costs of different intervention models may vary.

These and additional questions can be used as a checklist in preparing to request funds needed to initiate the service. Funds for nutrition services may be secured from a variety of sources. The more diverse the funding base, the more stable the program. The more diverse the funding sources used to maintain a public health nutrition program, the less dependent the program is on any one funding source. Single-source funding is a liability during budget reduction cycles. However, maintaining accountability for too many small funding sources ($<$ $10,000) may be time consuming and counterproductive.

Federal Funds

A variety of federal funds are available for use by state, local, and nongovernmental organizations or community-based organizations to operate food and nutrition programs. Federal agencies fund the major food assistance and nutrition service programs and demonstration projects that serve over 80 million Americans. These programs include the following:

- Department of Agriculture (USDA); Food and Nutrition Service
- Department of Health and Human Services (DHHS); Centers for Medicare and Medicaid Services (CMS)
- Department of Health and Human Services (DHHS); Centers for Disease Control and Prevention (CDC)
- Department of Health and Human Services (DHHS); Specific health block grant funds from the Title V, Social Security—Maternal and Child Health

Personal contacts with key administration in each of the major federal or state agencies are useful to obtain advance notice of requests for proposals (RFPs) and special project funding. Publications discussing available grants are listed on the Internet.

State Tax Revenue

State governments generate funds through state income taxes, sales taxes, various types of business taxes, and taxes on such products as alcoholic beverages and cigarettes. In recent years, some states have turned to lotteries and lawsuit settlement proceeds as revenue for public services. Local governmental units (cities or counties) have the authority to tax property owners for municipal services such as police and fire departments, schools, recreation facilities, and public health services. Tax levies are set annually based on the services needed, the priorities of policy makers, the demands of the taxpayers, and outside interests.

Most city, county, or state public health departments derive a portion of their income from this general revenue. Public health agencies generally seek their share of general revenue as a cornerstone of their operating income. There is keen competition for these funds in a health agency since they generally offer programs stable funding. If there is no general revenue in the budget for nutrition services, nutritionists need to discuss this funding source with agency administrators and business managers to prepare their request for future budget cycles. They may need to be persistent and assertive over several years to succeed. Some funding that is not restricted to a specific target population provides flexibility to plan more comprehensive and community-responsive programs identified in the community assessment.

State Grants and Other Funds

State departments of health, health and human services, aging, agriculture, and education usually allocate some funds for select food and nutrition services. The state funds may support statewide and/or local services. In many states a per capita or preestablished formula is used to allocate state and federal funds to local public health agencies. State agencies may have special legislated funding for nutrition programs. State agencies also serve as the conduits for federal funds earmarked for local program implementation. Specific federal project funds that state governmental agencies administer through a grants process include:

- Special Supplemental Nutrition Program for Women, Infants, and Children (WIC)
- Other supplemental food programs for targeted groups (farmer's market, summer food programs, special milk programs, day care programs, school lunch/breakfast programs, congregate dining, senior food program)
- Maternal and child health special projects
- Nutrition education special projects
- Health promotion special projects including obesity and overweight
- Chronic disease intervention and reduction special projects
- Targeted agricultural marketing special projects

Grant application procedures may have specific requirements that must be determined through the local agency administrator, state agency, or regional/central office nutrition consultants.

Contracts and Local Funds

A variety of tax-supported and voluntary local human or social service agencies, home health agencies, area agencies on aging, mental health agencies, developmental disabilities councils, school districts, correctional facilities, and community colleges frequently need nutrition services or have special initiatives or ongoing projects that require nutrition expertise. Agencies that do not budget and employ a full-time nutritionist on their staff often contract these services as the most efficient method for getting the short-term or long-term services they need. Those local agencies that need part-time nutrition services frequently maintain lists or files of available contractors and their specialists. It is important to cultivate contacts with planners and administrators with the local agencies who can advise on their needs, available funding, and interest in developing contracts.

Other voluntary health agencies, such as the heart association, diabetes association, cancer society, cystic fibrosis association, obesity association, or March of Dimes chapter or affiliate offices, also may need and contract for nutrition services or offer small competitive project grants. For short-term community projects, sometimes funds may be obtained from local businesses, banks, civic organizations, or churches.

Foundation Funds

Millions of dollars of private foundation projects are funded annually for specific priorities. The Internet is the most valuable resource for identifying these foundation funders. Foundation and grant information centers maintain information on the following:

- Names and contact persons for local, state, regional, or national foundations
- Information on past funding priorities and projects funded
- Dollar amount of awards for foundation projects
- Criteria and format for submitting funding requests
- Timeline for review of grant requests

Priorities of foundations change annually. Consequently, putting a new twist on an old idea or need may be required for the foundation to consider the proposal. Some foundations prefer that proposals be submitted on behalf of a nongovernmental, nonprofit agency. Nutritionists employed by a government health agency who seek a foundation grant might collaborate with a nonprofit agency that will submit the proposal and subcontract the professional nutrition work to the public health agency nutrition staff.

Charge Fees for Services

Recovering program costs through fees, adjusted for each target population, is another method to finance programs. A basic market analysis is useful to determine the range of fees appropriate to charge the various target populations or agencies. Fees must be based on actual costs, not guesswork. In presenting a plan to establish fees to administrators, government officials, the public, and coworkers, three alternatives might be offered:

- *Sliding scale fee-for-service*—The fee is based on the client's ability to pay, with the maximum fee being the actual cost of the service; this can be used for basic public health services.
- *Actual cost fee-for-service*—The actual cost of providing a service is calculated and is revised annually. It is charged for public health services where there are other private and nonprofit providers of the services within a community; a governmental provider does not put these service charges on a sliding scale due to the potential legal issues of unfair competition. A public agency will by design have few of these services because of need-based planning.
- *Cost-plus fee for-service*—This pricing model permits a nonprofit agency to recover the actual cost of a service in addition to a profit, which then can be used to subsidize another service within the agency. These "cash cows" may include innovative services or products (healthy grocery shopping tours for low-fat foods, diet and fitness classes, customized nutrition services, or weight management programs for employer groups) or long-standing, fully capitalized services such as individualized, physician prescribed medical nutrition therapy.

These "price" versus "cost" strategies are dependent on an accurate cost determination discussed later in this chapter.

PREPARE THE BUDGET

Generating the funds to cover the cost of delivering a nutrition service is an important part of fiscal management. Determining the real cost of a product or service is crucial to setting fees, collecting reimbursements, and writing grants. Preparing a budget for an array of services and then breaking it down into the actual cost of each product or service is the next step. The budget defines what services can be implemented with the amount of funding available.

An annotated budget is shown in Table 17–1.

REVIEW THE MONTHLY FINANCIAL STATEMENT

Controlling the budget requires a monthly comparison of projected income to actual expenses and encumbrances (items purchased, but not yet paid for). The agency's accounting staff should provide a monthly financial summary listing the

Table 17–1 Annotated Program Budget Income including the 8 Notes

A diversified income base is critical to a comprehensive nutrition program to meet priority needs that the community assessment identified. The only "fudge factors" are client fees and reimbursements that are projected based on past income-generating experience.

Healthy Weighs Nutrition Program

Grant A: Middle School Healthy Weighs		$ XXX
Grant B: Union Employee Weight Reduction Program		XXX
Client fees		XXX
Body Fit client fees	XXX	
Union client fees	XXX	
Third-party reimbursement—weight reduction		XXX
BC/BS United Medicaid/Medicare		
General revenue (local tax levy support)		-0-
State grant/allocation		-0-
Total income:		$XXXX

Healthy Weighs Nutrition Program Expenses

Salaries		$ XXX
Full-time (specify FTEs)	$ XXX	
Part-time (Specify FTEs)	$ XXX	
Fringe benefits		XXX
Mileage for local travel		XXX
Other travel		XXX
Telephone, local, long-distance		XXX
Internet connection, allocation		XXX
Postage		XXX
Printing		XXX

(continues)

Table 17–1   continued

Healthy Weighs Nutrition Program Expenses continued

Supplies		XXX
Office	$ XXX	
Food for demonstrations/clients	$ XXX	
Books		XXX
Subscriptions		XXX
Software upgrades		XXX
Space, rental/allocation		XXX
Equipment rental/allocation (1)		XXX
Copy machines	$ XXX	
Computers	$ XXX	
Telephones	$ XXX	
Video	$ XXX	
Equipment, purchase (2)		XXX
Computer/other hardware	$ XXX	
Other office equipment	$ XXX	
Utilities, actual/allocation		XXX
Staff training and continuing education		XXX
Out-of-town travel	$ XXX	
Lodging	$ XXX	
Registration fees	$ XXX	
Registrations, local	$ XXX	
Memberships	$ XXX	
Other		XXX
Indirect costs (3)		XXX
Central service charge (4)		XXX
Consultant fees (5)		XXX
Student stipends (6)		XXX
Equipment maintenance fee (7)		XXX
Contingent reserve fund (8)		
Total expenses (Total expenses that are ≤ total income)		**$XXXX**

Table 17–1   continued

Notes to Remember:

1. Carefully evaluate the rent versus buy decisions on all equipment.
2. Plan for life cycle replacement of equipment in each annual budget.
3. There may be an administrative overhead charge included as a percentage of each budget for overall agency indirect costs.
4. Additional overhead may be charged by the county, city, or state to cover the costs of attorneys, accountants, executive directors, and central purchasing that provide service but are outside of the nutrition or health department.
5. Include fees for graphic consultants, contract professional and technical assistance, external evaluation specialists, and auditor fees for federal funds received. Contract physician fees for grants/third-party reimbursement requirements especially if third-party reimbursement will cover the costs and result in nutrition services reimbursement.
6. Try to build in student stipends for internships if quality supervision can be provided for the students.
7. Fees are generally charged for some equipment rental based on volume or intensity of use for major equipment repair. Only contract if there is a good payback for high use or frequently broken equipment.
8. Have a carryover fund for emergencies.

Source: Chapter Author, Katherine Cairns.

current status of expenditures compared to the amounts budgeted. Table 17–2 displays an example of this analysis. The program manager must monitor this carefully so that all budgeted resources are wisely used. The monthly financial summary also enables the manager to determine when the income flow is inadequate compared to projections. Fund transfers between program accounts may be needed to balance the budget.

The monthly financial statement should be used to determine when there is a need for any of the following:

- Communicate with staff about the program's financial position.
- Trim discretionary costs (supplies, printing, and so on) or increase spending on consumable supplies.
- Increase or decrease staffing (overtime or voluntary reduction of hours, layoffs).
- Generate more income (find out why some health payers are slower to pay or rejecting billing claims and requiring more aggressive tracking).

A computer spreadsheet is a clear, time-saving tool to use to prepare the budget summary. There are many suitable financial software packages available. Most governmental agencies require all departments to use their purchased financial software.

Determining Program or Service Costs

Determining the costs for each specific service or product requires a slightly different adaptation of the program budget. The program manager must know the

Table 17-2 Monthly Financial Summary

	Months		Year-to-date (YTD)		
	Received this period	Budgeted this period	YTD received	YTD budgeted	YTD last year received
Income					
List all sources					
Total income:					
	Spent/ encumbered this period	Budgeted this period	YTD spent	YTD budgeted	YTD last year sent
Expenses					
List all expense categories					
Total expenses:					
Variance from projections:					

Source: Chapter Author, Katherine Cairns.

approximate utilization of staff and resources allocated to each service. Staff time is the largest expense in any service. Time studies or tracking of billable hours are frequently used to assess the amount of staff time each product or service requires. If a time study is not feasible (lack of time, staff issues, and so on), a quick, less precise method can be used to approximate the amount of staff time spent in each specific service area. This method is displayed in Table 17–3. Note that administrative time is factored into each service category.

The next step is to cost out staff, supplies, equipment, and other resources for each service area (Table 17–4), then divide the total cost by the number of clients or client visits (or relative value units, a productivity measuring unit used by some programs) expected to be served during the year. This yields a cost per contact, which is the actual cost to provide each unit of service.

Starting from the program budget, this cost determination analysis takes approximately two hours to calculate for each service. A program manager could devote about two hours each month to identifying the actual costs of one program a month and make needed adjustments in charges. More complicated systems of cost determination exist, especially for federally funded programs. These can be developed with the guidance of the agency's business manager or accounting department. Public health nutrition programs have been able to increase their operating income after doing this type of analysis. Health screening programs,

Table 17–3 Staff Time Allocation by Service or Cost Center for Cost Determination

Staff Member Name	Total FTE	WIC	Diabetes Clinic	Healthy Weighs Class	Group	Newspaper Column	Home Visit
Clerical							
Amy Jones	1.0	0.9	0.0	0.0	0.0	0.0	0.1
Xia Vang	0.8	0.1	0.1	0.3	0.2	0.1	0.0
Nutrition Assistants							
Tres Smith	1.0	1.0	0.0	0.0	0.0	0.0	0.0
Joli Harris	0.8	0.8	0.0	0.0	0.0	0.0	0.0
Sam Hicks	0.7	0.7	0.0	0.0	0.0	0.0	0.0
Blia Xiong	1.0	0.5	0.0	0.5	0.0	0.0	0.0
Nutritionists							
Mac Stokes	0.8	0.8	0.0	0.0	0.0	0.0	0.0
Tre Austin	1.0	0.0	0.0	0.1	0.3	0.1	0.5
Raj Bhajmer	1.0	0.0	0.0	0.1	0.3	0.1	0.5
Kate Conner	1.0	0.2	0.1	0.1	0.4	0.1	0.1
Total	9.1	5.0	0.2	1.1	1.2	0.4	1.2

Source: Chapter Author, Katherine Cairns.

medical nutrition therapy counseling, and group nutrition education programs are examples of programs for which this cost determination would be useful to document actual costs compared to reimbursed costs. The goal is to match reimbursed costs more closely to the actual costs of providing the public health nutrition service.

Divide the total cost of the service by the number of clients or client visits (or relative value units) expected to be served during the year. This provides a cost per contact or encounter, which is the actual cost to the program to provide each unit of this service. This can also be analyzed by the actual number of clients served in the most recent reporting period.

Analyze Service Productivity

A second stage of analysis for program managers concerned about the high cost of a given service is a service productivity analysis. Several references on how to conduct a detailed productivity analysis of program services are available. A simple analysis of service productivity levels involves multiplying the total full-time equivalents (FTEs) allocated to each service by 2080 (paid hours) or 1800 (billable hours) for each FTE position, then dividing by the number of clients or contact visits. See Table 17–5 for an example.

In Table 17–5, the budget for the Healthy Weighs classes is based on an actual reimbursed cost of $65.00 per class (and $13 a person for five class participants in another grant that funds this activity). If the number of classes can be increased from 650 to 792 with the existing staff, the program will generate an additional

Table 17–4   Cost Determination for Healthy Weighs Program

Service: Nutrition counseling/class   *Date of cost determination: 6-15-05*

Salaries		Comments
Xia Vang, .3 FTE	$ XXX	Full-time equivalent (FTE) by salary
Blia Xiong, .5 FTE	XXX	
Tre Austin, .1 FTE	XXX	
Raj Bhajmer, .1 FTE	XXX	
Kate Conner, .1 FTE	XXX	
Fringe benefit allocation	XXX	(Based on required allocation)
Mileage for site visits	XXX	Allocated or actual use
Telephone	XXX	Allocated on estimated/actual use
Postage	XXX	Allocated on estimated/actual use
Duplicating	XXX	Allocated on estimated/actual use
Supplies	XXX	Allocated on estimated/actual use
Office rental	XXX	Allocated based on space occupied
Equipment	XXX	Allocation based on use
Training/education	XXX	Allocation
Other	XXX	
Subtotal	XXX	
Indirect cost rate (___%)	XXX	Apply to subtotal
Total cost of service	**$ XXX**	

Source: Chapter Author, Katherine Cairns.

$9230 this year. Health care payers will not reimburse more than $65.00 a class this year. Suggest that staff initiate a quality improvement audit of existing clients to document outcomes. Documenting results with actual higher costs to health plans for negotiated reimbursement increases for serving high-risk Medicaid population in the next year.

Use of Cost-Effectiveness and Cost-Benefit Analyses

The third and final challenge of fiscal management is to evaluate the service or product once the costs and providers have been identified. Cost-benefit analysis and cost-effectiveness analysis are most commonly initiated. A cost-benefit

Table 17–5 Service Productivity Analysis

Service: Healthy Weighs Program	*Date of cost determination: 6-15-05*

1. How long *should* it take to provide one unit (visit) of this service?
   2 hours (includes direct service time, travel time, charting, case conference, and administration).
2. How long *does* it take to provide each unit (visit) of this service?
   Agencies may calculate this based on the following:
   - *2080 hours* (1.0 FTE paid with vacation/sick days included) or
   - *1800 billable hours* (1.0 FTE excluding vacation/sick/holiday hours)

Total FTEs: 1.1 X hours = 1980 billable hours
Total service units: 650 Healthy Weighs classes
1980 billable hours divided by budgeted classes = 3.5 hours per class

3. Explain difference between answers to 1 and 2.
   - 3.5 hours per class (actual) compared to 2.0 hours per class (estimate) is significant.
   - Thus, staffs take almost twice as long to prepare and teach the class compared to what they estimated during the budget cycle, *or* too many staff are assigned to this activity.
   - Suggest that staff adjust expectation to 2.5 hours per class and expect 792 classes this year or reduce staff to 0.92 FTEs to provide 650 classes. To break even financially for this service, staff must increase their productivity or be reassigned/reduced.

Source: Chapter Author, Katherine Cairns.

analysis is used in the planning process to decide if a program or service should be undertaken. A cost-effectiveness analysis is undertaken to determine the least costly way to provide the service or program. Cost-benefit and cost-effectiveness are discussed in more detail in Chapter 14.

Through the application of these analysis tools, the nutritionist can select services that generate income and become increasingly self-supporting. There is great risk in taking an innovative service idea, guessing at a charge for the service, providing the service, and later questioning why the staff time commitment is excessive in relation to the financial return. An analysis of the project, including the documented need, the population to be served, favorable pricing, and realistic income expectation could turn the innovation into a source of income. For other essential public health services, generating revenue may be less of an option.

Seek Sources of Third-Party Reimbursement

Income can be derived by billing insurance carriers such as governmental health care programs (Medicaid, Medicare), Workers' Compensation, health maintenance organizations (HMOs), managed care organizations (MCOs), and other special health insurance pools (catastrophic health, state-sponsored alternative care pools, organized employer groups). Each health carrier has its own billing procedures that the agency accounting office must determine and continuously update. It is most cost-effective for the agency accounting department to select

the three or four third-party reimbursement sources that cover the majority of the agency clients and bill these carriers. Clients not covered by those carriers would be treated as fee-for-service clients and advised to collect reimbursement from their own carrier. Some organizations contract with health care reimbursement firms that require an assignment of benefits from all clients and handle all agency billing for a predetermined fee.

Emerging opportunities for nutritionists and dietitians to generate income are developing in this area of third-party reimbursement. As discussed in previous chapters, nutrition services are increasingly being reimbursed for weight management, medical nutrition therapy, and chronic and acute care interventions. Nutrition and health programs are identifying ways to protect revenue raised from third-party reimbursements to permit carryover of these funds between fiscal years for program-specific initiatives.

Obesity-related interventions may be reimbursed by employer-sponsored health plans. The IRS Ruling 2002-19 allows a tax deduction to individuals who are advised by their physician to lose weight to treat obesity or as a part of recommended treatment for another diagnosis or disease. This is defined in Section 213, Medical/Dental Expenses, 26 CFR 1.213-1, and section 262; 1.262-1. Deductions for uncompensated expenses for medical care are permitted when the expenses exceed 7.5% of adjusted gross income. Expenses for prescribed diets or foods to alleviate a physical or mental defect or illness are deductible. The ruling includes the cost of special food if the food alleviates or treats an illness. This must be substantiated by a physician when the special food is not needed to meet the normal nutritional needs of the taxpayer. The IRS now refers to obesity as a disease based on the scientific and professional evidence published by the federal government.

Federal Medicare policy on obesity and therapeutic weight reduction is changing. Previously, only very narrow medical procedures related to bariatric surgery may have been approved for Medicare reimbursement. With the July 2004 policy change, Medicare is declaring obesity to be a disease that can be treated with medical, pharmacological, and medical nutrition therapy under the supervision of a Medicare-approved practitioner. This change in Medicare's coverage policy puts the focus on nutrition in public health. According to the Department of Health and Human Services, this policy change could include coverage of surgery, medical nutrition therapy reference, and exercise counseling.

Federal Medicaid policies may be reexamined based on the Medicare precedent. Reimbursement for primary prevention is usually considered to be part of well-child and preventive adult physician visits without additional reimbursement. It is necessary to examine each state's Medicaid policies for covering health education and clinical guidance services that are provided separately from clinical well-child and well-adult visits.

As always, seek the advice of the agency's reimbursement advisor to be sure to follow correct documentation, referral, coding, and billing procedures.

Sharpen Grant Writing Skills

Most public health nutritionists need to become grant writers to obtain outside income to support innovative services, reach new populations, develop and test creative interventions, and initiate special projects. Any or all of these may then turn into long-term, income-producing services.

Here are several hints for the successful grant writer:

- Keep a grant idea folder to file innovative ideas that would require external funding. Ideas noted as a 1-paragraph description can be contributed by staff members. The community needs assessment will help produce some ideas for needed public health nutrition services.
- Foster staff development by conducting a competitive internal seed grant program within the program or agency. Allocate a small amount of the annual budget to this research and development (R&D) fund.
- Find several grant writers and reviewers within the agency with whom to brainstorm ideas and advise on writing grant proposals.
- Reduce all grant proposals to a 1-page worksheet as an initial step. A sample worksheet is shown in Table 17–6.
- Network with potential project collaborators in the health agency or the community who can work on grant proposals of mutual interest, sometimes on short notice.
- Identify reliable people and organizations that can be counted on to write letters of support. Some of these individuals or agencies may prefer that the support letter be written for their signature.
- Plan to write three to four application grants for each grant funded.
- Practice writing concisely. If the idea cannot be conveyed in five to six double-spaced pages, (including needs statement, methods, objectives, budget, and collaborators), grant reviewers may be less likely to focus on the project idea.
- Maintain a file of standard agency information that can be quickly pulled for grant application attachments. Items, such as Agency Internal Revenue Tax Exemption 501 C-3 statements, audited budgets, lists of current agency board members, agency descriptions, federal identification numbers for the agency, and up-to-date personnel curriculum vitae, should be in this file.
- Maintain a file of grants submitted previously.
- Use word-processing and spreadsheet software to write the narrative and prepare the budget spreadsheet. This makes it easier to revise the proposal without introducing errors.
- Get on the mailing lists of every government and/or private agency and foundation that announces related grant and contract requests for proposals (RFPs) that can be identified.

Additional hints for grant writing will undoubtedly be added to and shared with other people in health agency. Sharing the work and the glory when a new

Table 17–6   Sample Grant Application Internal Worksheet

Project title (5 to 7 words): _____

Amount requested : _____ Total project cost: _____

Estimated in-kind support: _____

Project collaborators:

Project summary:

Statement of specific problem or need:

Target population:

Objectives— Measurable and time-specific	Methods	Evaluation— Tied to objectives

Budget, including in-kind contributions:

Letters of support to be sought from:

Source: Chapter Author, Katherine Cairns.

grant comes to the agency is the mark of a true professional. Researching grant funds and writing proposals take time. Alas, well-written proposals are not always funded. Even experienced grant writers receive rejections. It takes persistence. If a proposal is rejected, ask for a copy of the grant evaluation sheet to learn by experience and try again and again.

POINTS TO PONDER

- Given the staffing patterns described in Table 17–4 and 17–5, is the nutrition program using the best mix of staff and allocation of staff time to result in the desired outcomes? What additional information would be useful? What productivity-enhancing strategies would be useful for the nutrition staff involved in the Healthy Weighs class?
- Suggest a grant application idea to increase financial resources for the home visiting service. Complete a grant application internal worksheet (Table 17–6) for the idea and discuss.
- How should fees for nutrition services be established, and how should this income be most effectively allocated?
- Explore the health care billing and coding references used by the state Medicaid program, and identify two potential billing codes for public health

nutrition services. Identify the state and federal requirements (documentation, supervision, service provider, and eligibility) for use of these billing codes. Medicaid reimbursement rates paid by the state Medicaid agency should be public information. Request the reimbursement rate for the billing codes identified for different health care providers. Compare findings.

HELPFUL WEB SITES

Internal Revenue Service Revenue Ruling:
www.taxlinks.com/rulings/2002/revrul2002-19.htm

BIBLIOGRAPHY

American Dietetic Association. Nutrition services in managed care- an ADA position paper. *J Am Diet Assoc.* 2002;102:1471–1478.

Baker J, Baker RW. *Health Care Finance: Basic Tools for Non-financial Managers.* Boston, Mass: Jones and Bartlett Publishers; 2003.

Baker J. *Cost Accounting for Healthcare Organizations: Utilizing Information and Technology for Effective Decision Making.* McGraw-Hill Professional; 1999.

Conklin MT, Simko MD. Cost-benefit and cost-effectiveness analyses of nutrition programs. *Qual Rev Bull.* 1983;9:166–168.

Dever GEA. *Improving Outcomes in Public Health Practice: Strategies and Methods.* Gaithersburg, Md: Aspen; 1997.

Disbrow D. The costs and benefits of nutrition services: a literature review. *J Am Diet Assoc.* 89(Suppl):S4–S63.

Gapenski L. *Healthcare Finance: An Introduction to Accounting and Financial Management.* 2nd *ed.* Chicago, Ill: Health Administration Press; 2001.

Internal Revenue Service. IRS Revenue Ruling 2002-19. Available at: http://www.taxlinks.com/rulings/2002/revrul2002-19.htm.

Lighter D, Fair D. *Principles and Methods of Quality Management in Health Care.* Gaithersburg, Md: Aspen; 2000.

Obesity and employer health plans. In Focus. International Foundation of Employee Benefit Plans. May 2004;4.

Omachonu V. *Total Quality and Productivity Management in Health Care Organizations.* Institute of Industrial Engineers; 1991.

Schramm WF. WIC prenatal participation and its relationship to newborn Medicaid costs in Missouri: a cost/benefit analysis. *Am J Public Health.* 1985;75:851–857.

Thompson TG. Coverage of anti-obesity procedures by Medicare. July 16, 2004. *Health Plan and Provider Report.* 2004;10:744.

Warren C, Reeve J, Fess P. *Accounting.* Cincinnati, Ohio: South-Western College Publishers; 2001.

CHAPTER 18

Empower the Public to Choose Healthy Food

Marjorie Scharf and Sandra B. Sherman

Reader Objectives

- Describe the complex interacting factors that influence people's food choices.
- State some examples of nutrition intervention strategies based on social cognitive theory.
- Suggest opportunities for public health nutritionists to use the *Dietary Guidelines for Americans 2005* to advocate changes in policies to provide the public with greater access to healthy foods.
- Understand that planning and developing nutrition interventions needs to include consumers and members of community organizations.
- Define *health literacy* and its importance to design nutrition messages that are culturally relevant, age appropriate, and easy to understand.
- Identify multiple nutrition interventions that can be incorporated into a particular setting.

TODAY'S EATING PATTERNS

Overweight and obesity in the United States have increased dramatically over the last two decades. Americans now consume more and expend fewer calories than they need to maintain a healthy body weight. Americans confront a smorgasbord of food choices in corner stores, fast-food outlets, family restaurants, supermarkets, vending machines, street vendors, dollar stores, and even pharmacies. Most Americans need to eat fewer calories, make wiser food choices, and be more physically active.

Individuals who consume food or beverages sweetened with added sugar may consume more calories than they need. They are also likely to consume fewer vitamins and minerals. For children, sugars from processed foods or added to foods contribute an average of 20% of total food energy.[1] People of all ages consume more than 130 calories per day from sweeteners.[2] More than one out of every 10 calories in an adolescent's (ages 12–17) diet comes from soft drinks.[3] A positive association between drinking sweetened beverages and weight gain has been found. Nutritionists must educate consumers to reduce added sugars in their diets. Nutritionists must advocate for healthier beverages to be sold in schools, convenience stores, and at work places. *Dietary Guidelines for Americans 2005* recommends decreasing intake of sweetened foods and beverages to reduce calorie intake and help achieve recommended nutrient intakes.

Diets high in saturated fats, trans fat, and cholesterol may increase the risk of coronary heart disease. Studies show that Americans consume too much of all three of these types of fat. An intake of more than 35% of calories from fats is likely to increase saturated fat and calorie consumption. Adults and children need to decrease their intake of saturated fat and trans fat. Some also may need to decrease their cholesterol intake. Processed foods that contain partially hydrogenated oils provide approximately 80% of trans fat in the diet. Nutritionists educate consumers to reduce fat in their diets. More importantly, public health nutritionists advocate to food processors to reduce the amount of fats, especially trans fat and saturated fats, they use in processed foods. *Dietary Guidelines for Americans 2005* recommend a total fat intake between 20% and 35% of calories for adults. Most dietary fats should come from polyunsaturated and monounsaturated fats.[4]

Most Americans consume more sodium than they need. Decreasing sodium intake is recommended to reduce the risk of high blood pressure. Approximately 75% of sodium in the diet comes from salt added to foods in preparation and processing. Convenience foods and foods served by fast-food restaurants are often high in sodium. Nutritionists can educate consumers to use less salt. Food processors and food service personnel are advised to use less salt in foods they prepare for the public. The *Dietary Guidelines for Americans 2005* recommend that individuals consume less than 2300 mg (approximately 1 tsp salt) of sodium per day and eat more potassium-rich foods, such as fruits and vegetables.[4]

Americans of all ages are becoming more sedentary. In 1999, 65% of adolescents participated in some form of recommended athletics. In 2002, 25% of adults had not participated in any leisure time physical exercise during the previous month. A sedentary lifestyle increases the risk of obesity and diet-related diseases. Nutritionists must encourage Americans of all ages to increase their physical activity and decrease their sedentary lifestyle. Schools and places of work can be encouraged to provide the time and facilities so that both youngsters and adults can participate in physical exercise. The *Dietary Guidelines for Americans 2005* recommend that adults do at least 30 minutes of moderate physical activity most days, with an additional 30 minutes to prevent weight gain. A marked decrease in physical exercise combined with a diet of high-fat foods, served in supersized portions, contributes to the current obesity epidemic.[4]

FACTORS AFFECTING FOOD CHOICES

To guide and motivate people to choose and prepare foods that promote health and prevent obesity and related diseases requires understanding the many interacting and often competing factors that influence popular food choices. Nutritionists should identify the unique set of factors that influence the populations with whom they work. They can use this understanding to develop effective strategies to improve food choices.

Food choices are influenced by a complex combination of factors including biological, experiential, intrapersonal, and environmental.[5] See Figure 18–1.

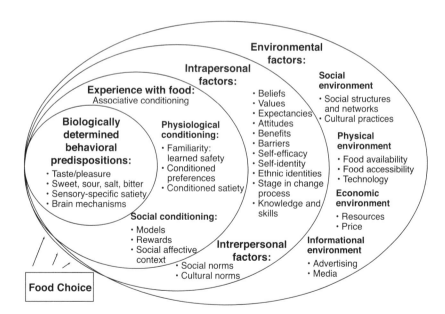

Figure 18–1 Social Cognitive Theory: A Multi-faceted Approach to Modify Food Choices. *Source:* Isobel R. Contento, Nutrition Education: to be published by Jones and Bartlett 2007, Sudbury, MA Publishers. www. jbpub.com. Reprinted with permission.

Biological determinants of food choices change slowly. Social and environmental determinants have changed dramatically over the past few decades. Advances in food processing have introduced thousands of new foods to supermarket shelves each year. As the numbers of these products increase, consumers need nutrition information to enable them to make informed choices. With more women working, families have increased their purchases of prepared foods and are eating more meals away from home. These prepared foods usually contain increased amounts of added sugar, salt, and fat. At the same time, advances in technology have created more sedentary entertainment including watching television, playing video games, and using computers. Nutritionists planning interventions must understand the many factors that influence food choices and physical activity levels. The extent to which nutritionists succeed in improving food choices depends on how well they understand these complex interacting variables. Personal, economic, and environmental factors influence what adults and children choose for meals and snacks.

Personal

- Parents' food preferences
- Religious practices or ethnic heritage of the family
- Family's preferred methods of preparing food
- Whether or not the family eats together
- Nutrition knowledge and cooking skills of the family members who prepare the food

Economic

- Family income
- Available operable equipment for food preparation and storage
- Transportation to a well-stocked supermarket
- Time available to spend on food shopping, cooking, and eating
- Food insecurity (limited access to safe nutritious foods (see Chapter 4)

Environmental

- Convenience of grocery store or supermarket
- Foods available during the day at school and place of work
- Foods available en route to the work place or school
- Access to fresh, locally grown fruits and vegetables

WAYS TO MODIFY FOOD CHOICES:
A MULTIFACETED APPROACH

Social Cognitive Theory

Improving the nutritional health of individuals and the people in the community requires 1) personal and family attitudes that prioritize health, 2) improved awareness that nutrition makes a difference, 3) obtaining knowledge and skills to choose healthy foods, and 4) altering the external factors, or environment, that affect the individual or family food selection. Social cognitive theory addresses the complex interacting factors that influence people's food choices and suggests methods to promote behavioral change.[6] Applying this theory, food choices are explained by the interaction of behavior, personal factors, and environmental influences. Behavior is not solely the result of the environment any more than environment is the result of the personal behavior. The three constructs influence each other to be able to design an effective intervention. Nutritionists must understand changes in the individual and families and their interaction with the environment.

Social cognitive theory emphasizes developing skills needed to improve the nutritive quality of diet and increase the value each individual places on good health and nutrition. A nutrition intervention based on this theory would provide individuals with repeated opportunities to taste healthy foods. Community leaders, health professionals, and others would work to overcome barriers to choosing nutrient-dense foods. Influential role models, including peers, would demonstrate healthy eating practices. Incentives would be offered to reinforce messages. Individuals would be encouraged to develop practical skills and self-confidence to read and understand food labels, plan meals, prepare foods, and choose healthy foods. Observation followed by hands-on practice develops social support for healthy food choices and preparation.

Two examples of health promotion programs using social cognitive theory are the Child and Adolescent Trial for Cardiovascular Health (CATCH) and the Gimme 5! Program. CATCH was designed to influence cognitive factors through classroom instruction and environmental factors. The program changes the food service and physical education programs in selected schools. Outcomes indicated improvement in cognitive and environmental variables and nutrition and physical activity.[7]

Gimme 5! Fruit and Vegetables for Fun and Health focuses on environmental, personal and behavioral factors.[8] It encourages children to ask their parents to purchase their favorite fruits and vegetables, and increase the availability of fruits and vegetables in meals and snacks. The program also encourages fast-food restaurants to offer more fruits and vegetables. It promotes taste testing of fruits and vegetables that are FaSST (fast, simple, safe, and tasty) in the classroom. The taste tests are associated with fun activities such as rap songs, preparing FaSST recipes in the classrooms, and sending the recipes with assignments to prepare them at home. Fourth- and fifth-grade students monitored their fruit and vegetable consumption, set goals, received rewards for achieving these goals, and identified the problems when goals were not met.

The success of nutritionists to improve healthy food choices depends on their understanding of these complex interacting variables; applying those models helps to design interventions to increase the probability of success.

Community Participation

The health of a community depends upon the health all of its residents. This depends on the physical and social aspects in the community that enable its people to live healthy lives. To improve the health of individuals and create healthier communities, individuals must work together.[9]

No agency, individual, or professional has the knowledge and resources to improve the food choices of everyone in the whole community, nor can they speak on behalf of a community. Representatives of the community, including residents, community organizations, health professionals and their organizations, concerned consumer groups, and the media work together to develop, implement, and evaluate nutrition interventions. Each partner contributes unique strengths. Residents and community groups offer insight and guidance as they identify the factors that affect their food habits and nutritional health. The population's priorities lead to acceptable, relevant, and culturally appropriate strategies. Consumer groups can contribute organizing and advocacy skills. The media and business partners offer expertise to tailor and market messages to specific populations. By working together to create interventions, the partners develop commitment and ownership of the project. When the partnerships mobilize and coordinate around strong, consistent health and nutrition messages, conflicting or duplicating efforts can be avoided. An important role of public health nutritionists is to facilitate active community participation and collaboration.

Nutrition interventions must address the multiple components of the social cognitive theory model affecting individual or population food choices. To improve the food choices of schoolchildren, an environmental approach means offering foods recommended in the *Dietary Guidelines for Americans 2005* in their school cafeterias and vending machines. In Los Angeles, New York City, and Philadelphia, parents, nutritionists, health professionals, and community leaders successfully collaborated to convince their school boards to remove soft drinks and artificially sweetened beverages from schools and to offer only bottled water, 100% fruit juices, and milk.[10] Many school districts have now developed a snack food and beverage policy. Nutrition standards are the basis to select foods that can be offered throughout the entire school, including those served in the cafeteria, school fundraisers, school stores, and classroom parties. Examples include replacing fried chips high in total fat and trans fat, candy, and cookies with low-fat whole-grain snack crackers or fruit and 100% fruit juices. Along with this environmental change, these interventions entice students to select healthy foods. They emphasize role modeling, developing practical skills, critical thinking, and offering choices of nutrient-dense new foods. Strategies based upon the social cognitive theory include:

1. Students taste a variety of healthy snack foods, and then vote on which foods to use as fundraisers and to be sold in the cafeteria. Students assist in promoting these healthy food choices. Teenaged role models shape the food choices of their peers and of younger children.[11]
2. Students survey their parents regarding their favorite healthy snack foods and create a shopping list made up of these choices.
3. Students design and survey neighborhood stores to determine and list the availability of 100% fruit juices, fresh fruit, and low-fat snacks.
4. Students critically analyze food marketing techniques used in television and radio and apply these techniques to promote the sale of the healthier snack foods.
5. Parents and teachers taste healthy new snacks at school meetings.
6. Teachers become role models when they choose the healthy foods in the school cafeteria and eat lunch with their students.

The same type of multilevel, participatory approach can be used to help people in a community achieve the *Dietary Guideline* of eating nine servings of fruits and vegetables a day. For example, The Food Trust, a nonprofit organization in Philadelphia,[12] helps to create farmers' markets in areas of the city where the people have limited access to fresh fruits and vegetables. The local farmers bring their fresh fruits and vegetables to the markets; they also provide information about preparation methods at the point of purchase. Some farmers offer samples for taste testing. Community health agencies publicize these markets and offer blood-pressure and other health screening along with samples to taste and related health and nutrition information. This initiative is mutually beneficial to the people in the community as well as to local farmers. Easy access to fresh, locally grown fruits and vegetables can improve the quality of the population's nutrient intake, while minimizing their need for individual action. Successful interventions must include partnerships and ongoing collaboration among many different resources.

Advocacy and Policy Development

Policies made at the national, state, and local levels, in private and public sectors, influence population eating habits. Chapters 5 and 6 discuss the process through which nutrition policy is established and highlight the role of the public health nutritionist. Advocacy, combined with community organizing, helps shape policy.

The *Dietary Guidelines for Americans 2005* provide many opportunities to advocate policies that require food processors, food marketers, food service establishments, policymakers, and legislators to promote food products that serve the best interest of health:

1. Federal and state labeling laws and regulations influence food quality and make ingredient information available to the public. Public health nutritionists join forces with others to ensure that the food industry is not allowed to make false claims in an attempt to take advantage of the attention received by the *Dietary Guidelines*.

2. Food processors, food advertisers, food distributors, and restaurants influence the ingredients, quality, and price of foods available in the markets through the formulation of products and their promotion. The *Dietary Guidelines* can be used to pressure the food industry to offer greater choices of products that do not contain trans fat, that contain less added fat, sugar, and salt, and that include more whole grains. This includes foods offered in vending machines, corner stores, work places, school cafeterias, and fast-food restaurants. Along with providing tasty, healthy foods, and nutrition education, product promotion must ensure consumers continue to purchase these new foods.

3. The food service industry needs incentives to produce a greater array of healthy foods and consumers may require incentives to purchase them.

4. Personnel policies and work schedules influence the amount of time employees have during a day to purchase and eat a healthy meal or snack and to exercise. The *Dietary Guidelines for Americans 2005* emphasize the importance of exercise in the prevention of overweight, obesity, and chronic diseases. In the *Guidelines 2005*, the recommended amount of daily exercise is increased to one hour per day.[4] Worksites can create safe places for employees to walk for exercise during breaks, and provide access to safe stairwells and possibly discounts to gyms.

5. School districts have enormous potential to improve the diet and overall health of children. Public Law 108-265 (June 30, 2004) requires that by June 30, 2006, each local education agency participating in the National School Lunch Act or the Child Nutrition Act of 1966 shall establish a local School Wellness Policy to promote student health and reduce childhood obesity.[13] See Table 18–1.

Table 18–1   School Wellness Policy

School wellness policies must include: 1) goals for school-based nutrition education and physical activity, 2) nutrition guidelines for all foods available on school campus during the school day, e.g., meals, snacks, fundraisers, parties and 3) other components identified as being part of a healthy school nutrition environment, e.g., parent education. In addition, this School Wellness Policy must be created with involvement from parents, students, teachers, school nurses, school board representatives, and other school staff.

Source: US Congress Public Law 108-265, June 30, 2004, 118 STAT. 729, Section 204, Washington, DC.

Combining heightened awareness of the *Dietary Guidelines for Americans 2005* and the requirement of a school wellness policy through a participatory approach can promote positive dietary changes.

Environmental Change

A community nutritionist assesses the environmental barriers to healthy food choices available in the target community and plans, implements, and evaluates effective nutrition interventions. By identifying barriers and overcoming them, nutritionists increase their success at influencing dietary change to improve health outcomes. Involving influential members of the community in designing assessment and interventions, then publicizing the results, can obtain greater support for change. Examples of assessment questions for high school students, parents, and community members collaborating with the public health nutritionist are:

1. Do people in the community have access to a corner store or supermarket that features a variety of affordable, high-quality, fresh fruits and vegetables? Are their supermarkets accessible by public transportation?
2. Are healthy food choices available and promoted in fast-food restaurants, work places, and school cafeterias? Do they offer choices of fruits and vegetables?
3. Are steps safe and available for students or employees to get additional exercise?
4. Is lunchtime in schools and workplaces long enough for students and workers to eat in a relaxing manner?
5. Are children rewarded for good work at school with fruits or whole-grain snacks or nuts instead of candy?
6. Do elementary schools have a safe place for children to play at recess or after school?

When the answer to any of these questions is no, environmental change supportive of healthy eating and physical exercise is needed. Some interventions that could overcome these environmental barriers include:

1. In neighborhoods that do not have access to fresh fruits and vegetables, work with a neighborhood group to bring in a weekly farmers' market.
2. Encourage schools, neighborhood stores, employee cafeterias, and fast-food restaurants to promote their healthy food items and serve smaller portion sizes. Encourage them to serve more whole-grain breads, cereals, and low- or non-fat milk products. Promote the purchase of healthier foods through taste testing, posters, and point-of-purchase nutrition information. Popular fast-food chains promote the substitution of apples for French fries in their "Happy Meals"™, providing a boost to the apple industry as well as encouraging

children to eat apple slices. The apples, however, were packaged and sold with low-fat caramel sauce for dipping, adding extra sugar and calories.[14]

3. Help a school district or local school to develop an alternative to using candy or cookies as fundraisers and to reward good work. Collaborate with the Parent-Teacher Association (PTA), principals, food service directors, and students to list appealing healthy foods and nonfood items that can be used.

4. Encourage worksites to suggest ways employees can incorporate exercise breaks into their workday. These might include a list of local fitness centers that offer a midday yoga or aerobic exercise class, create a walking club, ensure the steps between the floor are clean and safe to encourage midday stair climbing.

NUTRITION COMMUNICATIONS

Well-designed messages help individuals and communities understand their needs and take appropriate actions to maximize their health.[9] Environmental changes, such as introducing new healthy food products into the cafeteria and vending machines, cannot stand alone. Education and information are needed to promote the adoption of healthy environmental changes. While the *Dietary Guidelines'* recommendations reflect current research evidence, nutritionists must assist consumers by translating the *Guidelines* into advice they can act upon everyday.[15]

Written information is often the primary form of nutrition intervention. Public health nutritionists must select the essential content and put it into the relevant context. Effective messages motivate the intended audience to put the nutrition information into practice.

The term *health literacy* refers to an individual's ability to read, understand, and to follow evidence-based (see Chapter 2) nutrition-related health instructions and messages. These include warnings about food-drug interactions, how to understand interactions on prescription labels, nutrient labels on food packages, use of recipes and suggestions for low-fat food choices at fast-food or family restaurants. Based on research by the National Adult Literacy Survey, 90 million Americans or one-half of adults may struggle with health literacy.[16] Other authorities estimate that 27 million American adults, nearly one in five, may not be able to read a pamphlet. Literacy is a range, or continuum, of reading skills that help people function in daily life, with individuals falling at different places on the continuum.[17] Those who struggle to read do not usually use print materials for health information.[9]

To select or adapt existing educational materials or to create new ones, public health nutritionists must evaluate the appropriateness of written materials for their various target audiences. The Suitability Assessment of Materials in Table 18–2 offers clear direction for readability formulas, how to design visuals, and their effective use to prepare and pretest materials and use nonprint materials to reach low-literacy audiences. This Suitability Assessment of Materials (SAM) is useful

Table 18–2 Suitability Assessment of Materials—SAM Scoring Sheet

2 points for superior rating
1 point for adequate rating
0 points for not suitable rating
N/A if the factor does not apply to this material

Factor to Be Rated	Score	Comments
1. Content		
(a) Purpose is evident	_____	_____
(b) Content about behaviors	_____	_____
(c) Scope is limited	_____	_____
(d) Summary or review included	_____	_____
2. Literacy Demand		
(a) Reading grade level	_____	_____
(b) Writing style, active voice	_____	_____
(c) Vocabulary uses common words	_____	_____
(d) Context is given first	_____	_____
(e) Learning aids via "road signs"	_____	_____
3. Graphics		
(a) Cover graphic shows purpose	_____	_____
(b) Type of graphics	_____	_____
(c) Relevance of illustrations	_____	_____
(d) List, tables, etc., explained	_____	_____
(e) Captions used for graphics	_____	_____
4. Layout and Typography		
(a) Layout factors	_____	_____
(b) Typography	_____	_____
(c) Subheads ("chunking") used	_____	_____
5. Learning Stimulation, Motivation		
(a) Interaction used	_____	_____
(b) Behaviors are modeled and specific	_____	_____
(c) Motivation/self-efficacy	_____	_____
6. Cultural Appropriateness		
(a) Match in logic, language, experience	_____	_____
(b) Cultural image and examples	_____	_____
Total SAM score: _____		
Total possible score: _____, Percent score: _____%		

Source: Adapted with permission from Cecilia Doak, Leonard Doak and Jane Root, Teaching Patients with Low Literary Skills, 2nd ed. Philadelphia, J.P. Lippincott, 1996.

to evaluate the appropriateness of existing materials as well as to develop new materials.[17] The six categories included in the assessment are: content, literacy demand, graphics, layout and typography, learning stimulation, and cultural appropriateness. In addition to using this tool themselves, public health nutritionists should train others to use it.

For more sources and examples of easy-to-read nutrition education materials, go to www.nal.usda.gov/fnic/pubs/bibs/gen/lowlit.html. Readability formulas are also used to assess the reading level of text. The Fry formula is easy to use and well designed for fieldwork.

With the increasing ethnic diversity in the United States, public health nutritionists face the challenge of communicating with many non-English-speaking clients. Materials cannot just be translated into another language. They need to respect cultural differences. Effective translation of materials into another language includes:

1. Review of the draft by several health practitioners who are fluent in the language and understand the food practices and cultural health norms of the population
2. Translate the draft of the translated material back into English to ensure its accuracy
3. Field test and obtain feedback from the intended audience

Realistic colored illustrations of foods commonly eaten by the ethnic audience with captions will help convey the main messages and motivate both non-English-speaking and English-speaking audiences. Food models, pictures, and cartons of real food are useful educational tools to convey nutrition messages.[17]

Graphs and charts, commonly used in nutrition education materials, can be challenging for consumers to comprehend. Examples of information often conveyed through charts include foods allowed on prescribed diets, different levels of fat in foods, food label information, and seasonal availability of fruits and vegetables. Materials with information organized in this way should be pretested with the intended audience.

As in planning any intervention, it is essential to use consumer participation to develop, design, and pretest nutrition education materials. Members of the intended audience can offer insight and guidance. One method to obtain consumer input is through focus group discussions.

APPLY SOCIAL MARKETING TECHNIQUES TO PROMOTE HEALTHY FOOD CHOICES (see Chapter 15)

Providing information is not enough to change behavior.[18] Marketing experts do not use a one-dimensional approach of providing information to influence people to buy soft drinks, sugar- and fat-laden snacks, and fast foods. Food manufactures and chain restaurants use aggressive, sophisticated marketing techniques that attract attention, manipulate people's food desires, and coax them to buy their products. They use multiple communication channels such as television, radio, billboards, bus kiosks, incentives, discount coupons in circulars, and popular jingles. Studies demonstrate the influential role of advertising on children's food preferences, choices, and what they pester their parents to purchase.[19] A multidimensional approach must be used to promote healthier eating and physical activity choices and to balance the pressure of advertisers of foods of low nutritional value.

Audience augmentation often used in the marketing field assumes that different messages and communication approaches are required for different population groups. Audience-centered nutrition communications reflect what is important to the intended audience. Focus group discussions recommended for developing educational materials seek to understand the target population, including their preferred method to receive useful information.

Some examples of successful interventions that use social marketing techniques and collaboration to promote healthy food choices are as follows:

- *VERB*[TM] *It's what you do*—This national, multicultural, social marketing campaign is coordinated by the DHHS Centers for Disease Control and Prevention (CDC). The VERB campaign encourages "tweens" ages 9–13 to be physically active every day. The campaign combines paid advertising, marketing strategies, and partnership efforts to reach the "tween" audiences and their adults/influencers.[20]
- *"Got Milk?"*—This national campaign was developed by an advertising agency in 1993 for the California Milk Processors Board. Its message is simple, visually appealing, and does not require the ability to read English. The well-known slogan and famous people with the familiar "milk mustache" appear on billboards, sides of buses, bumper stickers, T-shirts, advertising for foods eaten with milk, and even tailing airplanes. The campaign includes recipes for foods using milk, photos of milk served with commonly enjoyed foods, contests, and partnering with health organizations promoting good dental health and the prevention of osteoporosis.[21]
- *5-A-Day Program*—This joint campaign of the National Cancer Institute, the National Center for Chronic Disease Prevention and Health Promotion (CDC), and the National Institute of Health of the US Department of Health and Human Services. The campaign promotes increased consumption of fruits and vegetables as stated in the *Dietary Guideline for Americans 2000*, eat 5 to 9 fruits and vegetables a day for better health. A companion message, Color Your Way to 5 a Day, uses vibrant colors to motivate and attract people to choose fresh fruits and vegetables. To reinforce the message, many collaborators provide a variety of teaching tools and marketing items.[22]
- *Healthy Lifestyles and Disease Prevention Initiative*—This campaign includes multimedia public service announcements (PSAs) and a new interactive Web site www.smallsteps.gov[23] to encourage people to make small activity as well as dietary changes, such as using the stairs instead of the elevator or taking a walk instead of watching television. The PSAs were developed for the US Department of Health and Human Services in cooperation with the Ad Council. The release of this educational campaign coincided

with the publication of the CDC study in the Journal of the American Medical Association on March 9, 2004.[24]

To eliminate conflicting or duplicative efforts, the health and nutrition promotion of community agencies, national organizations, professionals or organizations, concerned consumer groups, and the media should be mobilized and coordinated around strong messages. Public health nutritionists should collaborate with relevant campaigns and health observances of other organizations to maximize their messages. Examples of annual health and nutrition observances: 5 a Day for Better Health in September with the American Cancer Society; National School Lunch Week in October with the American School Food Services Association; World Food Day in October; and National Nutrition Month with the American Dietetic Association in March.

INTEGRATE NUTRITION INTERVENTIONS INTO EDUCATION AND COMMUNITY SETTINGS

Most nutritionists are employed by a specific agency or organization. While they might have some input or influence with the surrounding neighborhood or other organizations, their priority is to serve the people who are clients of their employing agency or institution. However, they can collaborate in program planning to ensure that interventions are appropriate. They can join with partners to maximize use and pool existing resources. Consistent, coordinated nutrition messages through schools, health care clinics and community centers, senior centers, faith-based organizations, and worksites increase the likelihood for success to improve personal and community health.

Examples of the opportunities to incorporate nutrition messages:

- *After-school programs*—US Department of Agriculture's Food Stamp Education Program funds many after-school programs that offer healthy foods as snacks, nutrition-related games and art projects, gardening and food growing activities, cooking and taste testing, to develop nutrition-related life skills.
- *Food and social services*—The federally funded WIC program (see Chapter 8) and elderly nutrition programs (see Chapter 10) offer vouchers to purchase locally grown fresh fruits and vegetables. Recipes and nutrition information often accompany the produce. Activities at food pantries and other sites in which food is distributed include food demonstrations, taste testing of foods that use ingredients available at most food pantries. Easy-to-use recipes may accompany the food bags. Other activities include healthy shopping tours of local supermarkets or farmers' markets, and home visits.
- *Recreation centers, community centers, libraries, senior centers*—Partners to provide nutrition interventions can use these community locations to

introduce and reinforce nutrition messages in many ways. Displays of nutrition literature can accompany an informational bulletin board with take-home healthy-eating tips, recipes, and snack and lunch ideas. Exercise programs targeted to a specific audience can make physical activity easy and fun and promote local contact with peers. All meals and snacks served should reflect the current Dietary Guidelines.

- ○ *Worksite*—Recognizing the value of physical activity and healthy food choices upon overall weight control, health, and work productivity, many employers offer employees discounts or reimbursement for gym membership with approved weight management programs, healthy foods and snacks in the cafeteria, and on-site health education programs. Philadelphia's Fun, Fit & Free! Trip is a promotion that challenges participants to take a series of 76-day trips to various fictitious locations around the country. Philadelphians go on trips to "Weightville," West Virginia; "Las Veggies," Nevada; "Pressureburg," Pennsylvania; and "Fitadelphia," Pennsylvania. The program offers Philadelphians a 10-week program that encourages them to visit local health clubs and participate in cooking and exercise classes.[25]
- • *Point-of-Purchase*—The Baltimore Healthy Stores Project is led by a research team from the Johns Hopkins Bloomberg School of Public Health in partnership with the Baltimore City Health Department and other interested community organizations. Using formative research conducted to understand the predominant influences on African-American adolescent diet in East Baltimore, programs will be developed to increase access to a nutritionally adequate diet, improve food security (see Chapter 4), and reduce the risk of diet-related chronic diseases. One of the project's initial steps included a Baltimore Healthy Stores Community Leaders Workshop, to build collaborations and rapport with organizations working to improve health in Baltimore city.[26]
- • *Faith-based*—Search Your Heart is a faith-based program for heart health and stroke prevention designed to reach African-Americans and Latinos. Bread for Life, one of several program modules offered through churches, is a heart healthy cooking and nutrition workshop.[27]

Extend the Message Through Other Health, and Related Professionals

One of the *Healthy People 2010* nutrition objectives is to increase to at least 75% the proportion of primary care providers who offer nutrition counseling or referral to qualified nutritionists and/or dietitians[9] (see Chapter 21). However, many health care and social service professionals as well as health education teachers have little or no training in current trends in nutrition, dietary recommendations, and cultural food preferences or medical nutrition therapy and education strategies. With the continuing high profile of the *Dietary Guidelines for Americans 2005* and the integral relationship between food choices and body weight to overall health and chronic disease, all health care professionals and educators must be attuned to the nutrition-related component of their specialty. Schools in some states are required to calculate body mass index (BMI), plot BMI on CDC's growth charts on all of their schoolchildren, and communicate these results to parents.[28]

Public health nutritionists join forces with others to empower the public to make healthy food choices. They work towards achieving this objective by educating members of the health care team, social services departments, and school district staff, most of whom are required to participate in continuing education to maintain their accreditation. Paraprofessionals, such as community nutrition aides, lay health advisors, and peer counselors, can be trained to provide up-to-date, evidence-based food and nutrition information to low-risk clients and groups, to extend the reach of public health nutritionists.

The nutritionist can also offer consultation to integrate nutrition screening and referral as part of overall public health and social services. Examples of appropriate sites are HIV clinics, family planning practices, school health programs, and the management of chronic diseases in health clinics. There are opportunities for public health nutritionists to develop nutrition education teaching tools and curriculum for use in schools. Nutritionists are responsible to ensure that all health care professionals use clear, candid, accurate, culturally and linguistically relevant nutrition messages.[9] By extending research-evidence-based nutrition messages through other health care and social service professions, public health nutritionists maximize their efforts and visibility.

NUTRITION SCREENING AND MEDICAL NUTRITION THERAPY

Follow-up of nutrition screening with individualized education, and counseling by a nutritionist in medical centers, outpatient clinics, fitness clubs, and private practices have been shown to have positive and clinically significant effects on food choices of persons with chronic and acute conditions.[9] This type of nutrition intervention requires partnering, communication, and collaboration with other health professionals (see Chapter 21).

Screening programs should be planned so that effective nutrition education for all participants begins at the first contact, continues according to the individual's needs and is coordinated with any medical intervention. Each client with an abnormal test result or body mass index (BMI) should be advised about its significance and how to follow up with diagnosis and treatment. Prior to conducting community-screening programs, plans should be made with health department and local physicians and registered dietitians to accept referrals. They must agree on the levels that define risk and know how to prescribe and implement treatments. Each patient who is referred should be followed to ensure that adequate and appropriate medical nutrition therapy is provided. Because follow-up activities are time-consuming and costly, some planners of screening programs omit follow-up, asserting that the client is responsible for following the recommendations given by the screening program. This philosophy defeats the aim of screening, which is to identify risk factors and empower and support individuals to remedy them. Before creating demands through a nutrition screening or referral program, an inventory should be made of community nutrition services offered by registered dietitians or qualified nutritionists, and those available should be assessed for quality. Additional services may need to be developed.[29]

Group nutrition education and individual counseling can be integrated into convenient locations, including schools, outpatient clinics, health centers, medical centers, recreation centers, worksites, and libraries. Group nutrition education is most effective when group members share a common need for nutrition information, and when sessions are culturally sensitive and relevant, interactive, skill building, and focus on need-to-know information. Nutritionists should understand the needs of group, the community in which they live, and potential barriers to obtaining a healthy diet. The *Dietary Guidelines for Americans 2005* challenge nutritionists to translate them into advice that clients can use everyday. Group sessions can be planned with public and voluntary health agencies. Sessions should be planned at convenient times and consider factors that may be obstacles to attendance, such as clients who need child care or transportation. Snacks highlight healthy food choices.

EVALUATION

What outcomes indicate success? Successful outcomes may be measured by achievement of desired changes in body weight and body mass index (BMI), normal blood chemistry values, and normal blood pressure. They also could include dietary changes that support the *Dietary Guidelines*, changes in personal beliefs and values about good health, and increased access to healthy foods and more opportunities for physical activity. The evaluation of a nutrition intervention may include measures that assess changes in the biological, experiential, intrapersonal and environmental factors outlined in the social cognitive model. While assessing changes in diet and health are the ultimate goals of a nutrition intervention, it is also important to measure changes in objectives related to the factors that influence these goals.

Seeking consultation from individuals and institutions with evaluation skills is an important component of evaluating a nutrition intervention. Evaluation is needed to measure the success of planned intervention, and to develop deeper understanding of the factors that contribute to success or to determine what needs to be strengthened in future efforts. Permanent change takes time and prescribed medical nutrition therapy may only partially influence health outcomes. In addition to providing information and motivation, nutritionists help people attain and sustain positive changes by continuing to assess, acknowledge, and overcome barriers to their population in choosing healthy foods.

POINTS TO PONDER

- How does the nutritionist balance the needs to serve high-risk target populations with those likely to generate income or political support?
- How does a nutritionist balance time spent in planning and delivering nutrition interventions with advocating for change at the policy level?
- How does the nutritionist translate complex scientific findings into simple, clear messages that motivate culturally diverse individuals to change their eating habits?
- How does the nutritionist compete with the professionally developed, audience-focused, high-budget messages utilized by companies to sell less healthy foods?

HELPFUL WEB SITES

Nutrition Education for Low-Literate Teens & Adults:
www.nifl.gov/nifl-health/2002/0291.html

NOTES

1. USDA. Foods sold in competition with USDA School Meal Programs, 2001. Available at: http://www.fns.usda.gov/cnd/lunch/CompetitiveFoods/report_congress. htm.
2. Hartsoe S. Fructose sweetener linked to obesity rise. *Associated Press*. March 25, 2004. Available at: http://story.news.yahoo.com/news?tmpl=story&cid=534&ncid= 534&e=1&u=/ap/20040325/ap_on_he_me/fit_fructose_obesity
3. United States Department of Agriculture. *USDA Continuing Survey of Food Intake by Individuals, 1994 to 1996*. Washington, DC: USDA;
4. United States Department of Agriculture, United States Department of Health and Human Services. *Dietary Guidelines for Americans 2005*. Available at: http://www. healthierus.gov/dietaryguidelines/

5. Contento I. *Strategies for Nutrition Education: Theory, Research, and Practice (need to check exact reference—not yet published)*

6. Glanz K, et al. *Health Behavior and Health Education, Theory, Research, and Practice*. San Francisco, Calif: John Wiley & Sons, Inc; 2002.

7. Luepker RV, Perry CL, McKinlay SM, et al. Outcomes of a field trial to improve children's dietary patterns and physical activity. The Child and Adolescent Trial for Cardiovascular Health (CATCH) collaborative group. *J Am Med Assoc.* 1996;*275: 786–776.*

8. Baranowski T, et al. Gimme fruit, juice and vegetables for fun and health: outcome evaluation. *Health Education & Behavior.* 2000; 27:96–111.

9. Office of Disease Prevention and Health Promotion, US Dept Health and Human Services. *Healthy People 2010.* Available at: http://www.healthypeople.gov.

10. The Food Trust. Healthy beverage toolkit. 2005. Available at: www.thefoodtrust.org

11. Hermann M. Teen role models can help shape new eating behaviors. *J Am Diet Assoc.* November 1, 2001:

12. The Food Trust. Available at: www.thefoodtrust.org

13. Wellness Policy. Public Law 108 -265-June 30, 2004. 118 STAT.729 Section 204.

14. You want any fruit with that, Mac? *New York Times.* February 20, 2005:Section 3.

15. American Dietetic Association January 12, 2005. Available at: http://www.eatright.org

16. American Medical Association Foundation. Available at: www.ama-assn.org/ama/pub/category/8577.html.

17. Doak C, Doak L, Root J., *Teaching Patients with Low Literacy Skills.* 2nd ed. Philadelphia, Pa: J.P. Lippincott Company; 1996.

18. Stuart T, Achterberg C. Education and communication strategies for different groups and settings. Available at: http//:www.fao.org/docrep/w3733e/w3733e04.htm

19. Center for Science in the Public Interest (CSPI). Pestering parents: How food companies market obesity to children. November 2003.

20. Available at: http://www.cdc.gov/youthcampaign.

21. Available at: http://www.gotmilk.com.

22. Available at: http://www.5aDay.com.

23. Available at: http://www.smallstep.gov.

24. US Dept Health and Human Services. Citing dangerous increase in deaths, HHS launches new strategies against overweight epidemic [News release]. March 9, 2004. Available at: http://www.jama.-ama.org.

25. fun fit and free

26. Baltimore Healthy Stores Project. Available at: http://www.healthystores.org.

27. Available at: www.americanheart.org

28. Available at: http://www.dsf.health.state.pa.us/health/CWP/view.asp?A=190&QUESTION_ID=236526

29. Kaufman M, ed. *Nutrition in Public Health: A Handbook for Developing Programs and Services.* Rockville, Md: Aspen; 1990:376–377.

BIBLIOGRAPHY

Clear and to the Point: Guidelines for Using Plain Language. (1994). National Institute on Health.

Clear & Simple: Developing Effective Print Materials for Low Literacy Readers (1994). National Institute of Health, National Cancer Institute

Beyond the Brochure: Alternative Approaches to Effect Health Communication. (1994). American Cancer Research Center and the Center for Disease Control and Prevention.

http://www.nal.usda.gov/fnic/pubs/bibs/gen/lowlit.html

http://www.nifl.gov

http://www.hsph.harvard.edu/healthliteracy/materials.html

http://www.nim.nih.gov/pubs/cbm/hliteracy.html

Healthy lifestyles & disease prevention initiative. Available at: http://www. adcouncil.org/campaigns/healthy lifestyles.

AMA Foundation. Health literacy overview. Available at: http//:www.ama-org/ama/pub/category/8577.html. Accessed

Center for Science in the Public Interest. *Dispensing Junk: How School Vending Undermines Efforts to Feed Children Well.* 2004.

Nestle M, Jacobson M. *Halting the obesity epidemic: a public health policy approach. Public Health Reports.* January/February 2000.

Nestle M. *Food Politics: How the Food Industry Influences Nutrition and Health.* University of California Press; 2002.

The National Alliance for Nutrition and Activity (NANA).From *Wallet to Waistline: the Hidden Costs of Super Sizing.* 2002.

National Literacy Forum. Adult and Family Literacy in the United States: Key Issues for the 21st Century [White paper]. 1999.

Food and Nutrition Information Center (FNIC). *Nutrition* education for low literate teens and adults. September 2002. Available at: http://www.nal.usda.gov/fnic/pubs/bibs/gen/lowlit.html.

CHAPTER 19

Develop a Qualified Public Health/Community Nutrition Staff

Betsy Haughton

Reader Objectives

- Describe the work to be accomplished by public health/community nutrition personnel.
- List and describe the three dimensions of public health/community nutrition practice.
- Compare and contrast public health nutrition personnel whose practice focuses on populations or systems versus community nutrition personnel whose practice focuses on individual clients and small groups (e.g., what they do, theoretical foundations for their practice, and their respective education and training requirements).
- Describe where public health/community nutrition personnel work, including their administrative structures and employment options.
- Recommend staffing ratios for population/systems-focused public health nutrition personnel versus those community nutrition personnel that provide counseling and education to individuals and small groups.

THE PUBLIC HEALTH/COMMUNITY NUTRITION WORKFORCE AS INFRASTRUCTURE

The public health/community nutrition workforce is a vital component of the public health infrastructure.[1] This workforce needs to be adequate in numbers and appropriately trained to support the essential public health functions and provide

443

essential public health nutrition services.[2] The public health/community nutrition workforce is defined as "all those who contribute to organized efforts to protect and promote health through better nutrition."[3]

Historically, the public health nutrition workforce has been primarily employed in official public health agencies funded by local, state, and federal tax dollars. Today, official public health departments working alone cannot adequately support the mission of public health and assure conditions in which people can be healthy.[4,5] Collaborations and partnerships of the public, private, and voluntary sectors are required for more successful action than can be achieved by any single sector working alone. This more comprehensive definition of the public health system embraces official state and local public health departments, working collaboratively with public health and health science academia, the health care delivery system, businesses and their employees, the media, and the people of the community at large with their schools, faith-based organizations, and other community groups.[6]

The public health/community nutrition workforce is employed in all of these sectors. Those who work in public health departments are federal, state, or local employees. Others work in private or voluntary agencies and institutions funded by philanthropic contributions from organizations and individuals. Some are self-employed in private practice and paid fees for their services, such as medical nutrition therapy counseling, nutrition education, staff training, or grant writing. All of these nutrition personnel participate in the broad view of the public health infrastructure as they work as partners across agencies and institutions in this system and within and across disciplines.

To build public health capacity requires public/community health nutrition workers to meet measurable objectives and perform effectively and efficiently.[7] The goals and objectives to be achieved are prescribed at the national level by *Healthy People 2010,*[8] and at the state and local levels by each state or local agency's current health improvement plan. Public health/community nutrition personnel practice should be driven by the nutrition services component of the state or local health improvement plan (see Chapter 14). Health objectives for the nation, state, or community should determine what public health/community nutrition staffs are required to do and how they practice.[9] This requires thoughtful analysis of the nutrition plan, considering the number and qualifications of public health/community nutrition personnel needed to implement the action plan and achieve the outcome objectives.

DEFINE THE WORK OF PUBLIC HEALTH/COMMUNITY NUTRITION PERSONNEL

The 1988 landmark Institute of Medicine report titled *The Future of Public Health* identified three public health core functions: Assessment, policy development, and assurance[10] (see Chapter 1). These population/systems focused functions are accomplished through 10 essential services.[11,12] *Assessment* means monitoring the population's health through surveillance and survey strategies and then using the data collected and analyzed to diagnose problems and identify assets as the basis for setting priorities. *Policy development* builds from assessment and includes setting priorities, program and strategic planning, mobilization of communities, formation of strategic partnerships, and use of data to inform, educate, and empower. *Assurance* involves establishing the legislative and regulatory mechanisms to promote health and prevent disease and evaluate the impact of public health plans and implemented programs. Assurance requires employing and supervising a workforce with the competence to provide the essential services. When necessary, this may mean referring or providing primary health care to individuals and families who cannot obtain it from other providers. Although assuring the essential services are the primary responsibilities of official health agencies, the broader public health system contributes to attainment of health goals by providing many of the essential services.

The core functions and essential services apply across public health. The essential public health nutrition services have been delineated by the Association of State and Territorial Public Health Nutrition Directors, the national organization that represents nutrition directors of state and territorial government health agencies.[13] These nutrition services can be categorized by the three core functions (Table 19–1). For example, the essential public health nutrition services for the assessment core function include assessing the nutritional status of specific populations or geographic areas, identifying target populations that may be at nutritional risk, and initiating and participating in nutrition data collection.

THREE DIMENSIONS OF PUBLIC HEALTH/COMMUNITY NUTRITION PRACTICE

How public health/community nutrition personnel practice and work in support of the core functions and essential services can be described along three dimensions as outlined in Figure 19–1.

Dimension 1: Life Cycle

Nutrition is essential to promote health throughout the lifespan. Historically, public health nutrition personnel focused on mothers and children, working with pregnant women to improve outcomes of pregnancy, and with mothers of infants, children, and adolescents to promote appropriate growth and development. This focus on the maternal and child population remains critical (see Chapter 8). However, research documents how important it is to maintain a health-promoting diet throughout life. For example, overweight and obesity are problems not limited to childbearing women and children; their relationship to chronic diseases must be addressed throughout all years of life.

Table 19–1 Essential Public Health Nutrition Services and Core Functions

Core Function	Essential Service
Assessment	Assess the nutritional status of specific populations or geographic areas.
	Identify target populations that may be at nutritional risk.
	Initiate and participate in nutrition data collection.
Policy Development	Provide leadership in the development of and planning for health and nutrition policies.
	Raise awareness among key policy makers of the potential impact of nutrition and food regulations and budget decisions on the health of the community.
	Act as an advocate for target populations on food and nutrition issues.
	Plan for nutrition services in conjunction with other health services, based on information obtained from an adequate and ongoing data base focused on health outcomes.
	Identify or assist in development of accurate, up-to-date nutrition education materials.
Assurance	Ensure the availability of quality nutrition services to target populations, including nutrition screening, assessment, education, counseling, and referral for food assistance and follow-up.
	Participate in nutrition research, demonstration, and evaluation projects.
	Provide expert nutrition consultation to the community.
	Provide community health promotion and disease prevention activities that are population based.
	Provide quality assurance guidelines for practitioners dealing with food and nutrition issues.
	Facilitate coordination with other providers of health and nutrition services within the community.
	Evaluate the impact on the health status of populations who receive public health nutrition services.
	Recommend and provide specific training and programs to meet identified nutrition needs.

Source: Adapted from Moving to the Future: Developing Community-Based Nutrition Services, p. 87, Association of State & Territorial Public Health Nutrition Directors, Prepared by Chapter Author, Betsy Haughton.

Dimension 2: Levels of Prevention

The levels of prevention range from prevention of risk factors (primary prevention), reduction of risk factors (secondary prevention), and treatment of disease (tertiary prevention). Most public health/community nutrition personnel focus on primary and secondary prevention, but some are involved in tertiary prevention. For example, the community nutrition educator who advises new mothers about how to feed their babies works on primary prevention, while the community dietitian who counsels overweight adults to control weight and reduce hypertension

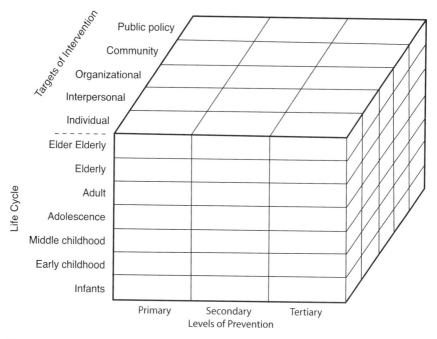

Figure 19–1 Dimensions of Community and Public Health Nutrition Practice. *Source:* Prepared by Chapter Author, Betsy Haughton.

is working on secondary prevention or risk factor reduction. The community dietitian who advises families of overweight children with Prader-Willi Syndrome practices tertiary prevention, or the treatment of this genetic disorder that includes hyperphagia, or overeating.

Dimension 3: Targets of Intervention

This dimension of public health/community nutrition practice is described by an ecological framework that includes five targets of interventions:[14,15,16]

1. Individual factors
2. Interpersonal factors
3. Organizational factors
4. Community factors
5. System or policy factors

When an individual receives prescribed medical nutrition therapy, the goal of the intervention is to change that person's nutrition knowledge, attitudes, and eating behaviors. This is accomplished by education and counseling. Interventions targeted at individual and interpersonal factors are referred to as *direct care* or *client-focused* services. Improved nutrition-related health outcomes are attained also by directing interventions to interpersonal factors, using families and friends as social support networks to maintain and reinforce individual dietary behavior change. Interventions to change interpersonal factors also may rely on peer support groups or enlist lay health advisers. Practice targeted at individual and interpersonal factors has become the foundation of many community nutrition programs and services.[17] Increasingly, since 1974 the vast majority of community nutrition personnel have been employed with funds from the Special Supplemental Nutrition Program for Women, Infants, and Children (WIC) (see Chapter 8). This program serves income-eligible pregnant and breastfeeding women, infants, and children up to age 5 years who are referred because of nutrition-related health risks. The women and caregivers receive nutrition education, coupons to purchase specified nutrient-dense supplemental foods, and referrals for health care. Individual factors are targeted when community nutrition educators and community dietitians provide this nutrition education and counseling, while interpersonal factors are targeted when they use facilitated group discussion.[18] Peer support groups help families adopt healthier eating styles.

Increasingly, the broader public health system requires public health nutritionists with graduate training in public health to work with population or system-level targets. Organizational factors are the target of interventions to improve the built environment or programs, practices, and policies within a specific organizational setting. A public health nutritionist might conduct a worksite wellness program to promote healthy eating practices by designing cafeteria menus that feature tasty, lower-calorie food choices labeled with nutrition information at point of purchase. The built environment includes the buildings and spaces that the community creates or modifies. It includes such places as greenways, workplaces, and parking lots. One example of how the built environment can be shaped to encourage more physical activity in the workplace is to place signs in stairwells and by elevators as point-of-decision prompts to encourage employees to use the stairs to increase the number of steps they take during each day.[19]

Community factors that extend beyond the worksite are also the goal of public health nutrition practice. For example, public health nutritionists may collaborate to develop, implement, and evaluate a communitywide media campaign to educate the public about healthy eating and regular exercise to prevent overweight and obesity. Another example would be to participate in launching a community coalition to promote breastfeeding.

Public health nutritionists also address nutrition-related health policy issues when they advocate for laws and regulations that impact what people eat, how much they eat, and where they eat. Media campaigns, coalition building, policymaking, and lobbying for new legislation are strategies at the fifth target of public health nutrition interventions. Public health nutritionists may recommend public policies to inform and encourage consumers to choose foods that contribute to a healthy diet that promotes health and prevents diet-related diseases.

Examples might include recommending that the sale of "competitive foods" be prohibited in public schools or that taxes be imposed on sales of sweetened soft drinks and confections and fat-laden snack foods in vending machines.

Figure 19–1 depicts the three dimensions of public health nutrition practice: 1) life cycle, 2) levels of prevention, and 3) targets of intervention. Public health/community nutrition personnel work with individuals, families, and communities at every stage of their lives and direct their interventions at the host of factors that influence how and what people choose to eat. The level of prevention defines the priorities of risk factor prevention or reduction and disease treatment. Table 19–2 provides some examples across the life cycle of public health nutrition activities that focus on the three levels of prevention and five targets of intervention.

PUBLIC HEALTH/COMMUNITY NUTRITION STAFF TO ACCOMPLISH THIS WORK

Public health requires a nutrition workforce that understands and applies all three dimensions of public health practice. A variety of public health/community nutrition personnel are needed. While each practices differently, all work together to improve nutrition-related health outcomes. Most of the currently employed public health/community nutrition staff provides nutrition counseling and education to individuals, families, and small groups. What follows differentiates the two broad categories of nutrition personnel who work in the community:[20] 1) those having a client-focus provide interventions targeted at individual and interpersonal factors, and 2) those having a population/system-focus provide interventions targeted at organizational, community, and policy factors.

Client-Focused Care

Community nutrition personnel who work face-to-face with individuals or families to direct their work to primary, secondary, and tertiary prevention across the life cycle. While job titles vary from one organization to another, in general, community nutrition workers include nutrition aides or assistants, nutrition technicians, community nutrition educators, and community dietitians. The distinctions between these personnel depend on their work with low- or high-risk clients, their academic nutrition preparation, and dietetics credentialing.

Nutrition assistants or aides work with low-risk clients and may be peer counselors or lay nutrition advisers. Their positions require on-the-job training, but do not require any academic training in nutrition. They know their neighbors and neighborhood and have real-life experience with the local food habits, including preferred cultural foods, usual food preparation methods, and other target behaviors, such as breastfeeding and family meal planning. They may be community

Table 19–2 Examples of Community and Public Health Nutrition Practice by Level of Prevention and Target of Intervention

Level of Prevention	Target of Intervention				
	Personal		Organization and Community		System
	Individual	Interpersonal	Organization	Community	Social Structure, Policy, Systems
Primary	Individual instruction on how to breast-feed	Buddy system to increase number of steps walked each day	Use of local produce in school lunch program	Local "5-a-Day" campaign in association with farmers' markets, schools, and grocery stores	Folic acid fortification of foods
Secondary	Nutrition counseling for high-risk pregnant women	Family counseling for weight control	Worksite wellness programs with screening and referrals	Health fairs with screening and referrals to primary care providers	Required food labeling for specified nutrients
Tertiary	Medical nutrition therapy	Medical nutrition therapy using family support network	Worksite incentives for improved glucose control	Diabetes classes offered at local health system	Insurance payment for medical nutrition therapy for diabetes nutrition education

Source: Prepared by Chapter Author, Betsy Haughton.

leaders who work effectively with the people from their community and speak their language.

Nutrition technicians have some academic preparation in foods and nutrition, usually have an associate degree, and are credentialed as dietetic technicians, registered (DTR). They too work with low-risk clients.

Community nutrition educators have bachelor degrees with some coursework in nutrition and food preparation. Nutrition technicians and community nutrition educators are primarily employed by local WIC programs to provide nutrition counseling and education to groups of low-risk pregnant or breastfeeding women and mothers of infants and preschool children.

Community dietitians work with high-risk clients and have academic preparation and training at the bachelor's level and they also have completed a specified program of supervised work experience to be credentialed as registered dietitians (RDs). An example would be a community dietitian who works with children with special health care needs. These members of the nutrition staff focus their work on outreach, screening, record keeping, teaching, education, counseling, care coordination/case management, and some consultation to other health professionals.[21]

Depending on the type of position, all public health/community nutrition personnel may perform some of the same broad categories of responsibilities, but at different levels and to different degrees of responsibility. For example, both nutrition aides or assistants and nutrition technicians may teach parents about how to feed their children to promote healthy weight. The community dietitian may help parents learn to feed their children and develop nutrition education materials and lesson plans that other personnel use in their teaching. The primary distinction between the roles of nutrition aides/assistants and nutrition technicians compared to community dietitians is the focus on primary prevention compared to secondary and tertiary prevention. Paraprofessionals and nutrition technicians focus on prevention of risk factors and low-risk nutrition education, while community dietitians usually focus on secondary and tertiary prevention. Community dietitians also may select or develop educational materials and programs and provide in-service education to prepare paraprofessionals and nutrition technicians to use these educational materials in their work.[22]

Since these community nutrition personnel focus on interventions at individual and interpersonal factors, intervention theories and models inform their practice accordingly.[23] For example, the community nutrition educator working with a teenage mother to help her choose healthy meals and snacks can use the stages of change model[24] to determine the adolescent's motivation to change. This model helps identify the readiness of the teenager to change behaviors, including eating habits. With this knowledge, a specific nutrition education pamphlet or lesson can be selected or tailored to the teenager's motivation level. Similarly, social cognitive theory[25] can be used to help individuals understand how their thoughts, interpersonal relationships, and environment shape their behaviors. For example, the community dietitian can help an overweight adult understand what triggers and reinforces overeating and then help develop self-management skills to develop self-confidence to make successful changes. This understanding of the relationship of thoughts, behaviors, and the environment helps target interventions at the interpersonal level.

Required academic preparation and credentials depend on the roles the various personnel perform. Credentialing as a dietetic technician (DTR) or registered dietitian (RD) requires specified academic preparation and supervised clinical training as stipulated by the Commission on Dietetic Registration.[26] In addition, community dietitians who work with select groups of clients may seek additional certifications, such as an International Board Certified Lactation Consultant (IBCLC) or Certified Diabetes Educator (CDE). To help staff maintain credentials and keep current on evidence-based theory and practice, community nutrition personnel should receive ongoing in-service education and on-the-job training, and participate in professional development. They should be offered opportunities to attend professional or academic short courses to enhance their skills in primary, secondary, and tertiary prevention across the life cycle and targeted at individual and interpersonal factors. Experience as a community dietitian can be the first step on the public health nutrition career ladder to be enhanced by a graduate degree in public health.

Population/System-Focused Personnel

The current epidemic of obesity and overweight and the resulting economic and social burden of diet-related chronic diseases require population/systems-focused programs and public policy changes directed to the wider community to reach many more people at much less cost (see Chapter 18). Interventions at the community and systems level shape the environment to support healthy eating practices of all of the community's individuals and families. Public health nutritionists who have a population/system approach work on interventions across the lifespan. They focus more attention on primary and secondary prevention and less on tertiary prevention. Their interventions address the organizational, community, and policy issues to support the population as a whole to choose health promoting eating practices.

Nutrition personnel who work at the population/system level also use theories to guide evidence-based practice. For example, public health nutritionists who intervene within organizations can apply organizational change theories.[27,28] One of these, Stage Theory of Organizational Change, suggests that organizations pass through different stages as they adopt new policies, programs, and services. To move from one stage to another, different strategies are used. Another organizational stage theory, Organizational Development Theory, focuses on human relations and the process of organizational change. Using these theories, a public health nutritionist first might use Organizational Development Theory and consult with a school system as it begins to formulate and adopt nutrition policies. Then, after the policies have been institutionalized, the public health nutritionist might use Stage Theory and consult with the school as it evaluates the impact of these policies and begins to establish new policy goals.

Public health nutritionists who work to improve community factors related to food and nutrition will find other intervention theories or helpful models. For example, using community organization theory,[29] a public health nutritionist would partner with concerned community members as equals and encourage them to identify their common problems, priorities, and goals, and then to develop programs that mobilize community resources to develop and implement strategies to address these priorities. Public health nutritionists who try to effect policy change draw upon this theory and others to make strategic use of media advocacy, for example, to promote public policy initiatives.

Usually public health nutritionists use multiple strategies to effect change. For example, the East Tennessee 2-Step Initiative[30] was designed to address the problem of overweight and obesity in a 16-county region. Community stakeholders, health department staff, and university researchers working together identified evidence-based strategies to promote healthy weight that would work within the region at the individual, organizational, community, and policy levels. Public health nutritionists were involved throughout the process, using their skills in planning and evaluation, management, fiscal control, and research. One public health nutrition-trained health department member provided leadership for the initiative overall, drawing especially upon skills in partnership and coalition building.

All public health nutritionists are the leaders responsible for the core functions. Specific roles performed by public health nutrition personnel vary depending on whether they are responsible for organizational, community, or policy factors and whether their practice also includes management and administrative responsibilities. They plan and evaluate programs and services at some level. The public health nutrition director works with the agency administrators and planners to integrate nutrition plans into the agency's health improvement plan. Other public health nutritionists may work with an assigned program director and staff, and plan and evaluate specific nutrition programs and services as part of the strategic plan for a selected public health program, such as maternal and child health, adult health, health promotion, food safety, or licensure of group care facilities. The primary roles of public health nutritionists and managers are policymaking, management, fiscal control, planning/evaluation, supervision, consultation, education, and care coordination/case management.[31] Public health nutritionists also may participate in research projects, particularly those related to evidence-based practice and its determination.[32] These personnel must be skillful communicators and able to work with populations from diverse cultures in their communities. They must be able to work effectively with a wide variety of community organizations in collaborations and partnerships.[33] To carry out their assurance function they plan for staffing and employ, manage, and supervise the community nutrition workforce that provides direct services to clients.

The titles used for nutrition personnel with population-system responsibilities vary depending on where they work and how they practice. Titles may include public health nutrition director, public health nutrition supervisor, public health nutrition consultant, and public health nutritionist. The use of *public health* in the title signifies the population/system responsibilities that require a master's degree (Master of Public Health [MPH], Master of Science in Public Health [MSPH], or Master of Science [MS]), which includes both graduate course work and supervised field experience in public health. The graduate public health course work includes biostatistics, epidemiology, public health policy, and administration, environmental and occupational health, and social-behavioral sciences. This background prepares public health nutritionists to work with the population/ system approach. The knowledge and skills required for graduate-level training in public health and advanced nutrition have been established by the Association of Graduate Programs in Public Health Nutrition, Inc. and published in *Strategies for Success: Curriculum Guide—Graduate Public Health Nutrition Programs.*[34] Credentialing as a registered dietitian (RD) is also important.[35,36] These knowledge and skills statements build on those required for dietetic registration as published by the Commission on Dietetic Registration.

SIZE OF THE PUBLIC HEALTH/COMMUNITY NUTRITION WORKFORCE

Responsibility for the public's health is shared by agencies and organizations in the public, private, and voluntary sectors.[37,38] Public health and community nutrition personnel work in all of these sectors. Unfortunately, there is no complete census of all of the nutrition personnel who work in all of these sectors. The Association of State and Territorial Public Health Nutrition Directors periodically conducts the most complete census. The most recent census in 1999–2000 mainly counted nutrition professionals or paraprofessionals in public health/community nutrition programs funded directly or indirectly by state or local health departments. This census enumerated almost 11,000 public health/community nutrition personnel. Almost 68% of these were government employees in state and local public health agencies. Over 25% of those counted were employed in private not-for-profit agencies. Less than 1% was employed in the for-profit private sector.[39] This census did not count the public health/community nutrition staff who work in the private sector or other federally funded programs, such as Cooperative Extension Services, or State and Area Agencies on Aging, who provide nutrition education for individuals, families, and communities.

Public health and community and nutrition personnel may be employed as budgeted or contract employees. In the 1999–2000 public health nutrition workforce census, most of the nutrition personnel were budgeted employees employed full-time or part-time by a health agency or institution. Less than 4% were employed on contract and paid an hourly rate.[40] Increasingly, there are public health nutrition personnel in private practice who contract for specific services. Private-practice nutrition consultants may contract to write grants for local health agencies for funding to support healthy weight initiatives or to develop and evaluate weight management programs for hospital systems or worksite wellness programs. Few of these nutritionists were included in the census.

ADMINISTRATIVE STRUCTURES FOR PUBLIC HEALTH/COMMUNITY NUTRITION PERSONNEL

Nutrition personnel work within the broad public health system and its variety of administrative structures. While nutrition personnel may be employed in one program or sector, increasingly they will work in partnership with those employed in other sectors and those living within the target community. This is particularly true of personnel who work with a population/system focus. Staffs need administrative support for this collaborative work and skills to work within their agency and across the public health system.[41]

In official state or local health departments, administrative structures are usually either discipline-specific or matrix organizations. In a discipline-specific administrative structure there is a nutrition program unit headed by a public health nutrition director or administrator. In this model, all nutrition personnel and related support personnel are "housed" within this nutrition unit. The public health nutrition director is responsible to the public health agency director, assistant or deputy director, or a director responsible for a generic program, such as community preventive health or local health services. All nutrition personnel report to the public health nutrition director, but they may be assigned to work across a variety of programs, such as WIC, maternal and child health, chronic disease prevention or health promotion, which may include a special "5-a-day" project to promote more fruit and vegetable consumption. There usually is a nutrition budget managed and controlled by the public health nutrition director to cover salaries and expenses of the nutrition personnel employed by the agency.

In a matrix organization, specialized nutrition consultants are responsible to and report to categorical program directors (e.g., maternal and child health, WIC, adult health, health promotion) rather than to their state's public health nutrition director. The health agency director may appoint a lead public health nutrition coordinator or consultant, who serves as the nutrition adviser to the agency director, program directors, and planners. This lead nutritionist does not supervise the specialized public health nutrition consultants. However, the lead public health nutrition consultant may coordinate and provide technical assistance and guidance to the specialized public health nutrition consultants, if they or their program director requests it.

Each administrative structure has strengths and weaknesses. Many nutrition personnel believe there is strength in the discipline-specific model, especially if the public health nutrition director manages and controls a budget. However, there have been few studies to document strengths and weaknesses of one or the other model, or even a hybrid model. Experienced public/community health nutrition personnel have learned that administrative structures change as public agencies frequently undergo legislated reorganizations. Staff must be flexible and learn quickly how to be effective in a variety of administrative structures and to maximize strengths and minimize weaknesses of the administrative structure in which they work.

FUNDING THE PUBLIC HEALTH NUTRITION WORKFORCE

The public health's nutrition workforce is usually funded from a variety of sources. The federal government, specifically the US Department of Agriculture (USDA) funds the WIC Program that supports more than 80% of personnel who work in nutrition programs affiliated with state and local health departments.[42] The eligible population for the WIC Program is written into the enabling legislation and regulations. Therefore, nutrition staff funded by WIC work predominantly with low-income pregnant and breastfeeding women, infants, and children up to 5 years of age. About 6% of nutrition personnel work in programs in state or local health agencies that are funded by the US Department of Health and Human Services, while just over 7% are paid with state and local general revenue.[43] Only this small number of public health/community nutrition personnel is available to serve adults or other populations identified as high nutritional risk by the community assessment and not eligible to participate in WIC.

Information about funding sources for public health/community nutrition personnel who do not work with programs affiliated with state health agencies is not available. However, these personnel are also part of the overall public health system and their funding sources and salaries make important contributions to the public's health.

A basic premise of public health/community nutrition practice is that the population's priorities and needs determine what is to be accomplished. If this premise is accepted, then these priorities and needs should drive how nutrition staff practice and what they do.[44] Data must show that nutrition personnel make a positive impact across the three dimensions of practice: 1) life cycle, 2) level of prevention, and 3) target of intervention. It also is important to demonstrate impact and the importance of this impact. Cost-benefit and cost-effectiveness analyses can support the need for improved salaries and increased numbers and types of public health/community nutrition personnel required[45] (see Chapters 14, 16, 17).

Staffing Ratio Recommendations

In the past few years there has been little work to study and evaluate staffing recommendations for public health/community nutrition personnel. Factors that determine the type of personnel required and their numbers relate directly to the work to be accomplished and the size of the target populations. Staffing for nutrition personnel mainly serving individual clients is determined by the size of the anticipated caseload and the need for staff to work across the life cycle with interventions that address individual and interpersonal factors. A general rule of thumb is one community dietitian to supervise two nutrition assistants or nutrition technicians for every 1000 high-risk participants in an ambulatory nutrition program. Other recommendations suggest one community dietitian to serve every 500 to 800 clients who need nutrition counseling.[46]

For population/system-focused work, the standard recommendation used by the Association of State and Territorial Public Health Nutrition Directors in its census survey is one public health nutritionist focusing on core functions for every 50,000 people in the community.[47,48] These are the public health nutritionists involved in primary and secondary prevention across the life cycle and who work on organizational, community, and policy factors that impact nutrition-related health. As the size of the target population increases or its assessed nutrition-related priorities increase, such as obesity and overweight, the number of public health nutrition personnel and their responsibilities must change. In a large metropolitan area, where a large number of nutrition personnel are required, there may be a need for a public health nutrition director, a public health nutrition supervisor, and a staff of public health/community nutritionists.

Professional Staff Development

A competent public health/community nutrition workforce must be well prepared to serve the population with whom they work. Many of the nutrition staff now employed by state and local health departments are well trained in nutrition and dietetics, but lack academic training in public health knowledge and skills.[49] Continuing professional development must address these areas. Recognizing the need for these skills and the barriers faced by existing staff in acquiring them, the Public Health/Community Nutrition Practice Group (PHCNPG) of the American Dietetic Association in collaboration with other professional associations developed Guidelines for Community Nutrition Supervised Experiences.

Public health nutritionists can use these guidelines to provide on-the-job supervised training for nutrition personnel who lack public health knowledge and skills.[50] Currently there is discussion within the public health field about the need for a public health credential for all professional public health disciplines.[51]

SALARIES FOR PUBLIC HEALTH/COMMUNITY NUTRITION PERSONNEL

Salaries for public health/community nutrition personnel vary widely across the country and across personnel types.[52] The type of agency or sector also influences how much nutrition staffs are compensated. When the American Dietetic Association conducted a salary survey of its members in 2002 it found that nutrition/dietetic personnel with more years of experience and supervisory and budget responsibility had higher salaries. Among registered dietitians, those who were self-employed and those employed in government agencies were paid higher salaries than those who worked in other areas.[53] Many of these dietitians are part of the overall public health system.

Salaries for nutrition staff who work in official health departments or government agencies are assigned to pay scales established for each position title and related to each position's qualifications and responsibilities. Pay scales should be comparable to those of other public health professionals who have equivalent responsibility, years of experience, and level of education. For example, the public health nutritionist who has a master's degree and is a registered dietitian should have a salary comparable to that of a public health nurse or health educator who performs work that requires graduate training in public health and professional credentialing. Similarly, community nutrition educators with bachelor degrees and limited experience should have salaries comparable to those of bachelor's degree health educators with limited experience.[54]

When there are concerns about competitive salaries, job audits, work surveys, and salary surveys can document the issues. For example, a metropolitan health department concerned with recruitment and retention of staff can conduct a work survey and job audit. The findings can be used by the public health nutrition director and agency administrators to justify salary adjustments to be competitive not only with other public health personnel within the agency who have comparable levels of education, experience, and job responsibilities, but also with other nutritionists and dietitians in the geographic area who have comparable levels of responsibility and required credentials. The public health/community nutrition census conducted by the Association of State and Territorial Public Health Nutrition Directors also includes salary information by state and position title.[55] Public health nutrition directors and administrators can use this information to determine how competitive their agencies' salaries are in relation to other states within the region and across the country.

POINTS TO PONDER

- What is required for the public health/community nutrition workforce to move from client-focused care and toward more population/system-focused work?
- How can the current public health/community nutrition workforce gain the public health expertise required to do more work with populations and systems?
- What is the career ladder in community and public health nutrition?
- How can public health/community nutritionists document that their work positively influences the nutrition-related health of individuals, families, and communities?
- What strategies can be used to educate public health agency administrators and personnel directors that differing competencies and educational preparation are required for nutritionists working with populations/systems and those who provide direct client care?

NOTES

1. US Dept Health and Human Services, Public Health Service. *Public Health Work-force*: *An Agenda for the 21st Century. A Report of the Public Health Functions Project*. Washington, DC: US Dept Health and Human Services; 1997:4–6,23–25. Available at: http://www.health.gov/phfunctions/pubhlth.pdf. Accessed October 10, 2004.

2. Probert KL. *Moving to the Future*: *Developing Community-Based Nutrition Services* (workbook and training manual). Washington, DC: Association of State and Territorial Public Health Nutrition Directors; 1997:87.

3. Hughes R. A conceptual framework for intelligence-based public health nutrition workforce development. *Public Health Nutr.* 2003;6:602.

4. Institute of Medicine. *Future of the Public Health's Health in the 21st Century* Washington, DC: National Academies Press; 2003:28.

5. National Association of County and City Health Officials. Mobilizing for action through planning and partnerships. A strategic approach to community health improvement. Available at: http://mapp.naccho.org/fulltextintroduction.asp and http://mapp.naccho.org/CommunityRoadmap.asp. Accessed June 17, 2004.

6. Institute of Medicine. *Future of the Public Health's Health in the 21st Century* Washington, DC: National Academies Press; 2003:28–31.

7. Beaglehole R, Dal Poz MR. Public health workforce: challenges and policy issues. *Human Resources for Health.* 2003;1. Available at: http://www.human-resources-health.com/content/1/1/4. Accessed June 17, 2004.

8. US Dept Health and Human Services. *Healthy People 2010*: *Understanding and Improving Health*. 2nd ed. Washington, DC: US Government Printing Office; 2000. Available at: http://www.health.gov/healthypeople. Accessed June 17, 2004.

9. Hughes R. A conceptual framework for intelligence-based public health nutrition workforce development. *Public Health Nutr.* 2003;6:600.

10. Institute of Medicine. *The Future of Public Health.* Washington, DC: National Academies Press; 1988:43–47.

11. Institute of Medicine. *Future of the Public Health's Health in the 21st Century* Washington, DC: National Academies Press; 2003:31–33.

12. US Dept Health and Human Services. Public health in America. Available at: http://www.health.gov/phfunctions/public.htm. Accessed June 17, 2004.

13. Probert KL. *Moving to the Future: Developing Community-Based Nutrition Services Workbook and Training Manual.* Washington DC, Association of State and Territorial Public Health Nutritional Directors. 1997:87.

14. Brownson RC, Baker EA, Lee TL, Gillespie KN. *Evidence-based Public Health.* New York, NY: Oxford University Press; 2003:170–174.

15. Gregson J, Foerster SB, Orr R, et al. Systems, environmental and policy changes: using the social-ecological model as a framework for evaluating nutrition education and social marketing programs with low-income audiences. *J Nutr Educ.* 2001;33(Suppl):S4–S15.

16. McLeroy KR, Bibeau D, Steckler A, Glanz K. An ecological perspective on health promotion programs. *Health Educ Q.* 1988;15:351–377.

17. McCall M, Keir B, for Association of State and Territorial Public Health Nutrition Directors. *Survey of the Public Health Nutrition Workforce, 1999–2000.* Nutrition Assistance Program Report Series. Washington, DC: Office of Analysis, Nutrition and Evaluation, Food and Nutrition Services, USDA; 2003:25. Available at:http://www.fns.usda.gov/oane/MENU/Published/WIC/FILES/Publichealthsurvey. pdf. Accessed June 17, 2004.

18. Abusabha R, Peacock J, Achterberg C. How to make nutrition education more meaningful through facilitated group discussions. *J Am Diet Assoc.* 1999;99:72–76.

19. Task Force on Community Preventive Services. Recommendations to increase physical activity in communities. *Am J Prev Med.* 2002;22:67–72.

20. Dodds JM, Kaufman M. *Personnel in Public Health Nutrition for the 1990's. A Comprehensive Guide.* Washington, DC: The Public Health Foundation; 1991:11–19.

21. Dodds JM, Kaufman M. *Personnel in Public Health Nutrition for the 1990's. A Comprehensive Guide.* Washington, DC: The Public Health Foundation; 1991: 18,36–48.

22. Dodds JM, Kaufman M. *Personnel in Public Health Nutrition for the 1990's. A Comprehensive Guide.* Washington, DC: The Public Health Foundation; 1991:36–41.

23. US National Institutes of Health, National Cancer Institute. *Theory at a Glance*: A Guide for Health Promotion Practice. Part II: Theories and Applications.* Bethesda, Md: National Cancer Institute; 1995: NIH Publication No. 97-3890. Available at:

http://www.cancer.gov/aboutnci/oc/theory-at-a-glance/page3. Accessed June 17, 2004.

24. Prochaska JO, Velicer WF. The transtheoretical model of health behavior change. *Am J Health Promotion*. 1997;12:38–48.

25. Bandura A. *Social Foundations of Thought and Action: A Social Cognitive Theory*. Englewood Cliffs, NJ: Prentice-Hall; 1986:18–22.

26. Commission on Accreditation for Dietetics Education, American Dietetic Association. *CADE Accreditation Handbook*. Chicago, Ill: Commission on Dietetic Registration; 2002:3–13.

27. Beyer JM, Trice HM. *Implementing Change: Alcoholism Policies in Work Organizations*. New York, NY: Free Press; 1978.

28. Porras JI, Robertson PJ. Organization development theory: a typology and evaluation. In: Woodman RW, Pasmore WA, eds. *Research in Organizational Change and Development* (Vol 1). Greenwich, Conn: JAI Press; 1987:1–57.

29. Rothman J, Tropman JE. Models of community organization and macro practice: their mixing and phasing. In: Cox FM, Ehrlich JL, Rothman J, Tropman JE, eds. *Strategies of Community Organization*. 4th ed. Itasca, Ill: Peacock; 1987:3–26.

30. Stephanie Welch, Personal Communication for *East Tennessee 2-Step Healthy Weight Initiative*. Knoxville, Tennessee, June 2004.

31. Dodds JM, Kaufman M. *Personnel in Public Health Nutrition for the 1990's. A Comprehensive Guide*. Washington, DC: The Public Health Foundation; 1991:21–34.

32. Brownson RC, Baker EA, Lee TL, Gillespie KN. *Evidence-based Public Health*. New York, NY: Oxford University Press; 2003:44–83,159–163.

33. Public Health Foundation, Competencies Project. Core competencies lists. Available at: http://www.trainingfinder.org/competencies/list.htm. Accessed June 17, 2004.

34. Association of Graduate Programs in Public Health Nutrition. *Strategies for Success. Curriculum Guide. Graduate Programs in Public Health Nutrition*. 2nd ed. Association of Graduate Programs in Public Health Nutrition, Inc; 2002:2–5. Available at: http://nutrition.utk.edu/resources/StrategiesForSuccess.pdf. Accessed June 17, 2004.

35. Association of Graduate Programs in Public Health Nutrition. *Strategies for Success. Curriculum Guide. Graduate Programs in Public Health Nutrition*. 2nd ed. Association of Graduate Programs in Public Health Nutrition, Inc; 2002:2.

36. Dodds JM, Kaufman M. *Personnel in Public Health Nutrition for the 1990's. A Comprehensive Guide*. Washington, DC: The Public Health Foundation; 1991:21–35.

37. Institute of Medicine. *The Future of Public Health*. Washington, DC: National Academies Press; 1988:42–51.

38. Institute of Medicine. *Future of the Public Health's Health in the 21st Century* Washington, DC: National Academies Press; 2003:28–33.

39. McCall M, Keir B, for Association of State and Territorial Public Health Nutrition Directors. *Survey of the Public Health Nutrition Workforce, 1999–2000*. Nutrition Assistance Program Report Series. Washington, DC: Office of Analysis, Nutrition and Evaluation, Food and Nutrition Services, USDA; 2003:1–4.

40. McCall M, Keir B, for Association of State and Territorial Public Health Nutrition Directors. *Survey of the Public Health Nutrition Workforce, 1999–2000*. Nutrition Assistance Program Report Series. Washington, DC: Office of Analysis, Nutrition and Evaluation, Food and Nutrition Services, USDA; 2003:30–31.

41. National Association of County and City Health Officials. Mobilizing for action. Available at: http://mapp.naccho.org/lphsa/index.asp.

42. McCall M, Keir B, for Association of State and Territorial Public Health Nutrition Directors. *Survey of the Public Health Nutrition Workforce, 1999–2000*. Nutrition Assistance Program Report Series. Washington, DC: Office of Analysis, Nutrition and Evaluation, Food and Nutrition Services, USDA; 2003:34–36.

43. McCall M, Keir B, for Association of State and Territorial Public Health Nutrition Directors. *Survey of the Public Health Nutrition Workforce, 1999–2000*. Nutrition Assistance Program Report Series. Washington, DC: Office of Analysis, Nutrition and Evaluation, Food and Nutrition Services, USDA; 2003:35.

44. Hughes R. A conceptual framework for intelligence-based public health nutrition workforce development. *Public Health Nutr*.2003;6:600.

45. Brownson RC, Baker EA, Lee TL, Gillespie KN. *Evidence-based Public Health*. New York, NY: Oxford University Press; 2003:56–67.

46. Kaufman M. Personnel for delivery of nutrition services. In: Sharbaugh CO, ed. *Call to Action. Better Nutrition for Mothers, Children, and Families*. Washington, DC: National Center for Education in Maternal and Child Health; 1991:278.

47. Peck E, ed. *Leadership and Quality Assurance in Ambulatory Health Care: What Is the Role of the Public Health Nutritionist?* Berkeley, Calif: University of California; 1978:132–133.

48. Kaufman M. Personnel for delivery of nutrition services. In: Sharbaugh CO, ed. *Call to Action. Better Nutrition for Mothers, Children, and Families*. Washington, DC: National Center for Education in Maternal and Child Health; 1991:46.

49. McCall M, Keir B, for Association of State and Territorial Public Health Nutrition Directors. *Survey of the Public Health Nutrition Workforce, 1999–2000*. Nutrition Assistance Program Report Series. Washington, DC: Office of Analysis, Nutrition and Evaluation, Food and Nutrition Services, USDA; 2003:37–50.

50. Mixon H, Dodds J, Haughton B. *Guidelines for Community Nutrition Supervised Experiences*. 2nd ed. Chicago, Ill: Public Health/Community Nutrition Practice Group, American Dietetic Association; 2003:1–2.Available at: http://www.phcnpg.org/GuideCommunityNutrSuperExp.pdf. Accessed June 17, 2004, 18–47.

51. Cioffi JP, Lichtveld MY, Thielen L, Miner K. Credentialing the public health workforce: an idea whose time has come. *J Public Health Management and Practice*. 2003;9:451–458.

52. McCall M, Keir B, for Association of State and Territorial Public Health Nutrition Directors. *Survey of the Public Health Nutrition Workforce, 1999–2000.* Nutrition Assistance Program Report Series. Washington, DC: Office of Analysis, Nutrition and Evaluation, Food and Nutrition Services, USDA; 2003:31–32.

53. American Dietetic Association, *2002 Dietetics Compensation & Benefits Survey.* Chicago, Ill: American Dietetic Association; 2003:11–17.

54. Kaufman M. *Nutrition in Public Health: A Handbook for Developing Programs and Services.* Rockville, Md: Aspen Publishers; 1990:397.

55. McCall M, Keir B, for Association of State and Territorial Public Health Nutrition Directors. *Survey of the Public Health Nutrition Workforce, 1999–2000.* Nutrition Assistance Program Report Series. Washington, DC: Office of Analysis, Nutrition and Evaluation, Food and Nutrition Services, USDA; 2003:31–33.

BIBLIOGRAPHY

Association of Graduate Programs in Public Health Nutrition. 2nd ed. Association of Graduate Programs in Public Health Nutrition, Inc.; 2002. *Strategies for Success. Curriculum Guide.* http://nutrition.utk.edu/resources/StrategiesForSuccess.pdf. Accessed June 17, 2004.

Dodds JM, Kaufman M. *Personnel in Public Health Nutrition for the 1990's.* Washington, DC: The Public Health Foundation; 1991.

Institute of Medicine. *The Future of the Public's Health in the 21st Century.* Washington, DC: National Academies Press; 2003.

Kaufman M. *Nutrition in Public Health: A Handbook for Developing Programs and Services;* Rockville, Md: Aspen Publishers; 1990.

Kaufman M. Personnel for delivery of nutrition services. In Sharbaugh CO ed. *Call to Action. Better Nutrition for Mothers, Children, and Families.* Washington, DC: National Center for Education in Maternal and Child Health; 1991.

McCall M, Keir B, for Association of State and Territorial Public Health Nutrition Directors. *Survey of the Public Health Nutrition Workforce, 1999–2000.* Nutrition Assistance Program Report Series. Washington, DC: Office of Analysis, Nutrition and Evaluation, Food and Nutrition Services, USDA; 2003. Available at: http://www.fns.usda.gov/oane/MENU/Published/WIC/FILES/Public-healthsurvey.pdf. Accessed June 17, 2004.

Mixon H, Dodds J, Haughton B, *Guidelines for Community Nutrition Supervised Experiences.* 2nd ed. Chicago, Ill: Public Health/Community Nutrition Practice Group, American Dietetic Association; 2003. Available at: http://www.phcnpg.org/GuideCommunity NutrSuper-Exp.pdf. Accessed June 17, 2004.

Probert KL, ed. *Moving to the Future: Developing Community-Based Nutrition Services* (Workbook and Training Manual). Washington, DC: Association of State and Territorial Public Health Nutrition Directors; 1997.

CHAPTER 20

Manage and Mentor Public Health Nutrition Personnel

Cynthia B. Bartosek

Reader Objectives

- List the primary roles of the public health nutrition program manager.
- Identify the overarching considerations in assigning employee workloads.
- Describe the components of the employee performance management process.
- Identify approaches to provide continuing education to meet individual and group needs.
- Describe the relationship between the employee's performance appraisal and career development plan.
- List the progressive steps when it becomes necessary to take disciplinary action.

ROLES OF THE NUTRITION PROGRAM MANAGER

More private and public sector organizations embrace performance excellence of their staff as the driving force to enhance their business. As such, the roles and responsibilities of program managers have evolved. Gone are authority figures, hierarchical reporting relationships, control-oriented supervision, and emphasis on extrinsic motivators such as pay, benefits, and job security. In their place are shared authority and responsibility; process and system-oriented continuous quality improvement; and focus on stewardship, making a contribution and a personal difference.[1]

Also fueling these changes is the diversity in the workforce. It is no longer a melting pot, but more of a stir-fry. Managers now seek to recruit staff that represent and speak the languages of the diverse populations they serve. Today's workers represent various races, ethnicities, cultures, ages, and both genders. For the first time, four generations share the workplace. This often-overlooked generational diversity can be a source of either conflict or synergy. Each generation contributes its own world perspective. As with other types of diversity, the key is to know each employee as an individual and respect each person's various values, motivators, assets, liabilities, and expectations.

In the book *Generations at Work: Managing the Clash of Veterans, Boomers, Xers and Nexters in Your Workplace*, Ron Zemke proposes the "ACORN Imperatives" as a key element to deal with inevitable intergenerational clashes. These are:

- *A*ccommodate employee differences
- *C*reate workplace choices
- *O*perate from a sophisticated management style
- *R*espect competence and initiative
- *N*ourish retention[2]

While Zemke focuses on generational differences, this sound advice improves any work environment.

Many debate the difference between *managers* and *leaders*. Which is more essential? In both the traditional and performance excellence business models, management involves four general functions: planning, organizing, leading, and controlling/coordinating activities. The difference between the two models is the amount of emphasis placed on each of these functions.

Planning (see Chapter 14) requires developing program goals with measurable objectives consistent with the organization's strategic or business plan. Determining the activities necessary to achieve the measurable outcomes, identifying resources needed, and making appropriate individual and team assignments are components of the planning process.

Organizing transforms program resources into services to achieve the goals and objectives. In addition to human resources, the program infrastructure includes budgets, information, facilities, equipment, office, and record systems.

Leading has recently taken on greater significance. The ability to set the direction for the public health nutrition program, communicate the stated goals, and influence others to work to achieve the objectives is critical for success. In the quest for excellence (see Chapter 24), the program manager is the champion for organizational performance.

Coordinating has changed from controlling people to coordinating work systems and processes to ensure that the program goals and objectives are achieved. Focus is on policies and procedures, managing individual and program performance, and taking some risks.

Both leadership and management skills are required to ensure that the public health nutrition program staff has the ability to respond to the rapidly changing environment and new challenges. Leaders create a new vision and ensure that each employee's individual efforts contribute to make the vision reality. Managers keep the complex systems and infrastructures running.

Successful program managers foster a work environment that inspires and motivates employees to feel important and dedicated. In their book on employee retention, Beverly Kaye and Sharon Jordan Evans cite the reasons people choose to remain in their current jobs. These include:

- Career growth, learning, and development
- Exciting, challenging work
- Making a difference and a contribution
- Congenial coworkers
- Feeling part of a team
- Recognition for work well done
- Fun on the job
- Pride in the organization and its mission[3]

Each person on the staff may have different motivators. Extrinsic or external motivators include money, benefits, rewards, and punishment. Intrinsic motivators satisfy the workers' desire to do something because of the satisfaction that it gives them. Intrinsic motivation is the more powerful force.[4] External motivators may have detrimental effects on performance. Examples include an overemphasis on "making the numbers," unwillingness to admit mistakes, and excessive competition among the staff mentors. Once the promised reward is gone, so is much of the incentive. The productive manager knows each employee and matches staff members with opportunities and challenges that will increase their job satisfaction and intrinsic motivation.

An opportunity now more often available to employees is the option to work part-time. This is an attractive benefit for parents with child care responsibilities, those furthering their education, or older workers who are not yet ready for full-time retirement. For both the employee and the employing agency, there are advantages and disadvantages to the use of part-time workers. While part-time workers can be scheduled to expand the staff during peak activity periods, they often miss staff meetings and training opportunities that occur during quieter periods. This is a particular problem when new procedures are introduced. Part-timers also may miss opportunities to participate in special events such as health fairs or community meetings. Some part-time workers complain that they do not feel that they are part of the team. Supervision can be challenging when the employee is available on a limited basis. Timely coaching or corrective action may be less possible.

Contract workers present similar benefits and challenges. Generally contract or temporary workers are employed to work for a limited time period on a special project, to meet short-term service demands, or to "fill in" for a permanent staff member who is on extended leave. Contract or temporary employees may work either full- or part-time depending on the nature of the assignment. Advantages include greater staffing flexibility since the number employed can vary. Contract workers may be needed to provide special skills for a specific project. Also there is a potential for saving the costs of fringe benefits. Disadvantages may include the lack of commitment to the organization's goals, and morale issues related to the lack of benefits. Permanent employees may resent temporary workers who may be paid at a higher hourly rate. Contract workers employed for a limited time may not be offered the same training and career development opportunities as the permanent staff. Depending on the nature of the work, the part-time employee may be required to attend the general agency orientation, but not ongoing in-service training. Most organizations require only the performance standards stated in the contract with the employee. The contract manager is accountable for ensuring that these performance expectations are met.

MANAGEMENT SKILLS

Problem solving and decision making are two skills essential to carry out supervisory functions. Every day thousands of routine decisions are made automatically using tacit knowledge. Many managers may not even be aware that they are making a decision. Complex or controversial problems require a more systematic approach.

The problem-solving model challenges the manager to address a wide range of issues, from personnel disputes to process flaws. First, the problem cannot be solved until it is fully and correctly identified. Enough information from a variety of sources is required to understand the potential causes and to prepare alternative solutions. Each option should be evaluated to choose the best alternative. Criteria must weigh the pros and cons, feasibility, and potential long-term results. An action plan can be developed to implement and monitor the results. Finally, it is important to verify that the problem has been solved.

Build the Team

Webster defines a *team* as "a group of people formed around a common goal." Chapter 21 describes the use of teams to leverage nutrition services in the community. Teams are most effective to manage and improve work processes, develop ownership of program changes, promote initiative and creativity, and spread evidence-based nutrition information to a larger population. Team members are no longer limited to those who work together in the same unit or physical location. Members may come from different geographic locations or work shifts, multiple disciplines, and represent several levels of the organization. Ad hoc teams with representatives from several different community agencies may be brought together to work on a single issue.

Public health agencies offer many opportunities for cross-functional or inter-disciplinary teams prepared to collaborate on cost-beneficial approaches to the community's health needs. A team brought together to implement and monitor a school-based obesity prevention project might include representatives from the county health department's nutrition and school health programs; the school's food service staff, curriculum development specialists, and physical education program; and faculty from the local university nursing and physical education programs. With more popular interest in food and nutrition-related health issues, other public agencies and local business leaders welcome opportunities to become partners in community-focused initiatives.

Regardless of focus, structure, or membership, every team must have a clear purpose consistent with its overall organizational goals. All teams depend on the work of each member to contribute to the measurable outcome.

Communicate Effectively

Complete, clear, consistent communication is essential for any organization but commonly identified as a problem by many employees. Correcting misunder-standings is time-consuming and stressful. When employees do not receive com-plete, accurate, and timely information, they make assumptions based on their limited information. Vague information is easily misinterpreted and passes quickly through the "employee grapevine." Rumors damage both individual and program performance. Stress increases, while motivation and morale decline.

How can the manager be sure that all employees clearly understand the pro-gram direction, expectations, and how they can contribute? Managers must share what they know and also the ambiguities. Feedback can be used to determine whether or not the message was understood. This provides the opportunity for the managers to clarify the information and correct misinterpretations. Staff meet-ings, memos, e-mails, and one-on-one discussions improve communication. The same information from multiple sources is more likely to be heard. Employees should be encouraged to ask questions and provided with lists of reliable resources.

Communication flows in two directions. Managers must listen to employees to understand and respect their concerns and perspectives. In programs with a large staff, managers may not be involved in the day-to-day work. Proposals for pro-cedures or program changes may overlook important details or create operational problems. Employees who carry out the routine work frequently are able to iden-tify potential problems and suggest solutions. Seeking employee input shows that managers value their opinions and consider their concerns seriously.

A variety of mechanisms can provide employees with the opportunities to pro-vide input. Examples include "town hall" meetings, suggestion boxes, coffee breaks used to provide informal opportunities for staff discussions with managers, setting a time for staff to "take ten" minutes with senior leaders. Most employees want to hear about plans for the future of the program and the organization, their role in that future, their value to the organization, and how any impending changes might affect them. They may also want to know how they can obtain the knowledge and skills to advance in the organization.

Conduct Productive Staff Meetings

Meetings offer opportunities to communicate and share vital information, gain feedback, and solve problems. When unnecessary or poorly run, meetings can be frustrating, boring, and a waste of time. Managing a productive meeting is a skill often overlooked or undervalued. Numerous books, workshops, and Internet resources are available to help managers sharpen their skills. Before calling a meeting, the manager must decide if it is necessary. Are there less time-consuming, or more effective, ways to reach the desired outcome? Alternative communication methods include fax, e-mail, one-on-one conversations, or viewing a video.

Meetings are best used to present new information or procedures and seek feedback, solve problems, or make decisions. The key to a successful meeting is to clearly define the type of meeting and its purpose. Why the meeting? What needs to be accomplished? The outcome or product could be an action plan, potential solutions to problems, consensus on issues, or to achieve common understanding of a new policy or procedure. Examples include a staff meeting to introduce a new program or procedures or a team meeting to review program monitoring results and plan for any needed corrective actions.

The next step is to identify who needs to participate to achieve the desired outcome. Many managers invite people who cannot be productive participants and who make little contribution toward achieving the meeting's goal. It is also easy to overlook someone from outside the usual group or work unit who may contribute valuable insights and expertise to the topics to be discussed.

The meeting location can be critical to its success. The room size and atmosphere should be conducive to the type and purpose of the meeting, the number of participants, and the agenda. Distractions to the participants should be limited. While a small conference room may be appropriate for a management team meeting, a group planning community-wide nutrition education activities may be more creative in a classroom setting with a blackboard or flip charts to record ideas as they are generated. Unusual locations stimulate creativity and identify potential partners for nutrition initiatives. Many parks, recreation centers, community agencies, and nonprofit organizations make meeting rooms available to public agencies.

A detailed agenda should be distributed to all participants in advance so that they can prepare for the meeting. Participants should be asked to list activities that need to occur for the group to achieve the desired outcome. A well-developed agenda includes the purpose of the meeting and expected outcome, a numbered list of topics to be discussed, the presenters, and the time allotted to discuss each agenda item. Helpful additions include a summary of any actions taken at a previous meeting and a list of any materials that participants may need to review and bring with them.

Chairing a productive meeting requires a fine balance between control and flexibility. The facilitator's role is to manage the meeting time, focus the group on the goal, and stimulate participation without appearing to be overbearing or stifling the group process. While each topic on the agenda should state a time period, the facilitator and the participants must be willing to modify the agenda if more discussion is necessary and productive.

Keys to managing a productive meeting include developing ground rules and obtaining group agreement to deal with conflict. It is essential to start and end the meeting at the scheduled time. This respects those who arrive on time and reinforces the importance of the meeting. Another useful technique is to open the meeting with a short icebreaker that encourages participants to relate on a personal level as well as to focus on the topics on the agenda. In every group there are quiet, less assertive participants. It is important to develop nonthreatening methods to make sure that all participants have an opportunity to contribute. Techniques such as round-robin brainstorming and providing note cards for written comments are effective.

An action register, or meeting minutes, lists each agreed-upon action, the person responsible for the follow up action and the due date. A written summary of the decisions or conclusions at the end of the meeting should, confirm participants' agreements, understandings, and areas of disagreement not resolved. The action register is included in the meeting notes, and should be distributed to participants shortly after the meeting.

A brief time scheduled at the end of each meeting might be used to evaluate the meeting process and discuss what worked well and what might have been improved. Participants might rank the meeting's usefulness on a scale of one to five and explain the reasons for their ranking. The program manager should speak last to avoid influencing the group. This information can be used to improve future meetings. For small groups each participant can be asked for input. In large groups a "popcorn" style evaluation works well.

Resolve Conflicts

When people work together in groups, conflicts are inevitable. Disagreements about how to complete work tasks, personality clashes, cultural differences, and differing ideas about how to bring a variety of disciplines to agreement about best work processes are becoming more common. When dealt with quickly and constructively, these challenges become opportunities to improve program performance.

While conflicts will never be eliminated from the workplace, managers can take some preventive measures. The manager must be aware of the group dynamics among the staff, within the organization, and among community partners. Everyone must know the goals to be achieved, their responsibilities, and ways to work together to achieve the goals. Conflicts must be resolved quickly to avoid negative affects on productivity and morale. Many managers who dread dealing with conflict try to avoid it, hoping it will just go away. It rarely does. Viewing conflict as an opportunity to exchange diverse approaches and points of view directs energy away from the anger fueling the situation and toward creative problem solving. The goal is to create open communication and ways to work together.

An increasing source of conflict among employees and between clients and staff is the growing cultural diversity in many communities. Each of these cultural groups may have different values, beliefs, and ways of interacting in work settings. Managing this diversity must recognize, respect, and capitalize on the different backgrounds of both employees and clients. Failure to listen and respect these differences can lead to discrimination complaints, high employee turnover, and a negative image of the public health agency in the community.

MANAGE PROGRAM STAFF

Two essential functions for managers are staffing and supervising. *Staffing* means determining what human resources are needed to achieve the program mission, goals, and objectives. Key staffing functions include:

- Identify essential job functions and the required knowledge, skills, and abilities (KSAs).
- Recruit and hire.
- Orient and train.

Supervision is managing productive performance (discussed in detail later in this chapter). Major supervisory functions include:

- Set performance goals and expectations.
- Create an environment that supports self-motivation.
- Observe each worker's performance and give constructive feedback.
- Conduct regularly scheduled performance reviews.
- Recognize and reward exemplary performance.
- Address identified performance issues immediately.

Staff Public Health Nutrition Programs

Most staffing decisions should be made at the times when the public health agency's nutrition program plan is developed, updated, expanded, or cut back. During the course of the year there will be vacancies and changes in funding; new mandates or technology may require assessing the need for one or more new or replacement positions. Two questions to answer may be: "Can the work be done without adding staff?" and "Are the skills and talents of current staff being used effectively?" If it is decided that a new position is needed or a vacancy must be filled, the functions and requirements of the job must be analyzed.

The first step is the job analysis. This critical step is often regarded as a tedious paper exercise. The complexity of the analysis varies. The basic components include the organization's mission and goals, a detailed description of the job duties; the mental, physical, educational, and licensing or certification requirements; the working conditions; and the minimum knowledge, skills, abilities (KSA) required.

The job analysis is a valuable tool to assess training needs, determine competitive salary ranges, develop interview questions and activities, recruit qualified applicants, determine what reasonable accommodations might be needed to employ disabled employees, and conduct performance reviews. The analysis must be based on the job requirements, not the person in the position.

With the analysis complete, it must be determined whether a full-time career service employee is necessary or a contract worker or volunteer would be appropriate. If the job is either short term or entry-level, a contract worker may be an option. If a career service position is to be established or filled, the job analysis is used to determine its salary level or range, including the fringe benefits. Other costs associated with the position, include training, equipment, furniture and space, and supplies required. These costs are often overlooked when budgeting new positions.

Write Position Descriptions

The position description uses the information from the job analysis. Focus is on the primary routine duties that support the program's mission and goals. While each organization may develop its own form and format, core components are found in all position descriptions. A brief summary overview of the nature, level, and purpose of the work. Information on roles, supervision and other relationships should be included. The essential duties, responsibilities, and accountabilities are listed in descending order by the percentage of time required. Duty statements should briefly describe the work to be performed. Descriptions should be outcome-based and use action words.

The KSAs required to successfully perform the essential functions must be stated clearly. Required credentials, education, and work experience are indicated. Some substitutions such as relevant work experience may replace an advanced degree to avoid eliminating a well-qualified and experienced applicant. All requirements listed on the position description must directly relate to one or more of the essential functions and are the primary selection criteria when filling the position.

Position descriptions should also include any special requirements of the position. These may relate to the work conditions, such as willingness to work nontraditional hours, ability to use specialized equipment, language proficiency skills to communicate with non-English-speaking clients, and access to transportation. The Occupational, Safety, and Health Administration (OSHA) requires documentation for any position that requires handling or exposure to human body fluids. Specific physical capabilities required to perform the duties should be noted, such as frequent bending and reaching, lifting, and carrying heavy items. Required mental capabilities may include calibrating measuring equipment, problem solving, or analyzing and interpreting data.

The list of duties should distinguish between methods and results. There may be more than one way to achieve the desired outcome. Nutrition education can utilize many different approaches—face-to-face, written materials, videos, using computer-based modules, individually, or in groups. A requirement to use only one specific method limits creativity. Flexibility encourages employees to grow and enhance their contribution to the organization.

To comply with the requirements of the Americans with Disabilities Act, it is necessary to identify the essential job functions and determine whether a disabled applicant can perform these duties with or without reasonable accommodation. The criteria for essential duties include:

- What is the importance of each function to the program operation; does the position exist to perform the function?
- How frequently is it done; does not doing it fundamentally change the job?
- How many other staff members are available to perform the duty?
- Can the task be redesigned or performed in another way or is it highly specialized, requiring special expertise?[5]

The position description also identifies the occupational classification for the position and includes the working or functional title. Most public and many private sector employers use the *Standard Occupational Classification* (SOC) system developed by the federal government. This comprehensive database promotes consistency by defining the usual duties and KSA requirements for job categories at both the provider and manager levels. O*NET is now being developed to be the primary source of descriptive occupational information, replacing the *Dictionary of Occupational Titles*.[6]

Successful Hiring Process

The goal is to hire the best applicant for the vacant position, to decrease turnover, and increase productivity. An often-unanticipated benefit is better performance as the supervisor gets to know employees better, recognizes their skills and talents, and understands what motivates them. Finding qualified applicants is often the most difficult part. Successful recruitment begins by discussing the new position with the existing staff. Current employees should be given the first opportunity to apply for any new or more advanced vacant positions. Building a talent pool starts by developing the knowledge and skills of existing staff. Word of mouth taps into employee and professional networks. Networking at conferences and meetings spreads the word through the local and state dietetic and public health associations. It may be necessary to advertise a position to reach beyond the organization's job listings and the local newspaper.

Use the Internet. Post job notices on the Web sites of professional associations and university alumni associations. There are numerous sites listing jobs available in public health agencies. Many newspapers list jobs on their Web sites. Private vendors that do not charge potential employers for listings should be used. The essential job functions, KSAs, and requirements should be included in the job announcements or Web site.

Highly qualified and desirable candidates for future jobs may not be currently seeking to change jobs. The agency's Web site can market the program as an exciting and rewarding place to work. It should clearly and effectively communicate the agency's mission, vision, and commitment to quality and customer and employee satisfaction. Hosting an open house or sponsoring a workshop can introduce potential qualified applicants to the agency's public health nutrition program. Interested candidates, former students, and interns should be sent periodic updates about openings and invited to visit when they are in the area.

Interview Applicants

Many employers screen applications to decide which applicants to schedule for formal interviews. The employer looks for evidence that the required KSAs, work experience, credentials, and education matches position requirements. Screening interviews may be conducted by telephone. This screening can identify "red flags" regarding the applicant's work history and general qualifications. A scoring system can determine which applicants are to be offered formal interviews. The formal selection interview may be one-to-one with the hiring authority or panel. The supervisor, a peer, and a representative from the human resources office make up the selection panel. Procedures should ensure consistency and objectivity. The selection should be made based on job-related qualifications, skills, and experience. Managers and supervisors should be trained to develop and use legal and informative interview techniques.

The interview is stressful to both the interviewer and the applicant. The interviewer should establish a friendly climate to put everyone at ease. The goal of the interview is to find "a good fit" between the applicant and the requirements of the job. Many interviewers overlook that the applicants are also determining if this agency is where they might like to work. An overview of the purpose and format of the interview informs the interviewer and interviewee of what to expect.

Probing questions assess the applicant's knowledge, skills, and abilities (KSAs) related to the job. Open-ended questions encourage the applicant to elaborate on experience and identify behavior patterns. Hypothetical questions can be used to determine how an applicant would handle some of the situations likely to occur on the job. When specific information is needed, closed-ended questions are appropriate. Leading, loaded, and multiple questions should be avoided. The applicant should be given enough time to think and fully answer each question. Ideally the applicant should do 75–80% of the talking during the interview. Listening attentively is one of the interviewer's most important skills.

Each applicant must be asked the same questions in the same sequence. Follow-up probing questions can be used to clarify an applicant's responses. It is permissible to ask applicants about:

- Knowledge and skills
- Education and experience
- Job required credentials
- Terms and conditions of employment such as willingness to work certain hours or access to transportation

Questions regarding the applicant's race, nationality, age, disabilities, marital status, family responsibilities, criminal record, or credit history are not permissible.

Applicants should also be asked to perform one or more tasks directly related to the position, such as analyzing a typical client case study, writing a client case plan using the SOAP (Subective & Objective indicators, Assessment, and Plan) note format or presenting a brief nutrition education class. The applicant might be asked to suggest how to resolve a problem that may be typical of the new job. Responses should be scored against set criteria for correct information and completeness. Performance-oriented activities provide a balance of questions to identify past behavior but may not always be a valid assessment of the applicant's ability to apply KSAs to the demands of this new position.

After all applicants have been interviewed, the most critical factors for their success must be considered. These include the skills of current employees and the additional needs of the agency. Each candidate must be compared to the job requirements, not to each other. When none of the applicants appears to be a good fit, it should be determined if the deficiencies are in attitudes or skills. Intensive training or education can raise skills to the level needed. Attitudes cannot be changed easily. Employing out of desperation to fill a position rarely works. Re-advertising the position may be wiser.

Applicant references must be checked. However, in the current litigious culture few previous employers will provide performance information. They may verify only employment dates, job title, and responsibilities. When hiring someone employed within organization, the applicant's personnel file may be accessed.

Orient New Staff

A well-planned orientation builds strong teams by exciting newly employed staff and their coworkers about each other. It introduces the new staff member to the agency and the staff, it gives them the information, targets, and goals expected and reduces barriers so they become productive more quickly. The mission, vision, and goals of the organization and how the new employee contributes to the "big picture" should be emphasized. The job description and performance standards and expectations should be discussed. The thoughtful manager makes the new employee feel welcome. Appropriate welcomes are stocking the office with essential supplies, personally introducing the new employee to coworkers and other key staff, assigning a "buddy," and arranging for a lunch group.

An orientation plan for each new employee speeds progress to productivity. It builds knowledge and skill areas that need to be developed. For each area, it develops an objective and action steps, and determines the sequence for completing the objectives. It monitors and documents the learning and provides ongoing feedback to the employee. For the training to be successful the plan should identify who is in charge of developing the plan, providing the training, and evaluating performance.

MANAGE EMPLOYEE PERFORMANCE

Changes in community demographics increase competition for staff and clients. There is increasing pressure to contain program costs. Unpredictable funding, new federal regulations, unfunded mandates increasing caseloads and service expectations, and greater emphasis on customer requirements all influence the ability to carry out public health program and organization missions. These changes are occurring throughout all business sectors. The focus on decision making and accountability at the level where the work is done demands a service culture that rewards team performance and integrates operations. A new human resource model has evolved to meet new demands.

Performance management is a systematic process to improve organizational effectiveness. Components include:

- Planning work and setting expectations
- Continually monitoring performance
- Developing the capability to perform
- Periodically rating performance
- Rewarding good performance[7]

This process supports the goals of the organization, linking the work of all employees to the mission of their work unit. It increases employees' job skills and competencies and develops their capacity to adapt to a variety of situations.

Any performance management system starts with the planning. With clear expectations and standards for individual staff members and groups, it is essential to direct the program's resources and efforts toward achieving the desired goals and objectives. Specifying measurement criteria to assess gaps in knowledge and skills completes the process. Necessary planning includes written and clearly understood policies and procedures, program plan objectives, job descriptions, performance standards, standards of conduct, and individual career development plans.

Policies and Procedures

Policies are guidelines to provide employees with a clear understanding of the organization's mission, goals, practices, and expectations regarding performance and conduct. Managers often fail to recognize the value of policy and procedure manuals as a performance management tool. In addition to policies specific to the public health agency and its nutrition program, various state and federal regulations must be addressed. These include Equal Employment Opportunity (EEO) Act, Americans with Disabilities Act (ADA), Family and Medical Leave Act (FMLA), and the Fair Labor Standards Act (FLSA). All managers and supervisors must understand the legal liability that can result when these rules are not followed.

Procedures derived from policies provide direction to deal with situations that may occur each day. Written agency and nutrition program procedures are an essential requirement when orienting new employees. Examples include clearing proposed news releases with an agency administrator, description of the process for scheduling a client visit, or conducting community nutrition education. Policies and procedures should be assembled into manuals or included in the employee handbook made available to each employee. Policies and procedures must be reviewed and updated periodically to ensure consistency with current "best practices."

Performance Standards

Most public health agencies have legal requirements that define expected employee performance standards and the conduct of regularly scheduled performance appraisals. The job description lists the essential functions and tasks assigned to the employee. The standards define how well these tasks must be performed to meet or exceed expectations. The standards are specific, measurable, verifiable, and achievable. Usually there is a set of core standards that apply to all employees in the organization. In addition there are job specific standards. To ensure that standards are consistent with the assigned work and the requirements of the job a periodic review process modifies the standards as program objectives and work assignments change. Employees should participate in developing and revising the performance standards for their positions. These standards are written for the position, not the person who fills it.

Performance standards should be reviewed with new employees as a part of their orientation. This provides an opportunity to establish a clear understanding of the expectations and the ongoing monitoring process. The standards also provide the basis for identifying employee development needs.

Assign Workloads

Arbitrary workload assignments can result in low morale and decreased productivity. High performers are often "rewarded" with more work. Unfair distribution of work frequently is reported as a problem on employee satisfaction surveys. A well-planned and implemented distribution of workloads increases productivity, enhances employee skills, and ensures that program objectives are achieved. Each program must develop its own method of deploying its staff. Assignments should make optimum use of each worker's skills and abilities to carry out the program mission and responsibilities within the available budget.

The framework developed must be equitable and consistent. It should give the highest priority to the work that is central to the agency mission and legislatively mandated goals; promote the visibility, status, and growth of the public health nutrition program; and give employees opportunities to use their talents. Time for creative community and personal development and service activities must be factored into the assigned workload. All functions need to be weighted and prioritized based on program goals and requirements. Work assignments are often based only on the number and type of client services that need to be provided and the required community and administrative functions.

Program responsibilities and capabilities change with increasing community nutrition program needs, new legislated mandates, and staff turnover. Fluctuations in funding require workload procedures to be reviewed regularly. This assessment is an integral part of budget planning. The process begins by identifying the key program functions and responsibilities. Requirements for participation in agency or community service activities and planned professional development also must be reviewed periodically. This includes the community programs and number and types clients to be served, minimum and maximum appointment requirements, and travel time.

The goal is to maximize productivity while encouraging staff members to fulfill all of their performance expectations. Assignments must be appropriate for the employee's professional competence and credentials. For example, medical nutrition therapy should be assigned to registered or licensed dietitians.

It is realistic to expect that workloads will vary to more effectively utilize each employee's strengths to achieve program goals. Assignments should demonstrate that each employee is expected to substantially participate and contribute to the entire essential and legally mandated functions of the program. Table 20–1 lists some usual functions for public health or community nutrition staff.

MONITOR AND APPRAISE PERFORMANCE

Regular feedback can close the gap between acceptable and outstanding performance. Observing employees as they carry out their daily assignments provides insights into their individual accomplishments, problems, concerns, and need for additional training. It provides a better understanding of employees' work and demonstrates their supervisor's interest in their success. In addition to direct observation, chart audits and peer reviews are routinely used to evaluate employees' work.

Frequent positive feedback reinforces behaviors that should be continued and developed. This is especially important when the task requires extra effort or challenge. For example, praising an employee who makes the effort to understand and deal with an upset client helps control frustrations in future difficult situations.

Feedback based on observation and other verifiable data has credibility and is more likely to improve employee behavior. Constructive feedback should be specific and descriptive rather than general or evaluative. It should be balanced, especially when problems are observed. Performance problems that are identified

Table 20–1 Examples of Work Load Functions for Public Health/Community Nutrition Personnel

Conduct community assessments.
Participate in health promotion events.
Develop and manage grants.
Participate on community advisory boards and task forces.
Serve as officer or committee member for a professional organization.
Participate in professional development activities.
Carry out administrative duties: budget, personnel, and facilities management.
Participate in a quality improvement team.
Facilitate group education classes.
Participate in school and community-based obesity prevention programs.
Develop nutrition education materials.
Assess and counsel clients in WIC and primary care clinics.
Coordinate breast-feeding peer counselor programs.
Conduct WIC outreach.
Provide training and technical assistance to community agencies and medical providers.
Train new nutrition program staff.
Offer field experiences for students and interns.
Develop program plans.

Source: Prepared by Chapter Author, Cynthia Bartosek.

should be addressed immediately rather than filed for the annual performance appraisal. Additional training, special assignments, or changes in work processes should be initiated to assist the employee to meet the expected standards. When managers provide ongoing feedback, nothing in the appraisal should surprise the employee.

Although often dreaded by both supervisors and employees, the performance appraisal is a valuable tool to improve the program's performance and productivity. How well employees perform their job duties and meet expectations is critical to the success of both the individual employee and the program. Properly implementing the appraisal system develops the employee and provides documentation to recommend pay increases and decisions regarding promotions, transfers, and on-the-job or academic training, demotions, or layoffs. The appraisal must be objective, use measurable standards, and be defendable.

Every organization has policies and procedures for conducting an assessment of each employee's work. The process typically includes a review and summary of available data to rank the performance against predetermined standards, discussing the assessment with the employee and providing an opportunity for the employee to respond and comment. Employees are encouraged to conduct a self-assessment that is incorporated into the rankings. The appraisal should be based on performance over the entire review period, not just the most recent weeks or months. In addition to summarizing performance related to the job functions and standards, the appraisal should note the employee's strengths and accomplishments during the review period. Areas that need to be improved are identified and agreement reached on how to accomplish the improvement. Sufficient time should be planned for productive discussion. This gives the employee the opportunity to comment and ask questions as each standard is reviewed. Most appraisal forms have a section for employee comments. The process, review, and update of the performance standards should reflect program changes or performance expectations. This is also an appropriate time to work with the employee to prepare career development plans.

When performance is deficient in any area, a performance improvement plan (PIP) may be required. Most organizations have policies defining when and how PIPs are used to measure and monitor activities to improve performance or modify behavior. The starting point is to determine whether the identified problem is a performance or behavior issue. The agency's human resources office can provide guidelines to make this determination and if documentation is required. Generally a PIP defines the specific duties or behaviors that must be improved and the standards to use to measure performance. An action plan is developed that includes specific goals, time frames for demonstrating change, and periodic review dates. At the designated intervals, the employee's performance is measured against the standards to determine if expectations are being met. If improvement is not observed, demotion or dismissal may need to be considered.

INDIVIDUAL CAREER DEVELOPMENT PLANS

In the rapidly changing work environment, professionals must be able to adapt to change and accept new responsibilities as programs evolve, new technologies, increased emphasis on teamwork, and process improvement. Development opportunities focus on strengthening performance in the current position as well as preparing for career advancement. While long-term career goals are considered, the plan is developed for the current performance review period. The typical plan should include any training and developmental activities that are: (a) required by agency or program regulations, (b) recommended by the supervisor based on the performance review, and (c) requested by the employee to prepare for advancement. In responding to the identified needs, it is important to consider workloads, budgets, and the potential affect if the training does not take place. The immediacy of the need is a prime factor when setting target dates. Once the plan is reviewed and agreed upon, both the employee and the supervisor sign it. Quarterly review of the plan maintains the focus, but provides for changes or modifications to be made as needed.

Performance development combines both formal and informal approaches. The traditional structured courses, workshops, and self-study programs are usually readily available and accessible. The manager can have the greatest influence by encouraging learning and growth-supporting activities to challenge the employees. It contributes to their increased understanding of the program and the community. Job rotations and special assignments provide employees opportunities to stretch their skills. Employee participation in professional organizations, cross-functional or interdisciplinary teams, community-based training, internships, management or leadership programs, and Web-based seminars should be encouraged and supported. Coaching, mentoring, and role modeling can also be used to develop a more competent work force.

IN-SERVICE EDUCATION

Consistent and rapid advances in nutrition and health care management, science, and technology require that learning be a lifelong process for all public health nutrition professionals. In-service education should support the program's mission, priorities, and initiatives, and provide learning opportunities for staff to keep their professional practice current. In a performance-focused organization, there are two aspects to continuing education. First, training designed to meet the broad needs of the organization. This includes training on new polices, procedures, or protocols; updates as nutrition knowledge advances; topics required to maintain state licensure; and subjects identified through a training needs assessment. Secondly, skill training may focus on areas such as computer and Internet applications, media, presentation skills, process management, or client-directed care.

A key component of the performance management system is the individual development plan. Professional development activities and studies to be completed during a specified time period are identified by each employee with the supervisor.

A continuing education plan is an integral part of the nutrition program plan and incorporates both training planned for nutritionists and for others, including public health and health care providers, child care workers, Head Start and schoolteachers and coaches, and other community organizations. As cross-functional and interdisciplinary teams become more of a way of life for nutrition programs, the needs of all team members must be considered when planning continuing education activities.

In developing continuing education plans and activities, these guidelines from Cornell University's Cooperative Extension Service can improve the quality and effectiveness of the training:

- Incorporate creative approaches focused on adult educational processes as well as subject matter content
- Integrate subject area related policy issues and applications; highlight model programs
- Demonstrate relationships among subject areas when delivering an interdisciplinary in-service
- Involve area specialists in planning and design, and when appropriate, as resource persons for teaching
- Provide information on program resources that are already available
- Focus planning to meet needs of the target audience (e.g., identify who should attend the in-service by focus of their program/organization responsibilities)
- Provide for evaluation and use results for future planning
- Recognize needs of diverse program audiences and differences in learning styles[8]

Methods of providing continuing education are only limited by imagination and perhaps budget. In addition to the traditional classroom-style workshops and seminars, interactive satellite and Web-based teleconferences, audio conferences, videotapes, newsletters, self-study modules, and train-the-trainer sessions can be used. Retreats, especially those held off-site, offer an opportunity to study a topic in depth.

Identifying existing academic and professional training resources reduces the work associated with providing continuing education. Many community agencies, as well as voluntary health and social agencies, have speakers' bureaus that provide programs on relevant topics at no or nominal charge. Colleagues in the dietetic or public health community may be willing to exchange training services, community partners can cosponsor training events of mutual interests. Other available resources are local community colleges and universities, culinary arts schools, and the area health education center. Adding variety to the in-service education-training plan keeps employees engaged and meets the needs of employees who have various learning styles.

BUILD CAREERS

In recent years, it is recognized that many people change careers at least three to four times in their working life, holding an average of seven jobs. Building career paths will be an invaluable tool in retaining a competent workforce.

Career pathing is defined as an organization's process for identifying specific job opportunities within its own structure and the sequential steps in education, skills, and experience that employees need to achieve their specific career goals. These goals do not necessarily mean promotions. A senior nutritionist may want to become a lactation consultant or a certified diabetes educator. Another may be interested in developing educational materials. Experienced employees can be assigned to train and mentor new staff. Consulting opportunities with other disciplines in the organization or other community agencies develop new skills in a particular area of interest.

Staff should be encouraged to develop clear and specific career goals. The individual portfolio development process developed by the American Dietetic Association for registered dietitians provides a basis for planning career-building activities. The manager can advise based on observation of each staff member's abilities and potential. Knowledge of requirements for advancement in the organization and potential opportunities to be available can be shared. Opportunities that help to advance skills include:

- Serve as an officer or board member in a professional, civic, or service organization.
- Represent the agency on a community coalition addressing health promotion issues.
- Write and submit an original article to a professional journal.
- Design and conduct applied research.
- Prepare a grant application.
- Develop a media campaign around nutrition and fitness.
- Create or update the agency's nutrition program Web site.

Creative managers identify available resources to assist employees develop their strengths to progress by arranging flexible or alternate work schedules, education leave with or without pay, tuition waivers or reimbursement for courses to work toward an advanced degree.

Internships are a key component of a career pathing program. In recent years several state health departments have established dietetic internships. These internships provide an opportunity for public health nutrition personnel to become registered dietitians. Many local agencies have found this to be a significant factor in their ability to recruit new graduates. If internships are a part of a career pathing plan, it is essential to plan for the employees' absence—their work still must get done—and to budget for any pay increases associated with resulting promotions or added duties when they return.

Creating career development paths for the employees aids both their recruitment and retention. An agency that offers a broad spectrum of learning opportunities, a work environment that supports professional development, and where employees can take "ownership" of their career and professional destiny is highly desirable to both keep current employees and to attract prospective employees.

MENTOR CAREER GROWTH

An inexpensive, highly effective way to foster career growth for nutritionists is by mentoring. The employee's personal growth and on-the-job effectiveness are enhanced through the relationship. Mentoring programs may be formal or informal. In a formal program mentors and protégés are matched based on their positions or the desired outcome. Informal mentoring is flexible, participation is voluntary, and the partners determine goals. The mentoring relationship may be limited to coaching on a specific skill, such as social marketing a family fitness program for the health agency. The scope may be more comprehensive, including career counseling and identifying professional leadership development opportunities. Clear, realistic expectations should be defined from the beginning. Research on mentoring relationships shows there is a set of particular skills that result in the most successful relationships. For the mentor these are listening actively, building trust, determining goals and building capacity, encouraging and inspiring.[9]

Successful mentoring programs have several features in common. Most critical is leadership buy-in and a supportive organizational climate. Another feature is program orientation for potential mentors and protégés to describe the concept. Clear expectations and goals must be agreed upon. As with any program, a mechanism for evaluating effectiveness is needed.[10]

Mentoring programs benefit the organization, the employee, and the mentor. When started as part of orientation, mentoring helps a new employee fit into the organization more quickly. For employees who are not meeting performance expectations, working with a mentor can reinforce training. Career coaching provides direction and links employees with available resources. For the mentor, the relationship often revitalizes enthusiasm for the job, resulting in increased productivity and motivation. Organizational benefits from a mentoring program can increase diversity in key positions, increase employee satisfaction, decrease staff turnover, and develop staff members to their full potential.[11]

RECOGNIZE EXCELLENCE IN PERFORMANCE

The final component of the performance management process is recognizing and rewarding performance that exceeds expectations. Organizational rules most often determine the criteria and policies for rewards programs and may limit the supervisor's resources to provide monetary rewards. However recognition itself is a powerful motivator. Employees who know that their supervisors are aware of their successes are inspired with a clearer idea of the agency's performance expectations. It is important for program managers as well as the immediate supervisor to provide verbal recognition. This recognition should focus on the successful actions that support the program goals rather than the employee's personal traits. This approach avoids perceptions of favoritism and reinforces the expected behaviors. A history of an employee's repeated recognition can support recommendations for pay increases, bonuses, or special awards when available.

There are important milestones and accomplishments in the life of the public health nutrition program—the highest WIC caseload ever, winning a productivity award, graduating a class of breastfeeding peer counselors, conducting a successful weight management program. Take a moment to celebrate. It is too easy to be caught up in the daily routine so that successes are often not recognized. Most organizations reward employees for:

- Length of service, especially landmark anniversaries, such as 1, 5, 10, and 20 years of service
- Attendance
- Productivity
- Customer service
- Superior performance awards
- Employee-of-the-month programs
- Retirement

Creative recognition of their successes shows employees that their accomplishments can lead to positive outcomes. Employees need to see how their work has improved lives. A community life bulletin board recognizes employees through letters, memos, pictures, thank-you notes, or WOW cards from clients and coworkers to give positive feedback. These are inexpensive ways to recognize employees. A year-in-review scrapbook with pictures and notes highlights employees' achievements throughout the year. A traveling trophy can go each month to the employee exhibiting the greatest overall performance. Rewards should go beyond paychecks. The agency budget might provide tuition reimbursement for work-related courses, registration fees for state or national professional conferences or short courses, or participation in a public health leadership program. For many nutritionists these opportunities mean more than a bonus or small pay increase.

Recognition activities can be formal, such as designating time at a regularly scheduled staff meeting to recognize achievements. Staff members appreciate being recognized for working hard or just "hanging in there." A personal note to the employee or a note sent to the employee's family might describe accomplishments that have contributed to achieving the programs goals and priorities. Variation in the types of recognition makes it "special."[12]

With current emphasis on measurable outcomes, it's easy to forget to recognize good effort, not just results. Sometimes hard work may not have the desired outcome or the results may be affected by external factors. Changes in staff, priorities, and work schedules may make it difficult to always meet goals. It is easy for employees to become discouraged and their productivity to decline. Knowing that their efforts are noticed and appreciated keeps them motivated and focused. When employees have had a frustrating week, a pizza party, balloon bouquet, or a personal thank-you card can get them back on track. "You help the marathon runner the most by offering encouragement and nourishment along the track, not just by waiting at the finish line with a trophy. Recognizing effort has a bigger impact than giving a prize at the end of the race. This also applies to employees, who are in a race every day."

DISCIPLINARY ACTION

Despite their best efforts to motivate staff, at some time all managers have to deal with a difficult employee. Common problems include frequent tardiness or absences, disruptive behavior, theft or misuse of agency property, insubordination, continuous violation of policies, substance abuse, or disclosure of confidential information. The challenge is to identify the cause of the problem and help the employee reverse the unacceptable behavior. It is essential to know the organization's standards of conduct and discipline policies and work closely with the human resources staff to assure compliance with applicable state and federal laws.

The first step is to determine whether the problem is a result of inadequate training or behavior. Often the symptoms are the same. Training is appropriate when the employee lacks competence to perform assigned duties, has inadequate skill to perform a new process, or infrequent practice in a specific task. Blatant violations of policy, safety threats, disruptive, unproductive, or negative behaviors that create a hostile work environment require corrective action.

Allowing negative behavior to continue implies that the behavior is acceptable, decreasing morale and productivity by the whole staff. In many organizations, the first level of corrective action is to meet with the employee to discuss the nature of the problem and explain why it is a problem. After clarifying any reasons for the problem, specific directions should be recommended to correct the problem within a stipulated time period. The employee's efforts to correct the problem will be supported. A written record of this discussion must be kept in an employee incident file. If the behavior does not improve, disciplinary action is required. A key factor in successfully dealing with problem behavior is complete and fair documentation to support any action that must be taken. It can be time-consuming to collect accurate information regarding events, actions, and results. However, it is crucial to defend the supervisor and agency from appeals, grievances, and legal actions that might be brought by the employee.

Most discipline systems list a progressive procedure that begins with an oral warning and can escalate to dismissal if the problem persists. An oral warning is used when there has been no change in behavior following the corrective action discussion and the violation is a minor infraction of the organization's policies. Supporting information is collected by interviewing those involved or who witnessed the incident. An oral warning must be "written up" and placed in the employee's personnel file. A summary memo signed by both the supervisor and the employee is completed for the file.

When an oral warning does not result in the desired behavior change within the specified time period or if there is a major rules infraction, a written warning is required. Beginning with a review of the oral warning, the details of the infraction must be clearly described with expectations for change and the disciplinary action that will occur if there is no immediate improvement. Organization guidelines should be used to complete a detailed written warning signed by both the supervisor and the employee. If the employee refuses to sign, a third-party witness can document the refusal.

Being "written up" can have a significant effect on an employee's behavior and motivation. At times, the situation is so serious that the employee must be removed from the workplace. In addition to failure to heed one or more written warnings, reasons for a suspension include violent or dangerous behavior or an infraction that requires an investigation that could result in dismissal. The discussion with the employee must stay focused on the problem and the supervisor must maintain control of the emotional climate. The format for the discussion is similar to that used with the less severe level of discipline. The seriousness of the situation must be emphasized and the possible outcomes, including the possibility of dismissal, discussed.

Most organizations have an appeals process. The procedures may be determined by agency policy, state law, or contracts negotiated by unions or collective bargaining groups. Employees may have the right to file a grievance in response to an oral or written warning. Governmental agencies generally grant an employee who has been dismissed the right to appeal. To be upheld, disciplinary actions must be progressive and consistent for all employees.

POINTS TO PONDER

- How does the traditional management role compare to the contemporary demands for supervising workers?
- How does having a multigenerational workforce affect the program? How must the management style be adjusted for each group?
- How is the performance appraisal used to plan future performance?
- How is conflict handled in the organization?

- What media does the organization use to disseminate information to employees? How could communications be improved?
- What developmental and career-building opportunities are available for agency nutrition staff? Are employees encouraged to take advantage of them?
- How has the public health agency addressed the increased diversity of clientele? Does the workforce reflect the community it serves?
- How can employee recognition and reward be tied to the organization's mission and goals?

NOTES

1. Florida Department of Health. *Basic Supervisor's Training Program Module 1, Roles and Skills of DH Supervisors, Participants Guide.* Florida Department of Health; 1999:3.

2. Rodriguez A. Managing generations at work. Sophia Associates Web site. 2003. Available at: http://www.sophia-associates.com/Managing_Generations_at_Work.pdf.

3. Motivating as a form of leadership. In: *The Supervisor's Toolbox for Leadership Development.* Human Resources Research Organization; 2004. Available at: http://www.humrro.org/toolbox2/motivation/index.html.

4. Motivating as a form of leadership. In: *The Supervisor's Toolbox for Leadership Development.* Human Resources Research Organization; 2004. Available at: http://www.humrro.org/toolbox2/motivation/index.html.

5. US Equal Employment Opportunity Commission. The ADA: your reponsibilities as an employer. US Equal Employment Opportunity Commission Web site. Available at: http://www.eeoc.gov/facts/ada17.html. Accessed February 2001.

6. The Occupational Information Network. What is O*NET? O*NET Consortium Web site. Available at: http://www.onetcenter.org/overview.html. Accessed August 2004.

7. Cornell Cooperative Extension Service. Guidelines for CCE in-service education courses. 2001. Cornell Cooperative Extension Service. Available at: http://staff.cce.cornell.edu/administration/. Accessed June 25, 2004.

8. profdev/inservice/guidel.htm

9. Office of Personnel Management. Performance management overview. Office of Personnel Management Web site. Available at: http://www.opm.gov/perform/overview.asp. Accessed June 1, 2004.

10. Center for Health Leadership and Practice, Pubic Health Institute. *A Guide for Mentors.* Center for Health Leadership and Practice, Pubic Health Institute; 2002:3.

11. Healthcare Financial Management Association. Corporate mentoring programs offer a competitive edge in labor markets. *HFMA Wants You to Know.* June 2003. Healthcare Financial Management Association Web site. Available at: http://www.hfma.org/publications/HFMA_WantsYouToKnow/060403_mentor.htm.

BIBLIOGRAPHY

Center for Health Leadership and Practice, Pubic Health Institute. *A Guide for Mentors.* 2002.

Center for Health Leadership and Practice, Pubic Health Institute. *A Guide for Protégés.* 2002.

Costello SJ. *Effective Performance Management.* The Business Skills Express Series. Boston, Mass: Business One Irwin/Mirror Press; 1994.

Hiam A. Employee recognition: why it matters: rewarding employees for a job well-done will do wonders for their performance—and your bottom line. June 24, 2002. Entrepeneur.com. Available at: http://www.Entrepeneur.com/article/0,4621, 301003,00. html. Accessed May 5, 2006.

Human Resources Research Organization. *The Supervisor's Toolbox for Leadership Development series.* Human Resources Research Organization Web site. Available at: http://www.humrro.org/ins_toolbox2/communication/allissues.htm.

Kouzes JM, Posner BZ. *Encouraging the Heart: A Leader's Guide to Rewarding and Recognizing Others.* San Francisco, Calif: Jossey-Bass Inc; 2003.

Kouzes JM, Posner BZ. *The Leadership Challenge: How to Keep Getting Extraordinary Things Done in Organizations.* 2nd ed. San Francisco, Calif: Jossey-Bass Inc; 1995.

McGill AM. *Supervising the Difficult Employee.* The Business Skills Express Series. Boston, Mass: Irwin Professional Publishing/Mirror Press; 1994.

McNamara C. *Staffing and Supervision of Employees and Volunteers, On-Line Organization Development Program Module #10.* Free Management Library. Available at: http://www.managementhelp.org/np_progs/sup_mod/staff.htm.

Murphy J. *Managing Conflict at Work.* The Business Skills Express Series. Boston, Mass: Business One Irwin/Mirror Press; 1994.

CHAPTER 21

Partner with the Public Health Team to Spread the Nutrition Message

Cynthia B. Bartosek

Reader Objectives

- Discuss the roles of various members of the public health team and how they can contribute to nutrition education.
- Describe the interdisciplinary team approach, and differentiate it from other care models.
- Describe the characteristics of a successful team.
- List some strategies to incorporate nutrition education into training for health professionals.
- Identify opportunities for using a team approach in a public health setting.

NUTRITION CARE THROUGH THE PUBLIC HEALTH TEAM

In public health, very little can be accomplished without teamwork. Whether it is advocacy, social marketing campaigns, community assessments, health promotion, or individual client care, the synergy resulting from collective effort is a key success factor.

The environment in which the nation's nearly 12,000 public health nutrition professionals and paraprofessionals[1] work continues to evolve to meet ongoing challenges and emerging threats. In today's world, the determinants of health for both individuals and communities are so complex that they are beyond the capacity of any one practitioner or discipline.

Changes in health care and public health priorities over the past decade have contributed to a resurgence of the concept of interdisciplinary collaboration. Well-coordinated collaboration across disciplines can be highly effective in dealing with the increasing complexity of public health and client care, meeting demands of funders and payers, keeping pace with new technology, and responding to public health threats. In public health, the interdisciplinary team model has the potential to be more cost-effective, and comprehensive by using population-based approaches that emphasize health promotion and disease prevention. The fundamental questions facing public health managers shift from "why and how to use a team" to "who is on the team?" and "how do the team members work together?"

In the collaborative model, the requirements of the population to be served determine the composition of the team. Members are chosen to provide the balance, diversity, and experience necessary to provide a broad range of perspectives and insights. Training and legal scopes of practice help to define the specific functions of each professional.

The public health nutritionist's role in the community is that of a consultant and educator to consumers, clients and other health professionals by translating scientific evidence into understandable, actionable information. In the primary care services, the nutritionist participates in case management conferences and team meetings, contributing information regarding the socioeconomic, cultural, and environmental factors that influence the community population and client food choices and dietary behaviors. This information, in concert with the medical assessment data, contributes to the team's efforts to establish realistic goals and intervention strategies and make appropriate referrals.

In the primary care setting, the core health care team may include physicians, nurses (including nurse practitioners and nurse-midwives), nutritionists, health educators, dentists, and social workers. The team includes not just the providers; support staff such as lab technicians, health support aides, medical records specialists, and clerical support staff play complementary roles in reinforcing nutrition education messages.

Each health professional on the team contributes to the client's understanding of the role of nutrition and diet in reducing risk factors and improving health outcomes.

- *Physicians*—Frequently the team leaders, physicians assess for and diagnose nutrition-related conditions and prescribe pharmacological and behavior modification interventions. Dietary recommendations may be given as anticipatory guidance, especially for infants or in relation to a specific medical issue such as diabetes or elevated cholesterol levels. High-risk clients are usually referred to a nutritionist for more in-depth nutrition assessment and counseling. Physicians and dietitians have been identified as being most influential in giving nutrition advice, making it imperative that they give consistent messages to clients, families, and the community.

- *Nurses*—In addition to screening and assessing clients, nurses frequently function as the case manager for the primary care team. They provide anticipatory guidance and basic nutrition and health promotion education. Nurses in home health or perinatal home visiting programs develop a rapport with the clients that makes them very effective in encouraging clients to follow nutrition plan recommendations. This relationship is also invaluable for identifying obstacles such as a lack of food resources or transportation to the grocery store, or a stove or refrigerator that is not working, or other family members who are adversely influencing the food choices. Nurses with advanced degrees or special credentials such as certified diabetes educators and international board-certified lactation consultants are able to provide more in-depth nutritional care for high-risk clients.
- *Health Educators*—These allied health professionals work closely with the nutritionist in developing and providing health promotion activities or chronic disease risk reduction and disease management. They work with individuals and groups in a variety of clinic and community settings including primary care clinics, schools, community recreation centers, and worksite wellness programs. Health educators also take the lead in reviewing and selecting or developing health and nutrition education materials that are culturally sensitive and in the language and at an appropriate literacy level for the populations being served.
- *Dentists and Dental Hygienists*—As more evidence implicates periodontal disease as a factor in poor birth outcomes and heart disease, there is an increasing recognition of the value of the dental professionals on the health care team. They focus on preventive practices to promote good oral health. In addition to screening and treating problems that interfere with chewing, nutritionists who work with mothers and their infants frequently partner with dental staff on initiatives to promote breast-feeding and appropriate cup use to reduce the incidence of dental disease among toddlers. Dental care is an essential component of many specialty clinics including diabetes, cardiovascular disease, and HIV/AIDS services.
- *Social Workers*—Many of the clients who receive care through public health primary care services cope with significant issues that affect their ability to access services initially and fully implement the care plans that are developed for them. Social workers assess these emotional and environmental obstacles and link clients with resources for assistance for housing, transportation, medications, food, and personal safety.

Health care teams in large agencies or those in specialty services may have additional disciplines represented. Physical therapists, occupational therapists, and speech therapists work with complex cases to help clients overcome physical limitations and improve functioning related to daily living skills. They collaborate with nutritionists to assess feeding and food preparation skills and recommend appropriate foods and adaptive equipment for self-feeding and food preparation. Nutritional needs and the client's chewing and swallowing abilities influence the types, amounts, and texture of the foods included in the nutrition recommendations. Clients may be referred to external providers for these services. In those cases, the nutritionist may need to initiate the contact to establish the collaboration.

Team Approach to Client-Focused Care

Most people have participated on teams at some time—in school or social clubs, playing a sport, or working on a project. As is the case with any team, the effectiveness of a health care team depends on the ability of its members to establish shared goals and work collaboratively to identify and meet client needs. Each member brings their personal insights, experience, and expertise to the discussion on how to best meet the client or population's needs. Collaboration among health care providers can improve client care while creating a satisfying work environment.

Capitation arrangements used by managed care organizations promote team-based care delivery. The financial incentives are for the group effort rather than the individual as is the case with fee-for-service. In an agency that is using a cost-based reimbursement rate for primary care services, the costs associated with providing nutrition counseling and education services can be included in calculating the rate.

Types of Health Care Teams

Health care teams are as different as the populations they serve and the environments in which they work. At one end of the continuum is the consultative model in which one provider, often the physician, retains central responsibility for the client's care, maintaining professional independence and consulting with other professionals as needed. Work is performed in sequence with limited communication between providers. In many cases, clients must move from one location to another to receive services from providers in different sites or in separate areas within a large facility. Although the providers consider each other a resource, there is little or no shared responsibility for client outcomes. Interactions may be limited to the physician completing a referral form containing limited information and the nutritionist returning a copy of the SOAP note or making a brief telephone conversation addressing specific questions about lab values or diet orders.

At a higher functional level, multidisciplinary teams are made up of individuals from more than one discipline in order to provide a broader scope of services. Each discipline is responsible for their own area only and functions independently to contribute its expertise and make its own recommendations. Team roles are generally determined by the organizational hierarchy, with the highest-ranking professional, most often a physician, being the team leader. The nurse on the team who ensures that referrals are made to appropriate resources may coordinate case management. Although there is often some sense of being part of a larger team, members have only a general understanding of the others' work and the degree to which it contributes to the care plan goals.

In this partially integrated system, team members usually work in the same location, although they may not necessarily work for the same employer. For example, a WIC office may be colocated in a migrant health clinic, a hospital, or a private medical practice office. This one-stop approach encourages better communication about client care and a better understanding of and appreciation for each discipline's contributions to the client's care. Without attention to team maintenance, however, this structure can result in fragmented care, duplication of services, poor communication among providers, and a loss of client focus. As the move to managed care has eliminated primary care services in many health departments, this team structure is often the one in which public health nutritionists must function.

Interdisciplinary teams are similar in that they are composed of representatives from different disciplines with varied and specialized knowledge, skills, and intervention methods. The differentiation is the level of interaction among team members who share a common client population and common client care goals. The members are interdependent as they coordinate, collaborate, and communicate with one another and with clients and their families to ensure that all aspects of the health care needs are integrated and addressed. Each discipline completes a comprehensive assessment and brings the findings to the team meetings where an integrated care plan is developed. The team monitors the care plan, making changes as needed. Some members of the team may not interact directly with the client, but contribute to the assessment and care process through consultation with other practitioners. Pharmacists frequently function in this capacity.

In this integrated model of care, client needs, rather than organizational hierarchy, determine how the disciplines interact. For example, it would be appropriate for a diabetes management team to be led by a certified diabetes educator regardless of whether their training is as a nutritionist, nurse, health educator, or physician. The expertise is more important than the job title. Because of the overlap in skills related to assessment, counseling, and planning, role blurring is common.

Although their success has been limited in general primary care settings, interdisciplinary teams are frequently used in specialty clinics such as those for maternal and child health, diabetes, cardiovascular disease, and HIV/AIDS. This structure promotes the inclusion of clients and their families as members of the team, helping them assume more responsibility for their own care.

This type of team is also very effective in implementing population-focused interventions. For example, the team developing a school-based obesity prevention initiative for students and their families might include school health nurses, physicians, school food service staff, health or physical education curriculum specialists, teachers, and parents in addition to the public health nutritionists.

Developing a comprehensive intervention program would be difficult without all of these perspectives.

Regardless of the type or composition of the team, members must work together to be successful. Evidence shows that being an effective team member requires the following:

- Recognizing other members' expertise, knowledge, and values
- Learning the individual roles and processes needed to work collaboratively
- Willingness to use group skills to work through differences and accomplish goals
- Coordinating and integrating care processes to ensure excellence, continuity, and reliability of care
- Communicating in a shared language[2]

Research also shows that effective teams share specific characteristics including the following:

- Patient-centered focus
- Common goals with measurable outcomes
- Flexibility in roles within professional standards of practice
- Effectively managed group dynamics, including communication, role clarification, and decision making
- Mutual responsibility and accountability
- Continuous learning through evaluation and feedback
- Celebration of small and large successes[3]

Consulting on Client Care

Nutritionists are integral members of the primary care team at both the program management level and as direct care providers collaborating on the integration of medical nutrition therapy or developing programs to implement necessary behavioral changes. Nutritionists have the ability to translate the science of nutrition into useful and actionable information, assisting clients to set realistic goals. Nutritionists also help other team members recognize the various cultural, environmental, and economic factors that influence food access, choices, and behaviors. By defining client care priorities, the team can put nutrition in perspective.

The methods for information exchange between team members vary with the formality of the team structure. The progress note, a problem list entry, or a note attached to the chart may be the most expedient ways to share client information in an informal structure. Journal articles with new or case-relevant nutrition information can be circulated or the Web site hyperlink sent via e-mail to other team members. Within the constraints of confidentiality policies, the nutritionist may also set an appointment with one or more members of the care team to discuss client assessment data and overall care goals and offer suggestions for interventions or referrals.

The formal interdisciplinary team approach uses scheduled case management conferences to review the medical record, identify additional information needed, and discuss possible intervention strategies. All team members work together to develop the care plan that includes overall and discipline-specific goals and assigns responsibilities for implementation.

Nutritionists contribute current scientific information to support the care recommendations and suggest culturally and linguistically appropriate education materials. They identify credible support resources in the community such as lactation consultants and peer counselors for breast-feeding women, weight management programs for adults and children, and physical activity opportunities, as well as facilitating WIC referrals for eligible clients.

Case conferences also provide an opportunity for the team to monitor the client's progress, discussing successes and barriers. This client-focused approach encourages family involvement in planning and implementation of the care plan. These discussions often provide a teachable moment for health professionals to learn more about each other's roles and expertise in screening, assessing, and counseling clients.

To be successful, integrated care systems require jointly developed infrastructure and tools including clinical pathways and protocols, care planning processes and tools, and client assessment tools. For nutrition services, this includes the following:

- Standards of nutritional care for low-, medium- and high-risk clients that are incorporated into the agency's overall clinical care standards.
- Delineation of the roles and responsibilities of the various health care providers for nutritional care, including criteria for referral to the nutritionist.
- Criteria for selection and use of nutrient or dietary supplements, infant formulas, and products for enteral and parenteral feedings.
- Criteria for selection and use of nutrition education materials and breast-feeding supplies, including breast pumps.
- Criteria for referral to WIC, community food assistance and nutrition education programs, and breast-feeding support services.[4]

Having these tools in place helps to ensure that appropriate and consistent nutrition recommendations and education are provided. An excellent resource for the health care team is *Bright Futures in Practice: Nutrition.* Developed by the Health Resources and Services Administration (HRSA) of the US Department of Health and Human Services in collaboration with other partners; this reference provides a thorough overview of nutrition supervision and recommendations for anticipatory guidance from infancy through adolescence. The book's guidelines highlight how partnerships among health professionals, families, and communities can improve the nutritional status of infants, children, and adolescents.

As the average age of the US population continues to rise—it is projected that by the year 2030 there will be disproportionately more elderly than young people—the adverse effects of current dietary patterns on chronic health conditions will have significant consequences for health expenditures and quality of life. Addressing the needs of large populations of the chronically ill will require greater collaboration among health professionals and an increased focus on prevention and the behavioral determinants of health.

In recognition of this need to focus on modifiable health determinants, one of the service objectives of *Healthy People 2000* was to "Increase to at least 75% the proportion of primary care providers who provide nutrition assessment and counseling and/or referral to qualified nutritionists or dietitians."[5] As shown in Table 21–1A, the Progress Report on Healthy People 2000 Nutrition Objectives, completed in 1992, showed a wide variation among primary care professionals who provided nutrition assessments, counseling and/or referrals.

For *Healthy People 2010,* this objective was revised to focus on those specific conditions for which nutrition intervention had been shown to be effective. The current objective is to "Increase the proportion of physician office visits made by patients with a diagnosis of cardiovascular disease, diabetes, or hyperlipidemia that include counseling or education related to diet and nutrition. The target remains 75% significantly higher than the baseline of 42% in 1997 as shown in Table 21–1B."[6]

The data from the two reports suggest both the types of practitioners and chronic conditions that would benefit most from a collaborative intervention teams effort. The reports also highlight the need for ensuring that all members of the health care team have enough knowledge of nutrition to be able to identify

Table 21–1A   1992 Progress Report on *Healthy People 2000* Nutrition Objectives

Percent of primary care providers who provided nutrition assessment and counseling and/or referral to 81–100% of patients		*Percent of primary care providers who formulated a diet/nutrition plan for 81–100% of patients who needed it*	
Pediatricians	53%	Pediatricians	31%
Nurse practitioners	46%	Nurse practitioners	31%
Obstetricians/gynecologists	15%	Obstetricians/gynecologists	19%
Internists	36%	Internists	33%
Family physicians	19%	Family physicians	24%

Source: Adapted from Satcher, David. *Healthy People 2000*, Nutrition Objectives.

Table 21–1B   Physician Office Visits That Include Ordering or Providing Diet and Nutrition Counseling for Three Conditions

Persons with Specific Conditions, 1997	*Any of the Three Conditions*	*Hyperlipidemia**	*Cardiovascular Disease**	*Diabetes**
TOTAL	42%	36%	65%	48%

Source: Adapted from US Department of Health and Human Services. *Healthy People 2010.* 2nd ed. With Understanding and Improving Health and Objectives for Improving Health. Washington, DC: US Government Printing Office; November 2000.

potential nutrition-related problems, provide appropriate nutrition education, and recognize when to refer clients to a nutritionist for more comprehensive nutrition services.

EDUCATING HEALTH PROFESSIONALS

The role of the local public health agency (LPHA) in assuring a competent public health and personal health care workforce is defined in the operational definition of a local public health agency developed by the National Association of County and City Health Officials (NACCHO). Specific expectations for carrying out this essential public health service include the following:

- Evaluate LPHA staff members' public health competencies, and address deficiencies through continuing education, training, and leadership development activities.
- Provide the public health workforce with access to the training and tools needed to do their job.
- Promote the use of effective public health practices among other practitioners and agencies engaged in public health.[7]

Core Competencies for Health Care Professionals

Following up on an earlier report on quality in health care, the Institute of Medicine's 2003 report *Health Professions Education: A Bridge to Quality* proposed five core competencies that all health care professionals should possess regardless of their discipline to meet the needs of this century's health care system. The "abilities to deliver patient-centered care, work as a member of an interdisciplinary team, engage in evidence-based practice, apply quality improvement approaches, and use information technology"[8] are equally applicable to both public and private health care settings.

Providing client-focused services through interdisciplinary teams depends on all team members having the ability to identify health risks based on assessment data, reinforce health messages, and recognize when to refer clients for more specialized care. Training for medical and allied health professions in the various aspects of nutrition care should be linked to the level of responsibility they have for carrying out key nutrition functions. The 1998 American Dietetic Association position paper, *Nutrition Education for Health Care Professionals*, outlined a framework, as shown in Table 21–2, for identifying nutrition-education training needs with anticipated job responsibilities.

A variety of approaches should be used to develop these nutrition competencies, keeping in mind the needs of adult learners. Traditional didactic lectures are

Table 21–2 Critical Aspects of Health Care Practitioner Education Programs

Aspect of Nutrition Care	Nutrition Education Responsibilities			
	Minimal[a]	Limited[b]	Broad[c]	Extensive[d]
Screen for nutrition risk.	X	X	X	X
Assess nutritional health.				X
Reinforce message of the importance of nutrition to health.	X	X	X	X
Reinforce that nutrient needs differ by person and at different points throughout the lifespan.			X	X
Educate about public health nutrition guidelines and the use of nutrition as a complementary therapy.			X	X
Prescribe diets, including enteral and parenteral nutrition.				X
Counsel on specific nutrition needs.				X
Educate on nutrition principles that relate closely to a specific discipline.			X	X
Refer to a registered dietitian for in-depth nutrition evaluation or counseling.			X	X

[a]Includes practitioners with beyond-high-school certificates such as home health aides and patient care assistants.

[b]Includes practitioners with a limited role in patient education such as diagnostic imaging professionals and vascular technologists.

[c]Includes practitioners with a large role in patient education such as physical and occupational therapists, nurses, and respiratory therapists.

[d]Includes primary care providers such as family practitioners, internal medicine physicians, obstetricians and pediatricians, midwives, nurse practitioners, and physician assistants and medical specialists such as cardiologists, oncologists, nephrologists, and surgeons.

Source: Adapted from *Nutrition education for health care professionals.* Former position paper of the American Dietetic Association. *J Am Diet Assoc.* 1998; 98:343–346.

not an effective means to teach the interpersonal dynamics needed for an integrated approach to client care. Clinical problem solving through case studies or computer-based simulations is invaluable for teaching health care practitioners. By working in small groups, participants learn to collaborate with each other to find creative solutions to a variety of types of problems. Collaborating with the nutritionist in a clinical setting provides the opportunity to challenge learners to work together to address real situations.

Other activities that can be used to foster awareness of and respect for the expertise of the nutritionists on the team include: grand rounds presentations, informal lunch-and-learn discussions, journal clubs, and interactive computer-based modules. Employee wellness programs offer another opportunity to introduce coworkers to nutrition screening counseling and education. When employees recognize the value of nutrition services for themselves, they are more likely to promote them for clients.

Continuing and In-Service Education Programs

Continuing education allows health care professionals to update their knowledge to stay current in their fields, enhance their technical skills, and meet requirements for state licensure and/or other credentials. Public health agencies can work with a wide range of groups to plan and cosponsor educational activities. Potential partners include academic institutions, governmental agencies, and hospitals or other health care facilities. Professional organizations such as the state or local dietetic and public health associations, the local medical society, and voluntary organizations such as the March of Dimes, American Heart Association, and American Cancer Society are actively involved in providing continuing education for health professionals. Most states have an Area Health Education Center (AHEC) network. In addition to supporting training and continuing education for health professionals, many of the AHECs provide access to the library resources of their affiliated academic centers giving providers a mechanism to investigate the body of health literature and other databases.

Advances in technology have made continuing education more accessible and convenient. Video and Web-enhanced teleconferences sponsored by universities and federal agencies such as the Centers for Disease Control and Prevention or National Institutes of Health bring nationally recognized experts to even the most remote location. Video streaming technology for Internet seminars and self-paced modules on DVDs make continuing education opportunities available at the participant's convenience. Incorporating small-group discussion or other interactive elements to these alternative approaches adds value to what could be a passive learning mode.

Planning continuing education events that promote multidisciplinary participation fosters teamwork and a collaborative mindset. Sessions can be marketed to a diverse audience including private practice, community health centers, hospitals, and community organizations. Offering continuing education units (CEU's), approved by credentialing agencies and state licensure boards helps to increase the perceived value of the activities.

Many professional journals, including the *Journal of the American Dietetic Association*, provide continuing education credits for other health professionals, including physicians. This interdisciplinary focus can be used effectively to increase the awareness of the multiple determinants of health and the value each discipline brings to the health care team. Nutritionists should also become familiar with the journals from other disciplines.

In service training differs from continuing education in that its primary focus is on the needs of the organization rather than the employee and it is usually designed to improve technical skills or introduce new procedures. Results from a training needs assessment based on the core public health and discipline-specific competencies may be used to develop an annual training plan for the agency. Many organizations use individual development plans to establish long- and short-term goals and identify training and experiential activities to increase employees' knowledge, skills, and abilities. Nutritionists can assist staff in other disciplines in identifying opportunities to enhance their skills in nutrition screening, assessment, education, and referral. Examples of developmental activities include "shadowing" a nutritionist, working with a mentor, and assisting WIC staff with an outreach event. Too often training is viewed as the only solution to increasing staff competencies.

Cross-disciplinary training is an effective but underutilized approach to strengthening the health care team by increasing both their scope of knowledge and its practical application. For example, an in-service training for a team designing and implementing a pediatric obesity prevention program would include an overview of the epidemiology of childhood obesity, the public health implications, the pathophysiology, current intervention philosophies, and available resources. The desired outcome for the training would be that the physicians, nurses, health educators, and nutritionists would have a common understanding of the current concepts related to the role of diet and physical activity in the prevention and treatment of childhood obesity. Interactive case studies could be used to illustrate interdisciplinary, client-focused strategies for addressing this issue.[9]

Every training and continuing education activity should be used as a "teachable moment" for promoting healthy behaviors. Health professionals, especially nutritionists, must ensure that both their messages and actions support a pattern of healthy eating and physical activity. Refreshments provided during continuing education activities should incorporate the key nutrition elements and be consistent with nutrition guidelines. Offering a variety of choices promotes adequate intake of essential nutrients and makes it easy to incorporate foods enjoyed by different cultural groups. Choose moderate portion sizes and serve just enough food for the number of people attending.[10] Incorporate stretching or walking breaks into the agenda to help keep energy levels high and support physical activity recommendations.

All education efforts should be evaluated to determine both participant satisfaction and effectiveness. Surveys at the end of the session can collect data regarding whether goals were met and the perceived value of the session. Subsequent follow-up can be used to assess changes in knowledge or practice resulting from the training. Feedback and suggestions are useful in planning future activities.

Team Training

Few disciplines include training on how to function as part of a team in their didactic course work. Successful collaboration between health care providers from different disciplines requires a unique set of teambuilding skills that includes understanding the responsibilities, skills, expertise of others, and their personal styles and temperaments. There are numerous resources and training courses on team building available to help teams develop these skills. Training is most effective if the team participates as a unit.

Team Opportunities in the Public Health Agency

The use of teams in public health is not limited to patient care. Teams are an effective means to engage staff at all levels in supporting the agency's mission, strategic goals, and performance improvement activities. Participation on the various teams, work groups, and task forces in the agency can be used to highlight the nutritionists planning and problem-solving skills. With their versatile skill set, nutrition managers frequently are called on to assume leadership roles in agency-wide teams.

LEADERSHIP TEAM

One of the significant changes in the operation of public health agencies has been the transition from an emphasis on management—"doing things right" to a focus on leadership—"doing the right things." As a result, the roles of the directors for the agency's discipline areas have changed. Although the leadership team still advises the agency director on policy issues, they more likely to be involved in planning and implementing the activities that directly support the 10 essential public health services including strategic planning, community partnership development, public health preparedness, and advocacy. With evidence-based practice being a priority for agency leaders, the nutrition director can provide data on the contributions of nutrition in addressing existing and emerging community health problems for consideration in strategic and budget planning.

QUALITY IMPROVEMENT

The shift in emphasis from quality assurance to systemwide quality improvement has created a broad range of opportunities for nutritionists to participate on teams. The peer review and chart audit are standard tools in evaluating quality of health care. The review team is composed of peers of those whose work is being examined. Interdisciplinary teams are the most cost-effective and least duplicative, as most disciplines base their assessments on many of the same measurements. The peer review process may look at care in general or focus on a practice area such as diabetes, pediatrics, family planning, or HIV/AIDs. In either case, the nutritionist is an essential member of the review team.

Other quality improvement teams may be established to address issues such as customer and employee satisfaction, process improvement, marketing, and safety. Addressing systemwide and program-specific issues around access to services, client flow and waiting times, cultural competence, or vending machine selections can help to ensure consistency in nutrition messages and in increased quality of care.

STAFF DEVELOPMENT

The interdisciplinary staff development team identifies the core competencies that all agency personnel should possess to meet the agency's current and future needs. Members collaborate to develop and promote processes and procedures to ensure that the agency's orientation, training, and continuing education activities give staff an understanding of all aspects of public health, including nutrition and health promotion. This team has a responsibility to align staff development activities with the mission, vision, and strategic goals of the organization.

EMPLOYEE WELLNESS

As evidence of the benefits of employee wellness programs mounts, more agencies are committing resources to implement health promotion activities for staff. The focus of these programs is the same as for external health promotion initiatives: reducing chronic disease risk factors and promoting healthy lifestyle behaviors. Changing food and physical activity behaviors is central to risk factor reduction. Involving nutritionists in the planning of the program is essential, and involving them in the implementation of the program is ideal.

TEAMWORK

Teams are often formed across work unit lines. These efforts may not work if there is turfism, competition for scarce resources, and lack of understanding about the goals of the organization and of each work unit. For cross-discipline and cross-unit teams to function effectively, there must be support from the administrators and supervisors, a clear indication of where the agency is headed, and why this effort is valued. There must also be a system that rewards team effort through the performance appraisal system and recognizes the amount of time required for the project effort. The team must have the authority to accomplish its mission. It must also have the resources it needs.[11]

Team Development

Many models describe the progression in team developmental. These models are similar and suggest that the process occurs in five predictable stages that are frequently referred to as: forming, storming, norming, performing, and reforming. Each stage is characteristically different and builds on the preceding one. As a team matures it faces specific interpersonal, leadership, and member behavior issues at each stage. Table 21–3 demonstrates the following matrix that integrates key characteristics of the most widely accepted team development theories.

Team Roles

Leadership skills are as important as professional expertise for team leaders. They must have a thorough understanding of the team assignment and skills in managing group processes. Leaders set the tone and direction for the team and must be able to adapt to a leadership style that is appropriate for the team's developmental stage. Because of the frequency of employee turnover, a significant challenge for team leaders are the changes in group dynamics as the team members come and go. Even mature groups may regress to an earlier stage as the participant mix changes.

Thinking styles and temperaments are as important as professional expertise when selecting team members.

Some individuals look at the big picture when approaching a problem; others think of the important details. Some individuals are skilled at reaching closure on issues, and some look at all of the alternatives. Some focus more

Table 21–3 An Integration of Team and Group Development Theory

Stage of Development	Leader Behavior	Member Behavior	Emotional Climate	Task Outcome
Forming	Directs	Dependence	Uncertain	Committing
Storming	Sells	Resistance	Conflict	Clarifying
Norming	Participates	Cohesion	Support	Rules develop, e.g., conflict, decisions
Performing	Delegates, negotiates	Interdependence	Pride	Achieving
Reforming	Evaluates, reviews	Maintaining	Satisfied	Consolidating, renewing

Source: Adapted with Permission from Ryan David. *Tools For Facilitating Health Care Teamwork: 2*, Workshops In Team Development, University Of Toronto, Toronto, Canada. Accessed February 14, 2006.

on people, others on ideas. Some people have critical thinking ability, and others are concerned with human values and interactions. All views are important when a group is working together to achieve common goals."[12]

The goal is to have a mix of styles that allow the team to perform at a high level.

Although diversity is valued in team composition, differences in values, attitudes, and perceptions can create conflict between members. Although conflict is most often viewed as a symptom that something is wrong, when it is managed in a positive way it can promote creative problem solving, innovation, and team growth and maturation. Conversely, poorly handled conflict can lead to an ineffective, dysfunctional team.

Effective collaboration and conflict resolution is built on a continual search for win-win solutions for achieving the team's goals. Strategies that can be used to resolve conflicts include the following:

- Establish standards to accomplish tasks and set the norms for team behavior.
- Create an environment that encourages each member to contribute.
- Listen carefully and respectfully to all opinions.
- Seek consensus in making decisions.
- Evaluate the team process and progress regularly.

Effective teams establish methods for setting priorities, assigning tasks, and managing meetings. A matrix can be used to map out the responsibilities of each team member, indicating the primary and secondary responsibilities and the priority level of the task. The individuals who must be informed or whose support is required can also be included.

One of the major reasons for failure of a team approach is poor communication among team members. Open, honest, and clear communication is essential for building the trust and respect that is necessary for teams to be effective. Many factors contribute to communication breakdowns: poor listening skills, inability to clearly and concisely convey relevant information, use of discipline-specific jargon, emphasis on hierarchy, and turf protection.

Benefits of Teamwork

As health care in both the public and the private sector becomes more complex and more expensive, there is a growing awareness that effective teams benefit the client, the health care team, and the organization.

The synergy that results within a highly functioning team leads to the development of more creative solutions to complex problems in all aspects of client care: access, delivery systems, and customer satisfaction. Quality can be enhanced resulting in increased efficiency, effectiveness, and reduction in medical errors.

Employee satisfaction and motivation are increased as practitioners learn new skills and innovation is encouraged.

From the client perspective, there are several benefits to receiving care from an interdisciplinary team. Increased coordination of care saves time, reduces anxiety, and provides a central point of contact for clients and their families. More communication that is open is possible, increasing the client's level of understanding and involvement in decision making. This environment empowers clients to be active partners in their own care, a key factor in chronic disease prevention and intervention.

Interdisciplinary teams' efficient delivery of care reduces duplication of effort or service and minimizes unnecessary interventions, resulting in lower costs. Other business benefits include reduced staff turnover and absenteeism, higher quality of care, reduced conflict, and better outcomes. The lack of nutrition professionals' involvement in interdisciplinary teams has been cited as a barrier to generating evidence of the effectiveness of medical nutrition therapy, an essential requirement for reimbursement for services.[13]

Using teams is not without its drawbacks. The process is time consuming and may take time away from other duties. One of the most difficult challenges is coordinating team members' schedules to allow sufficient time for discussion and planning. In the primary care clinic, precautions must be taken to ensure that clients do not become confused about who is the primary point of contact. Finally, successful teamwork requires ongoing attention to the process, interpersonal relationships, and a periodic reassessment of goals.

> Teamwork encourages a more comprehensive view of community health problems and is more likely to move an agency toward forward-looking health promotion and disease prevention strategies. For nutritionists, membership on teams extends their influence in the agency and the community since each member of the team becomes vested in the contributions nutrition makes in meeting public health goals.[14]

POINTS TO PONDER

- Despite a growing recognition of the value of working in teams, the traditional organizational models that promote silos of expertise continue to be common. How can public health nutritionists facilitate change?
- How well does training for public health nutritionists emphasize the skills needed to work effectively in teams? How can it be improved?
- What are the opportunities and challenges posed by interdisciplinary collaboration? How have you seen it work?
- What is the current impact and future potential of technology on collaboration among health professionals?

NOTES

1. McCall M, Keir B. *Survey of the Public Health Nutrition Workforce: 1999–2000.* Alexandria, Va: Association of State and Territorial Public Health Nutrition Directors, USDA Food and Nutrition Service; 2003. Available at: http://www.fns.usda.gov/oane/MENU/Published/WIC/FILES/Publichealthsurvey.pdf. Accessed April 2005.

2. Greiner AC, Knebel E, eds. *Health Professions Education: A Bridge to Quality.* The National Academy of Science; 2003:56.

3. Dixon DL. New perspectives on interdisciplinary teams in LTC. *Caring for the Ages* 2003; 4:19.

4. Kaufman M. *Nutrition in Public Health.* Rockville, Md: Aspen Publishers; 1990:225.

5. Satcher D. Healthy People 2000 Progress Review, Nutrition. US Dept Health and Human Services, Public Health Service; 1998. Available at: http://www.healthypeople.gov/data/PROGRVW/Nutrition/default.htm. Accessed May 5, 2006.

6. US Dept Health and Human Services. With Understanding and Improving Health and Objectives for Improving Health. In: *Healthy People 2010.* 2nd ed. Washington, DC: US Government Printing Office; 2000.

7. National Association of County and City Health Officials. *Operational definition of a functional local public health agency, draft* G4. Available at: http//www.NACCHO.org. Accessed April 2005.

8. Greiner AC, Knebel E, eds. *Health Professions Education: A Bridge to Quality.* The National Academy of Science; 2003:45–46.

9. Kaufman M. *Nutrition in Public Health.* Rockville, Md: Aspen Publishers; 1990:428.

10. The American Cancer Society. *Meeting well, a tool for planning healthy meetings and events.* 2000. Available at: http://www.hawaii.edu/foodskills/ACS/WellTraining Meeting.pdf. Accessed May 5, 2006.

11. Kaufman M. *Nutrition in Public Health.* Rockville, Md: Aspen Publishers; 1990:430.

12. Kaufman M. *Nutrition in Public Health.* Rockville, Md: Aspen Publishers; 1990:429.

13. Smith AR Jr, Christie C. Facilitating transdisciplinary teamwork in dietetics education: a case study approach. *J Am Diet Assoc.* 104; 962.

14. Kaufman M. *Nutrition in Public Health.* Rockville, Md: Aspen Publishers; 1990:435.

BIBLIOGRAPHY

Grant RW, Finocchio LJ, California Primary Care Consortium Subcommittee on Interdisciplinary Collaboration. *Interdisciplinary Collaborative Teams in Primary Care: A Model Curriculum and Resource Guide.* San Francisco, Calif: Pew Health Professions Commission; 1995.

Hall P, Weaver L. Interdisciplinary education and teamwork: a long and winding road. *Medical Education.* 2001; 35:872.

National Research Council. *Diet and Health: Implications for Reducing Chronic Disease Risk.* Washington, DC: National Academies Press; 1989.

Pew Health Professions Commission. *Critical Challenges: Revitalizing the Health Professions for the Twenty-First Century,* The Third Report of the Pew Health Professions Commission. The Center for Health Professions, University of California, San Francisco, 1995.

Ryan D. Tools for Facilitating Health Care Teamwork: 2, Workshops in Team Development, Sunnybrook Health Sciences Centre, Toronto, Ontario, Canada. Available at: http://ipe.utoronto.ca/resources/ryan2.html. Accessed February 14, 2006.

Scholtes PR, Joiner BL, Streibel B, Streibel BJ. *The Team Handbook.* 3rd ed. Madison, Wisc: Joiner/Oriel Inc; 2003.

Story M, Holt K, Sofka D, eds. *Bright Futures in Practice: Nutrition.* Arlington, Va: National Center for Education in Maternal and Child Health; 2000.

United States Department of Health and Human Services. *The Surgeon General's Report on Nutrition and Health.* Washington, DC: DHHS; 1988. DHHS Pub. No. (PHS) 88050210.

United States Department of Health and Human Services. *The Surgeon General's Call to Action to Prevent and Decrease Overweight and Obesity.* Rockville, Md: Department of Health and Human Services, Public Health Service, Office of the Surgeon General; 2001.

CHAPTER 22

Network/Internetwork for Public Health Nutrition

Mildred Kaufman and Charles N. Abernethy

Reader Objectives

- Define networking.
- Suggest public health and nutrition issues enhanced by networking.
- Compare and contrast the values of face-to-face networking *versus* Internet networking.
- State some tips for successful face-to-face and Internet networking.

DEFINE NETWORKING

Networking is defined as an interconnected or interrelated chain, group, or system. John Naisbett uses *network* as an action verb that links people to other people and clusters of people to exchange information, foster self-help, improve productivity and work life, and share resources.[1] Face-to-face networks, as envisioned by Naisbett, are structured to transmit information in a way that is quicker, more high-tech, and more energy efficient than any other process. Networks cut diagonally across institutions that house information and put people in direct contact with the resources they seek.[2] Naisbett forecasts networking to be one of the 10 new directions for the future.[3] Networking is also used effectively to advocate for changes in policies within an agency, and at the local, state, and national levels, as well as to influence legislation. The achievements of the *National Turning Point Initiative* implemented in 41 rural, urban, and tribal communities in 14 states has "produced evidence that partnerships between health departments and communities can transform a collection of categorical governmental programs into networks of public and private players, all of which participate in protecting against disease and promoting the health of the population."[5] For more see www.wkkf.org.

Recent development of the Internet and the World Wide Web provides a new tool to raise networking to another level utilizing the latest available technology. Face-to-face networking used in conjunction with high-tech Internet networking can extend the reach of public health nutritionists from their immediate neighborhood to a much wider, international world, and do it asynchronously (without the need to be "on" at the same time).

FACE-TO-FACE NETWORKING

Earlier chapters identified the growing number of complex nutrition-related public health issues facing localities, states, the nation, and the world. Expanding and diverse populations need more services at a time when official public health agency budgets are static, if not diminishing. *Healthy People 2010* proposes that "Partnerships are effective tools for improving health in communities" and emphasizes seeking out nontraditional partners.[6] Collaborating with other health and nutrition professionals in the community, building coalitions with professionals from public and private agencies and institutions, and enlisting citizen participation has been found to increase cost-effectiveness and productivity and to reduce duplicated efforts. Such collaboration also avoids imposing programs that do not meet the needs or conform to the cultures of the people who live in the community. Community partnerships empower the participants, earn their trust, and strengthen their commitment.[7]

The nutritionist who counsels an obese pregnant woman referred by the health agency's nurse-midwife reaches the client and perhaps her family. The nutritionist who convinces the county school superintendent to replace sugar-sweetened soft drinks with water, low-fat milk, and unsweetened fruit juices in the school vending machines reaches hundreds of students in the school district. The nutritionist who convinces corporate decision makers of a national fast-food chain to offer smaller portions of lower-calorie foods reaches millions of consumers. Nutritionists who use networking effectively can use the media to enhance the public understanding of current nutrition research findings and how food and exercise habits promote personal and family health. When nutritionists capture public attention, they can impact community values and norms. This process of exchanging and sharing food, nutrition, and health promoting information for the public benefit requires initiating, cultivating, and maintaining multiple and diverse networks both inside and outside the community. There is "power" when numbers of informed and respected health and nutrition professionals supported by their organizations join forces with consumer advocates to collaborate on any of the following:

- Promote healthy eating and exercise behavior change, which addresses national health promotion and disease prevention objectives.
- Ensure that evidence-based medical nutrition therapy is available as part of all federal and state tax-supported, employer-sponsored, and private health insurance plans.
- Promote nutrition and health status surveillance.
- Ensure food assistance to the hungry and homeless.
- Advocate legislation for a safe, health-promoting food supply.
- Combat health and nutrition fraud.
- Support standards for state licensure of nutrition and dietetic professionals.
- Generate public and private funding to expand evidence-based nutrition education for students in grades K–12, school teachers, health professionals, and consumers.

The ultimate networking challenge to knowledgeable, articulate public health nutritionists and their professional organizations is to be appointed to "seats at the table" of local, state, and national interdisciplinary and interagency advisory councils; commissions; or "blue ribbon" committees appointed to study and recommend health, food, and nutrition policy or propose legislation to appointed and elected officials. For example, obesity and overweight are second on the list of leading health indicators in *Healthy People 2010*[8] and are specified as important risk factors for high blood pressure, high cholesterol, type 2 diabetes, heart disease, stroke, gall bladder disease, arthritis, and certain types of cancers.[9] Nutritionists have extensive knowledge and experience in what works and what does not work to achieve appropriate weight loss. They are well prepared to participate in policy-making deliberations and recommend the integration of evidence-based nutrition, exercise, and behavioral interventions.

Participate in Community Networks

Figure 22–1 presents the complex web of interests within the community's health, social service, education, and business sectors which, in partnership with the public, should have a stake in food, nutrition, and health policy. The community assessment (see Chapter 3) describes approaches to setting community priorities among the current public health and nutrition issues. The community assessment identifies key individuals, families, committees, agencies, and organizations that have a stake in food, nutrition, and health issues for personal, family, and the public's health. Informal clusters of extended families, friends, neighbors, social cliques, schoolmates, and coworkers may be named in conversations with colleagues and community leaders. More readily identified are the social clubs, professional societies, health associations, service organizations, political parties, fraternities/sororities,

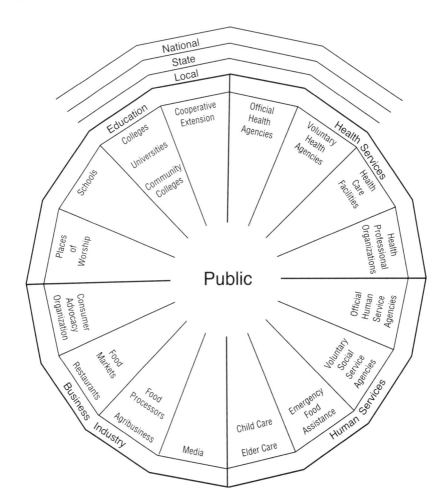

Figure 22–1   Building Community Networks to Address Nutrition Needs of the Population. *Source:* Prepared by Chapter Co Author and Editor, Mildred Kaufman.

religious congregations, that bring together people who share political views, professional expertise, ethnicity, or common values. Support groups join individuals and families who have a mutual health concern. The combined resources of all of these systems must address the priority needs.

Many communities support a regional planning council, a health and welfare council, an interagency coordinating council, or a coordinating office housed in the state or local official health and/or human service agency. This council brings together representatives of tax-supported (official) and nonprofit voluntary agencies providing multiple health and mental health services, children's and family services, aging services, food and financial assistance, housing assistance, vocational rehabilitation, and other health and human services, as well as the united giving organization and, most importantly, consumer and citizen representatives. Such a council may include religious or interfaith groups, educational institutions, and service leagues. This council identifies resources and community services that assist those who are dependent because of poor health, age, family stress, homelessness, social isolation, substance abuse, inadequate income, or education. Through an information and referral office and its printed directory or computer database, the council strives to help people in need find services and work through any eligibility requirements and "red tape." The directory or database provides detailed information on both the area population and the services in the community. Nutritionists should keep the database current on credible sources of nutrition education/counseling and food and financial assistance, including the contact person, the address, telephone number, e-mail address, geographic coverage, eligibility criteria for services, and fees charged.

Service organizations welcome members who share their causes, joining and actively volunteering time to work with civic, service, or professional associations concerned with health, nutrition, education, political, and social issues in the community. These activities open additional networks for nutritionists to educate the public, develop policy, and advocate for change. Providing nutrition and public health expertise and data from the community assessment can help service groups to document their public policy statements and advocacy positions to present to public officials. Professional nutrition expertise adds credibility to the organization's platform on health and nutrition issues.

Professional Networks

National, state, and the regional or local chapters of professional organizations provide a professional network for nutritionists who work in public or community health. The largest and most influential organizations that nutritionists should join as active participants are discussed here.

The American Public Health Association (APHA) provides a forum for workers who share interests in the broad practice of public health. Its sections represent areas of professional expertise, and its caucuses share concerns for current social or political "causes." APHA carries out a legislative program through its Washington headquarters. APHA offers continuing education through its annual meeting, monthly *American Journal of Public Health*, official newspaper *The Nation's Health*, special publications, short courses, and its Web site. Affiliated state associations conduct annual and regional educational meetings. APHA has a food and nutrition section where nutritionists from agencies, educational institutions, and industry work together on common concerns about public health nutrition programming and evaluation, nutrition monitoring, food safety, and nutrition education for professionals and the public. Active participation in APHA offers nutritionists the opportunity to network not only with nutrition professionals, but also with physicians, nurses, health educators, social workers, environmentalists, biostatisticians, epidemiologists, administrators, and others involved in promoting and protecting the public's health. For more see www.apha.org.

The American Dietetic Association (ADA) has established the educational and practice standards for nutritionists and dietitians. It provides extensive opportunities for continuing education through its annual national Food and Nutrition Conference and Expo, monthly *Journal of the American Dietetic Association*, and bimonthly *ADA Times* for members of the association. It offers a wide variety of educational publications for both professionals and consumers and position papers on a variety of timely issues in nutrition and dietetics. It maintains an active consumer and professional Web site at www.eatright.org. Through sponsorship of professional conferences and workshops it offers extensive continuing education opportunities. The ADA Center for Professional Development can be accessed at www.eatright.org/cpd.html. ADA conducts an active legislative program through its Washington office and an annual legislative symposium. The ambassador program of selected and trained regional media representatives provides a forceful image of qualified nutrition professionals in the national media. The peer professional practice groups network through numerous specialty practice groups within the national, state, and district associations. The ADA's Division of Community Dietetics includes a public health nutrition practice group which provides a "home" for nutrition workers interested in public health and community dietetics. Related ADA entities are the Commission on Dietetic Registration (CDR) and The American Dietetic Association Foundation and its National Center for Nutrition and Dietetics.

The Society for Nutrition Education (SNE) is an international organization of nutrition educators who promote healthy sustainable food choices. Members conduct research on nutrition behavior and communication, develop and disseminate innovative nutrition education strategies, and communicate information on food, nutrition, and health to students, professionals, policy makers, and the public. Members share ideas and resources through the *Journal of Nutrition Education and Behavior*, a newsletter, an annual conference, and a members-only e-mail list. Public policy and regulatory updates are disseminated to members through a monthly newsletter prepared by SNE's public policy consultant in Washington. Special interest divisions offer networking opportunities to members with similar interests and expertise including the public health nutrition division, communications division, social marketing network and weight realities division. For more see www.sne.org.

Tips for Face-to-Face Networking

There are at least three motivations for networking:

1. Professional development
2. Advancing and leveraging the profession, especially in public policy domains
3. Career development

Networking gains a broad base of support for food and nutrition issues, helps public health nutritionists achieve professional recognition, and earn opportunities to serve in leadership roles in the community, state, and nation. Building a larger, stronger network requires deliberate cultivation of casual contacts into involved colleagues. To enhance the process do the following:

- Prepare a written list of the most urgent community nutrition, diet, and health issues of significant concern to the public's health. List the desired outcomes to be achieved through networking efforts. Suggest some possible strategies to address these issues and the contacts and partners needed.
- Prepare a plan to communicate these issues and needs to a large number of influential "movers and shakers" in the community as well as at the state or national levels.
- Attend a variety of meetings, conferences, rallies, and social events attended by the identified community leaders. Prepare and rehearse an effective personal introduction that is compelling, memorable, and repeatable, designed to attract the attention and involvement of the listener.
- Mix among the conversation groups to meet and engage in friendly, but purposeful conversation and make useful connections. Always behave as a host not as a guest. Listen to the conversations to connect with those who have similar community concerns, values, and convictions.
- Always address contact persons by name, and remember their names. Exchange business cards with key contacts. File these cards noting when and why these individuals should be cultivated and contacted periodically.
- Follow up key contacts with a diplomatic note, e-mail, or friendly phone call. To maintain a continuing dialogue, always provide promised information, clippings, or references of mutual interest.
- Volunteer to work on community projects, and always do a good job.
- Be sincere in interpersonal interactions, always offering to help as well as to receive help.

Face-to-face networking is an active sharing process that involves professional expertise, interpersonal skills, diplomacy, political acumen, and integrity. If practiced and nurtured, face-to-face networking yields far-reaching results to benefit the community and the public's health. Those in the network feel empowered, competent, and self-confident. Although professional credibility is based on what you know, networking demonstrates the value of whom you know.

INTERNET NETWORKING

A variety of digital communication tools have arisen only recently; many did not exist for the general public 20, or in some cases, 10 years ago. Such means include e-mail, chat rooms, list server (or listserv or list-serv), Web sites, instant messaging (IM), teleconferencing, video conferencing, distance learning, and others (see

Table 22–1 for a more complete list, with comments). But the greatest hallmark of this digital communication form of networking, in addition to speed, is being both asynchronous in time and ageographic in location (saving travel time and fuel). Where once there was only post, telegraph, telephone, and fax, now many methods are inexpensively and conveniently available to the general public worldwide.

E-mail merges post with fax or telegraph and is easily copied and rapidly spread among an entire community.

Chat rooms provide an informal but written means to discuss a topic or series of related topics, and have an ongoing record of it available to all participants.

A list server (or listserv or list-serv) is set up by an organization, known as the host organization, as a means to provide to an identified community a somewhat formal document or document in development. A list server is a server computer on which a list of e-mail addresses becomes one overarching e-mail address. When a member of a particular list server group posts a message, the list server automatically forwards a copy of that message to every member on that list. A list server is used for e-mail newsletters, announcements, discussion groups, and opt-in e-mail marketing campaigns. The list server is a forum for discussion, questions, and knowledge sharing. Participation requires signing up at the listserv, so only those who have signed up and been accepted can receive these e-mails. This ensures limited membership and a level of privacy. An archive is created and updated every so often (usually hours). Participants are not to post messages that stray too far off the agreed-upon topic. And usually there are group norms about unacceptable personal attacks, flame wars (running arguments using inflammatory wording), or other inappropriate behavior. Such participants may have their e-mail address removed from the list server. The host organization usually also limits its responsibilities.

Web sites provide a means for wider access or a portal to a completely professional realm for nearly any interested party. Instant messaging (IM) provides a quick, quiet conversation. More educational material can be delivered through video conferencing, or for some material an electronic board is best for viewing.

A professional organization can now go beyond a simple Web site by transforming that Web site into a portal. A portal's goal is to become the first place on the Internet that people with interests in the profession turn to. The portal not only provides a place for the professional organization to place and update its own materials, but the organization can also provide links to other's Web sites, with annotations. For instance, the Web site of a local professional organization can be hyperlinked to local nutrition service organizations, and to accurate, credible nutrition information in answer to frequently asked questions (FAQs) from sources at the local, state, and national levels.

Distance learning is still developing. The goal motivating the current development of distance learning is to have an efficient means to educate ever wider and larger audiences, without the need to invest in real estate, build and maintain larger buildings, and require people to simultaneously converge at a single location. Several models of distance learning are in use today, including both synchronized or asynchronous totally Internet-delivered courses, or a mixed on-site and Internet course (University of Phoenix calls this form FlexNet), where students meet simultaneously with the course instructor face-to-face at a location (on-site) for an extended class at the course's beginning and end, while the intervening delivery is wholly by asynchronous Internet.

Table 22–1 presents a number of these Internet and other information tools organized by the various purposes of public health nutritionists, and includes comments and some examples. These examples are nonexhaustive and in no particular order. And an introduction to computer literacy written specifically for health care professionals, with descriptions of basic computer functions and their usages can be found in the recently updated edition of Joos and others.[9]

Nickerson reviews a number of these Internet and other information communications tools, some the same as listed above and some are variations, specifically e-mail, electronic bulletin boards, teleconferencing, telecommuting, computer-supported cooperative work (CSCW), and telepresence.[10] In reviewing these tools and their rapid evolution from the point of view of establishing a human factors research agenda, Nickerson raises a number of human interaction issues. For instance, e-mail is described as an "equalizer," because many prior existing social interaction cues are removed.[11] Electronic bulletin boards, unlike the board down the hall, are "accessed from essentially anywhere."[12] Teleconferencing seeks "to create a realistic impression of an actual gathering" although the actual dynamics of electronic "meetings" differ from those of face-to-face meetings in a variety of ways.[13] The human question for virtual or artificial realities is "how real (in appearance) is real enough." (Hearing, touch, smell can all be added to this question).

In a different review that approaches Internet utilization with more of a view towards development and maintenance of the professional health community, various Internet tools are rated along dimensions of bandwidth (delivery speed), latency (e.g., delay between sending an e-mail and its being received for viewing at its intended destination), availability (percentage of time actually usable), security (and privacy; protection from viruses, spam, spyware, and other forms of malware), and ubiquity (worldwide accessibility).[14]

Professional Education

Among the topics covered is professional education for not only basic sciences but also clinical education. The fact that basic science education in recent years has become "less didactic and more problem-oriented" has opened up professions to increase experimentation and use the Internet for such things as online textbooks, journals, interactive courseware, increasingly sophisticated simulations, and for clinical education and improved search and retrieval of information in its many

Table 22–1 The Internet and Other Information Tools

No.	Public Health Nutrition Professional's Purpose(s)	Time Dependency (All geographically asynchronous)	Internet and Other Information Tools	Comments/ Examples
1.	Communication, small numbers	Real time	Instant messaging (IM)	Chronological, little preservation, some attachments possible
2.	Audio, slow video, small numbers	Real time	Internet telephone	Voice over Internet Protocol (VOIP)
3.	Audio, slow video, larger numbers	Real time	Internet conference calls	Voice over Internet Protocol (VOIP)
4.	Communication, larger numbers	Asynchronous	E-mail, including attachments	Messages initially sorted in chronological order. Often manual filing to otherwise sort.
5.	Topical discussions	Asynchronous	Message boards	Maintains topic threads
6.	Document review	Asynchronous	List servers‡	Post protected documents
7.	Document development	Asynchronous	List servers‡	Post documents for group editing
8.	Research	Real time	Search engines	Very powerful/ efficient now. Many journals, publications now online. Google, esp. Scholar.
9.	Position statement(s)	Asynchronous	Web site	Not a printed publication, amenable to rapid real-time editing. Security an issue. Can be nonvolatile, e.g., .pdf image.
10.	Newsletters	Asynchronous	Web site	Not a printed publication, amenable to rapid real-time editing. Security an issue. Can be nonvolatile, e.g., .pdf image.

Table 22–1 continued

No.	Public Health Nutrition Professional's Purpose(s)	Time Dependency (All geographically asynchronous)	Internet and Other Information Tools	Comments/ Examples
11.	Education/ training	Synchronous	Blackboard, Net meeting	All participate at same time; lecturer controls or lecturer gives over control to questioner; all hear/speak.
12.	Education/ training	Asynchronous	Message boards	Outlook Express, and others. University of Phoenix Online and Flexnet Courses. Maintains topic threads, as opposed to chronological order.
13.	Opinions	Asynchronous	Blogs	Short for Web logs.
14.	Jobs			Either as job seeker or as employer of contract/ consultants or permanent hires
15.	Language management	Real time	Machine translation	Use with care, short sentences/ phrases, may have limited technical vocab- ulary. Examples are: Altavista Babel Fish Trans- lation, Google Language Tools
16.	Politics			See discussion

Source: Prepared by Chapter Co-Author, Charles Abernethy.

forms.[15] Continuing, continuous, and distance education are being increasingly explored and delivered using the Internet. Distance education has raised the issue of intellectual property protection, including rights of the faculty to retain the products of their intellectual work: is it a textbook to be copyrighted or software to be patented?[16]

Collaboration

Several instances of potential for enhanced collaboration are presented. For example, researchers in different locations can participate in the remote control of an experimental apparatus, utilize language translation among diverse geographically spread participants, and coordinate and conduct clinical trials at various locations.

Publishing

Not only can more information be included in any one article, including its raw data, but also the quality and acceptance of professionally respected articles on the Internet requires several protections for credibility: "(1) providing an enduring stamp of approval for documents, (2) allowing peer [review] groups to be defined and maintained, (3) searching the Internet to retrieve documents of interest [and acceptability], and (4) validating the authenticity of online documents."[17]

Professional Organizational Development

Professional organizations are encouraged to utilize the Internet for increased efficiencies to "convene groups that would develop standards and guidelines based on the experience and expertise of their memberships."[18] Proposed areas for guidelines development are: "(1) monitoring and conducting health-related chat sessions, bulletin boards, and forums, (2) remote education of health professionals, (3) disseminating information to a broad audience, (4) appropriate and inappropriate creation of provider/patient relationships, (5) assurance of the integrity and accuracy of patient-maintained health records, (6) means to assess trade-offs between security, confidentiality, and access, (7) direct marketing to patients of health care services (e.g., pharmaceuticals, prostheses), (8) communication across traditional boundaries (e.g., patient to provider), (9) clinical e-mail, (10) Web information services, and (11) privacy and security of electronic health information."[19]

Public Policy

This review raises the need for increased focus on public policy issues for the use of the Internet by professions in health care because the very rapid rise of the Internet has been impeded for professional usages by technical, practice, and legal issues based in the past. The huge volumes and speed of the Internet can magnify these kinds of issues. Less emphasis is placed then in the use of the Internet by a profession to manage its public policy programs.[20]

A caution: Experience with all of these information tools indicates that where trust must be established in order to take a risk and go forward, face-to-face communication is necessary. All of these methods provide for efficient and productive preparation and follow-up; they allow for communication of factual information and interpretations with some emphasis. Many of these electronic and other tools allow for thoughtful construction of ideas and maintain a written record to build upon.[20]

Experience also indicates that the trust built up through face-to-face networking can dissipate in the face of other, conflicting agendas without a deliberately conscious and disciplined follow-up using these Internet and other information tools.

POINTS TO PONDER

- How can the nutritionist select the community networks that will be most useful and receptive?
- How can networking be used to promote the public's health?
- How can nutritionists best coordinate face-to-face networking and Internetworking?

HELPFUL WEB SITES

American Dietetic Association: www.eatright.org
      Professional Development: www.eatright.org/cpd.html
American Public Health Association: www.apha.org
Society for Nutrition Education (SNE): www.sne.org
W.K. Kellogg Foundation: www.wkkf.org

NOTES

1. Naisbett J. *Megatrends: Ten New Directions Transforming Our Lives.* New York, NY: Warner Books; 1982:192–193.

2. Naisbett J. *Megatrends: Ten New Directions Transforming Our Lives.* New York, NY: Warner Books; 1982:192.

3. Naisbett J. *Megatrends: Ten New Directions Transforming Our Lives.* New York, NY: Warner Books; 1982:192.

4. Naisbett J. *Megatrends: Ten New Directions Transforming Our Lives.* New York, NY: Warner Books; 1982:193.

5. The Lewin Group. *Civic Partnerships with Health Departments Can Strengthen Public Health in America.* Battle Creek, Mich: WK Kellogg Foundation; 2001:5.

6. US Dept Health and Human Services. *Healthy People 2010, Understanding and Improving Health.* Washington, DC: US Government Printing Office; 2000:4.

7. Institute of Medicine. *Future of the Public's Health in the 21st Century.* Washington, DC: National Academies Press; 2003:180–181.

8. US Dept Health and Human Services. *Healthy People 2010.* 2nd ed. McLean, Va: International Medical Publishing; 2002:24.

9. US Dept Health and Human Services. *Healthy People 2010.* 2nd ed. McLean, Va: International Medical Publishing; 2002:29.

10. Joos I, Nelson R, Whitman N, Smith M. *Introduction to Computers for Healthcare Professionals.* 4th ed. Sudbury, Mass: Jones and Bartlett Publishers; 2005.

11. Nickerson R. Communication technology and telenetworking. In: *Emerging Needs and Opportunities for Human Factors Research.* Washington, DC: National Academies Press; 1995.

12. Nickerson R. Communication technology and telenetworking. In: *Emerging Needs and Opportunities for Human Factors Research.* Washington, DC: National Academies Press; 1995;188.

13. Nickerson R. Communication technology and telenetworking. In: *Emerging Needs and Opportunities for Human Factors Research.* Washington, DC: National Academies Press; 1995;190.

14. Nickerson R. Communication technology and telenetworking. In: *Emerging Needs and Opportunities for Human Factors Research.* Washington, DC: National Academies Press; 1995;191.

15. Committee on Enhancing the Internet for Health Applications. *Networking Health: Prescriptions for the Internet.* Washington, DC: National Academies Press; 2000.

16. Committee on Enhancing the Internet for Health Applications. *Networking Health: Prescriptions for the Internet.* Washington, DC: National Academies Press; 2000:102.

17. Committee on Enhancing the Internet for Health Applications. *Networking Health: Prescriptions for the Internet.* Washington, DC: National Academies Press; 2000:217.

18. Committee on Enhancing the Internet for Health Applications. *Networking Health: Prescriptions for the Internet.* Washington, DC: National Academies Press; 2000:117.

19. Committee on Enhancing the Internet for Health Applications. *Networking Health: Prescriptions for the Internet.* Washington, DC: National Academies Press; 2000:261.

20. Committee on Enhancing the Internet for Health Applications. *Networking Health: Prescriptions for the Internet.* Washington, DC: National Academies Press; 2000: 261–262.

Chapter 23

Win Administrative Support

Elaine C. Barnes

Reader Objectives

- List ways the nutritionist can ascertain an overview of the agency.
- Compare and contrast communication channels to interact with the administrator.
- List techniques to develop assertiveness skills.
- Specify strategies for working with the agency board.
- Discuss ways to gain support to expand nutrition programs and services.

UNDERSTAND THE ADMINISTRATOR'S PERSPECTIVE ON NUTRITION SERVICES

The nutritionists employed by the public health agency should keep in mind that the agency's nutrition program was envisioned, created, and justified by an administrator to meet a documented or perceived need. The program's existence indicates some degree of administrative support. Administrators may maintain or establish positions for public health nutrition personnel because of the following:

- Commitment to the expanding body of knowledge linking diet to health promotion and disease prevention and applications to community health.
- Requests from program directors or staff for nutrition expertise in the agency to complement and enhance their work, (e.g., maternal and child health, health promotion and chronic disease prevention, public health nursing, health education, school health, food safety and protection).
- Continuing tradition of a long-established, recognized nutrition program in the agency.
- Mandates of federal or state agencies that require nutrition personnel to be appointed to obtain categorical program funding.

The administrator who looks to the future and understands that nutrition is key to prevention of obesity and many costly disabling and debilitating chronic diseases will see the opportunities in the employing and expanding the nutrition program in the agency. The degree of support depends on the administrator's level of interest in nutrition, past experiences with nutrition personnel, and the rationale for their employment. The administrator who values the cost benefits of nutrition services in promoting health and preventing disease through the various agency and community programs will provide more enthusiastic support than the administrator who employs nutrition personnel only to conform to funding requirements. An administrator who has worked with an energetic, creative nutrition staff with a broad public health perspective will be more supportive than the one who has observed the passive nutritionist who functions solely as a technical expert.

DEVELOP AN AGENCY OVERVIEW

Nutritionists who understand the broad public health perspective and know the agency's mission, goals, constraints, problems, and challenges improve the probability for strong administrative support. By studying public health sciences, participating in public health organizations, and interacting with those public health colleagues who are familiar with the agency's internal and external environments, nutritionists create a basis to analyze and understand the employing health organization.

The Structure of the Agency

Understanding the agency's internal structure begins by studying its most recent table of organization. Informal connections between the organized units and individuals in the organization are often as important as the formal connections. Therefore, it is useful to write out a personal organization chart noting both types of connections. It is useful to update and review this chart, especially prior to embarking on a strategy planning session. It is important to note where public health nutritionists are placed in the structure and to whom they report in relation to the other disciplines and services.

It is informative to study carefully copies of the agency's official documents, including its mission and goals statements, strategic and operational plans, and annual reports. The more evidence there is that these statements of the agency are used, the more important these official statements are to the agency director and policy board. An indicator of the importance and acceptance of these official documents is their accessibility and use by program managers in the agency. If the search for such documents ends with the director's secretary retrieving a plan of work from a dead file or commenting that the plan is only prepared because the "feds" or state funding agencies require it, the document is not a vital, integral part of the agency's life. However, it is always useful to review it for background.

Even if the official agency documents are readily available and obviously utilized throughout the organization, developing an agency overview also requires an assessment of day-to-day agency operations. Sources of information to assess the agency's priorities and direction include the following:

- Staff conference agendas—Review the issues discussed most frequently over the past year and the decisions recorded.
- Agency budgets/financial reports—Compare the current year reports to last year and previous years to observe revenue shifts between federal, state, and local sources and between general revenue and third-party reimbursement and fees for services or external grants.
- Annual reports—Observe the report style, format, and organization. Note programs highlighted and accomplishments cited with pride and those programs that are given little or no mention.
- Informal conversations with colleagues—Discuss their plans, problems, hopes, dreams, morale, and frustrations. Ask colleagues to talk about their work histories, especially within the agency. Take note of any comments they make about their interest in nutrition and their assessment of the nutritionists on the staff.
- Press releases—Review the releases issued by the director and articles written about agency activities by staff to note their topics and content.
- Policy board meeting agendas and minutes—Often board meeting minutes are available on tape and in written format. Listen to or read at least the past year's minutes to note topics, discussions, and votes.

Understanding how the agency develops its policies is essential. Read written agency policies and procedures and note how and when each policy was adopted. Through conversations with peers, it is useful to find out if policies are known, respected, consistently administered, and how often they are changed.

A compilation of all this information is useful to develop an overview of the agency. An agency composite can be used as an important reference when structuring a strategy to develop administrative support.

SHARE THE AGENCY VISION

Basic to gaining the administrator's support is a shared vision of the agency, the contributions of nutrition and the nutritionists' staff to fulfilling the agency's mission, and its leadership role in the community. Developing a shared vision requires careful study of the agency's operational plans and review of the lead nutritionist's job description to determine its breadth and involvement in agency policy and decision making. Does the lead nutritionist attend and contribute to senior staff or agency management meetings where policy and budget are discussed? If not, how is information from meetings conveyed? Is it timely, accurate? If not, how can the lead nutritionist seek more involvement?

In studying the responsibilities, duties, and time allocations on all of the nutritionists' job descriptions, it is also useful to look at whether supervision is general or close. At the time of employment the scope of the job descriptions of all nutritionists should be discussed with the administrator, noting the degree of flexibility that might be anticipated and the opportunities for expanding nutrition services. Responses to questions should reveal the administrator's interest and long-term expectations for the nutrition services and the potential for adding new program areas that require additional nutrition personnel.

COMMUNICATE WITH THE ADMINISTRATOR

Some administrators welcome informal chats and frequent communication. Others encourage scheduled appointments with a structure. Others prefer written memos or e-mail messages, with face-to-face conferences reserved for crises or urgent issues. The administrator's approach to handling key issues, concerns, and conflicts should be discussed during the job interview or orientation. Utilizing appropriate methods of communication is another key to assuring administrative support.

Periodic conferences of the lead public health nutritionist with the administrator maintain dialogue and keep the administrator informed of current activities and accomplishments. Such conferences provide the opportunity to share successes and progress, convey information, and explore future program possibilities. Remember that the administrator's time is limited; so start with the most important issues. Ask the administrator for input when developing proposals for expansion of existing programs or development of new services or projects. The administrator may know of related activities and plans of others in the agency or community and may promote collaboration. Administrators enjoy positive interactions and usually encourage timely innovative plans that will contribute to the agency's public image.

Regularly scheduled dialogues that are positive in tone establish a trusting relationship for the occasions when it may be necessary to seek administrative advice on a crisis. Continuing dialogue that keeps the administrator informed forestalls surprises, which might cause embarrassment to the administrator or agency. Most administrators deplore surprises. When seeking advice or guidance on a crisis or conflict, the well-prepared manager will present several thoughtful alternative solutions. A key to earning respect as a responsible manager is the ability to succinctly outline the issues and delineate the several possible resolutions. Most administrators prefer to guide the decision making rather than to be the decision maker.

No matter how busy the administrator may appear, it should be remembered that the nutritionist's position was established because of administrative interest. Maintaining continuing positive, mutually satisfying communication with the administrator earns support and respect.

While maintaining open communication with the administrator, it is also useful to determine those individuals the administrator listens to on a continuing basis. Knowing the key people in the informal organizational channels helps gain access to vital information useful in developing strategies. The administrator's secretary or administrative assistant can be a key ally in finding out about the administrator's calendar and staff meeting agendas. Talking with staff that works most closely with the administrator is helpful to determine when to make a timely request for a new program and how to avoid a costly miscalculated strategy.

DEVELOP ASSERTIVENESS

An effective manager anticipates future directions, assesses the climate for change, gains support, and then proposes an action plan. Throughout the process, the plan is tested. Input from colleagues is sought to assure coordination and avoid duplication. Such input usually helps assure support from colleagues. In working for change, the nutritionist should recognize the inherent resistance to it. Moving in deliberate steps, monitoring feedback, negotiating, using suggestions, maintaining open communications, and sharing credit are strategies to overcome resistance. This may mean developing an idea and making plans in the background and letting the administrator claim the credit.

Nutritionists must diplomatically request information and resources needed to carry out management responsibilities. Financial information is critical in proposal development. As agencies streamline automated data systems, nutritionists should participate in planning, implementing, and evaluating enhanced management and client information systems.

Nutritionists are sometimes reluctant to speak out, fearing that they will be considered aggressive or self-serving. Learning to be assertive as a person and as a professional is an essential characteristic of leadership. To be assertive requires a sense of self-respect, self-worth, and self-confidence. The nutritionist must feel secure in an up-to-date knowledge base and be convinced that nutrition is a key factor in promoting health and preventing disease and that nutrition services have a significant place in existing and emerging public health programs, such as health promotion and chronic disease prevention and obesity and weight management. Viewpoints must be expressed with statements of conviction such as "I believe," "I am convinced," or "I feel strongly." Making forceful statements means taking risks. Others may not agree and may need to be won over with documented justification and persuasive arguments.

Guidelines for becoming more assertive include the following:

- Start with a situation that will result in success.
- Be persistent. Don't automatically take "no" for a final answer.
- Dress in business appropriate attire.
- Keep weight within normal limits, evidence of "practice what you preach."

- Be well groomed.
- Control emotions and always be courteous.
- Be forceful; speak with conviction.
- Maintain a sense of humor.

Many nutritionists are afraid to say "no" to requests for services that are more than they or their staffs can handle. Saying "no" diplomatically with an appropriate rationale is critical.

WIN WITH THE POLICY BOARD

In most public health agencies, the administrator is responsible to a board of health or board of directors. In tax-supported agencies, the elected officials usually appoint this board, and under statutes the membership must include designated numbers and kinds of health professionals, representatives of the public, and consumers. The board usually approves policies, programs, key personnel appointments, budgets, and legislative initiatives. The board members may have special interests that put pressures on the administrator and the agency. These pressures may place constraints on the administrator and on the availability of funds for some types of programs. To work successfully in the agency, it is useful to study backgrounds and interests and to observe the group dynamics of the board members as they interact at their meetings. Strategies for the lead nutritionist to work with the agency board include the following:

- Attend board meetings routinely, or whenever permissible, whether or not a nutrition issue is on the agenda. Attendance demonstrates the nutritionist's interest in the agency. This is particularly appropriate just after joining the organization and just after reading board meeting minutes from the previous year. Attendance assures the board members will know the lead agency nutritionist and will develop mutual respect with board members.
- Observe the interests and group dynamics in the meeting. Researching educational background of members is helpful. Note indications of their values, interests, concerns, and biases.
- Engage individual board members in conversation to learn about their views and priorities. When a board member expresses an interest in nutrition or asks for information, the appropriate materials or services should be offered. Prompt, helpful follow-up to these individual interests earns respect for the agency as well as its nutrition staff. It also provides an opportunity to inform and educate a board member who can become an advocate for the public health nutrition program.
- As appropriate, request the administrator to arrange a place on the agenda to report or orient board members to services and accomplishments in public health nutrition. Use graphics, pictures, and human-interest case studies to

stimulate understanding by the board. Microsoft PowerPoint presentations should be brief, factual, lively and to the point. Questions should be answered clearly, succinctly, and honestly.

- Justify requests for funds for new or expanded programs with graphics or visual aids that focus on quantitative, qualitative, and human-interest perspectives.
- Respect the judgment of the board members and treat them with the courtesy that goes with their office. If a request is not approved, be sure to understand the reasons for denial. This knowledge will help in reframing the proposal to try again at a later meeting. Being persistent is a key characteristic of successful managers.

In dealing with individual board members, listen more and talk less. Maintaining just the right balance of being personable with board members without being too familiar is critical. Never hesitate to ask the administrator for advice on the finer points of interactions with board members. Nevertheless, use every opportunity to tactfully educate board members to the role of nutrition in promoting the public health, providing data documenting successful nutrition interventions and suggesting opportunities to apply for external funds to develop expanded or new nutrition initiatives.

MOBILIZE COLLEAGUES

Colleagues and staff in other disciplines and programs are primary allies in creating a successful strategy. Developing mutual trust and respect of agency peers is the foundation of good working relationships. Being honest and dependable in dealing with colleagues is basic. Winners have broad support of others in the organization.

Usually a proposal for a new program prepared jointly by several service units or disciplines has broader impact than a proposal from a single unit. It may be useful to let a colleague take the lead in presenting a joint project. Individuals who always insist on being in the lead risk backlash from peers. Sharing lead responsibilities with colleagues is an excellent long-term strategy.

It is important to observe which projects and proposals gain support and which are not considered, and then try to figure out why. A collection of "whys" specific to the agency is valuable for developing future strategies.

PLAN THE STRATEGY

It is important to spend some time determining what agency support is needed today, tomorrow, next year, and in five years. Support takes many forms: more visibility and inclusion in agency policy making; invitations to participate on key committees; additional clerical support; additional public health nutritionist staff;

more space; a state-of-the-art computer system; or more adequate educational opportunities for staff. Once the needed support is defined, it is time to plan strategy. A successful strategy begins by asking these questions:

1. Why is this request necessary?
2. How does the community or public benefit? How does the agency benefit? How do other disciplines benefit? How does the nutrition staff benefit?
3. What information is available that supports the request?
4. What will the request cost? Will revenues be generated with the proposed plan? If not, what is the funding source? Are funds known to be available?
5. Who has the authority to approve this request?

Answers to each question should be written. By answering the questions a decision can be made about the real need and public interest. If there is uncertainty, the request should be set aside and given more thought. The needs and benefits must be supported by scientific evidence, such as population health in published statistics, before trying to convince the administrator.

If the need is affirmed, the arguments to be used to present the request should be prepared in writing and rehearsed. Someone, preferably a person not employed in the agency, should be asked to listen to the presentation of what is needed and why it is important. The listener should be encouraged to question any aspect of the proposal that is not completely clear. Those questions can be used to sharpen the written proposal, the justification, and the oral presentation.

The next step is to consider the background and management style of the administrator who is to approve the plan. In presenting a request to a budget-minded director, using a cost-benefit or cost-effectiveness analysis is a persuasive approach. For the director concerned with human values or public image, the presenter should stress how the plan would benefit people in the community.

The proposal and supporting documentation should be prepared in writing. It is important to decide whether to precede a discussion by sending the written request first or to discuss it first and follow up with the written proposal. The answer depends in part on what approach has been successful in the past. The analysis of the agency's mode of operation should provide guidance when experience is limited. The oral presentation should be rehearsed with a listener who is primed to challenge every aspect of the plan. The extra time to rehearse, revise, and rehearse again is critical to a well-developed presentation.

The nutritionist should always be prepared to negotiate. However, it is important to negotiate slowly—not to give up too much too soon. This means deciding what parts of the proposal are critical and what can be conceded. Develop a written negotiation plan, prioritize what can be given up, and draw a line above the absolute minimum requirements. Approval of an unworkable proposal is not "a win."

Despite the careful preparation, research, analysis, strategy development, persuasion, and negotiating, the request may be rejected. It is important to determine the reasons by asking thoughtful, unemotional questions, expressing genuine interest in understanding why the answer is "no." It is important to determine whether the negative response is due to a real budget deficit, lack of agency interest or potential priority, poor timing, opposition in the organization, the quality of the presentation, or other reasons.

Persist

If the initial strategy failed, develop an alternative strategy. If the proposal presents a documented community need, the development of alternative strategies should continue until the need has been fulfilled. Persistence pays off. For example, the nutrition department wants to establish a community-based weight management program in the local school system that involves nutrition, education, and physical activity components. First, the community need is documented. If a community assessment has been completed (see Chapter 3) the need to address the current youth obesity problem will be noted. If a community assessment is not available, the school system can provide helpful data to document the need.

Second, the cost-effectiveness of the program is calculated (see Chapter 14). A literature search will yield a model for developing the cost-effectiveness projections that result from disease prevention and associated reduction in medical costs. Collaborations or partners are asked for their support and endorsement.

Third, the proposal is written and presented to the agency director. The needs and benefits are recognized, but funds are not available for the project. As a compromise, a request of funding for a small pilot project is approved. Twice a year for the next several years, the pilot program is reviewed and results are documented. Using the results, a grant proposal is then developed to expand the program throughout the school system. The grant is awarded because of pilot program assessed community measurable results. Compromise and persistence accomplished two things: first, the need was addressed, and second, the success of this proposal lends credibility to the next one.

Empower

The enthusiastic support of the administrator and the board is vital to maintain and expand public health nutrition services. The desirable stance for nutritionists is fair treatment both during periods of expansion and in periods of downsizing. Some administrators make a sincere effort to be equitable in all matters. Others favor programs they understand, managers who curry their favor, services providing the most agency visibility, or programs that generate income. Public health nutritionists can learn lessons from those who have been successful.

To maintain or expand services, nutritionists must demonstrate their managerial skills. Program development means moving toward more comprehensive nutrition service to the community. Since the availability of federal funds for the Special Supplemental Nutrition Program for Women, Infants, and Children (WIC) in 1974, many public health agencies that had previously allocated multiple funding sources to support nutrition personnel transferred nutrition staff to WIC funds during budget crunches.

Such budgetary maneuvers have limited public health nutrition services to certifying low-income, high-risk pregnant or lactating women, infants and children, for specified foods, nutrition counseling, and education. Current interest in the obesity epidemic and health promotion and disease prevention objectives puts nutrition in the forefront. It is now urgent to educate administrators and policy boards about their obligation to provide nutrition services as part of health promotion and disease prevention programming directed to the general public and across the age and income populations in the community. Services to middle- and upper-income populations can generate income by charging fees and visibility for the agency. However, even these services require some startup funding. Nutritionists will earn the respect of administrators by proposing funding strategies to initiate new programs, (see Chapter 17) and new types of interventions to reach a broader community population (see Chapter 18).

Expanding program scope without adding nutrition personnel requires testing interventions that are more population based and rely less on labor-intensive, one-on-one interactions. When administrators demand more services without additional funding, nutritionists should study their operations, affect all possible economies, and enhance productivity. The economies that are implemented should be documented to the administrator. When more severe cuts in the budget will sacrifice quality or quantity of services or hours of operation, the administrator should be presented with the options, which may include reducing services, using auxiliary personnel, training volunteers, or developing income generators. Loading more work on already overburdened staff leads to low morale and costly staff turnover.

Interpreting nutrition service needs to the administrator is a responsibility of the lead public health nutritionist. "Power" is required to accomplish goals. Official power is attached to the administrative placement of the lead nutritionist position within an agency. Personal power rests on knowledge, skills, and the ability to develop successful strategies. Nutritionists are empowered by their competencies in health promotion and disease prevention. With the current focus on obesity and overweight, nutritionists have the knowledge and skills to lead in developing agency strategies to address the *Healthy People 2010* Objective 19-3, "Reduce the proportion of children and adolescents who are overweight or obese." In the agency, nutritionists must build personal power through integrity, diligence, persuasiveness, persistence, personality, and understanding agency politics.

Communicate and Work with Staff

The lead nutritionist is not just responsible for communicating with administrators and peers. Communicating effectively with nutrition division staff is imperative. Staff members are excellent sources of information, ideas, and solutions. Ask! In staff meetings or one-to-one conferences, seek input on a regular basis.

New proposals should involve the staff in planning. Seek staff assessments and suggestions. Revise the plan as needed and present again. Just as the administrator should not be surprised, do not spring surprises on staff.

Keeping staff informed, seeking staff input and rewarding staff for hard work and successes is a key to the lead nutritionist's success. The lead nutritionist and staff are a team. When important approvals are achieved, share the news and celebrate with staff. Assuring that staff hears division and agency news first is a key to gaining support and respect for their leader.

POINTS TO PONDER

- What is the right balance between agency and nutrition priorities? Is there conflict in one's priorities as a public health worker and as a nutritionist?
- How does a nutritionist differentiate between strategies that are ethical and appropriate from those that may be manipulative?
- What is the difference between being considered aggressive or assertive?
- What are the trade-offs between advancing interdisciplinary versus monodisciplinary projects or grant proposals?
- What are the best methods for communicating with and among staff?

BIBLIOGRAPHY

Kaufman M. *Nutrition in Public Health: A Handbook for Developing Programs and Services*. Rockville, Md: Aspen Publishers; 1990:455–465.

Puetz B. *Networking for Nurses*. Rockville, Md: Aspen Publishers; 1983:165–200.

Stone D, Patton B, Heen S. *Difficult Conversations: How to Discuss What Matters Most*. New York, NY: Penguin Books; 1999:185–216.

CHAPTER 24

Strive for Excellence

Harriet H. Cloud

Reader Objectives

- Define excellence in public health nutrition practice.
- List characteristics of professional excellence.
- Discuss legal obligations of an agency quality assurance system.
- Compare and contrast dietetic registration with state-legislated dietetic licensure.
- Discuss ethical issues in public health and nutrition practice.

PURSUE EXCELLENCE

Public health faces many challenges in this century; all need the knowledge and skills of the public health nutritionist. The pursuit of excellence standards defines a high level of competence and ethics in personal, professional, and organizational performance. A survey, to identify the training needs of public health nutritionists by the year 2005 identified the most important public health issues of the future and the knowledge and skills they will require.[1] The important issues were an increasing elderly population, increasing number of people living in poverty, prevention and control of chronic diseases with increasing focus on nutrition risk factors, health promotion, and disease prevention throughout the life cycle. Health professionals with cultural competency and sensitivity skills must serve increasingly diverse ethnic populations.

The public health nutritionist must pursue excellence as a leader, motivator, and a role model for the community, agency, staff, and peers. Achieving excellence requires the ability to foster and lead change to improve performance and outcomes. Leaders have been defined as visionaries with goals who work hard to achieve those goals, and who emanate optimism and creativity.[2] Some characteristics of leadership excellence derived from America's best-run companies apply to public health agencies and their nutrition programs:

- Well-defined values
- Commitment to quality
- Responsive to the consumer, client, and public
- Stimulating nurturing work environment
- Creativity and innovation
- Open lines of communication and sharing of information
- Inclusive process for decision making
- Ability to plan and foster meaningful change to achieve goals and improve performance[3]

Public health nutritionists should pursue excellence throughout their working experience. They must remain aware of changes in health care trends and they must be flexible and creative, responding to both changes as individuals and members of organizations. The pursuit of excellence is a continuing effort with legal and ethical obligations to the public, the agency, and the profession.

Personal Leadership/Excellence

Providing leadership is not just the responsibility of nutrition directors, managers, or supervisors whose titles denote positional power. Nutritionists in all areas of public health and at all levels of an organization can contribute to excellence through their personal leadership. On a personal level, leaders must understand themselves and actively maximize their strengths while addressing their weaknesses. Leaders in public health nutrition are skilled at solving problems, building trust, and are willing to take informed risks to foster and achieve change. When individuals demonstrate these leadership skills, organizations and programs flourish.

The public health nutrition professional must strive to serve their community and clients with credibility, integrity, and compassion. The committed professional is genuinely willing to promote and protect the health, safety, and welfare of the public. Self-responsibility requires commitment to planning and providing services that are ingenious and creative. These services must be sensitive to changing the client, community, and societal values and needs while also being cost-effective.[4]

Critical to developing personal excellence requires dedicating time and energy to periodic self-assessment and self-improvement. Each nutritionist should pursue a continuing education program based on a planned, periodic, written self-assessment. The individual's plan to improve professional knowledge and skills might include a variety of approaches including study of self-instructional materials, reading current journals, and participating in workshops, distance learning events, lectures, journal clubs, or graduate courses. Each individual's self-directed continuing education contributes to the strength of the profession and practice. Each nutritionist must participate in continuing education programs to keep pace with new knowledge and to overcome deficiencies in preservice training.

For example, to be knowledgeable and effective the nutritionist who aspires to develop new programs for children with special health care needs may need advanced academic course work in child growth and development and behavioral management principles. A nutritionist who works in health promotion and chronic disease prevention may need to develop more in-depth skills in epidemiology, community-based planning, coalition building, social marketing, group facilitation, and strategies to change eating and exercise behavior of diverse populations. New skills in the prevention and treatment of obesity, both for children and adults, have been identified and offered in educational packages such as certification in Adult Weight Management and Child Weight Management offered through the American Dietetic Association. All health care professionals are challenged to increase their skills in the use of informational technology.[5]

Several tools are available to assist with this process. The American Dietetic Association (ADA) has revised the continuing education requirements to maintain dietetic registration to focus on individual professional development through self-assessment and customized planning. For more go to the ADA Web site: www.eatright.org.

The Public Health/Community Nutrition Practice Group of ADA has developed two versions of a self-assessment tool for public health nutritionists. One tool addresses basic competencies, and the second tool provides guidance to assess advanced competencies in public health nutrition. These tools are designed to help nutritionists objectively assess their level of expertise in key areas of public health and nutrition practice and to guide each nutritionist to develop an individualized plan.

Another resource for developing public health competencies is "Guidelines for Community Nutrition Supervised Experiences," developed through ADA's Public Health/Community Nutrition Practice Group. It is available at www.phcnpg.org/CommunityNutrSuperExp.pdf.

This resource provides specific recommendations for personnel working in community nutrition programs who seek to enhance their level of practice, be they public health nutritionists, community nutrition educators, or clinical nutritionists and whether or not they are registered dietitians (RDs) or dietetic technician registered (DTRs). Enhanced education and training are critical to recruit and retain qualified community nutrition professionals. The resource is intended to strengthen practice in client-focused personal nutrition services as well as population/systems-focused nutrition interventions. The guide specifies expected target behaviors, work-related and learning activities, and presents examples of practical resources for each training area.

Professional Stature

Professional organizations striving to maintain excellence and respect for their discipline take responsibility by establishing a code of ethics, setting standards of practice, providing a system for peer review, and expanding continuing education opportunities. The basic academic preparation recommended for dietetic registration (RD) meets the standards of education established by the Commission on Accreditation in Education (CADE) of the American Dietetic Association. CADE sets the standards for entry-level nutrition/dietetic practitioners. ADA's code of ethics, includes standards of professional responsibility and principles reflective of health professional credentialing agencies, professional associations, and state dietetic licensure laws. It applies to credentialed dietetic practitioners, including both registered dietitians and dietetic technicians. It provides ethical guidelines; assists in protecting the nutritional health, safety, and welfare of the public; and enhances the profession's image.

To enforce the code of ethics and the standards of professional responsibility, the American Dietetic Association has established a review process for alleged violations. This process uses an organizational ethics committee, legal counsel, and an administrator of policy administration. The review includes investigation of the complaint, then hearings, followed by a decision for either acquittal of the respondent, censure, suspension, or expulsion. There is an appeals process that the complainant can initiate. The code of ethics and the published standards function as a peer review process with an educational tool and a review mechanism for alleged violations. The American Dietetic Association Code of Ethics is available at www.eatright.org.

STANDARDS OF PROFESSIONAL PRACTICE

Revised standards of practice for dietitians are on the ADA Web site at www. eat right.org/Public/GovernmentAffairs/98_9468.cfm.

These standards outline the expectation that all credentialed professionals and paraprofessionals will perform an annual self-assessment, set personal career goals, and prepare an action plan based on their assessed individual needs and career goals.

Standards of professional practice apply to the performance of individual dietetics professionals regardless of the setting, project, case, or situation. These statements define a dietetics professional's responsibility for providing services in all areas of practice. Although the standards describe the minimum level of performance expected of dietetic technicians registered (DTR) and registered dietitians (RD), they are also useful to assess the practice of public health nutritionists who may not be registered.

Registration and Licensure

The ethics code and standards of professional practice establish the criteria for both educational programs and professional practice. It is assumed that nutrition care provided by the credentialed practitioner protects the consumer from receiving inadequate care, misinformation, and inappropriate counseling. Two credentialing mechanisms to ensure client protection include registration through the nongovernmental Commission on Dietetic Registration and state licensure.

Registration by the Commission on Dietetic Registration requires educational and experiential preparation for dietetics as published by the American Dietetic Association (ADA) in their standards of education and standards of practice. At the entry level, ADA also requires the applicant to successfully pass a standardized examination. Maintaining dietetic registration requires completing 75 clock hours of documented continuing education in each 5-year period.

Dietetic licensure requires each state legislature to pass a dietetic licensure law and sets the criteria that a dietitian/nutritionist must meet to be licensed for practice in that state. The criteria for licensure are generally based on those established by the Commission on Dietetic Registration. The national dietetic registration examination is usually accepted as the state's licensure examination. Most state licensing laws provide waivers for nutrition practice by persons with other specified credentials.

Advanced-level dietetics practice was identified as a need for members of the American Dietetic Association through a survey of their practice groups in 1991.[6] A model of advanced level practice was developed. This model became the basis for certification in metabolic nutrition, renal nutrition, pediatric nutrition, and the development of a Fellow certification. These models require three to five years experience in practice for specialty certification and passing an advanced examination in the specific field. The Fellow certification requires the completion of a master's degree and completion of a minimum of eight years work experience while maintaining the Registered Dietitian status. It also requires evidence of accomplishment of one notable professional achievement, occupation of multiple professional roles with diverse and complex responsibilities and functions, and possession of a diverse network of broad, geographically dispersed professional role contacts. It also requires evidence of an approach to practice that reflects a global perspective, deals with a challenging practice situation as it evolves, uses innovative and creative solutions, is intuitive, and values professional growth and self-knowledge.[7]

Malpractice and Liability

Protection of the client is germane to the provision of quality nutrition care and medical nutrition therapy. By utilizing self-assessment, standards of practice, continuing education, quality assurance programs, and adherence to the code of ethics, the nutritionist protects clients and strives for personal protection against any liability for malpractice.

However, in any professional practice liability issues can arise inadvertently. It is advisable in today's litigious health care environment to make sure that the employing agency's insurance policies cover the nutritionist's practice or that the nutritionist carries an individual professional liability insurance policy. Although the possibility of lawsuits may seem remote, nutritionists have been cited. Liability insurance coverage for nutritionists is available. The American Dietetic Association can provide information on insurance carriers and costs. For more go to the ADA Web site: www.eatright.org.

ETHICAL ISSUES IN PUBLIC HEALTH NUTRITION

Ethics is defined as that branch of philosophy concerned with what is morally good and bad, right and wrong. Beyond the professional code of ethics, many health care practitioners face current ethical issues that were never anticipated in the past. Many of these arise from the apparent conflicts in prevailing individual, family, professional, and societal values, obligations, responsibilities, and rights in making critical decisions about the health and welfare of individuals, family members, special interest groups, and society as a whole. These ethical dilemmas reflect very different perspectives and values. These issues require serious soul-searching by thoughtful professionals who make policies and decisions intended to provide for the greatest public good.

Ethical behavior always requires objective study of the issues, careful weighing of the alternatives, consultation with administrators and other members of the team, seeking advice of outside experts, and searching for a negotiation strategy that will achieve the greatest good for the greatest number. Respecting rights and preserving confidentiality are essential elements when resolving ethical issues.

Agency and Legal Obligations

Many positions in official local, county, and state public health agencies are established through federal, state, or local legislation that provides the framework and funding for the nutrition services. Legislation is typically defined in more detail through regulations and guidelines from the funding agency, which outline the programs or services to be offered and the training and experience required for those who provide the services. The nutritionist employed with tax dollars must study the enabling legislation, regulations, and guidelines carefully and thoughtfully to ensure that funds are used as required by the law, that services are provided at the appropriate level, and that personnel and resources are utilized as mandated. The nutritionist must be committed to plan, implement, and evaluate services and programs that conform with the legal requirements and agency policy. Nutritionists must understand and respect both the intent as well as the letter of the law.

Legislation, regulations, and guidance materials from administering agencies define program purposes and expectations. These documents describe program content, plan requirements, appropriate use of funds, allowable budget items, staffing patterns, evaluation methods, and any requirements for submitting periodic written reports. A written statement of the policy of nondiscrimination in employment of staff and service to clients and the community is usually required.

Within the requirements of the law, there is usually opportunity to develop programs that meet the mandate while offering creative, cost-effective, evidence-based programs and services tailored to the assessed community needs. Nutritionists may need to provide rationale and documentation of effectiveness to implement innovative program ideas that may be new to the funding agency or the community.

When creative program implementation appears to be limited by law and regulations, consultation should be sought from the staff of the funding agency. If the law or regulations continue to be obstacles to implement an effective program, it is appropriate to bring this to the attention of the local, state, or federal legislators who passed the legislation and suggest changes using the legislative process (see Chapter 7).

STATE LEGISLATION

State legislation as documented in the public health statutes or codes using the general language, "to promote and protect the health of the public." Within this language public health nutrition services can be implied and thereby funded. Several state legislatures have gone further to include legislative language in their public health code that specifies specific nutrition services. Some states have enacted legislation to provide additional state funding to expand WIC services for perinatal care, for health promotion, for congregate meals for the elderly, or to conduct nutrition monitoring and surveillance.

State and local codes vary by jurisdiction, but usually specify nutrition and food service requirements as part of licensure for child day care and residential facilities for children, nursing homes, adult congregate living facilities, halfway houses for substance abusers, camps, and correctional facilities. These requirements usually mandate that nutritionists or dietitians participate in writing the regulations and guidance materials, serve on the agency inspection teams, and provide or arrange continuing education or technical assistance to group care facility staff. Food service sanitation codes are of particular importance in group-care facilities; nutritionists working with these facilities must maintain close contact with environmental health staff that inspect and certify these facilities (see Chapters 12 and 13).

FEDERAL LEGISLATION

The federal legislation that most often enables and provides federal grant funds for public health nutrition services in state and local health agencies includes the following:

- Social Security Act (Department of Health and Human Services)
  - –Title V Maternal and Child Health Block Grant
  - –Title XVIII Medicare
  - –Title XIX Medicaid
  - –Title XX Social Services
- Public Health Service Act (Department of Health and Human Services)
  - –Title X Family Planning
  - –Preventive Health Services Block Grant
  - –Alcohol and Drug Abuse Block Grant
  - –Chronic Disease Prevention Grants
  - –Nutrition and Physical Activity/Obesity Prevention Grants
  - –Community Health Services
  - –Migrant Health Services
  - –Indian Health Services
  - –Child Care
  - –Head Start
  - –Public Health Training
  - –STEPS to a Healthier US Initiative
- Older Americans Act (Department of Health and Human Services)
  - –Title III Meal Programs for the Elderly
- Child Nutrition Act (Department of Agriculture)
  - –Special Supplemental Nutrition Program for Women, Infants, and Children (WIC)
  - –Child Day Care Feeding
  - –National School Lunch Act (breakfast, lunch, summer feeding)
  - –Farmers Market Nutrition Programs
- Food Stamp Act (Department of Agriculture)
  - –Food Stamp Nutrition Education and State Nutrition Networks
- Education for the Handicapped (Department of Education)
  - –P.L. 94-142
  - –P.L. 99-457
  - –P.L. 102-119 (Individuals with Disabilities Education Act)

Legislation Change and Review

Laws, regulations, and guidance materials are periodically reviewed and amended in the legislatures and the federal, state, and local agencies responsible for their enforcement. Nutritionists are responsible for monitoring the laws and regulations that affect public health and nutrition practice. It is important to determine how the health agency reviews the *Federal Register.* For more go to www. gpoaccess.gov/fr/index.html.

It is also important to be alert to announcements of changes in state legislation and local ordinances. Procedures vary among state and local agencies, and it may require some research to locate the information. Monitoring the local newspaper, radio, and television news as well as maintaining dialogue with the administrator's office and with consultants from the appropriate state and federal agencies are ways to "stay on top" of constantly changing legislation and regulations. Read legislative pages in the public press, public health and dietetic newsletters and journals and publications.

QUALITY ASSURANCE

Community nutrition professionals must be involved in defining and assuring the quality of nutrition programs and services. Quality assurance is defined as a systematic program for assuring excellence in health care, including definition of indicators or criteria and thresholds or standards, devising methods for determining the degree to which standards are met and the mechanism to identify and correct deficiencies.[8] A quality assurance program should be an integral part of program planning and evaluation and deserves both agency and individual attention. The ADA has issued quality management principles that provide a useful framework for the development, implementation, and evaluation of guides for practice. These principles include the following:

Perspective of the customer—To the extent that guides for practice consider the needs of patients, clinicians, and employers they fulfill quality management objectives.

Commitment from the top—Organizational commitment to quality starts at the top. It has been shown that for the implementation of guides for practice to be successful, there must be commitment from the top, especially from the health agency administrators, program directors, and physicians.

Scientific evidence and methods—Quality management planning and implementation activities are grounded in scientific evidence and methods, as are rigorously developed guidelines.

Continuous improvement—Quality management is synonymous with commitment to continuous improvement rather than fixed goals. The principle is found whenever guidelines are monitored and outcomes are measured and evaluated repeatedly.

Systems defects—In quality management, errors are assumed to be the result of systems defects rather than individual mistakes. By definition, guides for practice are designed to influence general rather than individual patterns of patient behavior.

Ongoing feedback—Continuous improvement requires ongoing feedback. Feedback on the care processes and patient outcomes decreases variations in implementation while verifying what works and what does not work in practice.

Terms used in the quality assurance process are *criteria, indicators, outcome criteria, process criteria*, and *patient care* or *program audit* and are defined below.

Criteria: Predetermined elements of health care services or public health programming used for quality assessment; professionally developed statements of desirable processes or outcomes. Flexibility in such criteria allows for variations in methods and practices based on the setting.

Indicators: Predetermined elements of services that may or may not specify the exact method to be used for verification.

Outcome criteria: Predetermined elements demonstrating measurable and observable results of change in the health status or behavior of the client or population group.

Process criteria: Predetermined elements selected from key activities or procedures in the delivery of care or programs.

Patient care or Program audit: Process of surveillance and periodic monitoring of patient or program data using the predetermined criteria by the team of professionals.

The process of quality assessment compares existing structures, processes, and outcomes of care with predetermined standards to determine any discrepancies that may exist. Quality is assured when programs are developed and implemented to resolve the problems that led to the discrepancy. The three basic elements of quality assurance are (1) standards (criteria) and measures (performance levels), (2) monitoring and evaluation, and (3) control and remedial action.[9]

Standards for nutritional care provided in public health settings should be developed for each of the services offered by the agency. For each standard, criteria are developed to measure the elements of a program or intervention. Model standards of care with appropriate criteria have been developed by both state health agencies and professional organizations. Guidelines for clinical care have been published by several of the practice groups of the American Dietetic Association. These are based on current scientific knowledge and clinical practice. These models and guidelines can be individualized for specific care settings.

The following components must be in place in the agency quality assurance system:

- Staff commitment to a quality assurance system—Staff should understand that data collected can demonstrate the benefits of evidence-based nutrition services. Where deficiencies are found, data can be used to justify additional facilities or staff positions. The quality assurance process can generate enthusiasm and creativity among the staff—both strong motivators.

- Quality assurance chapter in the nutritionists' policy and procedure manual— The policy statements should state that periodic monitoring will occur, who is responsible for monitoring, and the commitment to follow up as necessary with remedial action. The procedure section includes the monitoring plan, the frequency of data collection, and the criteria used for each category of care (e.g., women's health; prenatal care; infant, well-child, or school child health; children's special health care; adult health promotion; weight management; geriatric services; group care facility consultation; home health services, and community programs).
- Information systems to collect objective statistics for the assessment process—Data collection systems should preferably be computer assisted. If a manual system is required, easy-to-use forms must be designed to meet the unique needs of the agency.
- Feedback or reporting system to communicate the results of data collection— Results should be compiled and disseminated quickly, usually once a month, so that remedial steps can be taken to maintain the quality of care. Because data are collected internally, corrections that can occur within the care unit can be initiated immediately.
- Written plan for remedial action that includes summaries of the data collected, findings, and remedial steps—This plan should be submitted to the authorized quality assurance coordinator in the agency and maintained in the unit's quality assurance file.

Remedial steps could include staff in-service education, budgeting for staff to attend continuing education courses, or seeking any needed consultation on program planning, staffing, and service delivery. Periodic review and discussion of findings with the administrator maintains agency support and budget needed for additional staff, space, and equipment.[10]

POINTS TO PONDER

- What are the arguments for and against access to genetic mapping of individuals to determine their risks for chronic disease and illness related to dietary behaviors?
- What issues must be considered when legislation is proposed to limit the purchase of high-calorie, low-nutrient foods by participants of federal food programs?
- What factors must be considered and who should be involved in deciding whether to deny or withdraw food and fluid from individuals who are

severely handicapped or terminally ill, whose quality of personal and family life is completely impaired, and for whom costs for care are overburdening for family and society?

- What are the considerations in deciding to legally charge a parent/caretaker with neglect/abuse when they do not comply with medical nutrition therapy recommendations that control/manage a child's health condition which, if untreated, can contribute to mental deficiency (e.g., inborn metabolic errors), disability (e.g., obesity), life-threatening conditions (e.g., renal disease), or costly medical care (e.g., complications of diabetes)?

- How should eligibility criteria for food assistance and nutritional care programs be established when serving a selected target population discriminates against others in the community who view themselves as equally needy?

- How should nutrition professionals decide about accepting hospitality, program sponsorship, grants, or honorariums from organizations that may appear to cause a conflict of interest in program policies or practices?

HELPFUL WEB SITES

American Dietetic Association: www.eatright.org
Federal Register (FR): www.gpoaccess.gov/fr/index.html
Public Health/Community Nutrition Practice Group: www.phcnpg.org

NOTES

1. Owen AL. The art and science of community nutrition. In: Owen AL, Splett PL, Owen GM, eds. *Nutrition in the Community: The Art and Science of Delivering Services.* 4th ed. Boston, Mass: WcB McGraw-Hill; 1999:22–55.

2. Useem M. *Leading Up: How to Lead Your Boss so You Both Win.* New York, NY: Three Rivers Press; 2001.

3. Useem M. *Leading Up: How to Lead Your Boss so You Both Win.* New York, NY: Three Rivers Press; 2001.

4. Owen AL. The art and science of community nutrition. In: Owen AL, Splett PL, Owen GM, eds. *Nutrition in the Community: The Art and Science of Delivering Services.* 4th ed. Boston, Mass: WcB McGraw-Hill; 1999:22–55.

5. Maillet JO. Future trends in dietetics: challenges in the next decade. *J Am Diet Assoc.* 2004; http://www.eatright.org/cps/rde/xchg/ada/hs.xls/governance_5079_ENU_HTML .html. Accessed May 5, 2006.

6. Bradley RT, Young WY, Ebbs P, Martin J. Characteristics of advanced level practice: a model and empirical results. *J Am Diet Assoc.* 1993;93:197–202. http://www.healthy people.gov/default.htm. Accessed May 5, 2006.

7. Bradley RT, Young WY, Ebbs P, Martin J. Characteristics of advanced level practice: a model and empirical results. *J Am Diet Assoc*. 1993;93:197–202.

8. Splett PL. Evaluating nutrition programs. In: Owen AL, Splett PL, Owen GM, eds. *Nutrition in the Community: The Art and Science of Delivering Services*. 4th ed. Boston, Mass: WcB McGraw-Hill; 1999:448–477. http://www.healthypeople.gov/default.htm. Accessed May 5, 2006.

9. Splett PL. Evaluating nutrition programs. In: Owen AL, Splett PL, Owen GM, eds. *Nutrition in the Community: The Art and Science of Delivering Services*. 4th ed. Boston, Mass: WcB McGraw-Hill; 1999:448–477.

10. Splett PL. Evaluating nutrition programs. In: Owen AL, Splett PL, Owen GM, eds. *Nutrition in the Community: The Art and Science of Delivering Services*. 4th ed. Boston, Mass: WcB McGraw-Hill; 1999:448–477. http://aspe.os.dhhs.gov/PIC/pdf/6179.PDF. Accessed May 5, 2006.

BIBLIOGRAPHY

Biesemeier C, Marino L, Schofield M. *Connective Leadership: Linking Vision with Action*. Chicago, Ill: American Dietetic Association; 2000.

Buckingham M, Clifton D. *Now, Discover Your Strengths*. New York, NY: Free Press; 2001.

Covey S. *Principle-Centered Leadership*. New York, NY: Simon & Schuster; 1991.

Helgesen S. *The Web of Inclusion—A New Architecture for Building Great Organizations*. New York, NY: Doubleday; 1995.

Kouzes J, Poser B. *The Leadership Challenge*. San Francisco, Calif: Jossey-Bass; 1995.

Mixon H, Dodds J, Haughton B. *Guidelines for Community Nutrition Supervised Experiences*. 2nd ed. Chicago, Ill: Public Health/Community Nutrition Practice Group, American Dietetic Association; 2003. Available at: http://www.phcnpg.org/Commnutr.html. Accessed February 14, 2006.

CHAPTER 25

Anticipate the Future

Meg Binney Molloy

Reader Objectives

- Understand the changing demographics in the United States and emerging health problems of the 21st century.
- Overview anticipated 21st century changes in global public health, US health care delivery, medical science, food supply, and information technology with potential impacts on nutrition practice.
- Discuss future roles, skills, and opportunities for the public health nutrition practitioner, specifically in leadership, policy making, advocacy, public awareness, and program evaluation.

EXPECT DEMOGRAPHIC CHANGES

Aging

The population of the United States will become increasingly silver and gray in the next decade as American's average lifespan extends beyond the 70s into the 80s, with an increasing number of centenarians.

The leading health problems of the future will certainly be linked to the graying population. Clearly there will continue to be an increase in obesity-related chronic diseases, such as heart disease, stroke, diabetes, sleep breathing disorders, as well as increased mental health and neurological diseases such as Alzheimer's and Parkinson's diseases.

Ethnic and Cultural Diversity

Continued immigration from other regions of the world, particularly Latin America, will significantly influence demographic language, and social conditions in the United States. Health care organizations and public health providers will be challenged to quickly gain insights into these new cultures and learn their languages to communicate with them.

Socioeconomic Status

During the last two decades, the US income gap between the "haves" and "have-nots" has steadily widened. Many lower-paying jobs have moved offshore. This has resulted in significant layoffs and cutbacks. New jobs have been created, but most offer a low wage and fall into the temporary, health care, and food service industries. Many of these jobs do not provide health care benefits. During this period, the costs of basic necessities have soared, particularly food, health care, fuel, and housing. Lower- and middle-class taxpayers shoulder a higher tax burden. Home ownership has become increasingly difficult for lower- and even middle-income families. The cost of public and private higher education has soared during a time when fewer lower- and middle-income families are able to save money. Wealthy citizens, on the other hand, have seen steady gains in their income through tax breaks and higher returns on their stock and other investments.

FUTURE PUBLIC HEALTH ISSUES WILL PUT NUTRITION AT THE FOREFRONT

Overweight and Obesity

Daily newspapers and weekly news magazines report the obesity epidemic in the United States. Nearly 20% of adults in the United States are obese, a 61% increase since 1991. Obesity is now the most prevalent childhood and adolescent nutrition-related disease in the United States.

Analysts dissect the cost, the causes, and lack of clear solutions. From community design where opportunities to be physically active have been engineered out, to surplus food commodities making the United States food supply the least costly in the world, the causes and solutions are complex.

Increasingly, Americans eat fewer meals prepared at home. In the 1970s, about 20% of the food budget was spent on food prepared and eaten away from home. In 1992, this had increased to 38% of the food dollar being spent on food prepared away from home. Many studies show a correlation between foods prepared outside the home and increased consumption of amounts of fat, sodium, and refined carbohydrates, as well as larger portions served to both adults and children.

During the 20-year period that diets have increased in these less healthful components, physical activity has decreased. In 1996, the US Surgeon General released a recommendation for either 20 minutes of vigorous physical activity at least three days per week, or 30 minutes of moderate exercise at least five days per week. In 2004, only 33% of adults met this recommendation, and youth fall short of *Healthy People 2010* objectives for engaging in vigorous activity. There has been a decrease in the number of youth and adults who walk or ride bikes to school and work. Overweight and obesity will continue to increase in the United States.

Medical care costs of chronic diseases attributed to obesity have passed the tipping point. These are now the leading contributors to medical care costs in the United States. Looking ahead, it is certain that these costs will increase over the next decades. It will take a significant shift in the focus of child care, K–12 schools, worksites, food companies, cities, states, and federal programs before this epidemic can be slowed and incidence stabilizes. It will require working with childbearing women to increase breast-feeding. More healthy, active lifestyles must be promoted through programs for young children, youth, adults, and seniors. It will take intensive efforts to reverse the epidemic to the point that the prevalence of obesity will decrease. Preventing and managing obesity is becoming and will remain the major focus of public health and health care in this century.

Bioterrorism

September 11, 2001, changed the lives of Americans and their institutions. The threat of terror has changed the way that many businesses operate. Before 2001, the possibility that the food and water supply could be intentionally tainted with organisms or poisonous chemicals was a faint concern. Post-2001, it is a central issue for municipal governments, state, federal, and international regulatory bodies, as well as private food and beverage manufacturers. Preparedness has become a prime focus for the food industry, and public health nutritionists will be a part of these teams in the many settings where food safety and security must be addressed.

FORECASTING FUTURE HEALTH CARE FINANCING AND DELIVERY

During the last 20 years, health care delivery systems have increasingly become more integrated. Academic medical centers and large hospitals are now health systems composed of multiple specialty hospitals, networks of health care professionals, affiliated diagnostic laboratories, pharmacies, rehabilitation facilities, and nursing homes, as well as training programs for the specialized health care professionals. This centralization of health care has grown in order to drive down costs and to increase profit. The health care sector, like many other service industries in the United States, is shifting to a for-profit administrative structure with shareholders and CEOs considering profitability as a their guiding priority. Health care insurance providers have also become large, integrated systems also driven to contain costs. Insurers are now beginning to shift the costs to employers and federal, state, and local governments, who subsequently shift the costs to consumers.

As health care financing challenges increase with a larger aging population and increasing burden of chronic diseases attributed to obesity, pressures will mount. Consumers, employers, and governments will demand a health care system that delivers better quality health care at less cost. Employer health insurance costs continue to rise at the same time that health systems and medical providers receive lower reimbursement rates from state and federal governments and private health insurers. Pressures mount for higher-quality care from health care providers, while consumers feel their pockets pinched for health care. There must be renewed discussion for national health care reform for a universal model of health care. In this discussion, the role of health promotion and disease prevention, spotlighting nutrition and dietary change of the population, will be significant to saving costs and improving the population's health outcomes.

ADVANCES IN MEDICAL SCIENCE

The Role of Genetics Within Medical Care

A health care visit may soon begin with blood being drawn for genetic analysis. The physician will review the profile and advise the patient of genetic risks for disease and how to prevent those risks through behavioral strategies such as diet, exercise, stress reduction, and other preventive care components. For any active diseases, the physician will prescribe drugs that will result in the best disease management for the patient's specific genetic makeup. The physician will also be able to advise patients of the specific type of diet that they will respond to favorably. The nutritionist can guide those dietary changes, with information about specific foods that will reduce health risks and control disease.

CHANGES IN THE FOOD SUPPLY

Agribusiness

While Europeans have loudly fought genetically modified (GM) foods moving into their markets, many Americans have been largely unaware of this trend. Most Americans have been unconcerned and are increasing their consumption of designer foods. As in Europe, the debate will likely become a central food quality issue to US consumers as questions and new issues arise.

Agribusiness will continue to develop and bring to the market genetically altered foods. Business interests will cite the benefits of increasing the growth of plants and animals, pest resistance, longer shelf life, and enhanced appearance, taste, and other desired qualities for agricultural products. Opponents of GM foods will continue to cite the negative consequences and potential risks, which include effects in nutritive quality, cause of allergies, and the effects on the environment, as well as pest and herbicide tolerance and corporate control over agriculture.

Organic Foods and the Slow Food Movement

Another growing group of American consumers have moved in the opposite direction in the food marketplace. These consumers are actively purchasing locally grown, organic foods. They are followers of the Slow Food Movement using natural foods, simply prepared and eaten in a nonrushed manner. They value quality cuisine and human connections at their mealtimes. These consumers are willing to pay a higher price for smaller, less perfect fruits and vegetables grown without pesticides or animals raised without antibiotics. They place high value on health and their interest in supporting local sustainable agriculture. Health and natural food stores and cooperatives are gaining market share as this group of health and nutrition-conscious consumers grows.

Restaurant Industry Responds to Market Demands

Fast-food outlets, family-style restaurants, and fine dining restaurants responding to consumer criticism, litigation, and market research, are increasingly offering nutrient labeling on their menus. The hospitality industry is recognizing that an increasing number of consumers are seeking home-quality meals when they eat away from home, and prefer nutritious meals for their families. Locally owned restaurants, as well as regional and national chains, are offering healthy lines within their regular fare to reach consumers who are weight and health conscious.

Fortification of Foods and Beverages

There has been a growing expansion of new foods and beverages offered by all of the food markets targeted to health and fitness conscious consumers. These new foods and beverages are lower in calories, fat, sodium, and simple sugars. Beginning in 2006, federal regulations require that the nutrition label include trans fats. A reduction in trans fats in processed foods has already begun. Many foods are being fortified with healthful nutrients including omega-3 fats, calcium, antioxidants, and fiber sources. Additional additives and herbs will continue to appear in the food supply as market research drives development of new products.

These food supply and food marketing issues require new areas of training and result in an increased scope of practice for nutritionists who work with the public. Nutritionists will increasingly integrate physical activity expertise by developing exercise prescriptions for clients and seeking personal training and other fitness credentialing. Some nutritionists will specialize in complementary and alternative medicine, including herbal medicine, yoga, meditation, natural foods, genetically modified foods, and related opportunities. Many nutritionists will also expand their behavioral health expertise into smoking cessation and other substance abuse counseling. Entrepreneurial nutritionists may open their own food markets or design their own line of vitamin and mineral supplements. Public health nutritionists will expand their employment by the food industry, guiding fortification with antioxidants and other nutrients in food products. Employment or consulting opportunities will increase in the restaurant industry as nutritionists are needed to guide nutrient labeling and recommend healthy menu choices to consumers who enjoy eating away from home but demand nutritious choices.

IMPACT OF INFORMATION TECHNOLOGY ON NUTRITION PRACTICE

Distance communication modalities such as telephonic and Web-based counseling, Web-based chat rooms, and support groups will flourish. Nutrition professionals will increasingly use these technology-supported methods to reach and counsel consumers. (See Chapter 22)

Telephone Counseling Services

Time constraints increasingly keep many consumers from seeking walk-in health care services. At the same time, pressures to decrease health care utilization and to keep consumers healthy has led to telephonic health information and advice services to consumers. More and more bilingual nutritionists, nurses, and health educators will be available around the clock. They will offer consumers individually structured and tailored protocols to increase their physical activity, improve their diets, and to offer weight loss and medical nutrition therapy advice. In the field of tobacco prevention and control, state and national Quit Lines have set the model for a science-based modality to reach and assist smokers who wish to quit smoking. Telephonic services for nutrition and diet issues will become a significant part of health care of the future.

Reaching Colleagues and Clients Through Listservs, E-Mail, and the Internet

Web sites will be developed for health professionals and consumers to sign up to receive information from nutrition and health listservs. These Web sites will guide list members to sites for information about topics of interest to them. Consumers will sign up for Web-streaming services where topics of their interest will be pulled from the World Wide Web and sent to their personal Web site or e-mail account.

Consumers will increasingly seek specialized Web sites for diet, exercise, weight loss, and disease management. Consumers can enroll by entering personal data and submitting queries in order to receive information via links, Web-based modules, and text. Consumers will be able to receive live instant messaging counseling and feedback from Web experts.

As consumers become more familiar with technology-supported approaches to obtain information and resources and use tools such as the Tufts Nutrition Navigator and CDC or US DHHS links to assess and use quality Web sites, a growing need for nutritionists with expertise in the technology forum will grow. Nutritionists will join large health care organizations such as health insurers, academic medical centers, health Web sites, and Internet service providers. They will become involved in the design side of these services. They will participate in communications to consumers by e-mailing responses, being the food and nutrition experts within live chat rooms, or as forum experts responding to a thread of communications coming in from the end users.

FUTURE ROLES FOR PUBLIC HEALTH NUTRITION PRACTITIONERS

Take Leadership in Partnerships, Collaborations, and Coalitions

As strategies to improve the nutritional health of the public have become increasingly complex and multidisciplinary, nutritionists will need to align their work with others to be effective participants on a comprehensive team. This may mean working in coalitions to change a public policy through advocacy and lobbying efforts. It may mean working through multiple channels (schools, worksites, faith community, and broad community settings, and within health care) to establish the infrastructure to deliver comprehensive and coordinated nutrition messages and resources. By combining resources and reach, private and public partnerships will increase the capacity to deliver effective nutrition messages and services. Public health nutritionists will require leadership skills to assure that within the powerful partnerships the nutrition and health messages are accurate and consistent.

Employment of nutritionists working with partnerships may shift from traditional salaried positions to reimbursement as through independent contractors, contracts with public health agencies, nonprofit organizations, or fee-for-service private practice.

Policy

Some of the greatest challenges to professional nutritionists lie where a profitable industry markets a product to the American public with little government regulation. Educational institutions and politicians accept funding and allow unregulated food and beverage marketing to reach school children and other consumer audiences. This and other food marketing issues will become a policy focus for nutritionists and advocates in the coming decades. It will remain to be seen whether voluntary partnerships can be established that support both the health of the public and the financial health of businesses, or if state and federal regulation will be required to enforce standards for all foods and beverages available through public education and other public service units. Nutritionists employed outside of government and industry must monitor and assure that the public's interest is met when industry partners with and influences government standards, regulations, programs, and guidelines.

Public Awareness and Communication

The public's confusion about fact and fiction in nutrition is ever-present due to the changing popular fad diets and the daily news quoting questionable studies that contradict the latest credible research. As public health and nutritionists turned the corner into this century, a common theme began to be heard from the field: that a national priority should put resources toward developing and consumer-testing a set of clear nutrition messages and promoting sophisticated media campaigns through appropriate channels to reach various audiences. Due to the growing influence of industry in the creation of government guidelines, there will be an increased response by consumer protection, academic, nonprofit, and watchdog organizations related to the science evidence base for consumer messages and guidelines.

It is anticipated that in the future, nutritionists will be increasingly involved in developing and implementing health promotion public awareness and educational campaigns. Nutritionists in other settings will support local and institutional implementation of key messages to reach diverse audiences. Skills in various channels of communication, as well as partnerships with the communication industry and members of the media will be critical. Academic nutrition training programs as well as leadership organizations such as the American Public Health Association and the American Dietetic Association will need to promote leadership and communications skills among professional nutritionists to counter celebrity physicians and fitness icons whose message may be alluring but lacks credible scientific evidence as its foundation.

Evaluation to Link Programs to Financial Return on Investment

The economics of health interventions is increasingly important as inputs and outputs are measured and the cost and cost-benefit of various approaches are weighed. Nutritionists must be equipped with skills and align themselves with colleagues to evaluate impact and financial outcomes.

For decision makers, being able to cite cost-benefit and cost-effectiveness analysis data about a program is essential. Nutritionists must provide supportive information about the cost burden to an employer for increasing prevalence of diabetes and heart disease among employees. Nutritionists can calculate the return on the investment of serving healthy food in the worksite cafeteria and determine the cost-benefit for alternative approaches to addressing obesity at the worksite. Nutritionists who can provide employers with data about the cost benefits of reducing a diet-modifiable health risk such as hypertension or moderate weight loss will document the economic benefits of nutrition and physical activity to their employees.

The last 20 years has seen an increase in the US population's reliance on convenience, technology, and privatization within the food, restaurant, transportation, information technology, medical, and health care industries. The nation, as well as the world, has seen a growing focus on security and a lack of trust in government. Chronic diseases have overtaken infectious diseases and maternal and child health issues as the most prevalent public health concern. Health promotion and disease prevention interventions have begun to grow within public and private health systems.

What will the next 20 years bring? An aging population is certain, and another baby boom is possible. Overweight and obesity and chronic diseases upward trends will begin to flatten as concerted efforts create changes. Will government or private health care systems become more prominent in the future? Will organic foods or genetically modified foods continue to receive consumer support from the marketplace? Will insurers rely on employers and local and state governments, or will there be a shift to a national health care system?

Although some future scenarios can be predicted, some are not possible to anticipate. It is clear that the public health nutritionists of the future will always require a comprehensive skill set that includes nutrition and behavioral science; the tools of epidemiology, biostatistics, and evaluation; program management, as well as personnel management, finance, and leadership. These skills will inevitably be applied within health care settings, communities, local state and federal government, the policy and communication arena, and coalitions and partnerships.

POINTS TO PONDER

- How will public health nutritionists emerge as leaders to address the obesity epidemic?
- Will nutritionists be involved in advocacy and information technology roles?
- Will the food and restaurant industry employ nutritionists to create a healthier food supply and access to healthy foods?
- How can nutritionists influence the marketers to increase the demand for health-promoting, locally grown foods?
- Where should public health nutrition be in the year 2010? 2030? 2050?

BIBLIOGRAPHY

Brownson RT, Kreuter MW. Future trends affecting public health, challenges and opportunities. *J Public Health Management Practice*. March 3, 1997:49–60.

Dietz WH. Health Consequences of obesity in youth: childhood predictors of adult disease. *Pediatrics*. 1998;101:518–525.

Harnack LJ, Jeffery WL, Boutelle K. Temporal trends in energy intake in the United States: an ecologic perspective. *Am J Clin Nutr*. 2000;17:1478–1484.

Institute of Medicine. *The Future of the Public's Health in the 21st Century*. Washington, DC: National Academies Press; 2003.

Ma Y, Bertone ER, Stanek EJ, Reed GW, Hebert JR, Cohen NL, Merriam PA, and Ockene IS. Association between Eating Patterns and Obesity in a Free-living US Adult Population, *Am J Epidemiol* 2003;158:85–92; doi:10.1093/aje/kwg117. Found online at: http://aje.oxfordjournals.org/cgi/content/full/158/1/85. Accessed February 14, 2005.

Progress Review of Physical Activity and Fitness, US Department of Health and Human Services, Public Health Service, April 14, 2004. Available at: http://www.healthypeople.gov/. Accessed February 14, 2005.

US Dept Health and Human Services, Centers for Disease Control and Prevention. National Center for Chronic Disease Prevention and Health Promotion. *Physical Activity and Health: A Report of the Surgeon General*. Washington DC: DHHS; 1996.

Appendix A— USDA Dietary Guidelines for Americans 2005

Dietary Guidelines for Americans 2005

EXECUTIVE SUMMARY

The *Dietary Guidelines for Americans (Dietary Guidelines)* provides science-based advice to promote health and to reduce risk for major chronic diseases through diet and physical activity. Major causes of morbidity and mortality in the United States are related to poor diet and a sedentary lifestyle. Some specific diseases linked to poor diet and physical inactivity include cardiovascular disease, type 2 diabetes, hypertension, osteoporosis, and certain cancers. Furthermore, poor diet and physical inactivity, resulting in an energy imbalance (more calories consumed than expended), are the most important factors contributing to the increase in overweight and obesity in this country. Combined with physical activity, following a diet that does not provide excess calories according to the recommendations in this document should enhance the health of most individuals.

An important component of each 5-year revision of the *Dietary Guidelines* is the analysis of new scientific information by the Dietary Guidelines Advisory Committee (DGAC) appointed by the Secretaries of the U.S. Department of Health and Human Services (DHHS) and the U.S. Department of Agriculture (USDA). This analysis, published in the DGAC Report (http://www.health.gov/dietaryguidelines/dga2005/report/), is the primary resource for development of the report on the guidelines by the departments. The *Dietary Guidelines* and the report of the DGAC differ in scope and purpose compared to reports for previous versions of the *Dietary Guidelines*. The 2005 DGAC report is a detailed scientific analysis. The scientific report was used to develop the *Dietary Guidelines* jointly between the two departments and forms the basis of recommendations that will be used by USDA and DHHS for program and policy development. Thus it is a publication oriented toward policy makers, nutrition educators, nutritionists, and health care providers rather than to the general public, as with previous versions of the *Dietary Guidelines*, and contains more technical information.

The intent of the *Dietary Guidelines* is to summarize and synthesize knowledge regarding individual nutrients and food components into recommendations for a pattern of eating that can be adopted by the public. In this publication, key recommendations are grouped under nine interrelated focus areas. The recommendations are based on the preponderance of scientific evidence for lowering risk of chronic disease and promoting health. It is important to remember that these are integrated messages that should be implemented as a whole. Taken together, they encourage most Americans to eat fewer calories, be more active, and make wiser food choices.

A basic premise of the *Dietary Guidelines* is that nutrient needs should be met primarily through consuming foods. Foods provide an array of nutrients and other compounds that may have beneficial effects on health. In certain cases, fortified foods and dietary supplements may be useful sources of one or more nutrients that otherwise might be consumed in less than recommended amounts. However, dietary supplements, while recommended in some cases, cannot replace a healthful diet.

Two examples of eating patterns that exemplify the *Dietary Guidelines* are the USDA Food Guide (http://www.usda.gov/cnpp/pyramid.html) and the DASH (Dietary Approaches to Stop Hypertension) Eating Plan.[1] Both of these eating patterns are designed to integrate dietary recommendations into a healthy way to eat for most individuals. These eating patterns are not weight loss diets, but rather illustrative examples of how to eat in accordance with the *Dietary Guidelines*. Both eating patterns are constructed across a range of calorie levels to meet the needs of various age and gender groups. For the USDA Food Guide, nutrient content estimates for each food group and subgroup are based on population-weighted food intakes. Nutrient content estimates for the DASH Eating Plan are based on selected foods chosen for a sample 7-day menu. Although originally developed to study the effects of an eating pattern on the prevention and treatment of hypertension, DASH is one example of a balanced eating plan consistent with the 2005 *Dietary Guidelines*.

Throughout most of this publication, examples use a 2000-calorie level as a reference for consistency with the Nutrition Facts Panel. Although this level is used as a reference, recommended calorie intake will differ for individuals based on age, gender, and activity level. At each calorie level, individuals who eat nutrient-dense foods may be able to meet their recommended nutrient intake without consuming their full calorie allotment. The remaining calories—*the discretionary calorie allowance*—allow individuals flexibility to consume some foods and beverages that may contain added fats, added sugars, and alcohol.

The recommendations in the *Dietary Guidelines* are for Americans over 2 years of age. It is important to incorporate the food preferences of different racial/ethnic groups, vegetarians, and other groups when planning diets and developing educational programs and materials. The USDA Food Guide and the DASH Eating Plan are flexible enough to accommodate a range of food preferences and cuisines.

The *Dietary Guidelines* is intended primarily for use by policy makers, health care providers, nutritionists, and nutrition educators. The information in the *Dietary Guidelines* is useful for the development of educational materials and aids policy makers in designing and implementing nutrition-related programs, including federal food, nutrition education, and information programs. In addition, this publication has the potential to provide authoritative statements as provided for in the Food and Drug Administration Modernization Act (FDAMA). Because the *Dietary Guidelines* contains discussions where the science is emerging, only statements included in the Executive Summary and the sections titled "Key Recommendations," which reflect the preponderance of scientific evidence, can be used for identification of authoritative statements. The recommendations are interrelated and mutually dependent; thus the statements in this document should be used together in the context of planning an overall healthful diet. However, even following just some of the recommendations can have health benefits.

The following is a listing of the *Dietary Guidelines* by chapter.

ADEQUATE NUTRIENTS WITHIN CALORIE NEEDS

Key Recommendations

- Consume a variety of nutrient-dense foods and beverages within and among the basic food groups while choosing foods that limit the intake of saturated and trans fats, cholesterol, added sugars, salt, and alcohol.
- Meet recommended intakes within energy needs by adopting a balanced eating pattern, such as the USDA Food Guide or the DASH Eating Plan.

Key Recommendations for Specific Population Groups

- People over age 50—Consume vitamin B12 in its crystalline form (i.e., fortified foods or supplements).
- Women of childbearing age who may become pregnant—Eat foods high in heme-iron and/or consume iron-rich plant foods or iron-fortified foods with an enhancer of iron absorption, such as vitamin C-rich foods.
- Women of childbearing age who may become pregnant and those in the first trimester of pregnancy—Consume adequate synthetic folic acid daily (from fortified foods or supplements) in addition to food forms of folate from a varied diet.
- Older adults, people with dark skin, and people exposed to insufficient ultraviolet band radiation (i.e., sunlight)—Consume extra vitamin D from vitamin D-fortified foods and/or supplements.

WEIGHT MANAGEMENT

Key Recommendations

- To maintain body weight in a healthy range, balance calories from foods and beverages with calories expended.

- To prevent gradual weight gain over time, make small decreases in food and beverage calories, and increase physical activity.

Key Recommendations for Specific Population Groups

- Those who need to lose weight—Aim for a slow, steady weight loss by decreasing calorie intake while maintaining an adequate nutrient intake and increasing physical activity.
- Overweight children—Reduce the rate of body weight gain while allowing growth and development. Consult a health care provider before placing a child on a weight-reduction diet.
- Pregnant women—Ensure appropriate weight gain as specified by a health-care provider.
- Breast-feeding women—Moderate weight reduction is safe and does not compromise weight gain of the nursing infant.
- Overweight adults and overweight children with chronic diseases and/or on medication—Consult a health care provider about weight-loss strategies prior to starting a weight-reduction program to ensure appropriate management of other health conditions.

PHYSICAL ACTIVITY

Key Recommendations

- Engage in regular physical activity and reduce sedentary activities to promote health, psychological well-being, and a healthy body weight.
  - To reduce the risk of chronic disease in adulthood: Engage in at least 30 minutes of moderate-intensity physical activity, above usual activity, at work or home on most days of the week.
  - For most people, greater health benefits can be obtained by engaging in physical activity of more vigorous intensity or longer duration.
  - To help manage body weight and prevent gradual, unhealthy body weight gain in adulthood: Engage in approximately 60 minutes of moderate- to vigorous-intensity activity on most days of the week while not exceeding caloric intake requirements.
  - To sustain weight loss in adulthood: Participate in at least 60 to 90 minutes of daily moderate-intensity physical activity while not exceeding caloric intake requirements. Some people may need to consult with a health care provider before participating in this level of activity.

- Achieve physical fitness by including cardiovascular conditioning, stretching exercises for flexibility, and resistance exercises or calisthenics for muscle strength and endurance.

Key Recommendations for Specific Population Groups

- Children and adolescents—Engage in at least 60 minutes of physical activity on most, preferably all, days of the week.
- Pregnant women—In the absence of medical or obstetric complications, incorporate 30 minutes or more of moderate-intensity physical activity on most, if not all, days of the week. Avoid activities with a high risk of falling or abdominal trauma.
- Breast-feeding women—Be aware that neither active nor regular exercise adversely affects the mother's ability to successfully breast-feed.
- Older adults—Participate in regular physical activity to reduce functional declines associated with aging and to achieve the other benefits of physical activity identified for all adults.

FOOD GROUPS TO ENCOURAGE

Key Recommendations

- Consume a sufficient amount of fruits and vegetables while staying within energy needs. Two cups of fruit and 2 1/2 cups of vegetables per day are recommended for a reference 2000-calorie intake, with higher or lower amounts depending on the calorie level.
- Choose a variety of fruits and vegetables each day. In particular, select from all five vegetable subgroups (dark green, orange, legumes, starchy vegetables, and other vegetables) several times a week.
- Consume 3 or more ounce-equivalents of whole-grain products per day, with the rest of the recommended grains coming from enriched or whole-grain products. In general, at least half the grains should come from whole grains.
- Consume 3 cups per day of fat-free or low-fat milk or equivalent milk products.

Key Recommendations for Specific Population Groups

- Children and adolescents—Consume whole-grain products often; at least half the grains should be whole grains. Children 2 to 8 years should consume

2 cups per day of fat-free or low-fat milk or equivalent milk products. Children 9 years of age and older should consume 3 cups per day of fat-free or low-fat milk or equivalent milk products.

FATS

Key Recommendations

- Consume less than 10% of calories from saturated fatty acids and less than 300 mg/day of cholesterol, and keep trans fatty acid consumption as low as possible.
- Keep total fat intake between 20% to 35% of calories, with most fats coming from sources of polyunsaturated and monounsaturated fatty acids, such as fish, nuts, and vegetable oils.
- When selecting and preparing meat, poultry, dry beans, and milk or milk products, make choices that are lean, low fat, or fat free.
- Limit intake of fats and oils high in saturated and/or trans fatty acids, and choose products low in such fats and oils.

Key Recommendations for Specific Population Groups

- Children and adolescents—Keep total fat intake between 30% to 35% of calories for children 2 to 3 years of age and between 25% to 35% of calories for children and adolescents 4 to 18 years of age, with most fats coming from sources of polyunsaturated and monounsaturated fatty acids, such as fish, nuts, and vegetable oils.

CARBOHYDRATES

Key Recommendations

- Choose fiber-rich fruits, vegetables, and whole grains often.
- Choose and prepare foods and beverages with little added sugars or caloric sweeteners, such as amounts suggested by the USDA Food Guide and the DASH Eating Plan.
- Reduce the incidence of dental caries by practicing good oral hygiene and consuming sugar- and starch-containing foods and beverages less frequently.

SODIUM AND POTASSIUM

Key Recommendations

- Consume less than 2300 mg (approximately 1 tsp of salt) of sodium per day.
- Choose and prepare foods with little salt. At the same time, consume potassium-rich foods, such as fruits and vegetables.

Key Recommendations for Specific Population Groups

- Individuals with hypertension, blacks, and middle-aged and older adults— Aim to consume no more than 1500 mg of sodium per day, and meet the potassium recommendation (4700 mg/day) with food.

ALCOHOLIC BEVERAGES

Key Recommendations

- Those who choose to drink alcoholic beverages should do so sensibly and in moderation—defined as the consumption of up to one drink per day for women and up to two drinks per day for men.
- Alcoholic beverages should not be consumed by some individuals, including those who cannot restrict their alcohol intake, women of childbearing age who may become pregnant, pregnant and lactating women, children and adolescents, individuals taking medications that can interact with alcohol, and those with specific medical conditions.
- Alcoholic beverages should be avoided by individuals engaging in activities that require attention, skill, or coordination, such as driving or operating machinery.

FOOD SAFETY

Key Recommendations

- To avoid microbial foodborne illness:
  - Clean hands, food contact surfaces, and fruits and vegetables. Meat and poultry should not be washed or rinsed.
  - Separate raw, cooked, and ready-to-eat foods while shopping, preparing, or storing foods.

- Cook foods to a safe temperature to kill microorganisms.
- Chill (refrigerate) perishable food promptly and defrost foods properly.
- Avoid raw (unpasteurized) milk or any products made from unpasteurized milk, raw or partially cooked eggs or foods containing raw eggs, raw or undercooked meat and poultry, unpasteurized juices, and raw sprouts.

Key Recommendations for Specific Population Groups

- Infants and young children, pregnant women, older adults, and those who are immunocompromised—Do not eat or drink raw (unpasteurized) milk or any products made from unpasteurized milk, raw or partially cooked eggs or foods containing raw eggs, raw or undercooked meat and poultry, raw or undercooked fish or shellfish, unpasteurized juices, and raw sprouts.
- Pregnant women, older adults, and those who are immunocompromised— Only eat certain deli meats and frankfurters that have been reheated to steaming hot.

Source: NIH Publication No. 03-4082, Facts about the DASH Eating Plan, US Department of Health and Human Services, National Institutes of Health, National Heart, Lung, and Blood Institute, Karanja NM, et al. *J Am Diet Assoc (JADA).* 1999; 8:S19–27. http://www.nhlbi.nih.gov/health/public/heart/hbp/dash/.

Appendix B—Ask Thomas!

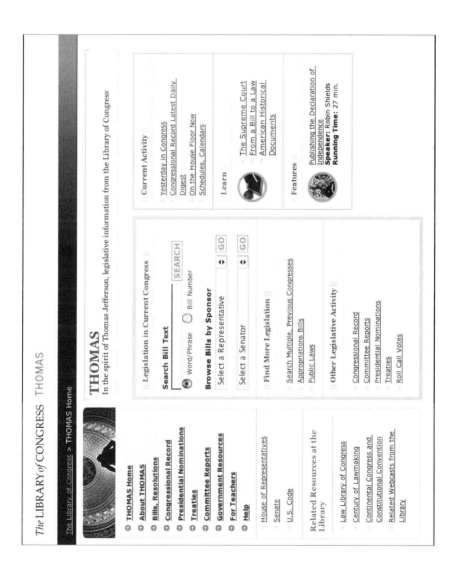

Appendix C—
Bookshelf for Public Health Nutritionists

Blumenthal DJ, DiClemente RJ, eds. *Community-Based Health Research*. New York, NY: Springer Publishing Co; 2004.

Boyle MA. *Community Nutrition in Action*. Belmont, Calif: Thomas Wadsworth; 2003.

Bronner F, ed. *Nutrition Policy in Public Health*. New York, NY: Springer Publishing Co; 1997.

Brownson RC, Baker EA, Leet TL, Gillespie KN. *Evidence Based Public Health*. New York, NY: Oxford Press; 2003.

Contento I. *Strategies for Nutrition Education: Theory, Research, and Practice*. Sudbury, Mass: Jones and Bartlett Publishers; 2006.

De Busk R. *Genetics: The Nutrition Connection*. Chicago, Ill: American Dietetic Association; 2003.

Detels R, McEwen J, Beaglehole R, and Tanaka H. *Oxford Textbook of Public Health*. 4th ed., New York, NY: Oxford University Press; 2002.

Endres JB. *Community Nutrition*. Upper Saddle River, NJ: Merrill; 1999.

Farley T, Cohen DA. *Prescription for a Healthy Nation*. Boston, Mass: Beacon Press; 2005.

Heaney RP, Dougherty CJ. *Research for Health Professionals Design, Analysis and Ethics*. Ames, Iowa: Iowa State University Press; 1988.

Gibney, Michael J., Margetts, Barrie M., Kearney, John M., "Public Health Nutrition," Nutrition Society Textbook Series, Blackwell Science, UK, (Iowa State Press, a Blackwell Publishing Co, Ames, Iowa) 2004.

Institute of Medicine. *Dietary Reference Intakes—Applications in Dietary Assessments* (2000) *Applications in Dietary Planning* (2003) Washington, DC: National Academies Press.

Institute of Medicine. *The Future of the Public's Health in the 21st Century*. Washington, DC: National Academies Press; 2003.

Issel ML. *Health Program Planning and Evaluation*. Sudbury, Mass: Jones and Bartlett Publishers; 2004.

Khoury MJ, et al, eds. *Genetics and Public Health in the 21st Century*. New York, NY: Oxford University Press; 2000.

Kleinman RE, ed. *Pediatric Nutrition Handbook*. 5th ed. Elk Grove Village, Il: American Academy of Pediatrics; 2004.

Leedy PD, Omrod JE. *Practical Research Planning and Design*. New York, NY: Macmillan Publishing Co; 2005.

Nestle M. *Food Politics*. Berkeley, Calif: University of California Press; 2002.

Neutens JJ, Robinson L. *Research Techniques for the Health Sciences*. San Francisco, Calif: Pearson Education, Inc; 2002.

Probert KL, ed. *Moving to the Future: Developing Community-Based Nutrition Services.* Washington, DC: Association of State and Territorial Public Health Nutrition Directors; 1996.

Stangl DK, Berry DA, eds. *Meta-Analysis in Medicine and Health Policy.* New York, NY: Marcel Dekker, Inc; 2003.

Timmreck TC. *Planning, Program Development and Evaluation.* 2nd ed. Sudbury, Mass: Jones and Bartlett Publishers; 2002.

Tulchinaky TH, Varavikova EA. *The New Public Health.* New York, NY: Academic Press; 2000.

Other:

For further reading and research, visit the American Dietetic Association's on-line index of position papers, supplements, and other publications at www.eatright.org.

Index